Fundamentals of Addiction

Fundamentals of Addiction

A Practical Guide for Counsellors

4th Edition—formerly published as *Alcohol & Drug Problems*

Edited by Marilyn Herie and W. J. Wayne Skinner
Foreword by Gabor Maté

camh

Library and Archives Canada Cataloguing in Publication

Fundamentals of addiction: A practical guide for counsellors / edited by Marilyn Herie and
W.J. Wayne Skinner; foreword by Gabor Maté. —4th ed.

Revision of: Alcohol & drug problems.
Includes bibliographical references and index.

ISBN 978-1-77114-147-5 (PRINT)
ISBN 978-1-77114-148-2 (PDF)
ISBN 978-1-77114-149-9 (HTML)
ISBN 978-1-77114-150-5 (EPUB)

1. Alcoholism counseling. 2. Drug abuse counseling. 3. Alcoholism counseling—Canada.
4. Drug abuse counseling—Canada. I. Herie, Marilyn, 1963–, editor of compilation. II.
Skinner, W.J. Wayne, 1949–, editor of compilation. III. Centre for Addiction and Mental
Health. IV. Title: Fundamentals of addiction.

RC564.15.A42 2013   362.29'186   C2013-902054-3   C2013-902055-1

Printed in Canada
© 2014 Centre for Addiction and Mental Health

This publication may be available in other formats. For information about alternative formats
or other CAMH publications, or to place an order, please contact CAMH Publications:
Toll-free: 1 800 661-1111
Toronto: 416 595-6059
E-mail: publications@camh.ca
Online store: http://store.camh.ca

www.camh.ca

This book was produced by CAMH Education.

4060/12-2019/P575

Contents

SECTION 3: SPECIAL ISSUES AND CONSIDERATIONS

SECTION 4: SPECIFIC POPULATIONS

SECTION 5: PROFESSIONAL PRACTICE AND SYSTEM ISSUES

Preface

Marilyn Herie and Wayne Skinner

Addiction treatment is often seen as a "black box" by clients and helping professionals alike. A popular perception of the process is something like this: 1) person hits "bottom" or is in the hot seat of an "intervention"; 2) person enters "rehab" (i.e., inpatient addiction treatment); 3) person gets "treated"; 4) person is "cured" (or drops out); 5) repeat as necessary. Although this portrayal of addiction and its treatment can make for a gripping storyline in film, television or fiction, it doesn't begin to reflect the reality of our current scientific understanding and the diversity of evidence-based approaches to addictions.

The fact is, not all people need or want specialized addiction treatment. Many clients are best served in community settings where they can receive services that are integrated into their overall care. The skills required to respond to addiction map well onto good clinical practice: listening to our clients with compassionate empathy, fostering trust and a positive therapeutic alliance, and respecting the innate autonomy of the people we serve. This book can be used by virtually any practitioner across the spectrum of care as a practical guide to helping clients overcome the harmful, sometimes devastating, effects of addiction.

For this fourth edition of *Alcohol & Drug Problems*, we decided on a new title, *Fundamentals of Addiction*, to reflect advances in the field extending beyond psychoactive drug use to include behavioural or "process" addictions. This iteration continues to build on a rich legacy of previous editions in providing practitioners with essential information and treatment models for diverse client populations.

As our knowledge and understanding of addictions increase, so does the complexity of the chapters in this edition. The content is divided into five sections. **Section 1: The Basics** lays the foundation and provides the theoretical framework for the book as a whole. The chapters cover a client perspective, diversity and equity competencies, harm reduction, motivational interviewing and the neurobiological and physical aspects of substance use. **Section 2: Clinical Interventions** examines screening and assessment, as well as a range of interventions and approaches, including brief interventions; relapse prevention; specific knowledge and skills relating to tobacco dependence, opioid misuse and dependence; family involvement; mutual support; and online interventions in the "digital age." **Section 3: Special Issues and Considerations** presents practical issues around treating people with concurrent disorders, trauma and neurobiological impairments, and discusses considerations for working with people in correctional settings and those with behavioural addictions. **Section 4: Specific Populations** examines diversity as it relates to women, youth, older adults, Aboriginal people and people with diverse sexual orientations and gender identities. Finally, **Section 5: Professional Practice and System Issues** shares invaluable knowledge about ethical issues in clinical practice, legal issues and tips for testifying in court, clinical supervision, and care pathways in an integrated addiction treatment system.

One challenge—as well as an advantage—of edited books is the diversity in authors' voices and writing style. We value this diversity, but also sought a consistent structure in order to give this edition a more cohesive look and feel and to amplify the practical nature of the information. To that end, most chapters begin with a short case example and conclude with key practice tips and recommended print and web resources. We, and sometimes the authors, struggled somewhat with the case examples. On one hand we wanted to provide real-world anchors for the content; on the other hand, no individual story can represent the rich complexity of human experience. These composite cases are offered in the spirit of each person being "like all others, some others, and no others" (to paraphrase Henry A. Murray and Clyde Kluckhohn in their 1953 book *Personality in Nature, Society, and Culture*).

This fourth edition has been wholly revised and updated, and as such has been a considerable undertaking. We wish, first of all, to thank our authors, who have contributed their expertise and many hours of their time with one goal in mind—to assist you in your important work of reducing the harm related to addictions. We are grateful to Dr. Gabor Maté for contributing the provocative foreword that challenges counsellors to consider early childhood experiences and trauma as significant risk factors for addictions, rather than the more commonly held and "misguided" view that genetics plays a major role in our predisposition to addiction.

We also wish to thank our reviewers for their careful reading of early drafts, and for their thoughtful and constructive feedback. In alphabetical order: Branka Agic, Paul Antze, Kirstin Bindseil, Myra Borenstein-Levy, Nick Boyce, Nicola Brown, Amer Burhan, Diana Capponi, Walter Cavallieri, Stephanie Cohen, Robin Cuff, Debbie Ernest, Margaret Flower, Cynthia Geppert, Christopher Hadden, Michelle Hamilton-Page, Patricia Hays, Dave Hedlund, Christian Hendershot, Kathryn Irwin-Seguin, Linda Jackson, Mattias Kaay, Milan Khara, Akwatu Khenti, Amy Krentzman, Sharon Labonte-Jaques, Wiplove Lamda, Lynn Lavallée, Bernard Le Foll, Michael Lester, Saul Lev-Ran, Myra Levy, Susan Morris, Ellie Munn, David North, Anna Palucka, Tom Payette, Mike Prett, Dan Reist, Núria Ribas, Janine Robinson, Lori Shekter-Wolfson, Debora Steele, Valerie Temple, Andrea Tsanos, Cristine Urquhart, Paulette West, Jodi Wolff, Martin Zack, Laurie Zawertailo and Sarah Zemore.

We are also immensely grateful to Julia Greenbaum, who co-ordinated the production of this fourth edition with grace, patience and persistence; Diana Ballon, for her masterful editorial skills; Hema Zbogar, for her laser-like copy editing precision; and Nancy Leung, for the simplicity and elegance of the book's design. CAMH's library staff helped many of the authors access the most current research on their topics, for which we are most grateful. To these contributors and many others behind the scenes, thank you for your help in bringing this project to completion.

We want to end our acknowledgments by returning to the beginning to honour the editors and authors of the book's previous three editions. Betty-Anne Howard provided the initial inspiration for the first edition, published in 1993, along with her co-editors, Susan Harrison and Virginia Carver. Susan and Virginia then edited and expanded the book through the second and third editions. Having done this once, we now have a deep appreciation of the commitment, dedication and skill they brought to doing this task three times! We have worked to hold true to the spirit and skill that Susan and Virginia (and their collaborators) brought to the formidable task of shaping this resource to become such a valued and respected guide on evidence-informed addiction treatment in the Canadian context.

With this book we have tried to shine a light into the "black box" of addictions, with a goal of increasing treatment capacity and access to services by those in need. To our many readers in clinical practice, we hope this guide continues to be valuable in your professional development and in your day-to-day work with clients.

We invite you to join our blog at www.porticonetwork.ca/web/addiction-fundamentals/welcome. This forum will provide an opportunity to promote and generate dialogue around various addiction issues informed by your reading of this book.

Foreword

Gabor Maté

> What is addiction, really? It is a sign, a signal, a symptom of distress. It is a language that tells us about a plight that must be understood.

—Alice Miller, *Breaking Down the Wall of Silence*

This fourth edition of *Alcohol & Drug Problems*—now the *Fundamentals of Addiction*—marks an important movement forward in the understanding of addiction. In taking notice of the behavioural addictions, it recognizes that the specific target of the addictive drive does not define the nature of addiction.

At the heart of addiction is what I'll refer to as the universal addiction process, which involves the same emotional dynamics no matter what the form of the addiction. These emotional dynamics are just as true of an addiction to a substance—whether ingested, inhaled or injected—as they are of compulsive Internet use, shopping, gambling, sexual roving or any number of behaviours that may even be valued and rewarded by society, such as excessive involvement with work, the acquisition of wealth or the attainment of power. More surprisingly, we now know that all addictive manifestations, substance-related or not, use and activate the same brain circuits and neurochemicals. These target behaviours may vary in their form, severity and consequences, but they are all expressions of a deeper and complex universal process whose templates are grounded in human psychological needs, emotional drives, neurophysiological functions, social and cultural influences and, if one may be permitted to utter the word in a scientific publication, in the *spiritual* nature of human beings.

According to the American Society of Addiction Medicine ([ASAM], n.d.), addiction is "a primary, chronic disease of brain reward, motivation, memory and related circuitry . . . reflected in an individual pathologically pursuing reward and/or relief by substance use and other behaviors" (p. 1). Considering addiction to be a "primary" disease implies that the addiction is unrelated to any previous condition or injury.

Yet to speak of addiction as a primary disease is to ignore the reality that an antecedent injury—if not of a physical nature, then at least of an emotional one—usually precedes the addiction. Emotional more than physical injury leads to long-term psychological and neurobiological consequences predisposing to addiction. People are quite resilient to surviving physical injury, much less so when that injury is psychic and occurs in the child's nurturing environment during the developing years.

When it comes to etiology, the ASAM, like much of addiction medicine practice, considers the major influence to be genetics. In fact, it asserts that "genetic factors account for about half of the likelihood that an individual will develop addiction"

(ASAM, n.d., p. 5). Yet this assertion is not supported by scientific evidence. Rather, trauma, the most important risk factor involved in the neurobiology and psychology of addiction, is listed very low among the ASAM's list of etiologic circumstances. It may be that, as a physician colleague in San Francisco once said to me, "The medical profession is traumaphobic."

For 12 years, I worked in Vancouver's Downtown Eastside, known as Canada's poorest postal code and notorious as North America's most concentrated area of drug use. Every female patient I ever interviewed offered or endorsed a history of sexual abuse in childhood, and all patients, male or female, had endured childhoods of abuse, neglect, abandonment and trauma. If this link to abuse had been something only I observed, one could easily dismiss it as subjective and unreliable. But large-scale population surveys have found a similar association.

Studies repeatedly find that extraordinarily high percentages of addicts have experienced childhood trauma, including physical, sexual and emotional abuse. Dube and colleagues (2003) remarked that the prevalence of childhood trauma among addicts was "of an order of magnitude rarely seen in epidemiology and public health" (p. 568). Their research, the renowned Adverse Childhood Experiences (ACE) study, looked at the incidence of 10 categories of painful circumstances, including family violence, parental divorce, family substance use problems, death of a parent and physical or sexual abuse, in thousands of people. The correlation between these experiences and substance use problems later in life was then calculated. For each adverse childhood experience, the risk for the early initiation of substance use problems increased between two- and fourfold. People with five or more such experiences had a seven to 10 times greater risk for substance use problems than those with no such experiences.

Dube and colleagues (2003) concluded that nearly two-thirds of injection drug use can be attributed to abusive and traumatic childhood events. In clinical practice with a heavily addicted population, I believe childhood trauma percentages may run close to 100 per cent. Although not all addicts have been subjected to childhood trauma, just as not all severely abused children grow up to be addicts, there is no doubt that most hardcore injection users have experienced childhood trauma.

According to a 2002 review by Harold Gordon at the U.S. National Institute on Drug Abuse:

> The rate of victimization among women substance abusers ranges from 50% to nearly 100%. . . . Clinic populations of substance abusers are found to meet the [diagnostic] criteria for post-traumatic stress disorder. . . . Those experiencing *both* physical and sexual abuse were at least *twice* as likely to be using drugs than those who experience either abuse alone. (pp. 116–117)

Alcohol consumption has a similar pattern: people who had suffered sexual abuse were three times more likely to begin drinking in adolescence than those who had not. For each emotionally traumatic childhood circumstance, there is a two- to threefold increase in the likelihood of early alcohol abuse. Dube and colleagues (2006) concluded, "Overall, these studies provide evidence that stress and trauma are common factors associated with consumption of alcohol at an early age as a means to self-regulate negative or painful emotions" (p. e8).

The salient psychological template for substance use or behavioural addiction is unresolved emotional pain. All addictive manifestations, substance-related or not, are an attempt, in the words of the former heroin-addicted Rolling Stones guitarist Keith Richards (2010), to seek oblivion: "The contortions we go through," the legendary musician writes in his autobiography, "just not to be ourselves for a few hours." And why? Because the emotional burden is too much to bear. It is not a linguistic accident that we speak of heavy drinkers as "feeling no pain." Abuse, neglect and even a simple lack of attunement owing to parents' stress will make children feel inadequate, empty and uncomfortable with themselves. The greater the environmental stress, as in the case of trauma, the greater that discomfort and the need to escape it. Although the addict's self-loathing is much exacerbated by the behaviours associated with addiction, the self-hatred long predates the addiction.

While the ASAM cites some of the cerebral circuits implicated in addiction, what it does not explain is that these brain circuits develop in interaction with the rearing environment and that under conditions of stress and trauma, key brain circuits of reward, motivation, emotional self-regulation, impulse control, stress response—all impaired in addiction—do not develop optimally. To quote a seminal article in *Pediatrics* from the Harvard Center on the Developing Child:

> The architecture of the brain is constructed through an ongoing process that begins before birth, continues into adulthood. . . . The interaction of genes and experiences literally shapes the circuitry of the developing brain, *and is critically influenced by the mutual responsiveness of adult-child relationships* [italics added], particularly in the early childhood years. (Shonkoff et al., 2012, p. 4)

Many studies have shown that trauma and neglect interfere with healthy brain development and thus create the neurobiological template for addiction. The hormone pathways of children who have been sexually abused are chronically altered (De Bellis et al., 1994). Even a relatively "mild" stressor such as maternal depression—let alone neglect, abandonment or abuse—can disturb an infant's physical stress mechanisms (Essex et al., 2002). Add neglect, abandonment or abuse, and the child will be more reactive to stress throughout life. A study published in *JAMA* concluded that "a history of childhood abuse per se is related to increased neuroendocrine [nervous and hormonal] stress reactivity, which is further enhanced when additional trauma is experienced in adulthood" (Heim et al., 2002, p. 117). A brain pre-set to be easily triggered into a stress response is likely to assign a high value to substances, activities and situations that provide short-term relief and show less interest in long-term consequences. In contrast, situations or activities that for the average person are likely to bring satisfaction, such as intimate connections with family, are undervalued, because in the addict's life, they have not been rewarding. This shrinking from normal experience is also an outcome of early trauma and stress, as summarized in a recent psychiatric review of child development:

> Neglect and abuse during early life may cause bonding systems to develop abnormally and compromise capacity for rewarding interpersonal relationships and commitment to societal and cultural values later in life. Other means of stimulating reward pathways in the brain, such as drugs, sex, aggression, and intimidating others, could become relatively more attractive and less constrained by concern about violating trusting relationships. The ability to modify behaviour based on negative experiences may be impaired. (Pedersen, 2004, p. 106)

Even when genetics play a role in predisposing someone to an addiction, the latest brain development data and, saliently, the findings of the literature on epigenetics, clearly show that genes are turned on and off by the environment, and thus are influenced by experience. For example, children with serotonergic gene abnormalities that may predispose them to addiction will not express those genes if they are brought up in a nurturing, supportive family. Reporting on a study published in the *Journal of Consulting and Clinical Psychology, ScienceDaily* (2009) highlights the importance of environment: "A genetic risk factor that increases the likelihood that youth will engage in substance use can be neutralized by high levels of involved and supportive parenting."[1]

If addictions are a response to pain and reflect the disordered neurobiology of childhood stress or trauma, they are also self-medications in the narrow medical sense. People with attention-deficit/hyperactivity disorder self-medicate with stimulants such as cocaine, nicotine or crystal meth; people with post-traumatic stress disorder with opiates; people with anxiety with benzodiazepines; and people who are depressed with cocaine and other substances. Of course, the addictive substances can damage the brain and cause further mental pathology, such as psychosis and depression. Concurrent disorders should not be seen as the exception, but the rule.

Many aspects of addiction theory and practice are covered in this book, and rightly so. Addiction cannot be understood from an isolated perspective. It is a complex human condition, a condition rooted in the individual experience of the sufferer and also in the multi-generational history of his or her family and—not least—also in the cultural and historical context in which that family has existed. The shameful statistics of addiction prevalence among First Nations people are not attributable to any genetic flaw, but to the historical trauma endured by the Aboriginal populations of North America; the horrendous multi-generational legacy of the residential schools; and the ongoing social, economic and cultural ostracization that continues to be their lot.

We see the same phenomenon with colonized peoples elsewhere. Beyond marginalized racial or economic groups, many suffer from the anomy and spiritual emptiness

---

1 For a refutation of the mistaken assumptions underlying the twin studies that seem to buttress the genetic hypothesis, see Maté (2008).

of a materialistic culture and its constant blandishments to fill our inner void with external acquisition or attainment, pursuits that themselves can become addictive. "It is impossible to get enough of something that almost works," the researcher and physician Vincent Felitti once aptly remarked.

To its credit, the ASAM definition of addiction recognizes the spiritual dimensions of the all-too-human problem of addiction. Spirituality in this context does not necessarily have a religious meaning, though for some people it may. More broadly, spirituality refers to people's innate capacity to connect to their own deeper consciousness, to a sense of innate value independent of external factors, to a confidence that we are more than just our rigidly reactive personality patterns and, finally, to a belief in a profound unity with all that exists. For addicts, one of the outcomes of suffering from early adversity is an alienation from these life-affirming qualities. When we recover, what do we find again but those inner truths? In finding them, we recover ourselves.

To recover, the addict surely does not need more punishment, more loss, more defeat. The addict has experienced those in sufficient measure already. On the contrary, according to the Catholic monk and mystic Thomas Merton, to find ourselves "we must know what victory is and like it better than defeat." Victory is the recognition of our humanness, that we belong, that we are not damaged goods after all.

Our society is far from understanding that addicts, having suffered since childhood, need our expertise, our support and, above all, our compassion. In that sense, addiction professionals need to be more than health care providers—they need to be social pioneers.

References

American Society of Addiction Medicine (ASAM). (n.d.). Definition of addiction. Retrieved from www.asam.org/for-the-public/definition-of-addiction

De Bellis, M.D., Chrousos, G.P., Dorn, L.D., Burke, L., Helmers, K., Kling, M.A., . . . Putnam, F.W. (1994). Hypothalamic-pituitary-adrenal axis dysregulation in sexually abused girls. *Journal of Clinical Endocrinology & Metabolism, 78,* 249–255.

Dube, S.R., Felitti, V.J., Dong, M., Chapman, D.P., Giles, W.H. & Anda, R.F. (2003). Childhood abuse, neglect, and household dysfunction and the risk of illicit drug use: The adverse childhood experiences study. *Pediatrics, 111,* 564–572.

Dube, S.R., Miller, J.W., Brown, D.W., Giles, W.H., Felitti, V.J., Dong, M. & Anda, R.F. (2006). Adverse childhood experiences and the association with ever using alcohol and initiating alcohol use during adolescence. *Journal of Adolescent Health, 38,* 444.e1–e10.

Essex, M.J., Klein, M.H., Cho, E. & Kalin, N.H. (2002). Maternal stress beginning in infancy may sensitize children to later stress exposure: Effects on cortisol and behaviour. *Biological Psychiatry, 52,* 776–784.

Gordon, H.W. (2002). Early environmental stress and biological vulnerability to drug abuse. *Psychoneuroendocrinology, 271,* 115–126.

Heim, C., Newport, D.J., Wagner, D., Wilcox, M.M., Miller, A.H. & Nemeroff, C.B. (2002). The role of early adverse experience and adulthood stress in the prediction of neuroendocrine stress reactivity in women: A multiple regression analysis. *Depression and Anxiety, 15,* 117–125.

Maté, G. (2008). *In the Realm of Hungry Ghosts: Close Encounters with Addiction.* Toronto: Knopf Canada.

Pedersen, C.A. (2004). Biological aspects of social bonding and the roots of human violence. *Annals of the New York Academy of Sciences, 1036,* 106–127.

Richards, K. (2010). *Life.* London, United Kingdom: Weidenfeld & Nicolson.

ScienceDaily. (2009, February 16). Genetic risk for substance use can be neutralized by good parenting [Press release]. Retrieved from www.sciencedaily.com/releases/2009/02/090210125437.htm

Shonkoff, J.P., Richter, L., van der Gaag, J. & Bhutta, Z.A. (2012). An integrated scientific framework for child survival and early childhood development. *Pediatrics, 126,* 460–472.

SECTION 1

THE BASICS

Chapter 1

Biopsychosocial *Plus*: A Practical Approach to Addiction and Recovery

Wayne Skinner and Marilyn Herie

This introductory chapter provides an overview of the key concepts and principles that shape and guide this book on the fundamentals of addiction. It is organized around several key questions: What is addiction? What can be done to prevent and treat addictions? How does change happen? And what does recovery mean?

The problem for the practitioner is how to organize the growing torrent of information and materials that threatens to flood our minds as we work to understand and help people affected by addiction. The domain of addiction appears to be expanding, from the well-defined space of substance use problems to a broader set of addictive behaviours. This expansion raises fears that the concept of addiction has become so general that it risks becoming meaningless and of little use as a concept. A truly contemporary approach to addiction must have a realistic understanding of the impact of addictive behaviours on individuals, families and communities. From a science-based perspective, sufficient knowledge and skill exist to be able to understand addictive processes and to constructively address the problems associated with addictive behaviours. It is both necessary and possible to build evidence-informed pathways that lead to better prevention, identification and treatment of addiction problems. If there is a foundational message guiding this book, it is this: addiction is something we can do something about. The compilation of expert knowledge this book gives us contributes to a comprehensive understanding of addiction and the problems related to it. And it asserts very clearly that there is much we can do to help people affected by addiction move toward the recovery and well-being they seek.

Understanding Addiction

Our approach to understanding addiction is based on a model that extends beyond the biopsychosocial (BPS) model originally proposed by Engel (1977) to what we refer to as a biopsychosocial *plus* approach. This evolving framework for understanding addiction builds on the three dimensions proposed by Engel to include culture and spirituality. We also extend the social dimension to emphasize socio-structural and macro-societal factors, especially those rooted in historical and contemporary socio-economic inequalities. These are essential considerations for understanding and addressing the social determinants of health.

We believe it is important to explicitly identify these additional aspects. We agree with Alexander (2008), Maté (2008) and others who argue that we should be open to considering other factors as well—from economic to anthropological to psychodevelopmental. Four decades ago, Engel's (1977) proposal was to move beyond a narrow, reductionist biomedical approach to health problems by including psychosocial factors, but that space needs to be widened even further for a fully evidence-informed, integrated approach to addiction. While there is a growing acceptance of the mind-body connection and its role in problems such as addiction, a primarily biopsychological model locates addiction as essentially a medical condition that requires medical treatment, a problem that is played out in the bodies and brains of people who have inherited or acquired vulnerabilities. While this does advance our understanding of addiction beyond the moral judgments that shaped its social perception for centuries, the expanded biopsychosocial *plus* (BPS+) framework offers the comprehensive scope needed for a more pragmatic, effective approach to preventing and treating the problems of addiction.

For people involved in the practical work of treating addictive behaviours, the BPS *plus* model is offered as a useful conceptual tool. First of all, this model is comprehensively *multi-dimensional*—BPS+ seeks to provide a full and rounded understanding of addictive behaviours and of their prevention and treatment. Second, the model is *integrative*: these dimensions do not exist as separate or disconnected vectors, but as intertwined and interdependent elements. A third element of the model is that it is *pluralistic*. BPS+ rests on a radical suspicion of explanations that reduce the essence of addiction to any one of these domains in ways that exclude the others. Instead, the model is open to the widest range of interventive approaches and methods that help clients to reduce the harms associated with addictive behaviours and to enhance their functioning and well-being. We expect the world of addiction theory and practice to be a contested space, where differences in approach are welcomed and critiqued, and required to prove themselves. We expect proponents in each area to make their strongest, most compelling cases for the merits of their fields of understanding and intervention, pointing out the limitations and the lacunae in knowledge and methods that apply to their particular approach. Since we want to ensure that clients have options and choices, we are bent on keeping open care pathways that include all these dimensions as clients and communities seek to thrive and flourish beyond the constraints of addiction.

If there is more to human beings than even a multi-dimensional, integrative, pluralistic model articulates, BPS+ at least draws us toward an understanding of the whole person. Having a non-reductive understanding of human beings means having an active understanding of the person affected by addiction by actively working to include all five dimensions in the practical work of preventing and treating addiction.

The BPS+ model draws on the empirical evidence and conceptual models that inform our understanding of psychoactive substance use disorders, as well as emerging knowledge about behavioural addictions that do not involve substance use. These behavioural addictions have as strong a biological dimension as those related to the use of psychoactive drugs, *plus* profoundly psychological, social, cultural and spiritual aspects.

What Is Addiction?

Addiction is the tendency to persist with an appetitive or rewarding behaviour that produces pleasure and sates desire, despite mounting negative consequences that outweigh these more positive effects. The person feels caught in this appetitive behaviour, and does not want to or cannot seem to moderate or stop it. Negative consequences include preoccupation and compulsive engagement with the behaviour, impairment of behavioural control, persistence with or relapse to the behaviour, and craving and irritability in the absence of the behaviour (Maté, 2008; National Institute on Drug Abuse [NIDA], 2010; Orford, 2000).

Perhaps the most common and archetypical example of a contemporary addiction is tobacco use: most people who smoke acknowledge that, given a choice, they wish they had never smoked or, more modestly, could stop. They certainly would not want their children or other family members to start. Most people who smoke have made at least one quit attempt over their lifetime but have been unsuccessful. Indeed, most successful ex-smokers had to make repeated attempts at cessation before they achieved a lasting result (2008 PHS Guideline Update Panel, Liaisons, and Staff, 2008).

Addictions are behaviours—they have to be enacted or performed: drinking alcohol, inhaling tobacco smoke, injecting heroin, snorting cocaine, pressing the button on a slot machine, buying a lottery ticket, eating food, having sex, shopping online. None of these behaviours is inherently addictive, but they all have addictive potential. They start out as behaviours that a person chooses to engage in, but become addictive when the person becomes caught up in them in ways that produce harmful consequences. A characteristic of addiction is the degree to which the person persists with the behaviour, reverting to it to feel pleasure and to find relief from pain and distress. In its more advanced forms, the person loses control over the behaviour. The feeling of loss of control is what people with more severe addictions commonly report as a defining characteristic of their problem.

Implicit in this model is the concept of addiction as occurring along a continuum. Addiction is not a binary either/or problem that you have or don't have. We are all on this continuum in terms of risk and harm. Depending on our situation, which can change depending on our physical health, emotional stress, social dislocation or other factors, we become more or less resilient or more or less at risk and "under the influence" of addiction.

Addiction as a "Disorder"

For the counsellor in a health care setting, the American Psychiatric Association's *Diagnostic and Statistical Manual of Mental Disorders* (DSM) has governed the way addiction has been constructed as "disorder." The DSM-IV, in effect from 1994 until the spring of 2013 (including a revision, DSM-IV-TR, in 2000), shaped diagnosis and the clinical perception of substance use disorders and other mental health problems. The new version, DSM-5 (APA, 2013), combines what were two levels of diagnosis—substance abuse and substance dependence—into one category—substance use disorders, or diagnoses that require specification of a particular substance (e.g., cannabis use disorder). The severity of the disorder is determined by the number and gravity of symptoms. Using a checklist, the clinician uses the number of symptoms to determine whether the client has no disorder, or a mild, moderate or severe addictive disorder. The term "addiction" was deliberately not used in DSM-IV, and was instead replaced by "substance abuse" and "substance dependence." However with the DSM-5, the term addiction has been reintroduced, and substance abuse and substance dependence have been removed. The overarching category becomes "substance-related and addictive disorders," which includes behavioural addictions that are not substance-use related.

The diagnosis of "pathological gambling" in the DSM-IV has become "gambling disorder" in the DSM-5. This allows gambling problems to be ranked along a continuum of severity, and acknowledges that problem gambling can be effectively understood in a paradigm of addictive behaviour. In doing so, it escapes the stigmatizing label that came with the term "pathological gambling." The DSM-5 also includes "behavioural addictions, not otherwise specified," a catch-all category for addictions that do not have a specific DSM diagnostic identity. The DSM panel did not include disorders such as Internet, sex and shopping addictions because of a current lack of scientific evidence to support these as clinical disorders.

These changes reflect a more dimensional understanding of addictions as occurring on a continuum. They also create a context for framing addiction within a broader context than substance use alone. By expanding the scope of what is considered an addictive disorder, there is the potential for more people to be identified with less severe symptoms, and for them to be helped earlier and with less intensive interventions than people whose problems have become more severe and require more involved services and supports.

Addiction as a Dimensional Problem

The move from a categorical to a dimensional understanding of addiction is evident not just in the DSM-5, but also in other attempts to understand addictive behaviours. For example, Miller and colleagues (2011) propose that addiction can be characterized by assessing severity along seven dimensions: use, problems, physical adaptation, behavioural dependence, medical harm, cognitive impairment and motivation to change. Each dimension is independent and all are interrelated, occurring along a continuum. On each dimension, a person can be evaluated on a gradient from low to high. This approach provides the counsellor with a fairly straightforward heuristic tool that maps out in a nuanced way the client's problems and progress toward meeting his or her goals without the more formal rigours of a DSM-5 diagnosis. The framework opens up a range of interventive options that can be drawn on to design treatment approaches that align with the level of care appropriate for each person in delivering client-centred care.

A Biopsychosocial *Plus* Model

To work therapeutically to address addictive behaviour, we need more than just knowledge about addiction: we need the skillful ability to apply knowledge to clinical practice in real-life situations.

Here we describe five dimensions that will not only help counsellors understand the nature of addiction problems, but will also open up essential pathways leading to change and recovery.

The Biological Dimension

The 1990s were dubbed the decade of the brain in medicine, ushering in the age of neuroscience. Advances in medical technology, such as neuroimaging and brain scanning, have had immense consequences for understanding addiction. In 1997, Alan Leshner, then head of the U.S. National Institute on Drug Abuse (NIDA), published a summative article on the neuroscientific view of addiction: "Addiction is a brain disease, and that matters" (Leshner, 1997, p. 45). Since then, the U.S. National Institutes of Health and the World Health Organization have pushed to get addiction seen as both a brain disease and a chronic illness. There are two main themes in this message: genetic differences explain the variability in people's vulnerability to addictive behaviour, and addictive behaviour, particularly the use of psychoactive substances, changes and disorders the brain in ways that are demonstrable using neuroscientific technologies.

These technological advances have encouraged the reductionist view that neurobiological approaches to addiction could win the war on drugs. The neuropathways of addiction lay the groundwork for pharmacotherapeutic solutions that promise to eliminate urge, counter and cancel the powerful euphoric effects of psychoactive substances, resolve withdrawal problems and eliminate the urges that lead to relapse that is so endemic to addiction. Even if some of these enthusiasms have not yet been proven, the advances of neuroscience have constructively elevated addiction from moral failing to valid health problem, not just needing treatment, but treatable by an emerging pharmacopoeia.

In addiction treatment today, it is vital to be aware of the biomedical nature of addiction problems and the ways that medicine intervenes, from overdose and withdrawal management to medication-assisted treatments to pharmacotherapies that reduce relapse risk. From the neuroscience perspective, three main factors contribute to addiction: genetics, environment and human development (NIDA, 2010).

It is important not to reduce the biological dimensions of addiction to neurobiology alone. Addiction is affected by and affects a person's biological functioning in many ways. Basic aspects of healthy functioning, such as diet, nutrition, sleep and self-care, are often compromised by addictive behaviour. Understanding the impact of these factors and considering them when addressing addictive behaviour can help people make positive changes and participate effectively in treatment and recovery. The biological dimension in that fuller sense is a key pathway, particularly to stabilizing and engaging someone whose life has been seriously disrupted by a chaotic lifestyle that has compromised physiological functioning. Addictive behaviours are profoundly biological in nature, and they require that we have an active and effective understanding of other dimensions, including the psychological.

The Psychological Dimension

The brain is to neuroscience what the mind is to the psychological dimension, guiding our understanding of addiction, and the ways that behaviour is shaped and moulded. Many psychological models, informed by science, govern our understanding of addiction, from classical and operant conditioning to social learning theory and the transtheoretical model (Kouimtsidis, 2010).

Heyman (2009) recently referred to addiction as a "disorder of choice." His views run counter to many popular views of addiction, including those held by people with addictions, who report that they have lost the ability to control their own behaviour. The element of choice and intention that might have existed early on is diminished and ultimately lost as a severe addiction develops. A behavioural perspective would argue that even the most mysterious behaviours are governed by laws of reward and reinforcement. Heyman and others show that when the operants (the positive and negative reinforcements) are altered, seemingly intractable addictive behaviour changes in response (Heyman, 2009; Pickard, 2012). They cite literature showing that when the setting is changed, as with American GIs in Vietnam, the rates of addiction normalize. In the extreme environment of a combat zone, soldiers used powerfully psychoactive substances to cope and self-manage, but when they repatriated, the rates of addiction reverted to what they would have been if these soldiers had not been in combat (Robins, 1973).

Other studies have shown that if the rewards are changed, the behaviour is affected. For example, people addicted to opioids who are paid not to use drugs or who are enrolled in token economies where they can earn rewards for not using are able to cut back or stop their use, even when the reward is quite modest. Heyman (2009) observes that in the modern industrial and post-industrial world, with the growth of appetitive commodities, people are being exposed to more addictive opportunities throughout the life cycle. He suggests that from childhood to old age, we tend to over-consume what we like best as part of our nature. As we live in more affluent circumstances and technology produces more and more appetitive products for us to consume, problems that were previously restricted to powerful drugs and a few other behaviours now can be evoked by an astonishing array of products, from the Internet to shopping to food. These psychological perspectives heighten our understanding of how we make choices and how the reward structure and abundance of modern life affect our appetites, desires, decisions and behaviours. Just as importantly, the psychological dimension allows us to understand and work with motivation, perception, expectancy, reward, meaning and maturation in helping to find solutions to addictive behaviours by developing behavioural alternatives that are more effective in helping individuals, families and communities thrive and flourish.

The Social Dimension

Leading thinkers in the biological and psychological sciences point to the decisive role of environment and how human development and life take place within an all-pervasive social surround (Leshner, 1997; NIDA, 2010). They point to the active and co-productive interplay among biological, psychological and social factors in addiction. While human biology and psychology are malleable, they also have limits and constraints. The problems of addiction emerge and can be more decisively resolved by the ways in which we are shaped by social realities, for example, by our socio-economic status, and depending on our access to housing, proper nutrition and health care.

A social-structural perspective

Typically the social dimension is considered to be the immediate interpersonal domain that is most proximal to the person who develops an addictive disorder. We think of the person's family and friends, workplace, leisure companions and faith community. These are all important in terms of how they increase risk or support resilience. However, we believe we need to take a broader view that includes macro-social factors. For example, issues related to class, race and gender are of great consequence in attempting to deal with issues related to addiction. This more comprehensive socio-structural perspective is essential to understanding the social underpinnings of addictive behaviour.

Seeing the social dimension as including broader socio-structural factors leads to a public health approach to social and health problems such as addiction. The social determinants of health are significantly correlated with addictive behaviours. In very direct ways, social disadvantage and social factors, such as access to employment, food and transportation, as well as stress, early life experiences, education opportunity, social exclusion and unemployment, shape the health outcomes of addictive behaviour. Not only is addiction in any community shaped by these factors, but addiction itself is a co-factor in the social determinants of health in that addictive behaviours compromise personal and community health even further (Wilkinson & Marmot, 2003).

Alexander (2008) presents an alarming view of the growth of addiction problems in contemporary society. He observes that, while social determinants contribute to addiction in predictable ways, more ominous forces cause what he describes as "the globalization of addiction." In his view, people and communities are more or less vulnerable to addiction depending on the degree to which they experience the alienating effects of dislocation.

Starting with psychosociological observations of the effects of colonization on Aboriginal communities on Canada's West Coast, Alexander (2008) has developed a comprehensive and dynamic model to explain some of the profound psychosocial problems of modern life. He posits that mental and community health require mature adults capable of independent agency and decision making who are at the same time socially integrated and engaged. Because of the power of free market society to produce enticing products, our appetites and desires become commodified, available for purchase in an ever-expanding and deepening web of products for sale. Addiction is not the problem; rather, it is what people who have been dislocated resort to as their lives become impoverished and dis-spirited. Alexander notes how habits grow and become overwhelming preoccupations requiring people's involvement at the cost of the balanced living that creates well-being. What emerges is not a single overwhelming habit, but a complex of addictive behaviours, all of which result in "overwhelming involvement . . . that is harmful to the addicted person and to . . . society" (p. 48). Alexander's concern is that addiction, understood this way, is not remedied by just improving the material conditions of existence. Indeed, as Heyman (2009) suggests, it is the profusion of consuming passions that leads to the growth of addictive behaviours in contemporary consumerist society. Alexander (2008) argues that we instead need to find other remedies for the dislocation that produces the "poverty of the spirit" from which people take refuge through addiction. Dislocation, classically seen in marginalization and disadvantage, now is a product of affluence in communities that are well off but dis-spirited and devoid of deeper purpose.

It is important not to assign an exclusively negative valence to addictive behaviour. Addictive behaviours are powerful for people who have given themselves over to them, which is what the word "addiction" means in the dictionary or etymological sense: to give yourself over, to award yourself to, to surrender yourself to the addictive behaviour. In that regard, the challenge in addressing addiction is not just to stop the behaviour, but to find alternatives that are meaningful to people, without the harmful consequences that characterize addictive behaviours.

Addictive behaviours occur in the social surround that gives shape and contour to our lives. This social dimension has a depth and range that encompass the proximal and local sphere of our immediate interactions and connections with family, friends, neighbours and others we encounter in our daily lives and the larger set of societal and socio-structural factors that forms the rules, assumptions, presumptions and norms, as well as the very conditions we experience in any society, on the basis of gender, race, class, age, education and countless other factors that shape our identities.

The Cultural Dimension

"Culture" needs to be allowed to carry the widest connotations possible. It refers to the essential importance that cultural rediscovery can have for indigenous people, refugees or members of often-marginalized communities who are able to speak their own language together, grieving, nurturing and celebrating their identities, the present and the future. It can refer to young people in a secular materialist culture who create ceremonies and rituals that evoke ecstatic experience and communal celebration. It can refer to people who feel marginalized by sexual orientation and preference.

Culture is that essential ingredient that is missing when considering people's vulnerability to addiction: culture may have been lost or not yet created, causing someone to suffer, as Alexander (2008) puts it, from dislocation. The more people find themselves in a cultural surround that respects them, that expects positive contributions from them (and rewards them for these) and that supports and protects those in need, the healthier the community and the members who compose it.

Even approaches that are usually criticized and challenged from the vantage point of those who emphasize the importance of culture acknowledge the need to have a culturally informed understanding of people affected by addiction. Both the DSM-IV and DSM-5 have tools to help the clinician make a cultural formation of the client's situation, reflecting a widespread awareness and acceptance of the importance of understanding the client's cultural belief system. Addiction as a concept is subject to interpretation through the lens of the culture—indeed the many cultures that inform and shape meaning for clients and counsellors alike. The question is not whether we should examine cultural factors, but how we will do so. This cultural dimension offers a powerful way of approaching addictive behaviours and is entwined with other key factors, including spirituality.

The Spiritual Dimension

If you listen closely to your clients who are struggling with addictions, you will hear about the importance of spirituality in their lives, whether religious or non-religious. Finding a personal "cure" for the crisis of meaning is a challenge faced by many people caught in addictive behaviours. Because this problem has to be resolved from the inside out, rather than prescriptively, it is important to respectfully keep the spiritual dimension as wide open as possible. This means keeping it open so that the therapeutic imagination respects the freedom of each person to find answers to their own questions in their own way. It involves supporting each client in searching for, connecting and making contact with the widest and deepest sources of wisdom and grounding that there are to be found.

We know that spirituality, in any form, can be protective of health and well-being, and is positively associated with lower rates of addictive behaviour. We also know that for many people devastated by addiction, spiritual affiliation and practice open up powerful paths for healing, recovery and growth. Many people seek escape and temporary transcendence through addictive behaviours, and many people draw on spiritual resilience and support to bring themselves out of the hopeless places they have wandered into. The power of mutual aid and peer support lies very much in the fellowship of others suffering in ways that are similar, working for solutions that are deeply personal and the result of the hard work of disciplined practice. But the quest for the peace and mindfulness that come with being spiritually centred is a common denominator in many healing journeys (Humphreys, 2004).

Gabor Maté (2008) provides a carefully constructed narrative of how addiction can be found in many forms of human behaviour. He found the most devastating levels of addiction in the lives of women and men living profoundly marginalized lives in downtown Vancouver. At the same time, he makes a much more comprehensive case for the BPS+ model of addiction, drawing out in detail the biological, psychological and social factors that co-construct addiction as a persisting human problem.

Each of the dimensions we highlight in the BPS+ opens up a key vector to an effective understanding of addiction for the practitioner, but even more importantly, these dimensions represent essential pathways to healthy functioning. Addiction treatment is the skillful ability to work with people affected by addictive behaviour, drawing on all of the resources that a comprehensive BPS+ approach offers, as needed in the stages and phases of the journey toward recovery and well-being.

FIGURE 1-1: Biopsychosocial *Plus* Model

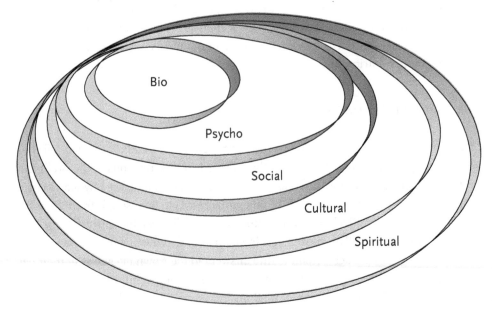

Addictive Behaviours Can Be Prevented

A BPS+ model sees addiction as existing on a continuum from absent to mild to moderate to severe. This approach also sees addiction as a variable: the presence or absence of addictive behaviours and their degrees of severity will vary over time, in both directions. In an ideal world, addiction would primarily be addressed through effective prevention. A growing evidence base now exists from which to design, deliver and measure prevention efforts (Canadian Centre on Substance Abuse [CCSA], 2007a; Health Canada, 2002; Heather & Stockwell, 2004; NIDA, 2003).

Because everyone is at some level of risk for addictive behaviours, universal prevention strategies are foundational for maintaining and enhancing health and well-being among the entire population. Prevention strategies can also focus on particular individuals and groups with identified higher risks for addictive behaviours, such as families with intergenerational histories of addiction, people who carry identifiable genetic vulnerabilities, and populations with identifiable deficits in parenting skills, neighbourhood resources and the social determinants of health. Counselling and educational efforts can help particular individuals, families and groups know their risks and support them in developing and using skills to avoid problems with substance use and other addictive behaviours.

Using the BPS+ framework, a comprehensive prevention strategy would look at all five dimensions we describe. Building healthy families and communities through effective health promotion policies and practices is the most fundamental step that can be taken to reduce addictive behaviours in a society. Advocates for each of the five dimensions are joined in endorsing that imperative (Alexander, 2008; Heyman, 2009; Health Canada, 2011; NIDA, 2010). Risk and protective factors for young people have been identified at the individual, family, peer and school levels (CCSA, 2007b). The evidence suggests that the early years are the most important for healthy human development (Sinclair, 2007). Intentional social policies that support children's development from conception through the early school years enhance the efforts parents and communities make to optimize their children's healthy development. Prevention efforts with families with young children are essential for developing not just a physically healthy child who grows into healthy adulthood, but a psychologically resilient child who matures into a socially intelligent and skillfully competent adult. The factors identified as affecting resilience include genetic profile, parental control, family cohesion, parental monitoring, drug availability, peer drug use, self-esteem, hedonistic attitudes and the balance between risk and protective factors (Karoly et al., 2005). How children are bought up shapes their physical and mental well-being, including their vulnerability to or resilience against addictive behaviours.

Because we know that prevention and health promotion efforts work, we know that the number of people with addiction problems can be minimized. In that sense, the high rates of addiction problems in contemporary society reflect the inadequacy of our prevention efforts (Alexander, 2008; Sinclair, 2007).

Addictions Can Be Treated with Early Interventions

If prevention is about reducing risk, treatment is about reducing harm. Treatment begins where prevention fails. The question with addictive behaviour is how soon can intervention be effective? The classic disease model asserts that addiction is a disease characterized by denial, and that people stop only when they "hit bottom"—when things get so bad that there are serious consequences. A BPS+ perspective argues that you can't start soon enough, and that even with prevention efforts in place, some people will have addiction problems. Sufficient evidence now exists to prove that addictive behaviours and their associated harms can be identified early, and that evidence-based strategies exist to guide how, when and where to intervene (CCSA, 2007a; Conrod et al., 2006; Mushquash et al., 2007).

Problems related to addictive behaviours typically manifest themselves as early as adolescence and in the early adult years, from age 16 to 24, when as many as three-quarters of these young people will have had previous mental health issues. For them, early intervention for mental health problems could well prevent addiction problems (Rush et al., 2010).

Effective, timely and urgent action is crucial, and has many advantages:

- The impact and effects of the addictive behaviour, in all BPS+ spheres, will be less.
- The length and intensity of the intervention needed will be less.
- The cost per case will be less, meaning reduced burden for health recovery services, so that more resources can be directed upstream to invest in health promotion and illness prevention.
- The technical clinical skills can be learned by a wide set of health and social service providers.
- The impact on the life of the client will be less disruptive.
- The client is supported to take responsibility for change, including making choices about goals and levels of support he or she wants to draw on.
- Action to make change can begin immediately.

Since most people have mild to moderate addiction problems, screening should be an inherent part of health and social service assessments. Eventually, this would mean that most addiction interventions would be offered outside the specialized addiction sector, in community and primary care settings, and in other specialized environments, such as mental health, physical health, criminal justice, and child and family services.

The evidence suggests that clients with mild to moderate addiction problems will have good outcomes with brief interventions that empower them to take a primary role in the change process. Not only can brief treatments be effective, but also they do not need to be delivered by specialists in the addiction treatment system. The work of early identification and early intervention is best syndicated across the full span of health and social services in a community. Another valuable factor is that clients tend to respond quickly to early intervention (within six or seven sessions) if they are going to do well, so that those who do not show improvement early on should be offered more support.

SBIRT: Screening, Brief Intervention and Referral to Treatment

Over the past decade, a number of techniques and tools have been developed and evaluated, enabling health care and social service professions to screen, treat and refer clients for problems related to addictive behaviours. Approaches for early identification and intervention include the Screening, Brief Intervention and Referral to Treatment (SBIRT) model developed by the Substance Abuse and Mental Health Services Administration (SAMHSA). It is "a comprehensive, integrated, public health approach to the delivery of early intervention for individuals with risky alcohol and drug use" (SAMHSA, 2011, p. 2). The model identifies six characteristics to be applied in all health care and social service settings:

- brief, quick screening and quick, short interventions
- universal screening (as part of regular intake processes)
- focusing on targeted behaviours (one or more specific problematic behaviours)
- providing interventions in non-addiction settings (e.g., public health settings, schools, doctors' offices, family agencies)
- having a seamless flow between screening, brief intervention and referral to specialized addiction settings
- providing research and experiential evidence to support the approach (using program outcomes to measure success).

Resources to do SBIRT are now widely available, for example, through SAMHSA and the College of Family Physicians of Canada.

While SAMHSA acknowledges that risky alcohol use has garnered the most attention in terms of the SBIRT model, enough evolving evidence exists to support its application to other problem areas. The model now applies to tobacco use, illicit drug use, depression, anxiety disorders and trauma (SAMHSA, 2011).

The SBIRT model (see Figure 1-2) starts with screening to allow for a quick calculation of risk. Risk is divided into low risk (no further intervention), moderate risk (brief intervention: one to five sessions lasting five to 60 minutes), moderate to high risk (brief treatment: five to 12 sessions) and severe risk (referral to specialized service for treatment).

FIGURE 1-2: The SBIRT Model

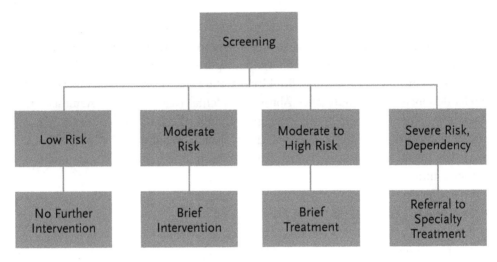

Source: SAMHSA (2011).

FRAMES: Six Features of Successful Brief Treatment

In their review of the literature, Bien and colleagues (1993) identified six key features linked to success in brief outpatient treatment. More than 20 years later, these six components remain salient and robust markers for the brief treatment of addictions. The mnemonic FRAMES has become foundational to evidence-based addiction treatment:

- **Feedback:** giving the client information that is relevant to his or her situation, particularly around the risks and negative consequences of the addictive behaviour.
- **Responsibility:** change is ultimately up to the client, from decision making to taking action to maintaining change, with the counsellor and other resources available to support, advise, guide and coach the client as needed.
- **Advice:** the counsellor guides the client on how to modify his or her addictive behaviour, drawing from clinical experience and the evidence base.
- **Menu:** the counsellor helps the client see that he or she has different options to choose from to work toward change.
- **Empathy:** the counsellor listens respectfully, supportively and attentively to the client's personal concerns and goals so the client experiences how the counsellor is compassionately working in the client's best interest.
- **Self-efficacy:** the counsellor works to enhance the client's belief that he or she can succeed at making change happen.

The services and supports provided by the health care and social services systems need to be more collaboratively connected to form a continuum of care if clients with addiction problems are to be seen as non-stigmatized consumers who are welcomed and supported in getting the help they need. Practitioners in the specialized addiction system need to share their expertise with other health and social service providers who lack this specialized knowledge. The National Treatment Strategy Working Group (2008) has produced practical approaches to identifying and treating addiction problems that can fit integrally in health care and other systems.

Addiction Treatment: Everything "Works," Except When It Doesn't

Again and again, the research literature on mental health and addiction treatment is proving to be rich in findings that report the null hypothesis: when well-trained thera-pists deliver two or more well-conceived interventions, both interventions produce better outcomes compared to those for clients who received no treatment at all, but there is no significant difference between either intervention. In fact, these findings apply generally to psychotherapy research (Asay & Lambert, 1999; Miller et al., 2011). Project MATCH (1997) offers a classic illustration: that research project, the most expensive random-ized control trial ever undertaken on addiction treatment, demonstrated that three very different interventions offered as brief treatments, plus extended research follow-up, all produced significant and persisting benefits for the clients receiving treatment, but with no significant differences among them. For adherents of particular models and approaches, this is disconcerting. But for clients, it might be encouraging to know that they could benefit from a range of evidence-based treatments. One factor that makes a difference when trying to determine best treatment practices is that some treatments have been more researched than others, and therefore have a stronger evidence base behind them. For other treatments, the evidence may be mostly practice based, derived from the knowledge and skills that come with years of direct front-line work and men-tors who share their clinical wisdom and savvy, without being formally researched. These two perspectives create tensions between researchers and clinicians.

Another dimension that enters the debate of what gets to count as knowledge comes increasingly from clients and consumers, people whose perspectives are often ignored or disqualified, especially if viewed from the stigmatizing perspective that peo-ple with addictions are in denial and cannot be relied on to speak the truth. However, in ways that are remarkably empowering, courageous and creditable, clients are insisting that they too have knowledge, which needs a place in the conversation about best prac-tices. Just as heroically and importantly, family members and concerned others are also realizing that they have a right to bring their knowledge and wisdom to the discussion of best practices. Marginalized for years, clients and families are still struggling to claim their full entitlement to be recognized as knowledge holders and as consumers who have the right to decide on the services they prefer and how they are provided.

That meaning is always shaped by and filtered through the fabric of culture is another factor contesting the narrow positivistic view that excludes knowledge that cannot meet strict methodological tests of truth. The recent document *Honouring Our Strengths,* developed by Aboriginal leaders and Health Canada (Health Canada et al., 2011), is an instructive example of a culturally shaped approach to knowledge and evidence.

The debate is and will continue to be about who is let on to the jury that arbitrates what evidence-based practices should be. This creates dilemmas for counsellors, researchers, clients, families and funders who have to defend the rationale for their decisions. As consumers, we expect the health care domain to be excellent, and we would be appalled if we or someone we care about were getting care of one sort when there was stronger evidence for another form of care.

There is much to work out in addiction treatment, from determining whether there are advantages to residential over outpatient care (and if so, for whom), to the merits of abstinence-only goals to harm reduction approaches, to whether to include significant others and family members in the treatment process. This debate needs to continue. As stronger evidence emerges, it is hoped that consensus will emerge among the constituents, all of whom have a stake in the process. In the meantime, addiction counsellors need a set of effective practices to guide them in the daily they work they do with people affected by addiction, in the reconstructed way we have described it here—existing on a continuum and extending to a wide range of addictive behaviours that carry the risk of harm. Our governing observation is that everything works in addiction treatment, except when it doesn't. Even doing nothing "works." A certain percentage of people who have identifiable addiction problems, including very severe ones, improve without seeking treatment, as do people who are on wait-lists for treatment (Granfield & Cloud, 1999; Miller and Carroll, 2006).

While we don't recommend doing nothing, when evaluating addiction treatments we need to determine whether the treatments are better than what happens when people take action on their own or are left on a wait-list. Evidence suggests that people who complete treatment do better, in general, than people who do not, and that the engagement skills of the counsellor are important in retaining clients in treatment (Miller et al., 2011). We also have evidence that confrontation produces worse outcomes in treatment than does motivational communication (Miller & Rollnick, 2013). There is also evidence that some medications work in some situations and have therapeutic advantages over psychosocial therapies alone. This is consistent with our BPS+ model, which indicates that we can be most helpful by exploring and identifying pathways in all five dimensions relevant to clients' present status and treatment goals.

We can also advise our clients based on our understanding of the evidence. For example, a doctor wanting to prescribe a drug to help a person with withdrawal symptoms would likely choose a drug that has the highest efficacy in addressing the person's symptoms. But the drug will not be effective in all cases, for one reason or another. What will the doctor do next? One option is to do nothing, because there is no other drug with comparable efficacy. Or the doctor could consider a second drug, with lower overall efficacy, but which does work with a smaller portion of the population. Ideally, the doctor will discuss with the person the pros and cons of each choice, so the two can arrive at a mutual decision.

In another situation, a counsellor offers a client cognitive-behavioural therapy (CBT) to treat severe alcohol use disorder. Although the evidence suggests that CBT is unsurpassed as the treatment of choice, the client has not responded well, and now is missing sessions. What does the counsellor do? One possibility is to prevail upon the client to keep going, knowing that if the client quits, the counsellor has at least offered the best intervention available. Or the counsellor could meet with the client and identify options to enable the client to make a choice. The counsellor could also encourage the client to visit other settings that offer different forms of care and check out mutual aid options. Sometimes our own biases and opinions, however well informed they may be, are the barrier that keeps a client from being aware of options in all of the BPS+ pathways to change and recovery. If our orientation were truly client centred and in the service of the client making informed choices, no doubt the respect and safety we offer would increase the likelihood of client engagement.

The How of Helping: Three Predictors of Success in Therapy

Meta-analyses and reviews by Lambert and his colleagues (e.g., Asay & Lambert, 1999) over several decades point to three ways in which counsellors influence the outcomes in therapy:
- the helping relationship
- the methods and techniques we use
- the hope and positive expectancy we support in the client.

Asay and Lambert (1999) also remind us that a fourth variable belongs totally to the client: the personal strengths and social supports they have to draw on.

The helping relationship

Of the three ingredients with which we work, it turns out that the helping relationship is the most powerful variable.

Clients of counsellors who are more empathic tend to have better treatment outcomes than those whose counsellors show less empathy. This suggests that the *how* of helping is at least as important in determining outcome as *what* method or model of treatment is used. In fact, Miller & Rollnick (2013) maintain that the ability of the counsellor to establish and maintain an empathic relationship is the best predictor of success in therapy. This extends beyond addiction to psychotherapy in general (Asay & Lambert, 1999; Miller et al., 2011).

Empathy is not just a state of mind, but a demonstrable and measurable skill that is integral to the work of therapy. Rogers (1951) recognized empathy as the heart of client-centred therapy. Along with highlighting genuineness and unconditional positive regard, Rogers felt that empathy promoted change and growth in clients. As an evidence-based practice in its own right, empathy has a place in any method of therapy, and is used in varying degrees in motivational enhancement therapy, CBT and 12-step facilitation.

The corollary to empathy is confrontation. Confrontation is a win-lose game you play with a client. If you convert the client to your position, you win. If the client opposes you and refuses to convert to the position you rightly hold, you lose. You can invoke stereotypical clinical language—the client is in denial or hasn't hit bottom yet. Sometimes you may win, and you get the client to convert, but this is not likely. It is easier on you and your client to work from a client-centred perspective, but it is skillful work, improving with practice, client feedback and supervision by peers and mentors.

Treatment methods and techniques

Even when one treatment is measurably better than another, it should not necessarily be the only option, just the one to start with. It is likely that the better intervention works for only a proportion of the clients who receive it, so that an intervention with a less effective overall success rate might be better for another segment of the client population. In that way, the better intervention appears to work with more people more of the time, but the worse intervention, while working for fewer people, does work some of the time. Efforts to give clinicians decision rules about best practices in addiction treatment still have a long way to go. That said, it is essential for optimal client care that counsellors and their agencies know what are the better and worse clinical practices in treating addiction.

Hope and positive expectancy

Expectancy—sometimes called the placebo effect or the ability to kindle and sustain the client's hope for a good outcome—is nurtured through therapist skill rather than a particular "method." It involves the willingness to work with the client and demonstrating an active and compassionate interest in the client's situation as he or she sees it, reflecting your sense of respect for the client and your commitment to putting your time into working together.

Client centred skills allow the counsellor to engage and work with the client on goals that are important to the client in ways that are negotiated between the client and counsellor. And the evidence, supported by what clients and counsellors alike have reported again and again, proves that the *how* of counselling is at the heart of therapy.

Figure 1-3 highlights the four factors in counselling that influence the outcome of therapy, as identified by Asay and Lambert (1999).

FIGURE 1-3: Therapeutic Factors Related to Improvement

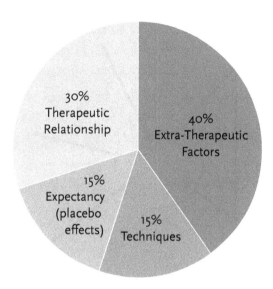

Source: Asay & Lambert (1999).

Treating Addictive Behaviours: Severity Predicts Complexity

Most of the population is at the low-risk or low-harm end of the addiction continuum. While only a minority will develop more severe addiction problems, they will usually require more intensive treatment and support. The likelihood of complexity grows proportionally with severity. People who meet criteria for a serious addictive behaviour have more symptoms or negative consequences, and more pronounced symptoms or negative consequences from their use. Their problems will exist on some level in each of the BPS+ dimensions, perhaps particularly significant in some, perhaps less so in others. They are also more likely to have physical and mental health problems. For example, the risk of certain cancers rises in direct proportion to the amount of alcohol use. To have an addictive disorder is to have a significantly elevated risk of having mental health problems, and that risk increases with the severity of the addiction (Health Canada, 2002; Skinner, 2005). This is another reason why a BPS+ approach is valuable: it helps identify the full range of issues that need to be understood to make an effective plan based on an accurate understanding of the client's needs, strengths and goals.

One way of representing the multi-dimensional aspect of addiction is by mapping out the problems areas, along with the client's readiness for change and the availability of social support, as in Figure 1-4.

FIGURE 1-4: Mapping Out the Multidimensional Aspects of Addiction

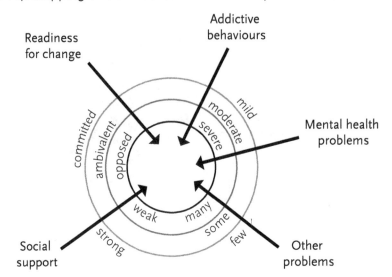

This mapping can be done with the client, as well as collaboratively with a multidisciplinary team. Tools like this allow tracking over time, as well as helping with the initial assessment, especially with clients with severe and complex problems, to help you find an area on which to focus your efforts. Be aware of your scope of practice—the orbit of things you can and cannot do. It is unrealistic for a single person to be able to address all of the client's problem areas and needs. The more severe and complex the situation, the more important it is not to be working alone. Ideally, the client and you have access to experts who can address both the client's immediate and long-term goals, and can tackle a shared plan together, one increment at a time.

Helping Change Happen: Building the Client's Recovery Capital

As many change narratives attest, most people with addiction problems—even some with severe addictions and those who do not participate in formal treatment—do solve or resolve their addiction problems.

A substantial literature on "natural recovery" or "recovery without treatment" now supports this scientifically, uncovering factors that play key roles in helping people change addictive behaviours.

While this change is not at all guaranteed, it occurs in significant enough numbers that clients themselves take note and are given the courage to take healthy risks to get there.

The reasons that people decide to change are diverse: some people's addictive behaviour is damaging their physical health, so that the behaviour is no longer the source of pleasure and reward it had been; for instance, they may have contracted HIV or hepatitis C. Other people may decide to change for psychological reasons because they don't like or can no longer recognize the person they have become. Sometimes the decision to change can be motivated by an embarrassing or worrisome social consequence of their addiction, such as being arrested, or humiliating public behaviour, such as becoming uninhibited and sexually compromised while intoxicated, or out of hand at a party. For others, the threat of losing a job or the breakup of a relationship is what makes them decide to change an addictive behaviour. Still others change with the desire to get in touch with their cultural roots and be guided by cultural values. And finally, feeling spiritually empty and bankrupt may be what propels someone to seek a stronger, more meaningful life. The birth of a child, the death of a parent, or another dramatic life event, such as surviving a life-threatening event, or getting a serious diagnosis, or seeing what has happened to someone else you care about or know—these are all examples people give as the precipitating factors for deciding to change an addictive behaviour without treatment (Cloud & Granfield, 2008; Granfield & Cloud, 1999; Klingemann et al., 2009).

People with addictive behaviours who can access social support have much better chances of a sustained recovery. Having problems that lead to low self-worth and an inclination to isolation or problematic interpersonal behaviour are precursors to addiction behaviours. The loss of social relationships and social standing that are often a consequence of addictive behaviour can contribute to the radical demoralization that comes with a life derailed by addictive behaviour.

In helping people with addiction, the goal is not just to get them to stop the addictive behaviour, but to develop alternatives that adequately meet their needs, without imposing the severe negative consequences that can come with addiction. Treatment, especially brief treatment, can only help the person prepare for or start that process of finding more positive alternatives to their addiction. It usually takes time for clients to feel that they have moved from the active state of addiction into the process of, or journey into, recovery.

Drawing on the theoretical work of French sociologist Pierre Bourdieu (Bourdieu & Wacquant, 1992) and on their own research on recovery without treatment, White and Cloud (2008) use the concept of "recovery capital," introduced by Granfield and Cloud (1999), which describes "the breadth and depth of internal and external resources that can be drawn upon to initiate and sustain recovery" from addictive behaviours (Granfield & Cloud, 1999, p. 1). Recovery capital reflects a paradigm shift in addiction treatment from a focus on problems and illness to one directed toward solutions and recovery. Cloud and Granfield (2008) define capital as "a body of resources that can be accumulated or exhausted" (p. 1972).

Cloud and Granfield (2008) divide recovery capital into four components:
- **Personal recovery capital**: either physical (e.g., safe shelter, physical health, clothing, food, transportation) or human recovery capital (e.g., values, education, knowledge,

skills, credentials, problem-solving abilities, interpersonal skills, self-awareness, self-esteem, self-efficacy, sense of purpose and meaning)

- **Family and social recovery capital**: close relationships with family and kin, and other connections that support recovery; non-addictive social networks, lifestyles and activities; and a positive sense of social inclusion and belonging in leisure, work, faith community or other value-based groups
- **Community recovery capital**: resources, policies and expressed attitudes that promote recovery, provide visible role models, provide mutual aid supports, offer access to treatment and continuing care resources, and actively support community reintegration
- **Cultural capital**: culturally based resources and connections that resonate with the person's positive sense of identity and belonging.

What is significant from a BPS+ perspective is the robust dimensionality this concept brings to the task of resolving the problems of addictive behaviours. Addiction solutions come not just from stopping the problem behaviours, but from cultivating healthy alternatives. The following recommendations have emerged from taking a recovery capital approach to addiction treatment (White & Cloud, 2008):

- Screen and offer brief interventions before clients use up their recovery capital.
- Reach out to connect with people who are marginalized and disadvantaged and have low recovery capital.
- Take a strengths-based approach to ongoing assessment of social capital.
- Determine levels of care on the basis of recovery capital.
- Mobilize resources in as many domains of recovery capital as possible to support recovery and well-being.
- Make changes in recovery capital a measure of how effective your efforts to help clients change are.

Conclusion

There are more things in heaven and earth, Horatio,
Than are dreamt of in your philosophy.

—William Shakespeare

Addiction treatment is ultimately about finding solutions to the problems that come with addictive behaviour. It is a very practical project that requires knowledge and values, and respect and compassion for each client. Most of all, it is skillful work. At its core is our ability to work empathically and respectfully with individuals, families and communities affected by addiction, often in extremely challenging circumstances. The BPS+ model allows us to construct a dynamic and evolving engagement with clients in the context of addiction and recovery. The biological, psychological, social, cultural and spiritual dimensions all contribute to a fuller understanding of clients' journeys into addictive behaviour, and each dimension opens up a care pathway that can be accessed at appropriate points in the phases and stages involved in that second journey toward recovery. The BPS+ model invites us to look beyond our particular approaches and scope of practice to the wider landscape of options that give clients the choices and resources they need to thrive in their communities. In that sense, it is a model that opens counsellors—that diverse, multidisciplinary group committed to finding the best solutions to the clients in their care—to supporting recovery in ways that are more fulsome and comprehensive, as well as practical and effective, than can be dreamt of—or accomplished—by any one approach alone.

References

2008 PHS Guideline Update Panel, Liaisons, and Staff. (2008). *Clinical Practice Guideline: Treating Tobacco Use and Dependence: 2008 Update*. Rockville, MD: Department of Health and Human Services. Retrieved from www.ahrq.gov/clinic/tobacco/treating_tobacco_use08.pdf

Alexander, B.K. (2008). *The Globalization of Addiction: A Study in Poverty of the Spirit*. Oxford, United Kingdom: Oxford University Press.

American Psychiatric Association (APA). (1994). *Diagnostic and Statistical Manual of Mental Disorders* (4th ed.). Washington, DC: Author.

American Psychiatric Association (APA). (2013). *Diagnostic and Statistical Manual of Mental Disorders* (5th ed.). Washington, DC: Author.

Asay, T.P. & Lambert, M.J. (1999). The empirical case for the common factors in therapy: Quantitative findings. In M.A. Hubble, B.I. Duncan & S.D. Miller (Eds.), *The Heart and Soul of Change: What Works in Therapy* (pp. 33–56). Washington, DC: American Psychological Association.

Bien, T.H., Miller, W.R. & Tonigan, J.S. (1993). Brief interventions for alcohol problems: A review. *Addiction, 88*, 315–335.

Bourdieu, P. & Wacquant, L.J.D. (1992). *An Invitation to Reflexive Sociology*. Chicago: University of Chicago Press.

Canadian Centre on Substance Abuse (CCSA). (2007a). *A Drug Prevention Strategy for Canada's Youth*. Ottawa: Author.

Canadian Centre on Substance Abuse (CCSA). (2007b). *Substance Abuse in Canada: Youth in Focus*. Ottawa: Author.

Cloud, W. & Granfield, R. (2008). Conceptualizing recovery capital: Expansion of a theoretical construct. *Substance Use & Misuse, 43*, 1971–1986.

Conrod, P.J., Stewart, S.H., Comeau, M.N. & Maclean, M. (2006). Efficacy of cognitive behavioral interventions targeting personality risk factors for youth alcohol misuse. *Journal of Clinical Child and Adolescent Psychology, 35*, 550–563.

Engel, G.L. (1977). The need for a new medical model: A challenge for biomedicine. *Science, 196*, 129–136. doi: 10.1126/science.847460

Granfield, R. & Cloud, W. (1999). *Coming Clean: Overcoming Addiction without Treatment.* New York: New York University Press.

Health Canada. (2002). *Best Practices: Concurrent Mental Health and Substance Use Disorders.* Ottawa: Author. Retrieved from www.hc-sc.gc.ca/hc-ps/alt_formats/hecs-sesc/pdf/pubs/adp-apd/bp_disorder-mp_concomitants/bp_concurrent_mental_health-eng.pdf

Health Canada, Assembly of First Nations & National Native Addictions Partnership Foundation. (2011). *Honouring Our Strengths: A Renewed Framework to Address Substance Use Issues among First Nations People in Canada.* Ottawa: Author. Retrieved from http://nnadaprenewal.ca/wp-content/uploads/2012/01/Honouring-Our-Strengths-2011_Eng1.pdf

Heather, N. & Stockwell, T. (Eds.). (2004). *The Essential Handbook of Treatment and Prevention of Alcohol Problems.* Chichester, United Kingdom: Wiley.

Heyman, G. (2009). *Addiction: A Disorder of Choice.* Cambridge, MA: Harvard University Press.

Humphreys, C. (2004). *Circles of Recovery: Self-Help Organizations for Addictions.* Cambridge, United Kingdom: Cambridge University Press.

Karoly, K.A., Kilburn, M.R. & Cannon, J.S. (2005). *Early Childhood Interventions: Proven Results, Future Promise.* Santa Monica, CA: Rand. Retrieved from www.rand.org/content/dam/rand/pubs/monographs/2005/RAND_MG341.pdf

Klingemann, H., Sobell, M.B. & Sobell, L.C. (2009). Continuities and change in self-help research. *Addiction, 105*, 1510–1518.

Kouimtsidis, C. (2010). Cognitive theories of addiction: A narrative review. *Psychiatrike, 21*, 315–323.

Leshner, A.I. (1997). Addiction is a brain disease, and that matters. *Science, 278*, 45–47. doi: 10.1126/science.278.5335.45

Maté, G. (2008). *In the Realm of Hungry Ghosts: Close Encounters with Addictions.* Toronto: Knopf Canada.

Miller, W.R. & Carroll, K.M. (Eds.). (2006). *Rethinking Substance Abuse: What the Science Shows, and What We Should Do about It.* New York: Guilford Press.

Miller, W.R., Forcehimes, A. & Zweben, A. (2011). *Treating Addiction: A Guide for Professionals.* New York: Guilford Press.

Miller, W.R. & Rollnick, S. (2013). *Motivational Interviewing: Helping People Change* (3rd ed.). New York: Guilford Press.

Mushquash, C.J., Comeau, M.N. & Stewart, S.H. (2007). An alcohol abuse early intervention approach with Mi'kmaq adolescents. *First Peoples Child & Family Review, 3* (1), 17–26.

National Institute on Drug Abuse (NIDA). (2003). *Preventing Drug Abuse among Children and Adolescents: A Research-based Guide for Parents, Educators and Community Leaders.* Washington, DC: Author. Retrieved from www.drugabuse.gov/sites/default/files/preventingdruguse_2.pdf

National Institute on Drug Abuse (NIDA). (2010). *Drugs, Brains and Behavior: The Science of Addiction* (rev. ed.). Washington, DC: Author. Retrieved from www.drugabuse.gov/sites/default/files/sciofaddiction.pdf

National Treatment Strategy Working Group. (2008). *A Systems Approach to Substance Use in Canada: Recommendations for a National Treatment Strategy*. Ottawa: National Framework for Action to Reduce the Harms Associated with Alcohol and Other Drugs and Substances in Canada. Retrieved from www.nationalframework-cadrenational.ca/uploads/files/TWS_Treatment/nts-report-eng.pdf

Orford, J. (2000). *Excessive Appetites: A Psychological View of Addiction* (2nd ed.). Chichester, United Kingdom: Wiley.

Pickard, H. (2012). The purpose in chronic addiction. *American Journal of Bioethics Neuroscience, 3* (2), 30–39. doi: 10.1080/21507740.2012.663058

Project MATCH Research Group. (1997). Matching alcoholism treatments to client heterogeneity: Project MATCH posttreatment drinking outcomes. *Journal of Studies in Alcohol, 58* (1), 7–29.

Robins, L.N. (1973). *A Follow-up of Vietnam Drug Users*. Special Action Office Monograph, Series A, No. 1. Washington, DC: Executive Office of the President.

Rogers, C.R. (1951). *Client-centred Therapy: Its Current Practice, Implications and Theory*. London, United Kingdom: Constable.

Rush, B., Urbanski, K.A., Bassani, D.G., Castel, S. & Wild, T.C. (2010). The epidemiology of co-occurring substance use and other mental disorders in Canada: Prevalence, service use, and unmet needs. In J. Cairney & C.L. Streiner (Eds.), *Mental Disorders in Canada: An Epidemiological Perspective* (pp. 170–204). Toronto: University of Toronto Press.

Sinclair, A. (2007). *0–5: How Small Children Make a Big Difference*. London, United Kingdom: The Work Foundation. Retrieved from www.centreforconfidence.co.uk/docs/Final_Report_0-5_How_small_children_make_a_big_difference.pdf

Skinner, W.J.W. (Ed.). (2005). *Treating Concurrent Disorders: A Guide for Counsellors*. Toronto: Centre for Addiction and Mental Health.

Substance Abuse and Mental Health Services Administration (SAMHSA). (2011). *Screening, Brief Intervention and Referral to Treatment (SBIRT) in Behavioral Healthcare*. Rockville, MD: Author.

White, W.L. & Cloud, W. (2008). Recovery capital: A primer for addictions professionals. *Counselor, 9* (5), 22–27.

Wilkinson, R. & Marmot, R. (2003). *The Social Determinants of Health: The Solid Facts* (2nd ed.). Copenhagen, Denmark: World Health Organization Europe. Retrieved from www.euro.who.int/__data/assets/pdf_file/0005/98438/e81384.pdf

Chapter 2

A Client Perspective

Cheryl Peever

For my money, memoirs written by addicts recounting their use are usually not what I would consider reliable accounts of that period in their lives. If anyone implies they can recall with perfect clarity the places, people, amounts and chronology of events surrounding their use, it's usually fiction. What I do trust are stories of treatment and recovery. People can recall with astounding detail the people they met, a look, a phrase or a gesture during the early phases of recovery. Your first experience with treatment professionals is an incredibly powerful moment. Your senses are heightened, your fear is acute and you are considering making the most profound change of your life. From the first moment you pick up the phone, walk into a meeting or attend an assessment, the circumstances of that moment and the days and weeks that follow become embedded in your memory. Even people who have relapsed many times and experienced multiple encounters with addiction professionals can relate important moments of every treatment experience.

I did not have good experiences with addiction facilities when I was looking for help, although in fairness to those I came into contact with, I would not have been considered a platinum client. The symptoms of my illness and the accompanying agitation, anxiety, depression and anger made it difficult for me to advocate appropriately for myself or ask the right questions. I found the system confusing and frustrating, and it seemed like there were more barriers than access points. As a professional, many years later, I have been critical of the way clients are often treated within the addiction and mental health systems and between those systems, although I admit great improvements have been made over the last 20 years. It would be wrong to only talk about the problems. In my career as a social worker, I have encountered incredibly skilled and innovative clinicians who are trying to do their best in spite of the challenges presented to them by clients with increasingly complex problems, higher demands for productivity and an underfunded system.

A chapter about consumer perspectives should not reflect only one voice or one time period. I decided that I needed to include the voices of others who had experience with substance use treatment. I began to ask everyone I knew who had been to treatment if they would speak to me about their experiences. They eagerly agreed. I also mentioned it to other professionals and asked if they had any clients who would be willing to talk to me. They did. At a talk I gave to an audience of both professionals and clients, I put it out there almost as an afterthought; yet I had a lineup of people wanting to be interviewed.

Initially, I thought I would ask a couple of people some pointed questions about their experiences with treatment. Instead I heard a chorus of about 40 people graciously and thoughtfully telling their stories of treatment, recovery and relapse, and offering suggestions for current and future professionals in the field.

Some people agreed to talk to me because they had negative experiences and wanted to suggest how clinicians and systems could do better. People who had positive experiences were equally as passionate about wanting to be heard; they wanted to talk about what worked and why, and to convey the importance their counsellors played in changing their lives. This was not a representative sample of all addicts by any means, but it was a decent cross-section of the population—people varied in age, gender, ethnicity and sexual orientation. Some people who spoke to me were using again; others were in early recovery; and some had been clean for many years. Several people had chosen to work in the addiction field because of their journey; others were in school or worked in other fields, and some were unemployed. People were surprisingly compassionate toward those who go into the helping profession and work with addicts, and they were incredibly savvy about the internal pressures faced by those who work within the system. Nevertheless, we think the system could work better; clinicians could be trained better, supervised better; and society could do a better job of understanding addiction and what addicts go through.

Throughout this chapter, I use the terms "addict" and "addiction" because those are the terms I use for myself. If this were an academic article, I would probably use terms like "people with substance use issues," or I would distinguish between people who are "substance abusers" and those who are "substance dependent." But this is a personal piece that conveys personal stories, so I choose to refer to myself and my comrades as addicts. Since alcohol is a drug, I include people who used alcohol as well as those who used chemical or herbal substances. I sometimes refer to "drugs and alcohol," even though alcohol is also a drug. Instead of distinguishing the drug addicts from the alcoholics and using another term for people who are cross-addicted, I use the word "addict" as an umbrella term, with apologies to those who may feel squeamish about it. Many of the people I talked to have a concurrent mental health issue. People don't refer to themselves as concurrent disorder clients, nor do they separate their mental health issues from their addiction issues. While clinicians may think of concurrent disorders as two disorders, those of us with personal experience generally think of it as one issue that affects our total experience. I don't distinguish between the groups.

No one is a textbook case.

The difficulty with papers, studies and books on addiction is that they have to distill addicts into traits, generalities and common denominators. Trying to place those templates onto the person in front of you misses the uniqueness and diversity of who they are, their experience and what they may be trying to tell you. By the nature of the lifestyle they have been living, and as a survival technique, most addicts are highly skilled at reading people. Some of us are used to walking into situations where we must complete a threat assessment in about 30 seconds, and we need to be able to spot the scam, the rip-off and the empty promises right away. So, we can spot phoniness and false bravado a mile away, and can detect weariness, but distinguish it from impatience, boredom or dismissiveness.

The client studies the clinician and tries to figure him or her out in much the same way the clinician studies the client—by looking at body language, tone, speech content, eye contact and so on. Clinicians often unknowingly telegraph their thoughts and attitudes during an encounter in subtle ways (Maté, 2008). A client can tell when someone is talking to them as a genuine human being and listening with compassion and empathy to what they are trying to say. A client can also tell when someone is making quick judgments or assumptions and slotting them into a category.

A clinician can ruin an encounter in only a few seconds, so that initial engagement with a client is incredibly important. Even if a client decides not to continue on into a program, that first experience with you can determine his or her feelings about treatment as a realistic possibility some time in the future. If clients know they will be treated with compassion and respect, they will feel comfortable about coming back. People who were initially unsure about entering treatment said they engaged in a program based on the first clinician they met. Overwhelmingly, what hooked people was being treated with dignity and feeling like that counsellor or that program could help.

At a recent talk I gave to professionals in a psychiatric program, I put this question to the audience: "Who would like to see clients treated with more respect?" Almost every hand in the room went up. When I asked "Who feels like they treat their clients with respect?" again, almost every hand went up. And therein lies the crux. Many clinicians think their interactions with clients are respectful, while others are consistently witnessing disrespectful encounters. If other clinicians can see it, you can bet your client can as well.

So how can you be sure you are treating clients respectfully? It's pretty simple. If you are talking to your client in the same way you would speak to your boss, a policeman, your bank manager or your doctor, you are probably being respectful. If you are talking to your client like a "street person," a "sick" person or as if you don't care how they interpret what you are saying, then you are being disrespectful. If when clients are not around you refer to them using terms like "junkie," "crackhead" or "drunk," chances are pretty good you will come across as disrespectful to your client. As Gabor Maté (2008) put it, "We see their reactions but don't realize that we ourselves may be creating what they are reacting to—not so much by what we say but by who we are being in the process" (p. 384).

I'm an addict. I'm not stupid.

Many folks I talked with expressed frustration that their intellect seemed to be put into question because of their substance use or substance of choice. Crack users and meth users in particular felt like they were treated as uneducated or just plain stupid.

Counsellors tended to convey this message by speaking slowly and emphasizing certain words with an infantilizing tone or repeating phrases and questions for emphasis. People with alcohol issues were sometimes treated to prepackaged slogans such as "just put a plug in the jug" (as if that hadn't already been tried). As a former cocaine user, I felt like I was treated as if I had just done a little too much partying until I mentioned dealing and intravenous use; then I could see in the clinician's face that my intelligence quotient plummeted and she was dropping me down a few notches on the seediness scale as well.

Having a substance use problem says nothing about your intelligence. It says nothing about who you are, your moral character, your family, your personality, your potential or your future. When I was at my worst, no one would have ever predicted I would someday be clean and sober with two degrees and a fulfilling career. Perhaps that's because societal stereotypes and media portrayals involving addicts can sometimes influence clinicians to set their expectations lower than they should. Additionally, some clinicians who are used to seeing people who are acutely ill on a daily basis can easily forget that those of us doing well in recovery are not an anomaly or the exception to the rule, but what professionals should be consistently striving for.

Some stereotypes are so common they influence our behaviour without our conscious awareness. We as a society, and sometimes health care professionals, tend to marginalize users or take a paternalistic tone based on some of those stereotypes. It may seem justified to treat addicts as people who need to be told what to do rather than as thinking, complex people who need help putting the pieces back together.

While some clients may not be well educated, others are, and many are quite intelligent regardless of how far they went in the education system. A good rule of thumb is to treat clients on the same level they think they are at, not the level you assume they are at. As one woman told me, "If I don't understand what someone is saying I will tell them; they shouldn't assume I don't know anything right from the start." Many counsellors have difficulty reconciling the discrepancy between a person who has the capacity to make good decisions for himself or herself yet has made poor decisions, at least by society's standards.

Using drugs, using certain drugs, using some drugs in certain ways, overusing alcohol and becoming dependent on substances are all usually seen as "stupid things to do." But addiction has nothing to do with smart or dumb. Smart and not so smart people can succumb to addiction, and all people make poor decisions at some point in their lives.

Addiction, when you are in the throes of it, doesn't feel like a decision at all; it feels like a necessity. It's a compulsion, a drive, an obsessive desire to acquire and use to obliterate unwanted feelings, destroy troublesome thoughts and cope with the pain of daily living. Addiction runs the control panel in your head and blessedly makes the small things seem meaningless and the important things trivial. But having your life run out of control and "needing" treatment doesn't mean you are ready for treatment, want treatment or can stick with it. Only a client can make that decision (unless, of course, the criteria are met for an involuntary assessment). Not the family, not the friends, not the employer. The drive overruns rationality sometimes (well, often), but that doesn't mean the person can't understand what is being presented to him or her, or what the options and consequences are. The counsellor does not own the destruction people do to their lives. The counsellor can't steal other people's lessons or take over their journey. And clients will never follow your timetable. Treat people as if you trust they can make a rational decision and chances are they will—eventually.

Being dependent on substances is scary. The idea of living without those substances is scarier.

By the time most people recognize they have a problem and need help, they don't remember their life before substances came into the picture. Those who do remember it may recall things like trauma, abuse, insecurity, social inadequacy, dysfunctional relationships, loneliness, self-destructive thoughts or mental health issues. The thought of dealing with those issues clean and sober seems impossible.

People build their lives around their use. The people, places and activities that make up their existence revolve around the substance of choice. Revamping and rebuilding a new life, when this may be all you've known, is like being asked to live in a foreign country. You don't know the language, the customs or the behavioural norms, and there is no map. You don't know how to go about normal daily activities because your former activities revolved around acquiring, using and recovering from your habits. When I first had a little clean time I asked another woman in recovery what she did with her day. She suggested going to the beach. What a revelation! I had forgotten there was a beach and that people sometimes just relax and enjoy things like water, sun and fresh air.

The idea of interacting with "straight people" on a regular basis is another source of stress. When you have a community of substance users, you have a culture, a lingo and a shared frame of reference. Learning how to make small talk and converse with people in situations that don't involve substances can feel extremely awkward. Feeling like you don't belong or don't know how to cope in the "straight world" can drive you back to what you know, even though it may be harmful.

It is not just the particular drug or beverage or what it can do for you that is addictive. Everyone develops little rituals that accompany their substance use. Those little rituals become a source of immense pleasure and comfort. To live without drugs or alcohol means living without the comfort of those rituals. Of course, new rituals can be developed, but that is hard to imagine when you are thinking about living your life without your substance of choice.

Clinicians may call the client "resistant" or "ambivalent." The correct term is "scared to death." Knowing you may have to abandon everything you know and get through the day without chemical assistance invokes terror in your soul. Although life may have been hard, nasty, dangerous and unhealthy, the fear can make you want to stick with the devil you know. Many people I spoke with said they wanted a "normal" life, but most admitted that at the time, they did not know what "normal" meant or what it would look like. One woman spoke of "wanting it but not wanting it," and wondering what it would mean to "become one of the pack." Recognizing and acknowledging that fear and what a multi-faceted, life-changing moment the client is facing is one of the best ways a clinician can help a client with choices and further the therapeutic relationship.

Getting help is step one of a thousand steps you have to take.

Recovery is more than learning to stop certain behaviours or learning to take medication regularly. People must transform many aspects of their lives and that may include where they live, who their support system is, their habits, activities and thinking patterns. No one developed an addiction quickly, so recovery takes time, lots of time, and can't be accomplished in 21 or 28 days. Treatment must be continuous, not fragmented, and must support people through the changes they are going to experience and see them through the inevitable setbacks. Learning to live and have a life without substances is a huge undertaking; yet programs don't always consider this when deciding what, or if, aftercare will be provided.

There is a huge demand for addiction treatment, yet few new programs. That places a huge burden on the supply side of the equation. Groups get bigger and more economical. Budget cuts require staff to do more with less. There is a push to get people through a program, but not necessarily to get them better. There isn't always staff to help with things like case management, finding appropriate housing and developing support systems and good coping skills. People risk relapse if they end treatment without any structure or systems in place to help them cope with the realities of their new lives.

Did you know what treatment was the first time you went?

A categorical "no." Treatment is a mystery to those who need it. If you pay attention to celebrity news, treatment seems like a resort in a remote setting with gourmet food, tennis courts, individual therapy and yoga classes. Generally speaking, that's not what it is unless you have lots of money. Many assume treatment is where you find a cure, and learn to become a different person. Again, that's not it. People I talked to were under the impression that treatment was going to "fix them." Some were looking for their problems to disappear; others wanted to understand why they were using, thinking that would solve the problem; and some simply wanted the desire for drugs and alcohol to be taken away. These misconceptions about what treatment will do for you are a recipe for disaster. Unless you truly understand what treatment is about and what you are supposed to get out of it, you are likely to be disappointed with the experience.

There are many kinds of programs, and there are many kinds of addicts and different ways to reach them. Some people require a structured program; others will cut and run as soon as a heavily structured rule-based program is imposed on them. Some addicts appreciate a standardized program, while others will label it "cookie cutter" and look for something more suited to their particular needs. Some find comfort in God, while others reject any form of religion or spirituality that is introduced. Some addicts respond positively to confrontation, and others would be traumatized by this approach. That isn't always made clear when a person walks into a facility, and he or she may not know what the best approach would be for them. They may not understand that finding a program that "fits" is an important component of recovery.

People need to know what is being offered and what other options are out there. If you want to cut down on your drinking or drug use, an abstinence-based program is not a good fit. If you are only interested in abstinence, and only want to be around others who are trying to stay abstinent, then a harm reduction program is going to be a source of irritation and cause resentment toward other clients. If you are looking for individual psychotherapy, a group-based program will leave you feeling like you are missing out on something. Many people who spoke with me felt they did not know what they were supposed to achieve in certain groups or programs. Finishing a group and being told you have "graduated" is nice, but it left many folks wondering what they were supposed to learn from it and how it was going to help them with recovery. These things should be discussed at the beginning and at the end of every group, so people know what it is they are supposed to take away and how they are to apply it.

Being in a program that is unclear or not suited to what you need can result in early attrition, early discharge, relapse and generally feeling like a failure. Many people don't know what they need because they have never done it before and may not know what suits them until it is not working. It is helpful to explain to someone who is not doing well that they may need a different type of program, rather than have them feel like a hopeless case. Turn it from "you aren't suited to our program" to "your needs are legitimate but we are having trouble meeting them in this kind of program." It would be helpful for clinicians to know where people can go to get a different type of program than what they offer if it doesn't seem to be a good match.

Remember that relapse is part of recovery. In fact, I've never heard of recovery happening without relapse. It sometimes takes many, many tries, but quite often a client who is trying recovery for the umpteenth time is labelled a "frequent flyer" and may experience a half-hearted effort by the staff. Yet think of how difficult that must be for that client. To keep relapsing is frustrating, confusing and frightening. It leaves people feeling like "it can't be done," or that they "don't have what it takes." Imagine the courage it takes to go back into treatment and face the same people, to hold your head up and say you are willing to try again.

Relapse, to people who don't understand it, is sometimes treated as if it is the end of the road rather than an indication that there is simply more work to do around managing the illness. Some programs "call people out" after a relapse and use punishment and humiliation as a technique. Making people feel worse about themselves than they already do is not therapeutic; it's cruel and unjustified (Kaplan & Broekaert, 2003).

Other chronic illnesses, such as diabetes, multiple sclerosis or rheumatoid arthritis, can also produce symptom relapse. Sometimes it occurs for no other reason than it is a remitting illness; other times the patient may have contributed to it through poor diet, medication mismanagement or too much stress. I can't imagine a medical professional handling this by any other means than compassion, education and getting the person back on track. Your doctor usually doesn't fire you for not following orders or making mistakes on the way to learning to manage an illness.

Yet learning to manage substance dependence is often not given the same leeway. An inexperienced clinician may take it personally and question whether they can continue working with the person because they feel let down or betrayed. Program leaders may view the person as "not ready" or as "flouting the rules." Things like motivation, commitment and competence are put into question. Clinicians often feel they should decide what they are going to do with the client, rather than asking the client what they want to do about the program. Professionals have a lot of power to shape a person's recovery journey. In some cases, that power is used to further the staff agenda, and the client is left out of the equation.

What does a great counsellor look like?

People who felt they had a great counsellor could not find enough words to express their gratitude toward that person who helped them through the most difficult period of their lives. They were likely to offer the bulk of the credit for their early recovery to their counsellor, rather than acknowledge any of the heavy lifting they themselves may have done. When asked what makes a great counsellor, everyone used the same adjectives.

The first was non-judgmental. Clients who felt like they were not being judged, sized up or critiqued were able to openly and comfortably discuss the full range of their issues, experiences and feelings. This was the most significant precursor to developing trust and respect in the therapeutic relationship. No one I spoke to mentioned respecting a counsellor based on credentials or years of experience. What inspired respect was a counsellor's ability to be non-judgmental. People who respected their counsellor listened to what they had to say and the suggestions they would offer, and remembered things they had said. Some quoted a particular line or phrase their counsellor had used that had an impact on their recovery. Even people who had relapsed would remember something their counsellor had said and take that phrase into their next recovery experience with a deeper understanding of what was meant.

In addition to being non-judgmental, a counsellor has to display humanity by being empathic and communicating an understanding of the client's experience. That may sound easy, but it really is a skilled practice. There is nothing worse than trying to explain your chaotic, messed up life to someone who has a blank look on their face or clearly is not relating to anything you have to say. That is not to say the counsellor has to be in recovery, or have had a chaotic life, although many people felt that clearly helps. A counsellor simply must be able to offer more than superficial responses and platitudes to be effective. Never use phoniness or fakery, and don't hide behind terms like "boundaries" or "professionalism." Boundaries are meant to prevent clinicians from becoming overly involved in a client's life to the point of being therapeutically detrimental. They were never meant to discourage humanity from entering into a therapeutic encounter. Being genuine and human is the only way to reach someone, and it can be achieved without sacrificing professionalism or violating any boundaries.

Addiction is more than a set of behaviours. It is accompanied by deeply personal, sometimes shameful, emotions and experiences. Demonstrating that you are hearing more than just the words and can put yourself in the client's life, without absorbing it, helps the client feel you are someone he or she can work with successfully.

When I was a student and first working with clients, I tried to emulate the counsellors I was shadowing. I spent so much time trying to sound smart and adapt to their way of doing things that I came across as awkward, detached and phony, which is pretty ironic. It was only when I realized that I just needed to be genuine and listen and respond to people as I would want to be spoken to that I was able to relax and be present for clients to hear their stories and meet their needs.

Given the heterogeneity of the client population, clinicians need to be flexible in their approach and include more than one style in their repertoire. Some clients are looking for factual information; others want to tell their story; some want to hear that the clinician can relate to what they are saying and give them validation, while others are looking for a more intellectual approach. Using the same methods with every client to obtain information, provide treatment options and conduct groups will only reach a small percentage of your client group. Being able to adapt to what is in front of you and what is needed for the situation is part of being a great clinician.

Many clinicians tend to overlook something that is often not included in text-books on technique or clinical practice but that is essential to recovery. Hope. It's incredibly important to instil hope in your clients. Not the phony "attaboy, you can do it" kind of hope, but the genuine offering that there is a better life out there and that sticking with it will pay off and that you will help the client get there. I am an example that it can be done, and I'm convinced that others can do it too. That's not to say it's easy, it's not, but it can be done, so I offer hope—always. Clients who said they had a great counsellor spoke about the hope they felt when they were with their counsellor. No matter how rough it got, their counsellor never let them forget there is hope and never stopped believing in them. All clinician/client interactions should be based on the expectation that the client can and will recover and have a better quality of life (Cherry, 2008).

I couldn't have done it without the others in the program.

Some people talked about having good counsellors who played a pivotal role in their recovery. Everyone talked about at least one other client, if not more, who was a significant part of the recovery journey. The power of a common experience cannot be understated. Going through something so difficult with others who were dealing with the same struggles played a monumental role in people's stories. Even if counsellors have had their own personal experiences of going through treatment, they are not going through it now; that is where other clients who are having the same feelings, thoughts, fears and irritations can be helpful.

Twelve-step programs have always capitalized on the power of fellowship and sponsorship (Narcotics Anonymous, 2004). Having another person to talk to who is also in recovery, who has time to talk and listen, and who can share lessons learned, steer you away from bad decisions and recognize warning signs if you are about to relapse is an essential part of the self-help movement. There will be times when clients may be fooling themselves, lying or overestimating their ability to stay clean. Other clients can point out those things in a way that clinicians may not be able to. Many programs that are not based on the 12-step model fail to capitalize on this valuable resource. Some outpatient programs have rules forbidding clients from socializing with one another or tell clients not to go for coffee or do things together after group. Sometimes clients are told they can go for coffee but they are not to discuss anything "personal" or talk about their recovery.

As a clinician, I understand the rationale. You don't want clients working on one another's problems and trying to rescue one another; you want them to focus on their own recovery. Clinicians also worry about clients triggering one another and taking it badly if someone relapses. The thing is, clients do it anyway. It would be better for people to have guidelines to adhere to when they socialize than to sneak around and worry about being discharged from a program for making a friend. Many addicts don't have people in their lives to talk to who aren't using and they don't know how to make friends with people who aren't in treatment. Those early steps toward making friendships while clean and sober are important steps toward a new type of social development.

Ah, the system!

It needs fixing. That was the general consensus among people who had been through treatment. It will come as no surprise to anyone in the addiction field that clients think it is difficult to find a treatment program and have to wait too long to get in. It would be useful if people seeking help had one phone number to call to get information about treatment programs and options. Many clinicians are familiar with the Drug and Alcohol Registry of Treatment (DART), but not many clients have heard of it. Making information more accessible and readily available would help clients or family members who need information about treatment. Some people felt it would be useful if all facilities pre-screened clients right away, rather than making them wait a week or more. When a client feels ready for treatment, there is usually a small window of opportunity. Any small frustration, such as waiting for an appointment, can close that window. Pre-screening clients when they first make inquiries about an appointment gives them the opportunity to ask questions and get information, and takes some of the mystery out of the process. This may help clients stay committed to keeping their assessment appointment, even if they have to wait.

Clients with concurrent disorders are still particularly disadvantaged when it comes to finding suitable treatment. Although they may be able to access more programs than they used to, it does not mean they receive holistic care that addresses all their issues. Even those who entered a concurrent disorders program felt their mental health issues were not addressed sufficiently and they were encouraged to get help for those issues within the mental health system only after they completed addiction treatment. If we conceptualize a concurrent disorder as two problems, treat it as if it is two problems and tell clients they need to get treatment in two different programs, what are their chances for recovery? They will either see the situation as overwhelming and not want to deal with any part of it, or they will think "I'll deal with this now and deal with the rest down the road" because that is often how staff present it to them. When a clinician minimizes one issue or the other, the client will too. But the fact is we don't flick a switch and shut off one part of our problems. Those problems interact and influence one another in powerful ways and can affect the treatment experience and outcome. Advising clients to address their mental health issues after they complete substance use treatment places the obligation on the client—the most vulnerable person in the equation—to be his or her own case manager. This simply sets clients up for failure.

Nothing about us, without us.

How often is client feedback sought in your organization? Aside from anonymous surveys that ask questions like "how satisfied were you with the group?" are there ways to provide genuine feedback about the program and the clinicians working within it? One person suggested that client feedback be incorporated into staff performance evaluations, which would certainly influence service delivery. Meaningful feedback can only be sought through one-to-one interactions or safe focus groups.

When I last managed a clinical program, I used to try meeting with clients when they were being discharged to ask about their experience and discuss suggestions for improving our program. Clients who were not comfortable talking about their experience could complete an anonymous survey that allowed them to voice any concerns or compliments, but usually they appreciated being able to talk to a person. In my experience, clients often made observations about clinicians that echoed opinions I had already formed from listening to clinicians speak in team meetings and rounds. The client voice confirmed what I already knew—that I had a superior clinician or I had some issues to address with training or supervision. Clients also offered suggestions for the program that were often easily implementable from an operations standpoint but that could only come from having experienced the program as a client.

Conclusion

There are probably few people working in the system who think it works perfectly. Most of us realize that the system often disadvantages clients in ways we feel we don't know how to change. But within individual programs, barriers can be lowered. How your program accepts clients, how quickly your program can accept clients and what your program offers can always be improved. Communicating with clients about what to expect and what the program is about will help them understand what they are entering into. Ensuring clinicians are well trained, well supervised and assisted with practice difficulties can improve outcomes and clients' perceptions of their experience. Asking clients about their experience and having a mechanism for them to offer feedback and suggestions can often uncover novel, inexpensive ways to improve a program.

When clients come to us, they are looking for help. They are experiencing a profound realization that life cannot continue the way it has been, but that doesn't mean it will be easy to change or that it will be easy for the clinician. Clients have the right to expect that clinicians will treat them with dignity, compassion and respect, and have the skills to see them through this life change. They will often challenge clinicians, but those who meet this challenge will have their clients' lifelong respect and often inspire some to enter the field. The clinician who can treat a client as capable and knowledgeable about his or her own life experience will be able to form a genuine partnership through the client's recovery journey. Clients will relapse—that is part of recovery—but your personal response to relapse should not be the deal breaker or your opportunity to make the client feel inadequate. No one I spoke with who has had success with recovery ever thought they would be successful. Usually, they had many failed attempts and were ready to give up. But someone gave them hope and eventually made them feel they could do it. To those people, whether professionals, laypeople or fellow members of the recovery experience: thank you—from all of us.

Practice Tips

- Remember that for your client, this is the scariest thing ever and it seems impossible. Help clients see that you understand that, and will help them get through it.
- Be non-judgmental and truly present for the client. Being mindful of your body language, your tone and the internal thoughts that may be coming to mind will help you do this. Remember, your client can read you.
- Learn as much about mental health as you have learned about addiction, and vice versa. Treat the whole person.
- Expect clients to recover and have a better quality of life. Offer them hope.
- Let clients know what they can expect from your program, and from you. Let them know what might be available in the community, should they be looking for something different.
- Have a mechanism for clients to offer open-ended feedback and suggestions about the program. Take their feedback seriously.
- Relapse means there is more work to be done and lessons to be learned. That's all.

Resources

Publications

Carr, D. (2008). *The Night of the Gun: A Reporter Investigates the Darkest Story of His Life.* New York: Simon & Schuster.

Maté, G. (2008). *In the Realm of Hungry Ghosts: Close Encounters with Addiction.* Toronto: Random House.

Internet

Canadian Harm Reduction Network
   http://canadianharmreduction.com
Drug and Alcohol Helpline
   www.drugandalcoholhelpline.ca
LifeRing Secular Recovery
   www.liferingcanada.org

References

Cherry, A.L. (2008). Mixing oil and water: Integrating mental health and addiction services to treat people with a co-occurring disorder. *International Journal of Mental Health and Addiction, 6,* 407–420.

Kaplan, C. & Broekaert, E. (2003). An introduction to research on the social impact of the therapeutic community for addiction. *International Journal of Social Welfare, 12,* 204–210.

Maté, G. (2008). *In the Realm of Hungry Ghosts: Close Encounters with Addiction.* Toronto: Random House.

Narcotics Anonymous. (2004). *Sponsorship, Revised.* Van Nuys, CA: Narcotics Anonymous World Services.

Chapter 3

Diversity and Equity Competencies in Clinical Practice

Janet Mawhinney

Marc, a relatively new counsellor at the agency, is disheartened when a client in a really vulnerable situation cancels his appointment. He is even more determined than ever not to lose his next client, Aleah. Aleah is a refugee who has been in Canada for less than a year. She arrived with her two children, age 4 and 6, after fleeing her home country due to civil war. Before arriving in Canada, Aleah and her children spent two years in a crowded refugee camp, where they witnessed many acts of violence. They are now struggling to adjust to a new life in Canada. Since arriving, Aleah has begun to rely on alcohol and the benzodiazepine Lorazepam (when she can get it) to deal with her difficulties, and she is struggling with her use.

In trying to engage with Aleah, Marc seeks out the advice of his colleague Nagin, who is well respected for her work with marginalized communities. Nagin encourages Marc to consider the social context in which Aleah was living, recognizing the impact of her life in her home country, and the effects of migration. Nagin suggests that Marc also think about how Aleah may have learned to mistrust authorities, and that she has clearly experienced trauma and may feel unsafe and unfamiliar seeking the help of a professional, particularly since she has substance use issues that she might fear will cause her to lose custody of her children.

Marc prepares by learning a bit about Aleah's home country and settlement issues to inform his engagement with her. He begins by listening carefully and allowing Aleah's trust to build gradually. He reflects back to Aleah her evident courage and resilience in managing the migration journey with her children, and her ability to get this far in the treatment system. Marc reflects on his own social location and cultural norms, and how being male, English-speaking, Canadian-born and part of the health profession may affect his rapport with Aleah and how to mitigate that impact to support Aleah in meeting her goals.

Diversity matters. It matters in the lives of clients, in the way services are designed and delivered, in how health systems are structured and in the very essence of how clinicians understand themselves and their work. The goal of this chapter is to understand how we can effectively integrate a diversity and equity lens into our professional practice as a core component of quality care. The chapter is an introductory road map to the specific skills and knowledge required to "do diversity" in addiction treatment.

Fortunately, there is a solid foundation of multidisciplinary research and practice literature, and several decades of dynamic debates about models, frameworks and approaches to draw on. The clinician is often highly motivated to "get it right," while at the same time fearful of getting it wrong. The question is, how do we move from intention to action, from research to practice? How do we bring the necessary knowledge and skills to bear to translate diversity and equity principles into clinical practice with diverse clients, applying a wide range of cultural perspectives on substance use?

Integrating diversity strategies into treatment and building equity and cultural competence into service models and systems certainly requires specific knowledge and skills. But implementing these concepts also builds on wisdom and capacities that are foundational for most clinicians. This work is about implementing the distinct but interrelated concepts of diversity, clinical cultural competence and health equity. In the practice literature, these concepts are often framed as relatively independent from one another, rather than as existing on a dynamic continuum, with each informing the other. In fact "doing diversity" in clinical practice draws on all three domains or concepts, applying a combination of awareness, knowledge and skills to achieve effective and equitable care outcomes. Rather than the onus being on clients to make themselves understood to the therapist, therapists can work to educate themselves and respond sensitively to the diverse needs of their clients, as the opening case study illustrates.

Diversity

At its weakest, diversity refers to differences removed from social context, a concept as banal as, "I like blue, you like yellow, we're all just people." From a social determinants of health lens, it's clear that diversity is not about "difference" per se, but about unequal power in society—both historically and today—operating across key social locations, including race, ethnicity, gender, class and socioeconomic status, sexual orientation, disability, language, accent and gender identity. Diversity in the health and human services context is about the impact of inequality on the health and well-being of marginalized individuals, communities and cultures.

Most health practitioners will be familiar with the significance of the social determinants of health to this definition of diversity. The categories of the social determinants of health are dynamic, but include income level and distribution, housing, employment, social exclusion and more recently, forms of oppression such as racism or ableism that in and of themselves are seen as social determinants of health (Mikkonen & Raphael,

2010). In the context of health, diversity is about how these characteristics of social locations affect and even largely determine health risks, access to service and overall health status. It is well recognized that populations with greater challenges in sustaining good health and in accessing housing and employment have a higher burden of illness and poorer health outcomes (Braverman, 2006). Plainly put, poverty, discrimination, social exclusion and stigma are bad for our health. Applied to addiction treatment, this reflects the need for a holistic approach that recognizes the effect of non-clinical factors on health and that acknowledges the many ways in which people view, understand and engage in recovery. A holistic approach also recognizes the importance of having access to adequate resources and life options.

The definition of diversity engaged here includes all the categories recognized by human rights codes and the Canadian Charter of Rights and Freedoms and related legislation, but is not limited to these. At the big-picture level of social structures, Canadian human rights laws are a vital component of "doing diversity," even if it is not always top of mind in clinical work. It is an under-appreciated fact that our highest level of law explicitly recognizes the need for the protection of minority rights and the de facto existence of histories of discrimination that have systemically disadvantaged specific groups in particular ways. (One need only do a quick Internet search for examples of systemic discrimination toward Chinese Canadians, Japanese Canadians, women, Aboriginal and First Nations Peoples,[1] various faith groups and people with mental health or addiction issues, for example.)

Entrenching the concept of "designated groups" and "prohibited grounds" of discrimination in human rights law creates a fairly unique system in which positive measures taken to redress historical wrongs and mitigate their current expressions are understood as acceptable and often necessary, and do not constitute bias or so-called reverse discrimination. For example, a positive measure such as hiring female clinicians to work with women victims of abuse or a program prioritizing Somali- or Arabic-speaking staff to work with members of the Somali community constitutes an expression of our human rights laws—not a breach of them. A structure or program design that is aimed at mitigating the impact of racism—for example, by integrating Aboriginal cultural practices within an Aboriginal addiction treatment program or prioritizing the hiring of skilled Aboriginal staff in a mainstream service—does not create a "reversal" of colonialism and racism. The perspective behind the term "reverse discrimination" grossly distorts the impact of decades-long systemic discrimination (including through formal government and institutional policies, laws and processes) and decontextualizes initiatives aimed at preventing and addressing discrimination. The term re-centres the focus on the status quo of established privileges and hierarchy (be it gender, race or class). If only a micro-level intervention such as priority hiring would actually reverse macro social and historical systems of oppression, full equality would

---

1 While the term "Aboriginal" is frequently used as an umbrella term for First Nations (status and non-status), Métis and Inuit, many First Nations reject the term as failing to recognize the distinct rights of each of these groups. This is particularly so since the Department of Indian Affairs and Northern Development was renamed the Department of Aboriginal Affairs and Northern Development Canada in 2011. For more information, visit www.chiefs-of-ontario.org/faq. The author generally uses the term "Aboriginal," but wishes to recognize the critique and the dynamic nature of debates around naming language.

be readily achievable! Surprisingly, federal and provincial laws are occasionally more progressive than some front-line staff and managers who may struggle with the notion of customized strategies in service design or delivery aimed at addressing barriers for specific populations or communities.

A core principle of diversity and health equity is the fundamental recognition that treating everyone the same does not result in equal outcomes. We don't begin from a level playing field and one size does not fit all. If the goal is to ensure equal opportunity for services and more equitable health outcomes regardless of identity or social location, then we need differential, customized treatment to address barriers to health care.

The demands of a broad human rights–based definition of diversity can seem daunting at first, but perhaps counterintuitively, this complexity is also one of its great strengths. Understanding diversity to include a range of social locations and identities means that each one of us has some wisdom, knowledge, expertise and lived experience of at least several of these identities: our ethnicity, gender, language and race, for example, inform our perspectives. Equally important, understanding diversity is about recognizing that each one of us has areas where we lack knowledge of different identities and social locations. Every service provider has a potential point of engagement with the issues of diversity and equity, some expertise and something new to learn. We are all multiply located. However, the integration of an analysis of systemic inequality, oppression and privilege is essential to this understanding of multiple diversities and human rights. When engaged effectively, these multiple points of knowledge assets and learning gaps can be a powerful component to a diversity competence strategy in clinical service.

This broad definition of diversity, which integrates anti-oppression rather than mere "difference," avoids the problems of a rainbow of identity relativism, which conveys that "we are all diverse," while absenting material inequality. This stance is expressed through comments that someone "doesn't see" race, colour, gender or ability, despite the evidence that such differences do matter. Rather, the broader definition enables us to reflect on the impact of unequal social power in each of these identities and makes visible the systemic, entrenched and institutionalized nature of privilege and marginalization. Practitioners and clients need to understand how inequality and inequity affect clients' health in order to develop meaningful strategies and interventions.

Understanding power dynamics is about mapping degrees of privilege and marginalization across and among each of these aspects of diversity. The fact that most of us have areas of privilege *and* areas of marginalization in our lives means that we have to pay particular attention to how specific power dynamics are expressed in any given situation, be it within a team, clinical service delivery or program design, or at the organizational level.

While each of us has experience with some unique combination of privilege and (for most of us) marginalization and multiple points of engagement with these issues, it is easier to remain blind to our own privilege, which by definition smoothes our pathways. Privilege is the absence of barriers, proximity to established norms and the accrual of unearned benefits. In clinical practice, it is important to recognize how our privilege is at play in the workplace and in the therapeutic relationship. In order to create safe spaces for clients, therapists may need to unpack the role of privilege and oppression in their relationships. At the very least, actions of the therapist must not reinforce or replicate oppressive patterns that may contribute to clients' presenting issues.

For the practitioner, this means that living with one or two points of marginalization, for example, female gender and lesbian sexual orientation, should not make one blind to or disengaged with points of privilege such as white skin, class and ability. In practice, these issues require a process of learning, critical reflection and a dynamic engagement within a complex social context. For example, a white middle-aged heterosexual nurse with 25 years of experience in addiction and sexual health work in large cities may have impressive skills and be highly culturally competent working from a harm reduction model with urban gay male communities, but will have a whole new learning curve in providing service for urban and suburban heterosexual women of colour at risk for HIV.

Bringing historically grounded evidence of inequality and current health equity data to our understanding of marginalization and privilege enables us to appreciate the particular salience of some issues or combination of issues to health status, such as intersections of gender, race, class and immigration. This information can be a powerful clinical tool. The last two national census results, for example, reveal that poverty is highly racialized, in that populations with the lowest income are recent immigrants (five years or less), Aboriginal Peoples, racialized people and people with disabilities. If we were to analyze the data further we would also see the gendered racialization of poverty within these communities (Block, 2010; Statistics Canada, 2011). This data can tell us which communities are at greater risk for poor health and can inform planning for health promotion, access to treatment and program design. "Doing" diversity means having the awareness of power and social location (of self, team, service and client or community), combining this awareness with knowledge of health data for specific populations and bringing that awareness and knowledge to bear in practice (the skills component). Health equity knowledge broadens the clinician's understanding of the client's social context to yield options that are realistic and meaningful for the client.

How we "see" and meaningfully practise diversity is both obvious and complex. Diversity can be both visible and invisible—the more visible often being race, sex, gender expression, age, some physical disabilities, ethnicities (at times) and some languages. Some diversities, including sexual orientation, class and socioeconomic status, may vary in visibility based on factors such as individual expression and the social context, including the class and gender norms in a service, organization or community. Working with front-line clinicians across the province, I have often been struck by the frequency with which diversity is assumed to refer exclusively or primarily to race and ethnicity (narrowly defined). Training in northern and northwestern Ontario, I have commonly heard "Oh, but we don't have much diversity here," as if the ethnoracial and immigration realities of southern Ontario and the Greater Toronto Area are the only true examples of diversity.

While it is essential to attend to the persistent relevance of race, ethnicity and immigration to health disparities, reducing diversity to these three issues can be limiting to inclusive service provision. For clients coping with addiction issues, a range of other challenges can also arise—around literacy; age-related issues (particularly for youth and older adults); stigma regarding mental health and addiction; sexism; marginalization of lesbian, gay, bisexual and trans people; barriers for people with disabilities (especially transportation and access to services); violence against women; marginalization of and racism toward Aboriginal and First Nations communities; and underlying poverty and social isolation. A well-prepared health professional needs to appreciate equity issues that intersect and span a continuum of identities and social systems. A systemic, broad and intersectional comprehension of diversity and power is thus critical to this work.

Health Equity and Its Relationship to Diversity

Having laid a foundation for a broad, intersectional and human rights–based understanding of diversity, it would be helpful to map out how this concept of diversity is related to health equity, a term less familiar to some, but increasingly central to the health sector, addiction services and equitable health strategies.

Many health and social services are adapting their diversity statements and policies to incorporate the language of health equity. Significant convergence exists between models of diversity I have outlined and the concept of health equity. One of the most cited definitions of health equity is "differences in health that are not only unnecessary and avoidable, but in addition unfair and unjust" (Whitehead, 1992, p. 431). Health equity addresses health outcomes that are not biological or genetic, but are the result of social systems and structures, and are thus avoidable and changeable, such as low birthweights for infants in poorer families, high rates of diabetes in Aboriginal communities or injury and trauma due to domestic violence.

Health equity is about understanding the ways in which disadvantaged social groups—such as the poor, racial and ethnic minorities, women, trans people, people with disabilities or other groups that have persistently experienced social disadvantage or discrimination—systematically experience worse health or greater health risks than more advantaged social groups. Health equity puts a focus on disparities in access to quality care and health *outcomes*—and thus has more of an emphasis on what can be measured and demonstrated than diversity strategies have tended to have. Pursuing health equity in clinical care means advocating for and working toward the elimination of such health disparities and inequalities. Broadly speaking, a health equity strategy would seek to measurably reduce gaps between the most socially advantaged and those who are not, including in incidence of chronic disease (e.g., diabetes, asthma, arthritis), premature death, injury, victimization by violence, as well as health system indicators, such as reduced wait times, accessing service before reaching an acute state, better specific health outcomes, and culturally and linguistically appropriate services. Strategies might focus on access issues, program design, clinical education and capacity, evaluation of service response, ensuring that service delivery is not contributing to the problem (health care inequities) and considering health outcomes for diverse clients.

Health equity in addiction services includes the willingness and capacity to work with and across identities one might not share. This includes the capacity to address one's individual bias, prejudice or ignorance of particular groups (e.g., refugees, a specific faith or ethnic group) or social issues (e.g., poverty, domestic violence) and ensuring these limitations do not affect clinical care. Working across diverse social locations involves the ability to navigate potential discomfort and awkwardness in our own learning. But if we take seriously the human rights foundation discussed earlier, we cannot simply rest with our biases and say "I am not okay working with 'x' population or community." Rather, we need to consider how we build capacity at the practitioner, program and system levels so that we are mitigating, not contributing to, health inequities. At the system level, population, community or issue-specific services are of course important, but we also need broad-based services that effectively provide care for all.

One example of how diversity and health equity knowledge might be applied in addiction service provision would be a readiness to work with lesbian, gay, bi, trans or queer (LGBTQ) clients regardless of one's own sexual orientation and gender identity. In this instance, the practitioner should have some knowledge of health equity research that shows higher rates of suicidality, addiction and some mental health issues (depression and anxiety) as a result of social exclusion and stigma toward the LGBTQ community (Buttery, 2004/2005). The practitioner might bring an awareness of the impact of gender and age differences within LGBTQ health disparities research, as well as awareness of the differences in prevalence rates among diverse LGBTQ people. Bringing health equity data and research to bear is of course not about projecting the socio-demographic health research onto the client, but about keeping this social context and health data in mind when learning about the client's specific life context.

For clients who are also minoritized on the basis of race or ethnicity, practitioners could explore how family, community and cultural resources are important in dealing with both racism and homophobia. When assessing resilience, risk and protective factors, social resources and sense of community, recognize that many racialized LGBTQ people are part of multiple communities and cultures and that these identities affect their wellness strategies. For some LGBTQ people, socializing in bars and clubs is an integral part of connecting with community—so strategies to deal with alcohol and other drug use must address questions of culture, identity and support in ways that are specific to the client's experience with the queer community. This exploration includes defining family and identifying where supports and social resources are found for the client. The client's other aspects of diversity also remain integral to the recovery process: disability status, mental health, literacy and socio-economic resources are all factors that shape the social determinants of health and identity strengths for clients. This is about bringing a diversity lens to the process, not assuming the primacy of diversity over other aspects of holistic identity, such as a person's interests and talents; being a parent, sibling or guardian; or their life journey and goals.

If we consider gender, another component of the diversity spectrum, the knowledge component for the clinician might include understanding that gender power relations are universal and vary only in the extent or degree of inequality and the specific expression or manifestation across geographic, cultural, generational, national and other lines. According to the Public Health Agency of Canada (Sen et al., 2008):

> Gender power relations are a root cause of gender inequality and are among the most influential of the social determinants of health. They determine whether people's health needs are acknowledged, whether they have control of their lives or their health and whether they can realize their rights. (p. 2)

This gender knowledge would include information about the clients and one's own beliefs and expectations about gender role norms. It could also include accessing epidemiological data about the impact of alcohol and other drugs on women compared to men; research on prevalence of trauma and linkages with substance use; risk of intimate partner violence or other potential impacts of sexism and gender inequality; and perhaps information about what groups are disproportionately represented among street-involved women and the criminal justice system (Aboriginal and First Nations women, lesbian, bisexual and trans women). Gender equity would also include moving beyond gender as solely binary male/female to include a spectrum of gender identities and expressions. This would include gaining knowledge about the trans community, the prevalence of barriers to accessing health and social services for trans people and the significantly heightened risk of violence and social isolation (and under what conditions this is most pronounced) (Trans PULSE Project Team, 2012).

This equity knowledge provides a rich social and political context for service provision, but it is never to be engaged in a deterministic or prescriptive way. In the face of this complexity, it is understandable to wish for a checklist or a single tool to help translate knowledge into practice. But there is a good reason to resist this impulse. Simply put, to reduce the realities of social location and power relations, histories of colonialism and resistance, or culturally specific knowledge to a checklist risks losing much of the meaning and knowledge needed to translate this information into effective practice. Minimizing the impact of culture, diversity and social location for an individual client in the face of the complexity of a person's actual life does a tremendous disservice to that person. Such an impulse is really asking clients to leave some parts of themselves at the door, with all the potential capacities and resiliencies therein, for the convenience or comfort of the service (or service provider). Yet who hasn't heard, "Can't we just focus on gender and deal with race somewhere else," for example, or "We're all here about our addiction issues. Your immigration issues are not the point." We want people to bring their whole selves to the recovery process and this means having some capacity at the system, program and practitioner level to integrate the multiple diversities each of us embodies.

The approach to diversity and health equity described here can act as a framework that can be applied in any context. The foundational concepts remain relevant across specific situations because at the core is the recognition that the issues of power, inclusion and diversity are never static, but are context dependent and dynamic. Thus, we need a foundational understanding of power and inequality and, at the same time, openness to the specificity of particular regions, communities and histories—and the unique ways in which an individual negotiates and navigates these realities. This is why there is no checklist for diversity inclusion and health equity, no recipe for cultural competency in clinical practice.

Cultural Competence in Clinical Practice

We all want to have the ability to respond sensitively, respectfully and effectively to clients and families in all of their diversity. The ultimate goal is for a practitioner, team and agency or service to apply equitable, effective and culturally appropriate knowledge and skills, in other words, competencies, into clinical work. This means we need a framework to understand how we do that and the engagement, creativity and organizational support to deliver services in a culturally competent and equitable manner. At its best, clinical cultural competence is a method to move this framework from idea to practice. Practitioners' genuine interest in meeting the needs of diverse populations is a positive driving force to tackle this potentially complex terrain.

Clinical cultural competence is about the *application* of culturally appropriate knowledge and skills in clinical work. More than 40 years of literature exists on cultural competence in the health field, while precedents in anthropology, behavioural sciences and organizational theory have been written about even before this time. Cross (as cited in Gilbert, 2002) offers the most widely cited definition in the literature: "Cultural competence is a set of congruent behaviours, attitudes, and policies that come together in a system, agency, or among professionals and enable that system, agency or those professionals to work effectively in cross-cultural situations" (Cross et al., 1989, p. iv).

One underlying premise of cultural competence is that most clinical encounters are cross-cultural in some way—especially if you consider a broad definition of culture and the diversity and marginalization and privilege within cultural groups (e.g., generation, income, disability, education, gender); furthermore, many people are in themselves "multicultural" and multiply diverse in heritage, ethnicities, nationalities, as well as cultures of youth/age/life stage. Culture in this view is not a single variable; rather, it is a dynamic concept, with multiple characteristics. Some researchers argue that many health practitioners have little training in the social and behavioural sciences in which concepts of culture and its reflection in attitudes, knowledge and behaviour are studied (Gilbert, 2002). And there are those who think that good technical skills are sufficient for clinical cultural competence. As we shall see, good clinical practice is a necessary foundation, but is not synonymous with or sufficient for clinical cultural competence. Clinical cultural competence requires good clinical skills, a diversity and power lens and cultural awareness applied to practice.

The fields of diversity in health and human services, health equity and cultural competence are dynamic and evolving. Multiple theoretical and practice frameworks exist within the cultural competence literature. It is beyond the scope of this chapter to delve into the differences between models of cultural sensitivity, humility, safety and awareness within, broadly speaking, the cultural competence field. But within the cultural competence field, a stream of clinical cultural competence work exists that centres power and inequality within the model and brings a rich non-static analysis of culture and meaning production to bear: this is the model engaged here. As with the terminology for diversity discussed earlier, we have to interrogate how the concept of cultural competence, or a particular iteration of it, is being applied. In particular, the term "cultural competence" has been critiqued for bringing an overly simplistic, ahistorical and depoliticized understanding of culture, effectively producing the very sort of cultural checklist and stereotypes I am warning against. This essentialist approach assumes an overly simplistic understanding of culture and indeed of individual and community negotiation of culture that is fixed and ahistorical. This simplistic model owes much to the world of global business, which seeks simple rules for customs, such as greeting by handshake or bow, or a trait list of how "x" people behave, eat, live or otherwise conduct themselves.

Remnants of an apolitical and essentialist lens on culture still linger in the equity literature, which is why some practitioners remain uncomfortable with the term. Others dislike the language of "competence" for its potential to quantify complex work as if one either is or isn't competent. Early models also focused exclusively on "the other" without a consciousness of the practitioner's (and the health system's) own cultures. Clinicians are now less likely to draw on these simplistic models, which have been heartily critiqued in the field of cultural anthropology, where paradigms of cross-cultural work originated (Carpenter-Song et al., 2007). It will be interesting to see how health and human services address issues of culture over the next few years as the research, application to practice and discussions continue. While it is vital to guard against a problematic essentialized version of culture and cultural competence, there is a robust body of work that does not operate from those paradigms.

Interestingly, a health care cross-disciplinary review of best practice literature and regulated health professional colleges (nursing, social work, occupational therapy, psychology and psychiatry) reveals that while there is a lack of an operationalized definition in the literature, there is significant overlap of understanding about clinical cultural competence (Harmaans, 2003). These health disciplines all recognize three main competence areas for clinical cultural competence: awareness, knowledge and skills. They also agree on several key features of clinical cultural competence, that it:
- is highly valued
- is understood as an ethical responsibility
- is developmental and requires ongoing learning
- ought to focus on client-system outcomes and client perceptions
- is a key aspect of client-centred care.

However, what is missing or less explicit across the disciplines is the need for social power relations and health equity to be central to clinical cultural competence. An explicit integration of power and equity within clinical cultural competence is a more recent iteration in the literature, but one that is central to this project.

ABCDE Framework for "Doing" Cultural Competence

Providing a framework for clinical cultural competence can enable us to understand the key domains in this project and help practitioners integrate this skill within their practice toolkit. This is necessarily a brief introduction and overview, not a substitute for a more sustained and extensive engagement with the literature.

Srivastava (2008) has reconfigured and expanded the widely recognized core domains of attitudes, knowledge and skills required for cultural competence as the "ABCDE" of clinical cultural competence—affective, behavioural, cognitive, dynamics of difference, and equity and environment. This is a brief introduction to these core domains.

The affective domain refers to cultural awareness and sensitivity, an understanding of culture and its impact on values, norms, world view and communications. This should be applied self-reflexively to one's own culture and social location and also to the culture of one's discipline, agency or organization and cultural view of health and illness. This domain is closely linked with the "cultural humility" model (Tervalon & Murray-Garcia, as cited in Kirmayer, 2012).

The behavioural domain refers to skills applied in practice at all stages of service provision, including engagement, negotiation, support, care planning, referral and closure, which enable the health care provider to integrate the client's cultural milieu, social power issues and self-reflective practice regarding the clinician's own "culture" (broadly defined), in order to engage with the client for the most appropriate goals and interventions. According to Srivastava (2008), "The behavioural domain of cultural skill is complex as it requires competency in the domains of awareness and knowledge along with 'knowing how' to provide effective care across cultures" (p. 27).

In the cognitive domain, Srivastava (2008) emphasizes two forms of knowledge essential for clinical cultural competence—*generic* cultural knowledge and *specific* cultural knowledge.

Acquiring both generic and culturally specific knowledge is one aspect of clinical cultural competence that has not overlapped significantly with the previous discussion of diversity and health equity. This domain of knowledge is essential to effective cross-cultural clinical work, and comprises one of the final key concepts for integrating "the how" of diversity in clinical practice.

Generic cultural knowledge

Generic cultural knowledge refers to universal components of culture and includes understanding what culture is; how it operates; what makes for culturally influenced communication styles (e.g., high context to reflect when unspoken information is being communicated implicitly versus low context, when information is being communicated explicitly); and predominant world views, such as independence/interdependence, autonomy/community, body/mind/spirit separation or integration, fatalistic/willful and so forth. Generic cultural knowledge can be learned and developed over time, but once a foundation has been learned, it can be applied across all cross-cultural work in a dynamic and reflexive way to understand the unique and myriad ways in which these components of culture can be expressed. This includes the necessary ongoing reflection of one's own culture and dominant norms, beliefs and practices within the health setting and system.

Culturally specific knowledge

Culturally specific knowledge is the ongoing process of learning about specific cultures (again broadly defined) and combinations of cultures that are relevant for the clients and communities you serve (e.g., Aboriginal urban youth, Tamil older adults). By definition, culture, communities and individuals are not static, so this is where the "work" of learning is never done. In "doing" cultural competence, just as with "doing diversity," it is not possible for any one individual, program or agency to become fully culturally competent for all cultures with the intersections of various diverse social identities therein, or even within one community. The practice of clinical cultural competence requires ongoing learning about specific cultures in varying social and historical contexts and exploring what this may mean for individual clients.

Where and how do we acquire culturally specific knowledge? This is really a question of how we learn about the people and communities we serve, but adding a focus on culture, diversity and equity. Health service providers typically use many strategies to learn about the communities and clients they serve; culturally specific knowledge acquisition is just an added component of that practice skill.

There are myriad avenues for learning about the nuances of cultures, including:

- reviewing existing research (population health studies, public health research, Statistics Canada health reports, advocacy research, epidemiological research)
- engaging with the community and community-based agencies or coalitions (partnerships, service agreements, formal and informal relationships)
- participating in structured education (courses, in-services, work exchanges)
- listening to your clients and their collaterals
- researching historical and current events affecting the community (e.g., awareness of the residential school system in Aboriginal and First Nations communities, cutbacks to refugee health resources, shifts in immigration patterns and settlement)
- exposing yourself to literature and film and participating in community events and festivals

- using team meetings, supervision and other existing forums within the clinical setting to share information and exchange knowledge to build capacity within the service.

Health care providers should not rely solely or primarily on the client for culturally specific knowledge. Marginalized clients and those whose identities are different from the clinician or from mainstream health care often experience the extra burden of educating the clinician in order to receive appropriate care. On a very practical level, this eats into the time the client has for himself or herself. As one client has said, "You only get 10 minutes at a physician for the most part and if you have to spend half of it explaining to them what's going on, you don't get your services" (Eady at al., 2008). Part of this project must be to develop strategies to support ongoing learning and knowledge exchange within organizations as part of the organizational competencies.

Srivastava's (2008) "dynamics of difference" and "equity and the environment" are about ensuring that principles of human rights, diversity and health equity are engaged with throughout the process at the client-clinician interaction level, the client-program/service level and the broader health system and societal level.

The cultural competence literature discusses multiple levels of engagement, including the micro or individual level, the meso team or program level and the macro level, both organizational and societal. As Srivastava (2008) emphasizes, clinical cultural competence cannot function without organizational support, no matter how motivated and informed an individual service provider may be: "Individual healthcare providers need organizational resources such as interpreter services and collaborative partnerships with community agencies for purposes of referral and consultation" (p. 29). This multi-level engagement comprises the equity and practice component of Srivastava's model.

Relationship between Diversity, Health Equity and Cultural Competence

The interconnections between the foundational concepts of diversity, health equity and cultural competence are critical to the conceptualization, system design and practice expectations of health services and have been a major focus of this chapter. Diversity includes the multiple and intersectional operations of power and privilege at the individual, institutional and systemic levels. Health equity then considers how diverse identities and social locations affect health status, which brings an emphasis on outcomes and measurement in how we deliver health services. Health equity provides a framework to bring diversity awareness into health deliverables. Clinical cultural competence, in turn, can be understood as a specific set of practices in service design and delivery, based on an awareness of culture, diversity and power, engaged to support equitable health outcomes. In other words, cultural competence is a practice strategy to reach health equity goals informed by a diversity lens.

Nuances in Practice

This chapter has provided an introductory map to the foundations and intersections of diversity, health equity and cultural competence in clinical work. At its core, this approach is about integrating a holistic approach that sees diversity and culture for both their potential risk and protective factors, viewing the client as the expert on his or her own life, demonstrating respect and regard for the client's world view, ensuring client-led treatment planning and being able to engage culturally specific and alternative therapies.

In practice, application of this approach will look different with every client. In the case example that opened this chapter, we were introduced to Aleah, who fled civil war with her two young children and came to Canada after two years in a refugee camp. In engaging Aleah and beginning to build a therapeutic relationship, her counsellor, Marc, considers the social context in which Aleah was living and the impact of pre-migration, migration and post-migration factors, including why Aleah might mistrust authority and state systems, the impact of trauma (including risk of sexual violence), the fear of losing custody of her children, her struggle to navigate the Canadian health system and perhaps her lack of familiarity with the role of the clinician in that system. Clinicians may also benefit by soliciting clients' explanatory models of their situation and addiction issues from a holistic perspective (Kleinman & Benson, 2006; Kleinman et al., 1978). In the case of Aleah, Marc reinforces Aleah's strength and resilience evident in managing the migration journey with her children, her parenting capacities, and her ability to engage with housing, income support and the treatment system. Marc also obtains specifics about Aleah's culture and socio-political realities to help build rapport and provide appropriate care, and to help her navigate Canadian health policy and systems issues, which have been affected by federal cuts to refugee mental health, preventative treatment and childhood vaccinations (under the Interim Federal Health Program in 2012). Marc also reflects on his own social location and cultural norms, and is mindful of the gender, linguistic, ethnic and other diversities at play in the treatment process. A fuller profile of equity engagement in practice would consider the structures and supports at the team, program and service levels as well. These are just a few of the many possible ways in which equity competencies could be applied with Aleah.

As discussed earlier, it is important to guard against stereotyping, essentialization or reducing a person to a cultural profile when working cross-culturally. A vigorous equity and client-centred orientation means that the clinician is always led by what is true for a particular client, not what might be a general truth for his or her culture or community. Lieninger (as cited in Srivastava, 2008) describes this culturally specific knowledge as "holding knowledge" of cultural patterns that the clinician has on hand to inform the engagement with the client, but not in a prescriptive manner. For example, the fact that some Aboriginal and First Nations cultures may communicate with pauses and less direct eye contact does not mean a particular client will. In the same way, the fact that some first-generation immigrants from a particular region may subscribe to traditional gender norms does not mean that your client or her husband from the same region will share these same perspectives. As a test of this, research your own cultural profile and reflect on the extent to which it resonates for you as an individual. Culture matters profoundly, but it is not deterministic.

For some dominant culture practitioners, learning about histories of colonization and racism may trigger an unhelpful guilt response that will need to be navigated in the therapeutic relationship. This can translate into counter-transference or boundary issues, such as needing the client to educate or absolve the clinician's sense of guilt. Newly acquired knowledge of histories of oppression occasionally translates to a focus on a static or rigid view of the impact of structural oppression on the client to the exclusion of the client's coping skills, resistance strategies and individual negotiation of the social and political world. This can be limiting to the client's sense of agency, autonomy and resilience and to the meanings the client has created in his or her own personal narrative, and risks slipping into a deficit model of marginalized cultures. There is a balancing act in bringing an awareness of the historic and systemic legacies of oppression and the self-reflection of one's own culture and contexts, while being led by the client's unique world view and orientation to the situation.

The integration of diversity and equity into clinical practice involves engagement at the micro or individual level, the meso or program/agency level and the macro or health-systems level. To be truly effective in this work, practitioners need adequate support and leadership. But at the same time, we can also break the work down into manageable goals. While this chapter is anchored in macro or big-picture issues of social inequality and health impacts, we also need to consider what is meaningful for a particular client. What are the things you can actually do something about? What is within the scope of your practice? This same question can be asked at the team or program level. This dynamic movement between big-picture analysis, concepts and knowledge and the unique particularities and specificity of clinical work is an important component of how diversity comes to life in clinical care. We should always be led and encouraged by the potential to have a positive impact when and where we can. And this, for many, is what also inspires and engages us in the health care and human services fields.

Organizational Considerations

Turning to the agency or organizational (meso) level, a useful strategy can be to consider the cultural and other diversity assets of the organization at the program design, policy, partnership and staff-capacity levels. Organizational competencies can include organizational values, governance, planning and evaluation, communication, staff development, organizational infrastructure and service interventions (Kirmayer, 2012).

Diversifying the staff complement and leveraging the wisdom and insights of staff from marginalized communities is one strategy to increase organizational capacity. Are staff from marginalized communities positioned to influence the agenda? Are their perspectives valued and heard within the agency or service? This of course does not mean hiring for identity per se, but for the skills and specific knowledge that is produced from the margins. At the same time, it is not feasible for services to continually match the shifting diversity of the populations they serve. Even when there is similarity of diversity (be it class, ethnicity, race or gender) between the service provider and the client, that does not create an inevitable similarity of perspectives or an optimal therapeutic match for that particular client. Further, staff from marginalized communities cannot be the sole bearers of the diversity and cultural competence agenda. Relying primarily on staff from marginalized communities places an undue burden on them while simultaneously letting staff from more dominant cultures or privileged identities off the hook for this important work. This is not a desirable situation and would eventually stall or sabotage efforts to provide more inclusive, equitable and culturally relevant services. A diversity asset audit would thus include the wisdom and skills of marginalized staff from their unique perspectives as the diversity and equity capacities and skills of more privileged staff, as well as the system and program design components. Thus education and capacity building of all staff is a core equity asset. The work of doing diversity and clinical cultural competence should be understood as an integral component of providing excellent care for all, and thus should be integrated within all aspects of service design and delivery.

Conclusion

This chapter has discussed the foundational concepts and critical skills for "doing diversity" in clinical practice, and framed these skills as essential to quality care. In thinking about "the how," we have seen that there is no single checklist for a clinical practice that integrates a diversity analysis and cultural competence in order to achieve equitable health outcomes for clients. However, this explication of concepts and frameworks provides markers along the way to guide us as we engage in the ongoing process of understanding core equity domains and their application to practice.

In practice, some of the skills required by the practitioner include critical self-reflection and an awareness of personal and cultural values, norms and biases, including concepts of health and illness and the health system. We have seen that it is important to bring an awareness of social location, power and privilege and a commitment to mitigating their impact in service delivery. In the therapeutic relationship with clients, the work requires knowledge of specific cultural norms and the historic and socio-political realities affecting the culture or community as both risk and protective factors. We need to genuinely appreciate clients' culture and diversity as assets and a source of resilience. This work also includes assessing the potential role of discrimination on health and well-being, and understanding the interactions between the service provider and client's cultural histories. For example, is the cultural history relatively neutral or does it resonate with a history of colonization? All of this may affect the process of cultural survival, particularly for clients who are multiply marginalized. An awareness of culturally specific interventions and strategies and the capacity to negotiate between conventional and culture-related definitions of problems and solutions are further assets in providing equitable care.

This overview of diversity and equity in clinical care aims to build on existing clinical competencies by providing (or refreshing) another set of skills to add to your clinical toolkit to achieve quality care. The practice of "doing diversity" builds on and integrates with core practice norms, such as client-centred care, self-reflective practice and the basic goal of providing excellent care, but also requires specific knowledge and skills. We have explored the linkages and fruitful overlap between the concepts of diversity, health equity and clinical cultural competence; diversity as descriptive of unequal power and social location; clinical cultural competence focused on capacities and skills applied to practice; and health equity with the aim of measuring and mitigating avoidable health disparities. If our objective is to achieve respectful, effective, culturally competent and equitable care, we need to engage with each of these paradigms at the individual, program, agency and health systems levels.

Practice Tips

- Critically reflect on your own personal and cultural values, norms and biases, as well as concepts of health and illness and the health system.
- Be aware of social location, power and privilege and commit to mitigating their impact in service delivery.
- Assess the potential role of discrimination on health and well-being.
- Learn about specific cultural norms and the historic and socio-political realities affecting the culture or community as both risk and protective factors.
- Engage the specific meaning of addiction issues and recovery for each client with a critical, not prescriptive, engagement with culture and diversity information.
- Navigate the interactions between the service provider and client's cultural and diversity histories.
- Review existing research (population health, public health, advocacy and epidemiological).
- Engage with diverse communities and community-based agencies or coalitions.
- Conduct an equity asset audit of your team program or agency and develop a strategy and action plan.
- Listen to your clients, and look for the signs they give you that suggest they feel heard and understood.

Resources

Publications

Agic, B. (2004). *Culture Counts: Best Practices in Community Education in Mental Health and Addiction with Ethnoracial/Ethnocultural Communities.* Toronto: Centre for Addiction and Mental Health.

Braverman, P. (2006). Health disparities and health equity: Concepts and measurement. *Annual Review of Public Health, 27,* 167–194.

Carpenter-Song, E., Schwallie, M. & Longhofer, J. (2007). Cultural competence reexamined: Critique and directions for the future. *Psychiatric Services, 58,* 1362–1365.

Leininger, M. (1996). *Transcultural Nursing: Concepts, Theories and Practice* (2nd ed.). Hillard, OH: McGraw-Hill.

Mikkonen, J. & Raphael, D. (2010). *Social Determinants of Health: The Canadian Facts.* Toronto: York University School of Health Policy and Management.

Patychuk, D. & Seskar-Hencic, D. (2008). *First Steps to Equity: Ideas and Strategies for Health Equity in Ontario 2008–2010.* Ontario Public Health Association.

Registered Nurses' Association of Ontario. (2007). *Embracing Cultural Diversity in Health Care: Developing Cultural Competence.* Healthy Work Environments Best Practice Guidelines. Toronto: Author. Retrieved from http://rnao.ca/bpg/guidelines/embracing-cultural-diversity-health-care-developing-cultural-competence

Sen, G., Östlin, P. & George, A. (2008). *Unequal, Unfair, Ineffective and Inefficient. Gender Inequity in Health: Why It Exists and How We Can Change It.* Final report to the WHO Commission on Social Determinants of Health. Retrieved from www.who.int/social_determinants/publications/womenandgender/en/

Srivastava, R. (2008). The ABC (and DE) of cultural competence in clinical care. *Ethnicity and Inequalities in Health and Social Care, 1,* 27–33.

Internet

Centre for Addiction and Mental Health Knowledge Exchange portal—Resources: Ethnocultural Communities / Cultural Competence
http://knowledgex.camh.net/policy_health/mhpromotion/culture_counts/Pages/culture_counts_ethno_resources.aspx#competence

Diversity Rx (U.S.)
http://diversityrx.org

Journey to Cultural Competence video (New Immigrant Support Network at The Hospital for Sick Children)
www.sickkids.ca/culturalcompetence/journey-to-cultural-competence-film/Journey-to-Cultural-Competence-Film.html

National Center for Cultural Competence (U.S.)
http://nccc.georgetown.edu

Statistics Canada Health Profile
   www12.statcan.gc.ca/health-sante/82-228/index.cfm
Toronto Community Health Profiles
   www.torontohealthprofiles.ca/index.php

References

Block, S. (2010). *The Role of Race and Gender in Ontario's Racialized Income Gap.*
   Ottawa: Canadian Centre for Policy Alternatives. Retrieved from www.
   policyalternatives.ca

Braverman, P. (2006). Health disparities and health equity: Concepts and measurement. *Annual Review of Public Health, 27,* 167–194.

Buttery, H. (2004/2005). Better dead than queer: Youth suicide and discrimination in a
   heterosexual world. *CrossCurrents: The Journal of Addiction and Mental Health, 8* (2),
   4–12.

Carpenter-Song, E., Schwallie, M. & Longhofer, J. (2007). Cultural competence reexamined: Critique and directions for the future. *Psychiatric Services, 58,* 1362–1365.

Cross T., Bazron, B., Dennis, K. & Isaacs, M. (1989). *Towards a Culturally Competent
   System of Care. Volume 1.* Washington, DC: Georgetown University Child
   Development Center.

Eady, A., Ross, L.E. & Dobinson, C. (2008). *Bisexual People's Experiences with Mental
   Health Services.* Toronto: Centre for Addiction and Mental Health & Sherbourne
   Health Centre.

Gilbert, M.J. (Ed.). (2002). *A Manager's Guide to Cultural Competence Education for
   Health Care Professionals.* Los Angeles: The California Endowment. Retrieved from
   www.calendow.org

Harmaans, M. (2003). *A Review of Clinical Cultural Competence, Definitions, Key
   Components, Standards, and Selected Trainings.* Toronto: Centre for Addiction and
   Mental Health.

Kirmayer, L. (2012). Rethinking cultural competence. *Transcultural Psychiatry, 49,*
   149–164.

Kleinman, A. & Benson, P. (2006). Anthropology in the clinic: The problem of
   cultural competency and how to fix it. *PLoS Medicine, 3* (10): e294. doi: 10.1371/
   journal.pmed.0030294

Kleinman, A., Eisenberg, L. & Good, B. (1978). Culture, illness, and care: Clinical lessons from anthropologic and cross cultural research. *Annals of Internal Medicine, 88,*
   251–258.

Mikkonen, J. & Raphael, D. (2010). *Social Determinants of Health: The Canadian Facts.*
   Toronto: York University School of Health Policy and Management.

Sen, G., Östlin, P. & George, A. (2008). *Unequal, Unfair, Ineffective and Inefficient.
   Gender Inequity in Health: Why It Exists and How We Can Change It.* Final report to

the WHO Commission on Social Determinants of Health. Retrieved from
www.who.int/social_determinants/publications/womenandgender/en/

Srivastava, R. (2008). The ABC (and DE) of cultural competence in clinical care.
Ethnicity and Inequalities in Health and Social Care, 1, 27–33.

Statistics Canada. (2011). *Women in Canada: A Gender-based Statistical Report:
Introduction*. Ottawa: Author. Retrieved from www.statcan.gc.ca

Trans PULSE Project Team. (2012). *Improving the Health of Trans Communities:
Findings from the Trans PULSE Project*. Retrieved from http://transpulseproject.ca/
research/improving-the-health-of-trans-communities-findings-from-the-trans-pulse-
project/

Whitehead, M. (1992). The concepts and principles of equity and health. *International
Journal of Health Services, 22*, 429–445.

Chapter 4

Working within a Harm Reduction Framework

David C. Marsh and Dale Kuehl

Fred is a 47-year-old man with a long history of problems with alcohol and other drugs. He started drinking alcohol at age 9 after many traumatic experiences in foster care. By age 15, he had started regularly using cocaine and dropped out of school. He first injected heroin when he was 17, and was soon involved in property crime and drug dealing to fund his addiction. Over the next 20 years, Fred was incarcerated several times and continued to use injection heroin daily. He has been infected with hepatitis C but has managed to avoid acquiring HIV.

In the community, Fred routinely accesses a needle exchange program and tries to avoid sharing injection equipment. He has been enrolled in methadone maintenance treatment four times, but each time dropped out within a year because his ongoing cocaine use caused him to miss multiple doses without ever getting to a stabilized dosage. Fred began to use a supervised injecting facility when it opened in his town so he would not have to inject in public, especially just after he was released from jail and had not found an apartment where he could use in private. The nursing staff at the facility referred Fred to a heroin-assisted treatment project designed for long-term heroin injectors who had not benefited from existing treatment options.

Over a year of receiving prescribed doses of heroin, which he injected in a supervised clinic, along with receiving counselling and medical services, Fred was able to stop using street heroin, decrease his illegal activity and obtain stable housing. He subsequently transferred to methadone maintenance treatment and has stopped injecting drugs and has dramatically decreased his cocaine use. The social stability that has resulted from these changes has allowed Fred to begin getting treatment for hepatitis C in conjunction with his ongoing methadone treatment.

Traditional service delivery approaches to working with people with substance use problems require them to abstain from all substances to be eligible for treatment. This one-size-fits-all approach is rooted in the belief that people with substance use problems are motivated to change by the adverse consequences of their behaviour. Continued substance use is viewed as a sign that the person is unmotivated to change and thus will not benefit from services. Moreover, providing services to someone who continues to use is considered potentially harmful to the user by reducing adverse consequences and thus delaying the person's commitment to abstinence.

Providing services using an abstinence approach is often based on a mutual understanding between the practitioner and the service user: the client agrees to an abstinence goal, and non-compliance is grounds for termination from a program or service. The assumption is that all substance use is problematic, that moderation or reduced use is not a viable option, and that failure to comply calls into question the person's motivation and readiness to change.

From the perspective of people who use drugs, the limitations of an exclusively abstinence-based approach are apparent. For people who are not interested in cessation but want to remain healthy, treatment requiring abstinence deprives them of the right to services. This includes refusing treatment to people who recognize they have a problematic relationship with one substance but are able to control their use of other substances. Certain subpopulations, types of substance and substance-using behaviours hold greater individual, economic and public health risks and may require specific targeted interventions beyond the "just say no" mantra. Harm reduction policies, programs and practices are alternative approaches that address those shortcomings by allowing for more flexible service delivery and greater individual autonomy. They are grounded in evidence-based research and draw on collective wisdom and knowledge from the lived experiences of people with substance use problems. Ironically, many people who use drugs can harbour the longing to be abstinent and drug free in the same way that many of us may have long-term goals that are currently out of reach. But we can take steps that move us toward that goal. Whether or not we get there, that we do things to reduce risks to our health and well-being, and that of others, describes the focus of harm reduction work. Indeed, as has been shown, clients who are given choices about their substance use goals actually have a higher likelihood of achieving abstinence goals than clients who have abstinence prescribed for them as the only allowable outcome (Sanchez-Craig & Lei, 1986).

In this chapter, we focus primarily on harm reduction interventions for people who inject drugs, particularly opioids. The discussion highlights Canadian research and evaluation of these interventions. While harm reduction has acquired an evidence-based scope that applies not just to substance use, but also more broadly to addictive behaviours, such as problem gambling, and behavioural addictions, such as eating disorders, these topics are covered in other chapters in this book. Here we focus primarily on harm reduction practices for injection drug use, which is how harm reduction first emerged. However, we recognize that this framework is now applied more broadly to preventing and treating addiction, and guided by evidence-informed policies and practices (Centre for Addiction and Mental Health [CAMH], 2002; Erickson et al., 1997; Kleinig, 2008; Marlatt & Donovan, 2005; Marlatt & Witkiewitz, 2002; Miller, 2008).

Definition and Principles of Harm Reduction

The manufacture and sale of illicit drugs is among the world's leading industries, affecting more than 200 million people and costing $2.1 trillion annually (United Nations Office on Drug and Crime [UNODC], 2011a, 2011b). As a result of worldwide injection drug use, 2.8 million people are HIV positive and 8 million are infected with hepatitis C (UNODC, 2011a). In Canada, the social cost of illicit drug use accounts for $8.2 billion and more than 1,600 deaths annually (Patra et al., 2007; Rehm et al., 2006). In the face of these dramatic harms to the health and welfare of Canadians, strategies for reducing the harms of illicit drug use have been studied and implemented.

However, harm reduction continues to be a controversial and often misunderstood concept, particularly in North American politics, where a change of government, especially at the national levels, creates almost tidal shifts in attitudes toward addiction—from moral to criminal justice to health-based models. Paradoxically, at the same time, acceptance of harm reduction as an integrating framework for both explicitly and implicitly addressing issues related to addictive behaviour treatment has grown (Miller et al., 2011). Key to understanding and applying harm reduction is embracing its widely accepted definition:

> "Harm reduction" refers to policies, programmes and practices that aim primarily to reduce the adverse health, social and economic consequences of the use of legal and illegal psychoactive drugs without necessarily reducing drug consumption. Harm reduction benefits people who use drugs, their families and the community. (International Harm Reduction Association [IHRA], 2010a, "Definition")

This definition and the accompanying position paper (IHRA, 2010b) clearly make the point that there is no conflict between harm reduction interventions and treatment. In fact, many harm reduction interventions are designed to facilitate entry to treatment. A CAMH position paper on harm reduction incorporates into its definition the statement that "harm reduction programs and policies must demonstrate that they have the desired impact without producing unacceptable unintended consequences" (CAMH, 2002, p. 1). This statement emphasizes the underlying expectation of rigorous evaluation built into harm reduction programs to demonstrate their effectiveness. It also locates addiction treatment within the prevailing paradigm of clinical pragmatism that guides health care in general: health care is not contingent on the client's moral standing. In other words, how clients may have contributed to their own health problems, which may have resulted in their needing health care, should not affect the treatment they are offered. Behaviours such as driving under the influence or eating excessively and developing health complications due to obesity or poor diet should not influence the care provided. Indeed, harm reduction can be offered when it becomes all too clear that worse things can happen to people than to have substance use problems; for example, acquiring infectious diseases that have health consequences not just for the individual but for the public health of the community. With harm reduction, addiction prevention and treatment have joined the paradigm of clinical pragmatism that makes modern health care, at the personal and community level, a distinguishing and envied feature of western societies.

The focus on rigorous evaluation explains why harm reduction discussions frequently focus on injection drug use. For practical reasons, evaluation of an intervention is more readily conducted when the end point is clearly defined, cheaply detected and occurs with sufficient regularity that a study of several hundred people over a period of months or a few years can detect a statistically meaningful difference. In many settings, HIV infection or overdose death among people who use injection drugs meets all these conditions: HIV infection, which still happens to at least one per cent of people who inject drugs each year in parts of Canada and at much higher rates in other parts of the world, can be cheaply and easily detected using a blood test. Because the effects of injection drug use can be easily evaluated, and due to the overwhelming public health argument for preventing the spread of HIV and hepatitis C, funding is available and interventions can practically be designed and evaluated. Rigorous evaluations of harm reduction interventions targeting tobacco-related cancer or alcohol-induced liver disease would require substantially larger numbers and longer time frames, based on the natural course of these illnesses. Therefore, the research literature is less well developed for harm reduction interventions with these substances. In this chapter, we look at examples of harm reduction interventions that have been subjected to rigorous scientific evaluation and have been shown to reduce harm.

The Emergence of Harm Reduction

The Netherlands was one of the first countries in Europe to adopt a harm reduction framework in its national drug policy. In fact, the first methadone clinic opened in Amsterdam in the late 1970s (Riley et al., 2012). Dutch drug policy has been described and criticized by some for its laissez-faire approach to drug use. However, from its inception, the focus has been to reduce the social and health consequences of substance use on the user rather than concentrating on drug use itself. Dutch policy also distinguishes between "soft" drugs, such as cannabis and psilocybin mushrooms, and "hard drugs," such as cocaine and heroin. The legalization, sale and taxation of cannabis remain regulated through "coffee shops." However, since 2005, there has been a shift in policy direction, with more restrictive regulations introduced to reduce the number of outlets able to sell cannabis and to prevent sales to foreigners visiting the country. The United Kingdom has also had a long history of harm reduction. In the 1920s, the Rolleston Commission brought forward recommendations to allow narcotics to be prescribed as a form of treatment, but these recommendations never resulted in widespread practice.

Harm reduction gained in popularity in the 1980s, particularly in the Netherlands, United Kingdom and, later, Australia and Canada, in response to the rates of blood-borne viruses being contracted by people who inject drugs. Although the guidelines and regulations varied among these countries, the philosophy remained the same. The harms associated with injection drug use, namely through sharing needles and other paraphernalia, placed people at high risk of HIV/AIDS and hepatitis C. Pragmatic approaches to address HIV as a public health problem evolved over time to include needle exchange and distribution programs, prescription heroin, mobile and street outreach services, the extensive use of peer staff, methadone maintenance treatment and drug consumption rooms. In the past two decades, some Canadian municipalities have distributed crack pipe kits, a practice that has been incorporated into Ontario's "best practices in harm reduction" (Strike et al., 2006), and Vancouver opened the first supervised injecting facility in North America.

As harm reduction strategies become more widespread, the substance use treatment field continues to evolve from its traditional "all or nothing" abstinence-based framework to client-driven interventions that match the goals of the person. As we begin to understand the multiple confounding factors that contribute to substance use problems, the chronic relapsing nature of drug use, the process of behaviour change and how to provide services to people who have not benefited fully from the treatment system, harm reduction remains an integral way to balance a person's right to self-determination within a broader public health model.

In addition to the expectation for rigorous evaluation and a focus on reducing harm, harm reduction programs frequently share common principles and values. These include pragmatism, prioritization of goals, flexibility to lower the threshold for entry to and retention in treatment, valuing the autonomy of people who use drugs to make their own decisions and their involvement, where feasible, in designing and delivering programs (Centre for Addiction and Mental Health, 2002; IHRA, 2010b).

Canada has a long and rich tradition of contribution to the international development of harm reduction and continues to be recognized as a world leader (Stimson et al., 2010). From 1988 until 2008, the federal government's national drug strategy incorporated recognition for reduction of harm as a component of the federal response to illicit drug use. Most recently, this was articulated in the *National Framework for Action to Reduce the Harms Associated with Alcohol and Other Drugs and Substances in Canada* (Canadian Centre on Substance Abuse & Health Canada, 2005). As of 2011, this framework for action has been endorsed by 44 organizations across Canada, despite a shift in federal government policy and funding away from harm reduction over the same period (Cavalieri & Riley, 2012).

Needle Exchange and Supervised Injection

Early on in the HIV epidemic, needle sharing was recognized as posing a significant risk for the spread of blood-borne viruses, and public health officials began investigating providing sterile injection equipment as a means of preventing HIV infection (National Institutes of Health, 2002). One of the first needle exchange programs to open in North America was initiated in Vancouver in 1988: that program has since distributed between two million and three million needles per year (Strathdee et al., 1997). Many national and international organizations have endorsed needle exchange programs as a mechanism for reducing the spread of HIV—a recommendation supported by scientific evaluation (Gibson et al., 2001). For example, a careful analysis of discarded syringes prior to and following the introduction of a needle exchange program in New Haven, Connecticut, demonstrated a reduction in the number of times each needle was used and in the likelihood of finding HIV in the discarded syringe (Heimer et al., 2002).

Critics of needle exchange programs frequently refer to a study conducted in Vancouver that demonstrated increased incidence of HIV infections among people who most frequently accessed the syringe exchange program (Schechter et al., 1999). However, careful evaluation of the data has shown that the increased risk of HIV infection was accounted for by frequent injection of cocaine and injecting in public spaces, while use of the needle exchange program reduced HIV-risk behaviour (Wood et al., 2002). More recent evaluations of needle exchange programs have demonstrated other changes in service delivery leading to reductions in HIV-risk behaviour: the expansion of the number and type of service locations (e.g., primary care clinics, drop-in centres and peer-run outlets); peer involvement in service provision; and abandonment of a one-for-one exchange policy (one clean needle for each dirty one) in favour of an unlimited distribution model, in which the person gets as many needles as he or she wants (Kerr et al., 2010).

Despite the well-documented benefits of needle exchange programs, researchers have demonstrated several limitations in their effectiveness. For example, people may continue to inject drugs in public spaces, thus increasing their risk of overdose death. Injecting in public may also cause users to inject as quickly as possible, thus increasing the risk for local tissue damage and infection (Broadhead et al., 2002; Dovey et al., 2001; Wood, Kerr, Montaner et al., 2004). Supervised injecting facilities (SIF), where they are available, address these harms by providing a safe and supervised environment where people who use drugs may inject them, and in some places smoke them. These facilities provide benefits beyond the scope of what can be provided by syringe exchange programs: injecting facilities reduce risks in the drug-taking environment, allow for professional staff to intervene in the event of an overdose, and enhance opportunities for providing primary care and referral to addiction treatment.

Extensive evaluation of an SIF that opened in Vancouver in 2003 has demonstrated a broad range of benefits both for injection drug users who access the facility and for the community (Wood, Kerr, Lloyd-Smith et al., 2004). The SIF has been shown to attract drug users at higher risk of acquiring HIV and having an overdose (Wood, Tyndall, Qui et al., 2006). After the facility opened, public injecting in the neighbourhood around the facility decreased (Wood, Kerr, Small et al., 2004). Regular use of the safe injection facility is associated with changes in behaviours that are linked to reduced risk of acquiring HIV, such as less syringe sharing and increased use of sterile water (Kerr et al., 2005; Stolz et al., 2007). Professional SIF staff can refer clients to addiction treatment: these referrals have increased the rate of admission to withdrawal management, led to subsequent enrolment in addiction treatment, and resulted in reduced drug use (Wood, Zhang & Montaner, 2006; Wood et al., 2007). These successful referrals have also produced an increased rate in the cessation of injection drug use among people using the SIF (DeBeck et al., 2011). Nurses at the SIF can also intervene in the event of overdose: their role and the overall functioning of the site have led to significantly reduced overdose mortality in the neighborhood around the facility (Kerr et al., 2006a; Marshall et al., 2011).

The evaluation has also sought to verify potential negative impacts of the facility. It found no increase in drug-related crime (Wood, Tyndall, Lai et al., 2006) and no negative impact on the likelihood of either relapse to injection drug use among those who had stopped injecting or prolonged drug use with a lower rate of cessation (Kerr et al., 2006b). Independent evaluation has shown that SIFs are cost-effective because of reduced health care costs from blood-borne infections (Bayoumi & Zaric, 2008). Overall, the SIFs provide a range of positive benefits for people who use drugs, for the health care system and for the broader community, and therefore are an example of how many other harm reduction interventions could be rigorously evaluated to show a broad range of benefits.

Medication-Assisted Treatment: Methadone Maintenance

According to Health Canada (2002), methadone maintenance treatment (MMT) is the most widely studied and most effective treatment for opioid dependence. (For a more detailed discussion of opioid addiction treatment, see Chapter 12.) MMT is the leading evidence-based intervention for people with severe opioid addiction. Its importance is easy to understand from a harm reduction perspective, in part because of strong evidence for MMT reducing the likelihood of HIV infection and other infectious diseases (Gowing et al., 2004). People who see abstinence from all psychoactive substances as the only purpose of addiction treatment are still prejudiced against clinicians who offer medication-assisted treatment such as MMT and clients who receive this treatment. However, most acknowledge the efficacy and pragmatic advantages of offering medication-assisted treatments to people with an opioid addiction. Patients with opioid addiction who take their daily dose as prescribed find their lives stabilized and more productive without the problems associated with withdrawal, sedation or intoxication (Dole et al., 1966). MMT has a long history in Canada. The first Canadian methadone program started in Vancouver in 1959 (Halliday, 1963; Paulus & Halliday, 1967). The

Addiction Research Foundation, now part of CAMH, in Toronto, has operated a MMT program since 1968 (Brands et al., 2000). However, in 1972, Health Canada introduced new regulations requiring physicians to have an exemption from the federal narcotic laws in order to prescribe methadone. This requirement led to declining availability of MMT in Canada, to the point where fewer than 600 people were in treatment across the country in the mid-1980s (Peachey & Franklin, 1985). In the mid-1990s, national and provincial governments took steps to increase the availability of MMT in response to the burgeoning HIV crisis among people who inject drugs (Brands et al., 2000). Since 2005, MMT programs have been available in all Canadian provinces, with particularly dramatic increases in treatment availability in Ontario and British Columbia (Brands et al., 2000; Nosyk et al., 2010).

MMT involves providing daily doses of methadone within a structure that should ensure patient safety and medical and psychosocial services (Health Canada, 2002). Several factors affect the effectiveness of MMT, including the availability of counselling services as a component of methadone treatment (Amato et al., 2004). MMT is more effective when methadone is prescribed in higher doses, a finding confirmed by a large review of the British Columbia MMT program, which showed that higher doses were correlated with improved retention in treatment and therefore better patient outcomes (Nosyk et al., 2009). However, despite these findings, many patients continue to receive doses below the optimal range of 60 to 120 mg per day (Nosyk et al., 2009), and the availability of ancillary psychosocial and counselling services is limited. Gaps in the system of services and supports in most jurisdictions continue to be a major challenge, as the discrepancy between actual practices and the evidence base continues to plague a domain that is under-resourced.

When prescribed within the context of appropriate services, MMT leads to a range of benefits, not only for patients, but ultimately for the community. Benefits include:
- reduced use of other opioids (Brands et al., 2003)
- reduced use of other drugs (Brands et al., 2002)
- improved mental and physical health (Health Canada, 2002)
- reduced illegal activity and incarceration (DeBeck et al., 2009)
- reduced risk of acquiring HIV infection (Gowing et al., 2004)
- improved outcomes of pregnancy (Health Canada, 2002)
- improved quality of life (Dazord et al., 1998).

In addition to being an effective addiction treatment, MMT also provides an opportunity for integrating primary care. This has been linked to improved patient outcomes, such as earlier initiation of treatment for HIV infection (Uhlmann et al., 2010).

Despite the large evidence base for the effectiveness of MMT, not all people with opioid addiction are attracted to or retained in MMT (Nosyk et al., 2010; Strike et al., 2005). Because treatment retention is correlated with many of the positive outcomes of MMT, the system needs to include MMT options with a low threshold for enrolment and to support patients remaining in treatment as long as they continue to benefit (Health Canada, 2002). Premature discharge from MMT is linked to a high risk of relapse to illicit opiate use and an elevated risk of overdose death (Woody et al., 2007). When MMT is not successful, other treatment options should be explored.

Heroin-Assisted Treatment

Heroin-assisted treatment (HAT) has been studied in many European countries as well as Canada (Ferri et al., 2011). HAT involves prescribing individualized doses of pharmaceutically pure heroin, which the patient self-administers under nursing supervision up to three times daily. Like MMT, HAT couples pharmaceutical treatment with comprehensive counselling and medical and psychiatric care. This treatment is typically reserved for people who have injected opioids long term, and not benefited from other treatment options (Oviedo-Joekes et al., 2008).

Many in the addiction treatment community may find the concept of providing heroin to those whose lives have been devastated by opioid addiction to be counterintuitive. But providing the drug in a clinical and supervised context allows the person who uses drugs to disengage from the illicit market, avoid illegal activity and stabilize their social situation (e.g., housing, income support) in ways that support recovery (Ferri et al., 2011).

Many of the harms associated with heroin injection arise not because of the drug itself, but the context of drug use (e.g., an illicit source resulting in unknown purity; an illegal market driving costs, and resulting in criminal activity for obtaining drugs; unsafe injection practices) (Ferri et al., 2011). The North American Opiate Medication Initiative (NAOMI) was a multi-site randomized clinical trial conducted in Canada to evaluate the effectiveness of HAT compared to optimized MMT (Oviedo-Joekes et al., 2008). This study recruited people with opioid addiction who, on average, had been injecting heroin for 17 years, had attempted treatment 11 times and were currently outside the treatment system (Oviedo-Joekes et al., 2008). Patients were then treated with either HAT or MMT for one year: those who received HAT were more likely to stay in treatment and to reduce their illicit drug use and illegal activity than people treated with MMT (Oviedo-Joekes et al., 2009). This clearly demonstrates that, within Canada, people most severely affected by opioid injection use could benefit from having heroin-assisted treatment as an option.

Harm Reduction Approaches for Alcohol

So far this chapter has focused on harm reduction interventions primarily for people who inject drugs. However, many other harm reduction interventions are also possible. To illustrate the spectrum of harm reduction interventions, we can consider approaches to alcohol.

The National Alcohol Strategy in Canada aims to promote a culture of moderation, which includes using several harm reduction strategies (National Alcohol Strategy Working Group, 2007). For example, public policy measures that limit the availability of alcohol, through reduced late-night bar hours or fewer alcohol sales outlets, have been demonstrated to reduce alcohol-related harm without requiring cessation of alcohol use (National Alcohol Strategy Working Group, 2007). Another effective public policy measure would be to establish a standard minimum price per standardized drink of alcohol. Using this approach, raising the minimum standard price by 10 per cent would lead to a six per cent reduction in related harms, including alcohol-related deaths (Stockwell et al., 2012). Server training interventions aimed at reducing the likelihood that bar patrons become excessively intoxicated are another strategy for reducing the harms of drinking without requiring cessation (Ker & Chinnock, 2008).

Public Policy

As described above, many harm reduction interventions have been shown to reduce the risk of HIV infection or other negative health outcomes for people who use drugs, while having positive benefits for the community through reduced criminal activity, improved public order and cost savings to the health care system. The recognition of these benefits, combined with the limited evidence for success of legal prohibition approaches, has led to increased global calls for a move away from prohibition and toward a public health approach to substance use (Global Commission on Drug Policy, 2011; Vienna Declaration, 2010). Portugal has made the most significant shift toward a public health approach: possession of drugs for personal use has been decriminalized since 2001, resulting in decreased drug use, reduced crime and increased admissions to addiction treatment (Domoslawski, 2011). These are paradoxical effects when seen through the stereotypical perception that it is necessary to criminalize drug use to reduce its prevalence. By changing the paradigm from interdiction to intervention using public health approaches, a range of interventions from primary prevention through early intervention and tertiary prevention are used, with problematic substance use being seen as a health problem mediated by social determinants of health. Policing and law enforcement are still directed at drug importation and distribution, while the individual user is seen as someone who is entitled to health care and social support whether or not he or she stops using drugs.

Despite the proven benefits of harm reduction strategies, global spending on harm reduction programs is estimated to amount to less than three cents per day for each person who injects drugs (Stimson et al., 2010). For a more detailed Canadian perspective on the possible public health approaches to substance use, refer to the recent discussion paper by the Medical Officers of Health in British Columbia (Health Officers Council of British Columbia, 2011).

Harm Reduction Psychotherapy in Clinical Settings

Patt Denning (2000) and Andrew Tatarsky (1998) have written clear and instructive texts about the use and clinical relevancy of integrating a harm reduction philosophy and principles into the psychotherapeutic relationship with people who have substance use problems. Their writings reflect a significant paradigm shift in the field of addiction treatment because they are based on the premise that people can engage in and be successful at psychotherapy without requiring abstinence as the eventual goal. The therapeutic relationship between client and clinician is at the core of this approach, and is what influences the change process.

Harm reduction psychotherapy draws on a variety of therapeutic modalities, including psychodynamic, cognitive-behavioural, humanistic and biological approaches to understanding and responding to individual risk factors and consequences associated with substance use (Tatarsky & Kellogg, 2010). Harm reduction psychotherapy allows the client and clinician to engage collaboratively during the initial assessment of substance-using behaviours and together devise a comprehensive treatment plan that is pragmatic, flexible and achievable.

Tatarsky and Marlatt (2010) recommend the following 12 clinical principles of harm reduction psychotherapy as a framework for building a collaborative therapeutic relationship between the client and clinician, and as a guide for the clinician to determine when to use certain interventions:

1. Substance use problems are best understood and addressed in the context of the whole person and environment.
2. Meet the client as an individual.
3. The client has strengths that can be supported.
4. Challenge stigmatization.
5. Substances are used for adaptive reasons.
6. Drug use falls on a continuum of harmful consequences.
7. Don't hold abstinence as a precondition of therapy before really getting to know the individual.
8. Engagement in treatment is the primary goal.
9. Start where the patient is.
10. Look for and mobilize the client's strengths in service of change.
11. Develop a collaborative, empowering relationship with the client.
12. Goals and strategies emerge from the therapeutic process (pp. 120–121).

These 12 principles serve to enhance the therapeutic relationship, allow for client self-determination and foster an open and honest dialogue between the client and clinician. Similar to other therapeutic interventions, harm reduction psychotherapy is focused on developing the therapeutic alliance and the subsequent reparative nature of this relationship and on capitalizing on this relationship to promote self-reflection, goal setting and the acquisition of new skills and strategies to address substance use (Tatarsky & Kellogg, 2010).

Since harm reduction psychotherapy is an integrated approach, it draws on evidence-based interventions and practices used in the addiction field. For example, the therapist may use motivational interviewing to promote change talk and positive changes in drug use or high-risk behaviours. Or the therapist may draw on Denning and Little's (2012) transtheoretical model of change, particularly at the assessment phase. Alternatively, the therapist can weave cognitive-behavioural approaches, such as structured relapse prevention, into the skills-building activities while also engaging in a thoughtful discussion with the client about the implications that making those changes may have on the client's thoughts, feelings and behaviours.

Conclusion

Harm reduction encompasses a broad range of public policy and public health interventions that all seek to reduce harm related to substance use. We have reviewed several approaches to highlight the range of options available, with a focus on evidence-based interventions studied in Canada. To see harm reduction and abstinence as opposites is to misunderstand the nature of addiction and the ways in which it can be treated. Within an overall philosophy of harm reduction, abstinence goals and abstinent-oriented services are seen as foundational, not exclusive, elements. Indeed, most people who seek addiction treatment, especially those with more severe problems, will continue to have their own goals for abstinence. The reality is that many of these people will have trouble achieving or maintaining these goals. Harm reduction as a public health approach assumes that neither abstinence goals nor abstinent behaviour should determine access to addiction treatment or other health care services. Instead, these resources need to offer evidence-based service and innovate new approaches to help people with moderation goals.

The spirit of a treatment system embracing harm reduction is that of open doors. A harm reduction approach challenges and inspires health care practitioners not to take only those clients who can benefit from care and support with non-abstinent goals. Finally, harm reduction compels us to find ways to do outreach and connect with those at greatest risk of harm from problems related to addictive behaviour: those who have tried and not yet succeeded at addiction treatment, and those who are so socially marginalized and demoralized that they have become radically alienated and dislocated. Harm reduction provides a philosophical framework and a set of pragmatic practices that allow the use of effective strategies to address all three of these populations: people seeking to abstain; those with non-abstinent goals; and those who remain disengaged from and unhelped by treatment services, and who need to be the focus of continuing concern.

Practice Tips

- Recognize that the client is the expert on his or her life, while you are the expert on the process—two expertises that complement each other.
- Be respectful and non-judgmental about the person's substance use and other addictive behaviours. Explore the benefits and costs as the client sees them. Show the client that you understand his or her point of view, issues and desired solution.
- Ask the client what he or she needs, including what he or she would like from you. Drug use may not be the primary concern for the client—and should not be for you.
- Consider what practical things you can do to help the client improve his or her situation, reduce risk exposure, enhance well-being and increase the likelihood of coming back to see you, or connect the client with other resources that provide the necessary help and support.
- Optimize your environment so that it is welcoming to visitors, particularly those you are working with, be they youth, single mothers, people who are homeless, Aboriginal people, members of diverse ethnicities or people involved with the criminal justice system.
- Identify the practical things you can reasonably provide or help the client access (e.g., condoms, clean needles, safer crack use kits, medical triage, clothing, housing support, income support, legal support). Take a Maslovian approach, looking at the client's need hierarchy from safety to social support to meaningful activity.
- Have protocols for intervening in a range of crisis situations, including contingencies for everything from overdose to disruptive behaviour to suicidal and self-harm behaviours.
- Always work on trying to connect with the person, and seek feedback about whether what you are doing is helpful to the person on his or her own terms.
- Employ, train and support peer workers.
- Ensure that harm reduction programs are open during hours that reflect clients' needs.
- Offer food and clothing as a way to entice people to use your services.
- Demonstrate respect for clients. More important than having the full range of supplies needed to provide services is the attitude of staff toward service users. A good and honourable relationship is very curative.

Resources

Internet
Canadian Harm Reduction Network
   www.canadianharmreduction.com
Drug Policy Alliance
   www.drugpolicy.org
Harm Reduction Therapy Centre
   www.harmreductiontherapy.org
Trip Project (Queen West CHC)
   www.tripproject.ca
Vancouver Area Network of Drug Users
   www.vandu.org

References

Amato, L., Minozzi, S., Davoli, M., Vecchi, S., Ferri, M. & Mayet, S. (2004). Psychosocial combined with agonist maintenance treatments versus agonist maintenance treatments alone for treatment of opioid dependence. *Cochrane Database of Systematic Reviews, 2004* (4): CD004147.

Bayoumi, A.M. & Zaric, G.S. (2008). The cost-effectiveness of Vancouver's supervised injection facility. *Canadian Medical Association Journal, 179*, 1143–1151.

Brands, B., Blake, J. & Marsh, D. (2002). Changing patient characteristics with increased methadone maintenance availability. *Drug and Alcohol Dependence, 66*, 11–20.

Brands, B., Blake, J. & Marsh, D. (2003). Impact of methadone program philosophy changes on early treatment outcomes. *Journal of Addictive Disorders, 22*, 19–38.

Brands, J., Brands, B. & Marsh, D. (2000). The expansion of methadone prescribing in Ontario, 1996–1998. *Addiction Research, 8*, 485–496.

Broadhead, R.S., Kerr, T.H, Grund, J.C. & Altice, F.L. (2002). Safer injection facilities in North America: Their place in public policy and health initiatives. *Journal of Drug Issues, 32*, 329–355.

Canadian Centre on Substance Abuse & Health Canada. (2005). *National Framework for Action to Reduce the Harms Associated with Alcohol and Other Drugs and Substances in Canada.* Ottawa: Author. Retrieved from www.nationalframework-cadrenational.ca

Cavalieri, W. & Riley, D. (2012). Harm reduction in Canada: The many faces of regression. In R. Pates & D. Riley (Eds.), *Harm Reduction in Substance Use and High-Risk Behaviour: International Policy and Practice* (pp. 382–394). Oxford, United Kingdom: Wiley-Blackwell.

Centre for Addiction and Mental Health (CAMH). (2002). *CAMH and Harm Reduction: A Background Paper on Its Meaning and Application for Substance Use Issues.* Toronto: Author. Retrieved from www.camh.ca

Dazord, A., Mino, A., Page, D. & Broers, B. (1998). Patients on methadone mainte-nance treatment in Geneva. *European Psychiatry, 13,* 235–241.

DeBeck, K., Kerr, T., Bird, L., Zhang, R., Marsh, D., Tyndall, M. et al. (2011). Injection drug use cessation and use of North America's first medically supervised safer injecting facility. *Drug and Alcohol Dependence, 113,* 172–176.

DeBeck, K., Kerr, T., Li, K., Milloy, M.J., Montaner, J. & Wood, E. (2009). Incarceration and drug use patterns among a cohort of injection drug users. *Addiction, 104,* 69–76.

Denning, P. (2000). *Practicing Harm Reduction Psychotherapy: An Alternative Approach to Addictions.* New York: Guilford Press.

Denning, P. & Little, J. (2012). *Practicing Harm Reduction Psychotherapy: An Alternative Approach to Addictions* (2nd ed.). New York: Guilford Press.

Dole, V.P., Nyswander, M.E. & Kreek, M.J. (1966). Narcotic blockade. *Archives of Internal Medicine, 118,* 304–309.

Domoslawski, A. (2011). *Drug Policy in Portugal: The Benefits of Decriminalizing Drug Use.* New York: Open Society Foundations. Retrieved from www.opensocietyfoundations.org

Dovey, K., Fitzgerald, J. & Choi, Y. (2001). Safety becomes danger: Dilemmas of drug-use in public space. *Health & Place, 7,* 319–331.

Erickson, P.G., Riley, D.M., Cheung, Y.W. & O'Hare, P.A. (Eds.). (1997). *Harm Reduction: A New Direction for Drug Policies and Programs.* Toronto: University of Toronto Press.

Ferri, M., Davoli, M. & Perucci, C.A. (2011). Heroin maintenance for chronic heroin-dependent individuals. *Cochrane Database of Systematic Reviews, 2011* (12): CD003410.

Gibson, D.R., Flynn, N.M. & Perales, D. (2001). Effectiveness of syringe exchange programs in reducing HIV risk behavior and HIV seroconversion among injecting drug users. *AIDS, 15,* 1329–1341.

Global Commission on Drug Policy. (2011). *War on Drugs: Report of the Global Commission on Drug Policy.* Rio de Janeiro, Brazil: Author. Retrieved from www.globalcommissionondrugs.org

Gowing, L., Farrell, M., Bornemann, R. & Ali, R. (2004). Substitution treatment of injecting opioid users for prevention of HIV infection. *Cochrane Database of Systematic Reviews, 2004* (4): CD004145.

Halliday, R. (1963). Management of the narcotic addict. *British Columbia Medical Journal, 5,* 412–414.

Health Canada. (2002). *Best Practices: Methadone Maintenance Treatment.* Ottawa: Author. Retrieved from www.hc-sc.gc.ca

Health Officers Council of British Columbia. (2011). *Public Health Perspectives for Regulating Psychoactive Substances: What We Can Do about Alcohol, Tobacco, and Other Drugs.* Vancouver: Author. Retrieved from http://drugpolicy.ca

Heimer, R., Clair, S., Teng, W., Grau, L.E., Khoshnood, K. & Singer, M. (2002). Effects of increasing syringe availability on syringe-exchange use and HIV risk: Connecticut, 1990–2001. *Journal of Urban Health, 79,* 556–570.

International Harm Reduction Association (IHRA). (2010a). What is harm reduction? A position statement from the International Harm Reduction Association. *IHRA Briefing.* London, United Kingdom: Author. Retrieved from www.ihra.net/what-is-harm-reduction

International Harm Reduction Association (IHRA). (2010b). *Global State of Harm Reduction 2010: Key Issues for Broadening the Response.* London, United Kingdom: Author. Retrieved from www.ihra.net/contents/245

Ker, K. & Chinnock, P. (2008). Interventions in the alcohol server setting for preventing injuries. *Cochrane Database of Systematic Reviews, 2008* (3): CD005244.

Kerr, T., Small, W., Buchner, C., Zhang, R., Li, K., Montaner, J. & Wood, E. (2010). Syringe sharing and HIV incidence among injection drug users and increased access to sterile syringes. *American Journal of Public Health, 100,* 1449–1453.

Kerr, T., Stoltz, J., Tyndall, M., Li, K., Zhang, R., Montaner, J. & Wood, E. (2006b). Impact of a medically supervised safer injection facility on community drug use patterns: A before and after study. *British Medical Journal, 332,* 220–222.

Kerr, T., Tyndall, M., Lai, C., Montaner, J. & Wood, E. (2006a). Drug-related overdoses within a medically supervised safer injecting facility. *International Journal of Drug Policy, 17,* 436–441.

Kerr, T., Tyndall, M., Li, K., Montaner, J. & Wood, E. (2005). Safer injection facility use and syringe sharing in injection drug users. *The Lancet, 366,* 316–318.

Kleinig, J. (2008). The ethics of harm reduction. *Substance Use & Misuse, 43,* 1–16. doi: 10.1080/10826080701690680

Marlatt, G.A. & Donovan, D.M. (Eds.). (2005). *Relapse Prevention: Maintenance Strategies in the Treatment of Addictive Behaviors.* New York: Guilford Press.

Marlatt, G.A. & Witkiewitz, C. (2002). Harm reduction approaches to alcohol use. *Addictive Behaviors, 27,* 867–886. doi: 10.1016/S0306-4603(02)00294-0

Marshall, B., Milloy, M., Wood, E., Montaner, J. & Kerr, T. (2011). Reduction in overdose mortality after the opening of North America's first medically supervised safer injecting facility: A retrospective population-based study. *The Lancet, 377,* 1429–1437.

Miller, W.R. (2008). The ethics of harm reduction. In C. Geppert & L. Roberts (Eds.), *The Book of Ethics: Expert Guidance for Professionals Who Treat Addiction* (pp. 110–123). Center City, MN: Hazelden.

Miller, W.R., Forcehimes, A.A. & Zweben, A. (2011). *Treating Addiction: A Guide for Professionals.* New York: Guilford Press.

National Alcohol Strategy Working Group. (2007). *Reducing Alcohol-Related Harm in Canada: Toward a Culture of Moderation. Recommendations for a National Alcohol Strategy.* Ottawa: Health Canada. Retrieved from www.nationalframework-cadrenational.ca

National Institutes of Health. (2002). *Management of Hepatitis C: 2002. Consensus Statement.* Bethesda, MD: Author. Retrieved from http://consensus.nih.gov/2002/2002hepatitisc2002116html.htm

Nosyk, B., MacNab, Y.C., Sun, H., Fischer, B., Marsh, D.C., Schechter, M.T. & Anis, A.H. (2009). Proportional hazards frailty models for recurrent methadone maintenance treatment. *American Journal of Epidemiology, 170*, 783–792.

Nosyk, B., Marsh, D.C., Sun, H., Schechter, M.T. & Anis, A.H. (2010). Trends in methadone maintenance treatment participation, retention, and compliance to dosing guidelines in British Columbia, Canada: 1996–2006. *Journal of Substance Abuse Treatment, 39*, 22–31.

Oviedo-Joekes, E., Brissette, S., Marsh, D.C., Lauzon, P., Guh, D., Anis, A. & Schechter, M.T. (2009). Diacetylmorphine versus methadone for the treatment of opioid addiction. *New England Journal of Medicine, 361*, 777–786.

Oviedo-Joekes, E. Nosyk, B., Brissette, S., Chettiar, J., Schneeberger, P., Marsh, D.C. et al. (2008). The North American Opiate Medication Initiative (NAOMI): Profile of participants in North America's first trial of heroin-assisted treatment. *Journal of Urban Health, 85*, 812–825.

Patra, J., Taylor, B., Rehm, J.T., Baliunas, D. & Popova, S. (2007). Substance-attributable morbidity and mortality changes to Canada's epidemiological profile: Measurable differences over a ten-year period. *Canadian Journal of Public Health, 98*, 228–234.

Paulus, I. & Halliday, R. (1967). Rehabilitation and the narcotic addict: Results of a comparative methadone withdrawal program. *Canadian Medical Association Journal, 96*, 655–659.

Peachey, J.E. & Franklin, T. (1985). Methadone treatment of opiate dependence in Canada. *British Journal of Addiction, 80*, 291–299.

Rehm, J.D., Baliunas, S., Brochu, B., Fischer, W., Gnam, J., Patra, S. & Taylor, B. (2006). *The Costs of Substance Abuse in Canada 2002.* Ottawa: Canadian Centre on Substance Abuse. Retrieved from www.ccsa.ca/Eng/Priorities/Research/CostStudy

Riley, D., Pates, R., Monaghan, G. & O'Hare, P. (2012). A brief history of harm reduction. In R. Pates & D. Riley (Eds.), *Harm Reduction in Substance Use and High-Risk Behaviour: Internation Policy and Practice* (pp. 5–16). Oxford, United Kingdom: Wiley-Blackwell.

Sanchez-Craig, M. & Lei, H. (1986). Disadvantages to imposing the goal of abstinence on problem drinkers: An empirical study. *British Journal of Addiction, 81*, 505–512.

Schechter, M.T., Strathdee, S.A., Cornelisse, P.G., Currie, S., Patrick, D.M., Rekart, M.L. & O'Shaughnessy, M.V. (1999). Do needle exchange programmes increase the spread of HIV among injection drug users? An investigation of the Vancouver outbreak. *AIDS, 13*, F45–51.

Stimson, G.V., Cook, C., Bridge, J., Rio-Navarro, J., Lines, R. & Barrett, D. (2010). *Three Cents a Day Is Not Enough: Resourcing HIV-Related Harm Reduction on a Global Basis.* London, United Kingdom: International Harm Reduction Association. Retrieved from www.ihra.net/files/2010/06/01/IHRA_3CentsReport_Web.pdf

Stockwell, T., Auld, M.C., Zhao, J. & Martin, G. (2012). Does minimum pricing reduce alcohol consumption? The experience of a Canadian province. *Addiction, 107,* 912–920.

Stoltz, J., Wood, E., Small, W., Li, K., Tyndall, M., Montaner, J. & Kerr, T. (2007). Changes in injecting practices associated with the use of a medically supervised safer injection facility. *Journal of Public Health, 29,* 35–39.

Strathdee, S.A., Patrick, D.M., Currie, S.L., Cornelisse, P.G.A., Rekart, M.L., Montaner, J.S.G. et al. (1997). Needle exchange is not enough: Lessons from the Vancouver injecting drug use study. *AIDS, 11,* F59–65.

Strike, C.J., Gnam, W., Urbanoski, K., Fischer, B., Marsh, D.C. & Millson, M. (2005). Factors predicting 2-year retention in methadone maintenance treatment for opioid dependence. *Addictive Behaviors, 30,* 1025–1028.

Strike, C., Leonard, L., Millson, M., Anstice, S., Berkeley, N. & Medd, E. (2006). *Ontario Needle Exchange Programs: Best Practice Recommendations.* Toronto: Ontario Needle Exchange Coordinating Committee. Retrieved from www.health.gov.on.ca

Tatarsky, A. (1998). An integrative approach to harm reduction psychotherapy: A case of problem drinking secondary to depression. *In Session: Psychotherapy in Practice, 4* (2), 16–29.

Tatarsky, A. & Kellogg, S.H. (2010). Integrative harm reduction psychotherapy: A case of substance use, multiple trauma, and suicidality. *Journal of Clinical Psychology: In Session, 66* (10), 123–135.

Tatarsky, A. & Marlatt, G.A. (2010). State of the art in harm reduction psychotherapy: An emerging treatment for substance misuse. *Journal of Clinical Psychology: In Session, 66* (10), 117–122.

Uhlmann, S., Milloy, M.J., Kerr, T., Zhang, R., Guillemi, S., Marsh, D. et al. (2010). Methadone maintenance therapy promotes initiation of antiretroviral therapy among injection drug users. *Addiction, 105,* 907–913.

United Nations Office on Drugs and Crime. (2011a). *World Drug Report 2011.* Vienna, Austria: Author. Retrieved from www.unodc.org

United Nations Office on Drugs and Crime. (2011b). *Estimating Illicit Financial Flows Resulting from Drug Trafficking and Other Transnational Organized Crimes.* Vienna, Austria: Author. Retrieved from www.unodc.org

Vienna Declaration. (2010). *The Vienna Declaration.* Retrieved from www.viennadeclaration.com

Wood, E., Kerr, T., Lloyd-Smith, E., Buchner, C., Marsh, D.C., Montaner, J.S.G. & Tyndall, M.W. (2004). Methodology for evaluating Insite: Canada's first medically supervised safer injection facility for injection drug users. *Harm Reduction Journal, 1* (1), 9.

Wood, E., Kerr, T., Montaner, J.S., Strathdee, S.A., Wodak, A., Hankins, C.A. & Tyndall, M.W. (2004). Rationale for evaluating North America's first medically supervised safer-injecting facility. *The Lancet Infectious Diseases, 4*, 301–306.

Wood, E., Kerr, T., Small, W., Li, K., Marsh, D.C., Montaner, J.S.G. & Tyndall, M.W. (2004). Changes in public order after the opening of a medically supervised safer injecting facility for illicit injection drug users. *Canadian Medical Association Journal, 171*, 731–734.

Wood, E., Tyndall, M.W., Lai, C., Montaner, J.S.C. & Kerr, T. (2006) Impact of a medically supervised safer injecting facility on drug dealing and other drug-related crime. *Substance Abuse Treatment, Prevention and Policy, 1*, 13.

Wood, E., Tyndall, M.W., Qui, Z., Zhang, R., Montaner, J.S.G. & Kerr, T. (2006). Service uptake and characteristics of injection drug users utilizing North America's first medically supervised safer injecting facility. *American Journal of Public Health, 96*, 770–773.

Wood, E., Tyndall, M.W., Spittal, P.M., Li, K., Hogg, R.S., Montaner, J.S. et al. (2002). Factors associated with persistent high-risk syringe sharing in the presence of an established needle exchange programme. *AIDS, 16*, 941–943.

Wood, E., Tyndall, M.W., Zhang, R., Montaner, J.S. & Kerr, T. (2007). Rate of detoxification service use and its impact among a cohort of supervised injecting facility users. *Addiction, 102*, 916–919.

Wood, E., Zhang, R. & Montaner, J.S.G. (2006). Attendance at supervised injecting facilities and use of detoxification services. *New England Journal of Medicine, 354*, 2512–2514.

Woody, G.E., Kane, V. & Thompson, R. (2007). Premature deaths after discharge from methadone maintenance: A replication. *Journal of Addiction Medicine, 1*, 180–185.

Chapter 5

Motivational Interviewing

Marilyn Herie and Wayne Skinner

Self-assessment: How would you respond?

How would you respond to the following client statements? Before you read this chapter, take a couple of minutes and write down a sentence or two. Imagine that the client is sitting across from you and you have to respond right away, so write down the first thing that comes to mind. You will have a chance to review these questions and your answers when you finish this chapter.

Client: *It's easy for you to tell me all these things I have to do. When was the last time you had someone on your case all the time?*
Counsellor: _____

_____

Client: *I've tried everything and nothing seems to help. What's the point?*
Counsellor: _____

_____

Adia is a 27-year-old single parent who attends school part-time while looking after her two young kids. Child protection services were called to her home when a neighbour discovered that the children were left unattended overnight. Adia has had previous involvement with police and child protection for drug-related offences and drug use. She is now mandated to attend addiction counselling in order to maintain custody of her children. She feels angry that "people are interfering in my business." She maintains that she no longer has a drug problem, and that her past drug use has never affected her parenting or her other responsibilities. Adia currently expresses that she does not want to attend treatment.

She is given an ultimatum from child protection services to go to addiction treatment or have her kids removed from the home. From Adia's perspective, the worker is unfairly using her power to force Adia into a treatment program she does not want or need. However, because she loves her children, she says she will "do what I have to do."

When Adia presents at the addiction treatment centre for her intake interview, she appears hostile and unco-operative. She answers the counsellor's questions in monosyllables, seems distracted and impatient and repeatedly asks how much longer the interview is going to take. When the counsellor points out that Adia has a history of drug-related offences and drug use, Adia becomes angry and defensive. After the session, the counsellor notes that Adia is "in denial," has no insight into her drug problems and is unmotivated to change.

This case example illustrates a common issue in addiction treatment: many clients seemingly attend treatment only because of extrinsic pressures rather than from any intrinsic motivation to change. Adia likely feels coerced into attending treatment, rather than taking part because she wants to. Yet in a way, she "chooses" to co-operate, or at least goes along with this demand.

Adia's case also illustrates how easy it is for practitioners to find themselves in an adversarial dynamic with their clients. On the one hand, clients often feel coerced into stopping or changing their substance use, are skeptical that substance use is really a problem and feel ambivalent about attending treatment. On the other hand, the practitioner may regard substance use as a major issue, work hard to engage with clients in a meaningful way and establish trust and rapport, and work collaboratively toward positive change. How can these seemingly dichotomous perspectives and goals align?

This chapter outlines the underlying philosophy and core skills of motivational interviewing (MI), a client-centred approach that can help build engagement and foster readiness to change among people who are ambivalent. Each skill is illustrated with various examples. We review the "spirit" of MI and the theoretical and empirical literature supporting the use of this approach in addiction treatment (and other behavioural change domains). We also discuss evidence and ways of adapting MI with diverse client populations. The chapter concludes with an outline of eight processes in learning and practising MI, and some key practice tips. The overarching theme we explore is captured in the metaphor of "dancing versus wrestling," and how MI can help us join with our clients and promote their autonomy and empowerment (Miller & Rollnick, 2013). It can be all too easy to fall into the trap of trying to persuade or coerce clients to accept our own agenda for change, which often leads to an adversarial or even confrontational dynamic that is generally counter therapeutic.

Defining MI

MI was developed in the 1980s by William Miller and Stephen Rollnick as a client-centred approach to enhancing motivation for change. The focus and skills of MI are a counterpoint to traditional approaches in addiction treatment, which emphasize breaking down "denial" through confrontation, direct advice and warnings or threats if change does not occur.

MI has been variously defined since its first conceptualization, and it has evolved over the years, reflecting advances in theory and research. The earliest definition focuses on MI as a directive but non-confrontational approach to helping clients explore and resolve their ambivalence about changing: it is a "client-centered, directive method for enhancing intrinsic motivation to change by exploring and resolving ambivalence" (Miller & Rollnick, 2002, p. 25). More recently, Miller and Rollnick (2009) described MI as *directional* as opposed to *directive*. This means that the client and counsellor work toward one or more specific and agreed-upon goals (directional), and the counsellor uses non-directive (client-centred) strategies to get there.

Three definitions of MI

A layperson's definition:
MI is a collaborative conversation style for strengthening a person's own motivation for and commitment to change.

A practitioner's definition:
MI is a person-centred counselling method for addressing the common problem of ambivalence about change.

A technical definition:
MI is a collaborative, goal-oriented style of communication with particular attention to the language of change. It is designed to strengthen personal motivation for and commitment to a specific goal by eliciting and exploring the person's own reasons for change within an atmosphere of acceptance and compassion.

Source: Adapted from Miller & Rollnick (2013), p. 29.

Rollnick and colleagues (2008) use the action term *guiding* to make a distinction between simply *following* the client non-directively and *directing* the client prescriptively. These definitions highlight that at its core, MI is a *way of being* with the client. It is a clinical approach that focuses on interpersonal communication, informed by a particular "spirit," incorporating complex relational and technical skills that need to be learned and practised over time (Miller & Rollnick, 2013).

The "Spirit" of MI

Using the skills of MI without embracing the underlying spirit is like listening to the lyrics of a song without the music. Just as the music is essential to any song, the philosophy or "spirit" of MI is an essential foundation to the practical strategies. The goal is to evoke the client's own reasons for change (and his or her ideas about how change should happen).

Spirit is a fundamental component without which any specific skill or strategy will "fall flat." Yet many counsellors are unable or unwilling to let go of the traditional expert role, and may even believe that it is dangerous to clients to do so. After all, what if a client, like Adia in the case example at the beginning of the chapter, refuses to change? It seems paradoxical that abandoning an attempt to push for change can actually promote change; yet anyone who has had the experience of being pressured into a behaviour or a course of action can attest to the truth of the axiom that people are most able to change when they feel free not to. In motivational interviewing, expertise is measured by the ability of the therapist to form effective helping relationships that guide clients toward healthy behavioural change, rather than dispensing technically correct advice to clients who are not inclined to change.

The four elements of the spirit of MI are partnership, acceptance, compassion and evocation of the client's ideas and goals toward change. Drawing on the work of Carl Rogers, MI spirit represents an egalitarian relationship characterized by unconditional acceptance and positive regard; compassionate and empathic understanding; and a stance of evoking versus installing ideas, goals and deep wisdom.

In MI, the counsellor actively fosters and encourages power sharing in interaction with the client, such that the client strongly influences the conversation in the context of a working partnership. Further, the concept of acceptance encompasses Rogers' therapeutic stance of unconditional positive regard, accurate empathy, support for clients' autonomy and affirmation of clients' strengths and efforts. Compassion, the third component of MI spirit, means actively promoting the welfare of the client and putting his or her needs first. Finally, evocation implies, "You have what you need, and together we will find it" (Miller & Rollnick, 2013, p. 21).

Evocation of the client's own reasons for change is more compelling than simply trying to educate and instruct the client about what objectively needs to be done to improve the situation:

> When clients are viewed primarily from a deficit perspective (e.g., being in
> denial; lacking insight, knowledge, and skills), it makes little sense to spend
> time eliciting their own wisdom. Instead, the counselor would be inclined to
> confront denial, explain reality, provide information, and teach skills. Within
> this perspective, consultation is clinician-centered, and it revolves around
> the counselor providing what the client lacks: "I have what you need." It
> can be quite a cognitive jump from this expert stance to MI, wherein the

counselor instead communicates a respect for the client's own perspectives and autonomy. The MI counselor seeks to evoke the client's own motivations for change ("You have what you need") rather than installing them. A willingness to entertain this client centered perspective is a starting point in learning MI. (Miller & Moyers, 2006, p. 6)

In general, counsellor behaviours and MI skills can be classified as *MI consistent* or *MI inconsistent* (Martino et al., 2006). MI-consistent behaviours relating to the spirit of this approach are summarized in Table 5-1, and are contrasted with MI-inconsistent behaviours. Note that MI inconsistent does not necessarily mean wrong for all clients in all circumstances; rather, this categorization is useful in assessing whether a practitioner who intends to use an MI approach is actually doing so.

TABLE 5-1

MI-Consistent and MI-Inconsistent Behaviours Relating to MI Spirit

MI CONSISTENT	MI INCONSISTENT
Emphasizes and respects client's autonomy	Asserts authority about what is best for this client, pursues own agenda in the session
Actively collaborates with client	Mandates specific goals (e.g., abstinence)
Elicits client's perspective, ideas, hopes, concerns, etc.	Provides unsolicited advice, feedback or information without client's permission
Demonstrates non-judgmental acceptance and conveys empathy through words, body language and tone of voice	Confronts or threatens client with negative consequences if change does not occur

The Four Processes of MI

In their recently updated edition of the MI "textbook," Miller and Rollnick (2013) outline four recursive processes of MI:

Engaging: Client engagement is essential to the helping relationship. Without engagement, it is not possible to proceed, as the client makes a decision about whether to join with the practitioner and actively participate in treatment. The skills of engagement must also continue throughout all stages in the helping relationship.

Focusing: With the client as equal partner, this "strategic centring" process hones in on the possible targets or directions for change. At all times, client autonomy is respected—

it is for the client to determine what he or she would like to address or work toward in treatment. Periodic "refocusing" may be needed as goals evolve or change over time.

Evoking: Once the client is engaged in treatment, and both client and practitioner have agreed on areas of focus, it is the practitioner's task to evoke from the client his or her ambivalence about changing, reasons for change and strategies for change. In this stage, the skills of MI become strategic in guiding the client in the direction of change by paying special attention to evoking change talk.

Planning: The process of planning can occur when (and only when) the client is ready to make a commitment to change. The skills of evoking commitment language, as well as the client's strategies and ideas for change, are key in this process.

Note that these processes follow a logical sequence, with each one building on the one that precedes it. However, practitioners may return to earlier processes throughout the helping relationship. It can be helpful to visualize the processes as steps on a staircase:

FIGURE 5-1: Four Processes of MI

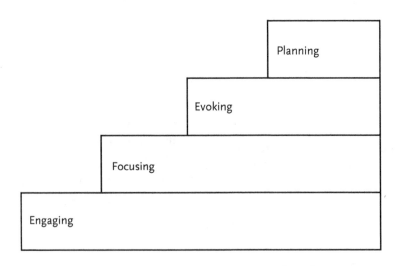

Source: Miller, W.R. & Rollnick, S. (2013). *Motivational Interviewing: Helping People Change* (3rd ed., p. 26). New York: Guilford Press. © Guilford Press. Reprinted with permission.

The core skills of MI described in this chapter are used throughout these four processes, although certain skills may be more applicable to specific processes. A detailed explanation of the skills and processes is beyond the scope of this chapter (which highlights practical approaches that may be helpful to counsellors beginning to learn about and apply MI in practice). For a more robust and nuanced exposition of MI processes and skills, see Miller and Rollnick (2013).

Theoretical Foundations

MI has been strongly influenced by Rogers' humanistic psychotherapy (Rogers, 1980), particularly in its emphasis on accurate empathy and unconditional positive regard. Prochaska and DiClemente's transtheoretical model ([TTM], 1984) was also an early influence on MI as it was first developed—so much so that the two approaches have been termed "kissing cousins who never married" (Miller & Rollnick, 2009, p. 130). In the second edition of their influential motivational interviewing book, Miller and Rollnick (2002) purposely omitted any references to TTM (also known as the Stages of Change model) in order to help correct the perception that MI is based on TTM.[1] Essentially, TTM outlines a process of change and different therapeutic tasks within each stage, whereas MI is an evidence-based intervention (or communication style) with techniques that can be used with anyone who is resistant or ambivalent about changing, or who is struggling with making a change. The main point is that an MI approach seems to work best with people who are not yet committed to—or continue to remain ambivalent about—change (Miller & Moyers, 2006); however, a client does not need to be assigned to a specific stage of change in order to benefit from MI (Miller & Rollnick, 2009, 2013).

Miller himself has acknowledged that he developed MI in the absence of a strong theoretical framework:

> When pressed I can usually come up with a reasonable theoretical ratio-
> nale, but the truth is that I usually start from curiosity and experience, and
> from a general interest in finding what works best for people in pain. With
> enough experience I start coming around to theory development. (Miller,
> 1999, p. 2)

It is only in the past few years that a cohesive theory base for MI has started to take shape. Self-determination theory, which posits that autonomy support, autonomous motivation and perceived competence predict health and behavioural outcomes, appears especially congenial to the spirit and strategies of MI (Vansteenkiste & Sheldon, 2006; Williams et al., 2006). In addition, cognitive dissonance theory (e.g., the gap between current behaviours and future goals) is relevant to some aspects of MI, especially the clinical skill of developing discrepancy (Draycott & Dabbs, 1998; Lundahl & Burke, 2009). Self-perception theory, which posits that hearing oneself argue for change affects motivation, relates to MI's focus on eliciting client change talk (the elements in clients' speech that favour change) (Lundahl & Burke, 2009).

Miller and Rose (2009) reviewed the past three decades of MI research in order to understand the "mechanics" of how this approach works to influence behaviour change. They highlight two specific types of components that work together to effect change: the *relational* (or empathic, interpersonal) components and the *technical* components that

---

[1] A detailed discussion of the critiques of TTM and how the Stages of Change model fits—or, more accurately, does not fit—with MI is beyond the scope of this chapter. See West (2005) for a summary of theoretical and empirical issues with TTM.

elicit and reinforce clients' own reasons for behaviour change. An emerging causal chain model for MI links together therapist training, MI skills, client responses and treatment outcomes (Miller & Rose, 2009).

These various theoretical strands are still being debated and discussed in the literature, and further iterations of MI will no doubt be grounded in more robust models and frameworks.

The Evidence Base for MI

The evidence base for MI is strong and compelling: since the 1980s, the number of research and clinical articles has doubled every three years, with more than 1,000 publications and more than 200 randomized clinical trials (Miller & Rollnick, 2009, 2010). Two recent meta-analyses (Lundahl & Burke, 2009; Lundahl et al., 2010) support the efficacy of MI in addiction and in other health behaviour change areas (e.g., mental health problems, diabetes, obesity, hypertension, criminal justice, homelessness, HIV/ AIDS). In particular, research supports the use of MI to enhance treatment engagement and retention, client goal setting and behaviour change, motivation and treatment outcomes (up to three years post-treatment). MI has also been researched in a variety of formats, including as a stand-alone treatment intervention (Miller & Rose, 2009); as a brief (i.e., a few minutes) counselling intervention (Herie & Selby, 2007); in combination with other approaches (Miller & Rose, 2009); and in groups (LaBrie et al., 2006).

Of course, there are numerous challenges in evaluating the efficacy of MI interventions in controlled trials. These are not all specific to MI research, but they should be considered in critically assessing the evidence. The following questions raise possible limitations:

- Did the study compare "pure" MI with another intervention? Many practitioners—and research studies—use an eclectic approach, combining MI with other evidence-based interventions, such as cognitive-behavioural therapy or contingency management.
- How was MI fidelity on the part of counsellors ensured? There is evidence that practitioners' self-reports of the interventions they offer may not correspond with what they actually do in a clinical session (Miller et al., 2006).
- What were the studies' inclusion and exclusion criteria? Many research trials exclude the most complex or severely dependent individuals, with positive results that may be statistically, but not clinically, significant (i.e., the results may not reflect the client population seen in real-life practice).

In general, treatment trials tend to find that no one intervention is innately superior for all clients under all conditions—this includes MI (Prochaska & Norcross, 2007).

Keeping these caveats in mind, when MI has been compared with other interventions (treatment as usual), outcomes in the MI condition were found to be effective 75 per cent of the time, with 50 per cent of clients gaining small but meaningful effects, and 25 per cent gaining moderate to strong effects (Lundahl et al., 2010). These results are consistent with research findings for other clinical interventions. However, an added benefit of MI over other treatments is that a smaller dose of treatment may be needed; on average, studies have found that MI treatments take an average of 100 fewer minutes, yet produce equal effects (Lundahl et al., 2010).

The body of research evidence helps to answer the question "Does MI work?" A recent study goes on to address an important related question: "*How* does MI work?" (Moyers et al., 2009). Moyers and colleagues (2009) micro-analyzed audio recordings of MI interventions to investigate the degree to which client change talk plays a role in treatment outcomes. Based on session recordings from the U.S. multi-site Project MATCH study (Project MATCH Research Group, 1999), therapist and client speech were classified using a validated MI coding instrument, the Motivational Interviewing Treatment Integrity (MITI) code (Moyers et al., 2003). Therapist utterances were coded as either MI consistent or MI inconsistent, and then further classified into subcategories (e.g., simple reflections, complex reflections, open-ended or closed questions).

Moyers and colleagues (2009) found that, overall, MI-consistent statements resulted in increased client "change talk" (i.e., demonstrating desire, ability, reasons, need or commitment to change), whereas MI-inconsistent statements led to counter-change or "sustain talk" (reflecting clients' investment in maintaining the status quo). Examples of MI-inconsistent statements include directing, informing, warning, reassuring and confronting clients. Furthermore, counselling sessions characterized by a high proportion of MI-consistent statements and a corresponding high rate of client change talk were associated with lower levels of weekly drinking post-treatment than were sessions that featured MI-inconsistent statements and lower levels of change talk. Gaume and colleagues (2009) found that clients whose therapists exhibited better MI-consistent skills had more positive alcohol treatment outcomes at one-year follow up, lending some preliminary support to Moyers and colleagues' (2009) research.

The causal chain for MI proposed by Moyers and colleagues (2009) can be illustrated as follows:

therapist MI-consistent speech → increased client change talk → improved treatment outcomes

Reflective listening, in particular, emerged as a very potent and important micro-skill in MI. The researchers found that reflecting change talk back to clients elicits even more change talk, and reflecting sustain talk elicits more sustain talk; in other words, "What therapists reflect, they will hear more of" (Moyers et al., 2009, p. 1122). These findings suggest that reflecting sustain talk may be a risky strategy, and lend empirical support to the emphasis in MI on listening for and eliciting change talk (change talk is discussed in the next section).

MI Core Skills and Strategies

The Spirit of MI

The spirit of MI guides how we use the skills described in this section. Often when counsellors come to supervision stating "Motivational interviewing doesn't work with this client," it is because the counsellor is using the skills without emphasizing partnership, acceptance, compassion and evocation—the components of MI spirit. Of course, it may be the case that MI is not appropriate for a particular client, but it is always worth reflecting on whether the skills were practised from a place of open curiosity about the client's situation and goals, and with a shared "agenda" (e.g., the counsellor is not implicitly or explicitly communicating "I know what is best for you").

This is easier said than done, as counsellors often feel a sense of urgency to "get" the person to change. Miller and Rollnick (2013) call this the "righting reflex," and note that avoiding our reflexive response to "fix" the client is key. In other words, suppressing counter-motivational behaviour (like the righting reflex) is often harder—and more important—than how much or how well we use the specific skills.

There are various ways we behave therapeutically, all of which can be based in genuine concern for the client. Wanting to correct or instruct the client usually has this compassionate base of concern. But the test of whether we are holding to the MI spirit can often be measured by empathy—not the counsellor's self-rating of how attuned he or she is to what the client is struggling with, but through feedback from the client that this client values and appreciates our efforts to understand how things are with him or her, on the client's terms, not ours.

With that in mind, the following section provides brief descriptions of MI skills. A more detailed description and examples can be found in Miller and Rollnick (2013), Rollnick and colleagues (2008) and Rosengren (2009).

Client-Centred Counselling Skills: OARS

The four OARS skills are fundamental to MI practice. Even in a brief conversation, they can build collaboration and enhance motivation for change. OARS is an acronym for:

- **O**pen-ended questions
- statements of **A**ffirmation
- **R**eflective listening
- **S**ummary statements.

Open-ended questions invite the person to elaborate further. Closed questions, on the other hand, generally limit the person's reply to "yes" or "no." Table 5-2 presents examples of closed versus open-ended questions.

Closed and Open-ended Questions

CLOSED QUESTIONS	OPEN-ENDED QUESTIONS
Did you have any cravings in the last week?	Tell me about your cravings last week.
Have you ever injected drugs?	What is your experience with injecting drugs?
Would you like to come back for another appointment?	We're at the end of our appointment—where would you like to go from here?

In general, open-ended questions are preferred over closed ones because they are more effective at eliciting the client's thoughts, feelings, preferences and goals.

Top 10 open-ended questions

What changes would you most like to talk about?
What have you noticed about . . .?
How important is it for you to change . . .?
How confident do you feel about changing . . .?
How do you see the benefits of . . .?
How do you see the drawback of . . .?
What will make the most sense to you?
How might things be different if you . . .?
In what way . . .?
Where does this leave you now?

Source: Rollnick, S., Butler, C.C., Kinnersley, P., Gregory, J. & Mash, B. (2010). Motivational interviewing. *British Medical Journal, 340,* p. 1244. © BMJ Publishing Group. Reprinted with permission.

Statements of affirmation acknowledge a client's efforts, willingness to engage or ability to make a change. Using these statements periodically throughout the conversation can help build self-efficacy and communicate the counsellor's regard for the client and the work he or she is doing. Note that statements of affirmation go beyond a counsellor's praise or positive judgment of the client (e.g., simply "handing out a good grade"). Rather, statements of affirmation emphasize clients' strengths, particularly those that are important and relevant to that person. The following exchange illustrates how positive judgments may be counterproductive:

Counsellor: *Please tell me about any times that you have been able to stop drinking in the past.*

Client: *Well, I was abstinent from alcohol for about four years when I was in my 30s.*

Counsellor: *Wow! Four years—that's really great!*

Client: *Actually, I was miserable. They were the worst four years of my life!*

Of course, not all clients would respond in this way, but the example illustrates the perils of inserting our own assumptions and judgments into the conversation. A more fruitful response might have been something along the lines of "You were able to stop drinking for quite some time. How were you able to do that?" The practitioner could then explore what led the client back to alcohol use, as well as relapse prevention and coping skills issues and current goals.

Here are some examples of statements of affirmation:

I appreciate your taking the time to come and talk to me today.

You have really been doing some thinking about this.

You are committed to making the best choices for yourself, including what types of goals you want to set in treatment.

Reflective listening is the most central of the OARS skills, and can also be the most challenging to learn and practise effectively. Many counsellors assume they already know and practise reflective listening; yet when their interviews are recorded and reviewed, it becomes clear that they default to some combination of questioning, advising and affirming. For example, go back to the self-assessment at the beginning of this chapter: Would either of your responses to the challenging client statements meet the following criteria for reflective listening?

There are two types of reflective responses: (1) *simple reflections* essentially repeat back to a client the explicit content of something he or she has said; (2) *complex reflections* include the client's unspoken (implicit) meaning, feelings, intentions or experiences. In general, complex reflections are more effective at continuing and deepening the conversation. One way to understand the difference between these two types of reflection is to imagine an iceberg (see Figure 5-2). The tip of the iceberg (above the water) represents the content (or the words the client speaks); a simple reflection focuses on the tip of the iceberg. The huge mass of the iceberg below the water represents all the thoughts, feelings and meanings that lie behind the client's words; a complex reflection focuses below the waterline (Miller & Rollnick, 2013).

FIGURE 5-2: Simple and Complex Reflections

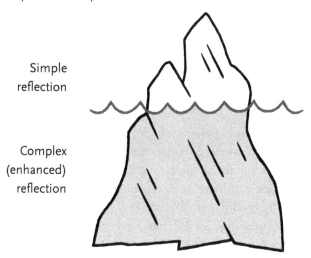

Simple
reflection

Complex
(enhanced)
reflection

Done well, reflective listening on its own can help open up new ground with clients and convey understanding and empathy. Table 5-3 provides examples of simple and complex reflections in response to different statements.

TABLE 5-3
Examples of Simple and Complex Reflections

CLIENT STATEMENT	SIMPLE REFLECTION	COMPLEX REFLECTION
I don't think I have a problem with drugs.	Using drugs is not a problem for you.	Your drug use is not something to be concerned about, so you aren't sure that coming here is going to be helpful for you.
I can see that I need to stop using crack, but smoking a joint now and then is no big deal.	You don't see a problem with the cannabis.	You're feeling like people don't understand that it's not the cannabis that's causing you all these problems, it's the crack use.

CLIENT STATEMENT	SIMPLE REFLECTION	COMPLEX REFLECTION
Things are way too stressful right now for me to deal with giving up cigarettes.	I am hearing that this is not a good time for you to quit smoking.	You intend to quit smoking at some point—it's finding the right time to do so that is a challenge.

The last component of the OARS skills involves periodically summarizing what has been discussed in the interview. *Summary statements* bring together key points and content and offer these back to the client in order to help reflect on where the conversation has led. Summarizing can be used strategically—since an important objective in MI is to elicit change talk, practitioners who are skilled in the approach are able to offer selective summaries, emphasizing the different kinds of change talk they hear from clients. Miller and Rollnick (2010) call this offering "bouquets of change talk" (with sprigs of sustain talk). Referring back to Adia's case from the beginning of this chapter, here is an example of what a summary statement might sound like if Adia's counsellor had used MI during the initial assessment:

> *Let me make sure I understand what you've been saying so far. (Adia nods.) Okay, so you have been forced to come for treatment, even though you are very clear that you don't have any problem with drugs. I'm also hearing that you came today because your kids are the most important things in your life, and you'll do whatever it takes to keep your family together. You acknowledge that drugs have caused some problems for you in the past, and you've worked really hard to stop using and to stay quit. It's feeling like no one recognizes the efforts you've made and how far you have come, and feeling respected is important to you. What did I miss?*

In this summary statement, the counsellor focuses primarily on the client's change talk (positive client comments about change) as opposed to the "sustain talk" (client comments that endorse the status quo). Change talk includes the following types of client statements, summarized in the acronym DARN CAT:

Desire for or **A**bility to make a change (what Adia has been able to accomplish with respect to her past drug use)

Reasons to come for treatment (Adia's children)

Need to change (problems with drug use in the past)

Commitment, **A**ctivation or **T**aking steps toward change (e.g., "I will do whatever it takes to keep my kids with me").

Counsellors need to use the OARS skills (open-ended questions, statements of affirmation, reflective listening and summary statements) with the spirit of MI front and centre (i.e., emphasizing partnership, acceptance, compassion and evocation at all times). Indeed, learning to listen for change talk is a skill in itself. These different types of change talk are discussed in the next section.

Recognizing and Reinforcing Change Talk

Change talk in general refers to clients' statements about their desire, ability, reasons and need for change, whereas commitment language represents a more assertive declaration about commitment/actions to change. Research shows that change talk is associated with enhanced motivation for change, and motivation is associated with increased likelihood of actual change. This supports the emphasis that MI places on listening for, and eliciting, change talk as key counselling skills (Miller & Rollnick, 2013; Moyers et al., 2009). Sustain talk is the opposite of change talk; these terms reflect two sides of a person's ambivalence about changing (two sides of the same coin). The skillful counsellor understands that difference and guides the client away from sustain talk and toward change talk, listening especially for statements that show commitment. Table 5-4 provides examples of change talk and sustain talk.

TABLE 5-4
Examples of Change Talk and Sustain Talk

CHANGE TALK	SUSTAIN TALK
I really need to quit smoking because of the bad example I am setting for my kids.	But I love to smoke; it is so much a part of my life.
I have started an exercise program, and things are going well.	But I know I will go back to my old ways once the cold weather comes.
My gambling is totally out of control.	But betting is the only way I can de-stress and forget all my problems for a while.
I know I should take my medication every day.	It's just that I hate the side-effects so much.

Expanding our understanding of what constitutes change talk can help us to know that we are on track—if we hear change talk, that means we are headed in the right direction. Reflecting change talk—and moving away from reflecting sustain talk—keeps the momentum of the conversation toward enhancing motivation for change. The acronym DARN CAT summarizes different kinds of change talk and commitment language:

Desire: "I want to be a good parent."

Ability: "I can quit any time I want."

Reasons: "I think I'm getting too old for this lifestyle."

Need: "They will take away my kids unless I go to this program."

Commitment: "I am going to get help with my drug problem."

Activation: "I've erased the dealers' phone numbers from my contact list, and I am getting a new phone number so they can't call me anymore."

Taking steps: "I've started taking a fitness class at the community centre twice a week in the evenings."

DARN statements tend to predominate when people are still deciding to make a change, whereas CAT statements indicate that a client is ready to take action. DARN statements on their own are insufficient or do not necessarily predict change. For example, Miller and Moyers (2006) point out that two people exchanging wedding vows "ideally respond with commitment language ('I do') rather than just change talk ('I hope so,' 'I could,' 'I have good reason to' or 'I need to')" (p. 11). Commitment language signals that a client is ready to actively plan for change or is already making some positive changes.

Evoking and Strengthening Change Talk

The strategies to elicit and strengthen change talk and commitment language build on the basic OARS skills. The following are effective ways to evoke change talk and help guide the conversation toward increased commitment:

Ask open-ended questions: "What are some of the less good things about drug dealing?"

Listen empathically and selectively reflect back: Client: "Don't get me wrong—I know my crack use is out of hand, but the dealers are everywhere in my neighbourhood." Counsellor: "Things are really difficult, and you are worried about how much crack you are using."

Look forward, look back: "Where would you like to be five years from now? How does that fit with where you are now?" "Tell me about what things were like for you before all of these difficulties started."

Link behaviour with values and develop discrepancy: "Your kids mean more to you than anything, and being a good parent is a high priority. Yet you also mentioned that they were scared when you left them alone in the house that time. How do those things fit together?"

When all else fails, the easiest way to elicit change talk is to listen carefully for any example of change talk (Desire, Ability, Reasons, Need), and then respond with "Tell me more about that." Asking for elaboration encourages more conversation about change.

Responding to Sustain Talk

Even the most highly skilled and experienced counsellors encounter sustain talk and discord; they are often manifestations of the client's ambivalence. It helps if we regard them as feedback pointing to a need for us to change our intervention strategies, as invitations to respond differently, especially by returning to reflective listening. In MI, discord and sustain talk have distinct meanings. Miller and Rollnick (2013) note that discord refers to client statements about the intervention process or relationship to the counsellor, particularly the direction in which the client perceives things are going (e.g., "But you don't understand what I'm going through" or "I am not ready to go there yet, if ever"). Discord is a normal human response to feeling pressured or challenged to do something about which a person is ambivalent. It often comes in the form of a "yes, but" statement (e.g., "Yes, but I tried that before"). Note that MI frames discord as an interpersonal process, which often occurs as a natural response to a counter-motivational statement or a directive or authoritarian stance on the part of the counsellor (MI-inconsistent responses).

Sustain talk, on the other hand, focuses on the client's behaviour and simply represents the opposite side of change talk (e.g., "I don't have a problem with drugs" or "There are some things about my drug use that I still really like"). Sustain talk represents the other side of a person's ambivalence about changing. It can be an expression of the client's desire for the way things are, feeling unable to change, having reasons for keeping things the same or needing to keep things the way they are—a kind of reverse DARN CAT (Rosengren, 2009).

While in earlier years MI made heavy use of the concept of resistance, the more recent introduction of the terms "discord" and "sustain talk" has seen a shift in our understanding of these concepts as the logical complement to change talk. Both terms underline the continuing challenge of working with ambivalence in helping clients move toward healthy behaviour change. Before and after we make decisions to change, we still experience ambivalence. Humans, especially when the stakes are high and the outcome is uncertain, tend to "ambivilate."

MI is especially interested in the ways that discord and sustain talk can be by-products of how we engage the client. However we think of these issues, we surf the waves of sustain talk using the same skills. Three types of reflective listening can be particularly helpful ways to respond to discord and ride the wave of sustain talk. The following strategies can open the door to a more productive conversation—that is, dancing versus wrestling.

Simple reflection: empathically reflecting the client's statement. This sometimes includes a small shift in emphasis or selectively reflecting a particular element of what the person is saying. For example:

> Client: *I couldn't change even if I wanted to.* (sustain talk)
>
> Counsellor: *You don't see how it would be possible to change.*

Amplified reflection: reflecting back what the client has said in an amplified or slightly exaggerated form (there should be no sarcasm in the counsellor's tone when using an amplified reflection). For example:

> Client: *I have no intention of quitting smoking* (sustain talk)*, and you can't make me!* (discord)
>
> Counsellor: *Smoking is something that you never see yourself changing.*

Double-sided reflection: acknowledging what the client has said and adding to it the other side of the client's ambivalence, using material the client has offered previously. For example:

> Client: *I don't drink any more than most of my friends. What's wrong with a few beers now and then?* (sustain talk)
>
> Counsellor: *So it's kind of confusing. On the one hand, you've told me you're concerned about how alcohol affects you, and on the other hand, it seems you're not drinking any more than your friends.*

We can respond by *shifting focus*; that is, shifting the conversation away from what seems to be a stumbling block to progress. Essentially, this means changing the subject when talking about an issue has become counterproductive at that moment. An example of shifting focus might sound like "That doesn't seem like a problem to you right now. What are some of the things you're dealing with that you feel are a challenge?" Finally, simply *emphasizing the client's choice and control* (autonomy) can help minimize resistance and move the conversation away from sustain talk. This means explicitly stating something along the lines of "It really is your choice what you will do about _____."

Remember that sustain talk, in particular, is to be expected in any conversation about change, especially when a person is feeling ambivalent. The counsellor's response can provide the forward momentum in the client's process of exploring and resolving his or her ambivalence and ultimately making a decision to change. However, we should always be open to—and accepting of—the possibility that a client may very well decide not to change despite our best efforts. If we have respectfully and empathically stayed with our clients through to this decision, it is more likely that they will come back and re-engage with us if or when their circumstances or perceptions change.

Developing a Change Plan: Agenda Mapping

Many clients present with multiple, co-occurring problems of varying degrees of concern or importance, and practitioners may identify additional issues based on their observations or assessments. It can sometimes be overwhelming for both client and clinician to sift through the many possible targets for intervention and come to a consensus around what to address. In the worst-case scenario, client and counsellor become sidetracked into an adversarial dynamic, where each advocates addressing issues that are differentially perceived to be the highest priority. Agenda mapping provides a structure and a process for joint problem identification and decision-making that still reflects the spirit of MI. Note that the OARS skills are used throughout the agenda-mapping conversation.

Collaborating to set an agenda for change is a way of guiding—versus prescribing—the work that client and counsellor will engage in together. The agenda-mapping worksheet in Figure 5-3 is like a roadmap of possible treatment destinations. It can be used as a way to open the conversation about change, and later on when considering next steps and developing a plan for change. There are different ways to introduce agenda setting to clients, but in general, the counsellor opens the conversation with some variation of a statement along the lines of:

> *If you like, we can talk about some of the things that you might find helpful to work on together. Here are some areas that you noted during your assessment.*

Follow-up questions might include:

> *How does this fit for you?*

> *What else is missing?*

> *What would you most like to work on?*

The case example of Adia outlined a number of possible areas that a counsellor could note on an agenda-mapping worksheet. These include child care and Adia's efforts to complete her high-school diploma. In addition, Adia may identify other concerns, such as housing, stress or financial problems. If Adia states that she has been successful in stopping her past drug use on her own, then the practitioner could suggest relapse prevention as a possible treatment goal. The question marks on the sample worksheet indicate other possible areas that Adia might identify as part of the agenda-setting conversation. Note that the agenda is the client's, and the counsellor works to ensure that action to produce positive change will be successful. Agenda setting gives a shape to the work the client and counsellor will do together.

FIGURE 5-3: Agenda-Mapping Worksheet

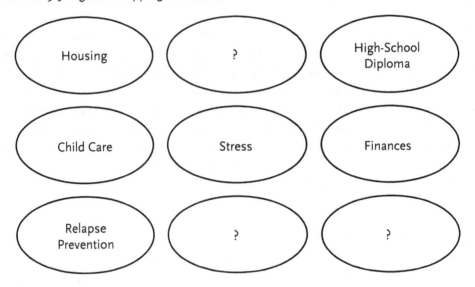

Source: Miller, W.R. & Rollnick, S. (2013). *Motivational Interviewing: Helping People Change* (3rd ed., p. 110). New York: Guilford Press. © Guilford Press. Adapted with permission.

Once the client and the counsellor agree on the presenting issues, it is up to the client to identify priorities and target areas. The objective in agenda setting is to work collaboratively and support the client's commitment to both the end point *and* the starting point, and then proceed to identify and explore the specifics. Small incremental changes in one area can lead to continued and growing commitment to work on change in other areas. Like assessment, agenda mapping is an ongoing process that evolves with increasing trust, rapport and engagement.

Consolidating Client Commitment and Planning

The Readiness Ruler is a useful tool to check whether clients are ready to take the important step of making a commitment to change. In general, higher ratings for importance, confidence and readiness signal that it is time to make a transition in MI strategies toward actively planning for, and consolidating client commitment to, change.

FIGURE 5-4: Readiness Ruler

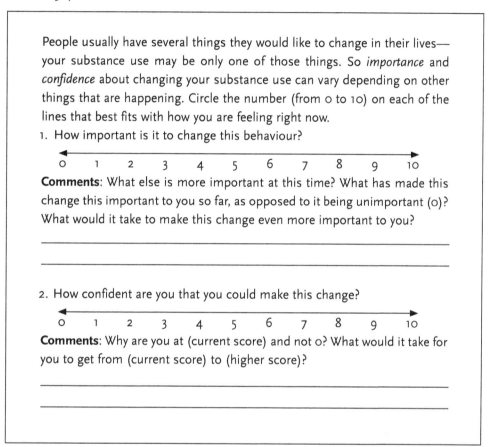

People usually have several things they would like to change in their lives—your substance use may be only one of those things. So *importance* and *confidence* about changing your substance use can vary depending on other things that are happening. Circle the number (from 0 to 10) on each of the lines that best fits with how you are feeling right now.

1. How important is it to change this behaviour?

0 1 2 3 4 5 6 7 8 9 10

Comments: What else is more important at this time? What has made this change this important to you so far, as opposed to it being unimportant (0)? What would it take to make this change even more important to you?

_____

_____

2. How confident are you that you could make this change?

0 1 2 3 4 5 6 7 8 9 10

Comments: Why are you at (current score) and not 0? What would it take for you to get from (current score) to (higher score)?

_____

_____

A useful follow-up to the Readiness Ruler is asking a key question to help facilitate the client's explicit commitment to making a change. The key question essentially invites the client to talk about "What's next?" with respect to making the change. Different ways to ask a key question include:

Given what we have talked about, what do you think you will do?

Where would you like to go from here?

What is your next step?

Once the client has expressed a preferred course of action, the counsellor can work collaboratively to help the person come up with a concrete plan. At this point, it is appropriate to be a bit more directive in the session. In fact, continuing to elicit and explore a client's desire, ability, reasons or need for change can be frustrating for clients who are ready to take action. Clients will often ask for advice or suggestions at this time, so continuing to rely primarily on the OARS skills may be less helpful. However, it is still important not to underestimate ambivalence and to be ready to cycle back to reflective listening and the other MI skills if the client seems unwilling or hesitant to commit to a goal or a plan of action.

After working collaboratively with a client to develop a plan for change, it is a good idea to consolidate commitment by asking an open-ended question that allows the client to clearly articulate why the change is so important to him or her. Questions like "What made you decide that now is the time you must do this?" "or "What are the reasons that make succeeding at this so important to you?" help the client hear himself or herself express out loud the necessity and salience of the change.

Asking permission is a useful way to invite "conversational consent" before providing information or making suggestions. There are three types of permission:

1. The client asks the counsellor for advice, information or suggestions—this is implied permission.
2. The counsellor asks the client for permission (e.g., "Can I share some of my thoughts about this treatment plan?").
3. The counsellor asks permission to present a menu of options, and asks for the person's choice (e.g., "Would you like to hear about some of the different kinds of treatment we offer here, including . . .? What do you think would work best for you?").

One helpful framework for providing information is "ask/tell/ask" or "elicit/provide/elicit" (Miller & Rollnick, 2013; Rollnick et al., 2008). In other words, begin the conversation by asking for the client's understanding of the problem or issue; follow up by briefly sharing relevant key information; then ask for the client's response to—and understanding of—the information. This cycle (or "MI sandwich" approach) can be repeated throughout a session or consultation, and can be especially useful when time is limited.

Throughout the process of negotiating a change plan and consolidating clients' commitment to change, it is important not to move too quickly. Listening for examples of sustain talk and discord helps ensure that we stay beside the client, not ahead of him or her. The Change Plan worksheet in Figure 5-5 gives a sample framework for a conversation about action planning. The worksheet can be completed with the client during one or more sessions focused on planning for change, and helps clients develop a concrete roadmap of strategies and supports. Note that it is important to periodically reassess the client's confidence and importance ratings of the stated goal in developing and implementing the change plan.

FIGURE 5-5: Change Plan Worksheet

The changes I want to make are . . .

_____

_____

The most important reasons why I want to make these changes are . . .

_____

_____

The steps I plan to take in changing are . . .

_____

_____

The ways other people can help me are . . .

_____

_____

I will know that my plan is working if . . .

_____

_____

Some things that could interfere with my plan are . . .

_____

_____

Source: Ingersoll, K.S., Wagner, C.C. & Gharib, S. (2002). *Motivational Groups for Community Substance Abuse Programs.* Rockville, MD: Center for Substance Abuse Treatment. © Center for Substance Abuse Treatment. Reprinted with permission.

Switching between Motivational Interviewing and Other Counselling Methods

The most advanced skills of MI relate to a practitioner's flexibility in switching between various counselling approaches or integrating MI with other treatment models. As Miller and Moyers (2006) point out, "MI was never meant to be the only tool in a clinician's repertoire. It was developed primarily to help clients through motivational obstacles to change" (p. 11). For example, clients who present as ready and committed to changing may benefit more from other, more directive evidence-based interventions; however, client commitment often fluctuates over the course of treatment. Practitioners' ability to cycle in and out of MI approaches as the need arises can enhance clients' engagement and retention regardless of the type of treatment they are receiving. In addition, the spirit of MI—emphasizing client autonomy, collaboration and evocation—is at the core of any client-centred approach.

Table 5-5 gives an example of how an integrated MI plus cognitive-behavioural therapy (CBT) approach differs from CBT alone. In this example, MI provides a "platform" for delivering the ingredients of the CBT intervention, and actively addresses any ambivalence or resistance that arises during treatment.

TABLE 5-5

MI to Enhance CBT

CBT	MI + CBT
Treatment begins with overview and rationale for treatment followed by functional analysis of target behaviour. (Functional analysis explores relationships between antecedents, or triggers, to the problem behaviour and consequences of the behaviour.)	Treatment begins by evoking client's view of the problem and increasing motivation for change by eliciting and reinforcing change talk.
Functional analysis of target behaviour is completed by asking a series of questions.	Functional analysis is completed in the context of an OARS conversation (open-ended questions, affirmations, reflective listening and summary statements).
Practitioner selects skill-building modules based on functional analysis of triggers and consequences.	Practitioner elicits client's thoughts and ideas about how to manage triggers, and guides client toward skill-building modules that meet client's change plan goals.
Homework is assigned with a rationale provided by the practitioner.	Practitioner asks permission to suggest homework that meets client's goals using a framework of (1) eliciting client's perspective; (2) providing information; (3) eliciting client's response to the information.

Source: Naar-King, S. & Suarez, M. (2011). *Motivational Interviewing with Adolescents and Young Adults* (p. 78). New York: Guilford Press. © Guilford Press. Adapted with permission.

As we noted at the beginning of this chapter, MI is primarily a way of being with clients that incorporates a set of specific learnable skills. Ongoing practice and clinical reflection are needed in order for counsellors to be able to practise MI with fluency and facility. Clients are our best teachers in this endeavour, since they provide immediate, proximal feedback about our effectiveness. Increased resistance and sustain talk signal that MI is not taking place and that the practitioner may be pushing for change prematurely or attempting to direct the client toward a course of action that he or she does not find helpful. This is a sign that we should probably switch strategies. On the other hand, change talk and commitment language tell us that we are "doing it right" and are heading in a positive direction.

MI with Specific Populations

Research on MI with specific populations has focused primarily on gender, age and ethnicity, and on working with people with diverse behaviour change target areas (Lundahl et al., 2010). In general, evidence supports the use of MI with both men and women, and with people from early adolescence to old age. Because MI is a cognitively based intervention, it has not yet been proven to be effective with pre-adolescent children (whose skills of abstract reasoning are not well developed). A recent book, *Motivational Interviewing with Adolescents and Young Adults* (Naar-King & Suarez, 2011), gives a wealth of practical suggestions for how to adapt MI for younger clients.

Martino and colleagues (2002) propose adaptations for people with cognitive impairments, such as those that often accompany severe psychiatric illness:

- Simplify reflective statements and open-ended questions.
- Use metaphors to anchor abstract material in reality (e.g., using the metaphor of a three-legged stool to illustrate the importance of three key areas of focus in recovery from concurrent mental health and substance use problems: 1) maintaining abstinence; 2) taking prescribed medications; and 3) participating in a concurrent disorders treatment program).
- Integrate strategies of repetition, simple verbal and visual illustrations, and breaks within sessions.
- Reduce reflective statements that focus explicitly on disturbing life experiences.
- Use a decisional balance to identify the positives and negatives of being abstinent from problematic substances, and the positives and negatives of attending concurrent disorders treatment.
- Assess the need for other interventions to promote psychiatric stability, logical reasoning or safety.

MI may also be a useful approach with people with acquired brain injury (Medley & Powell, 2010). In particular, the spirit and techniques of MI can help promote clients' self-awareness, goal setting and engagement in treatment and rehabilitation.

Research with different ethnocultural groups has been encouraging: a meta-analysis by Hettema and colleagues (2005) concluded that ethnospecific populations may benefit more from MI than from other mainstream addiction treatments (i.e., CBT and 12-step facilitation). One possible explanation is that the "client centered, supportive, and non-confrontational style of MI may represent a more culturally respectful form of psychotherapy for some ethnic groups" (Lundahl & Burke, 2009, p. 1241). Specific populations are heterogeneous in themselves, so any generalizations are potentially problematic. Nonetheless, these preliminary findings support MI as at least a promising practice with populations that have been traditionally ignored or under-represented in treatment research.

Learning MI: Eight Processes

Miller and Moyers (2006) hypothesize eight stages or processes through which clinicians progress in developing MI skills. This model draws on more than 10 years of research on MI training outcomes and strategies, providing a set of general guidelines for structuring MI training, as well as for practitioners to assess their own level of proficiency and progress.

1. The Spirit of MI

This is a key starting point. As we stated earlier, the spirit of MI is the most important prerequisite to practising the approach. Practitioners who sincerely convey their belief in the inherent human potential for growth and development in their clients, and who work in a collaborative, evocative and respectful way, are more able to acquire the skills of MI. Workers who can convey empathic regard to their clients are manifesting MI spirit in action.

2. Client-Centred Counselling Skills

These skills are not unique to MI, and are captured in the OARS approach described earlier: **O**pen-ended questions, statements of **A**ffirmation, **R**eflective listening and **S**ummary statements. These skills are all part of a meta-skill, accurate empathy, which is actually quite complex and never fully perfected by even the most seasoned, experienced clinicians.

3. Recognizing and Reinforcing Change Talk; 4. Eliciting and Strengthening Change Talk

Change talk, as we have seen, is predictive of behaviour change and positive treatment outcomes. Selectively listening for, eliciting and reflecting change talk builds motivation and reinforces clients' readiness to change. Recognizing and reinforcing change talk and eliciting and strengthening change talk are posed as distinct skills because it generally takes some practice for counsellors to be able to accurately distinguish and respond to change talk. Actively eliciting change talk is a more advanced skill.

5. Rolling with Resistance

Client resistance is inevitable, even in the most skillful motivational interventions. Resistance and sustain talk can also be a product of how we engage the client. Learning and practising the strategies to "roll with" resistance instead of opposing it can be a challenge.

6. Developing a Change Plan; 7. Consolidating Client Commitment.

Developing a change plan and consolidating client commitment are closely related, since a common pitfall for practitioners new to MI is pushing for change prematurely. Developing a change plan relates to knowing when a client is ready to commit to making a change and then transitioning to strategies to help develop a concrete plan. Consolidating client commitment requires that the practitioner support clients in actually committing to the change plan.

8. Switching between MI and Other Counselling Methods

The final process is probably the most challenging. MI can be used to build client motivation to enter other kinds of treatment programs, or it can be combined with other evidence-based interventions (or both). In addition, there may be clients for whom MI is not appropriate at all. The complex skills and clinical judgment to flexibly move between MI and other approaches, and to decide which approach to take, characterize this process of learning and development.

Evaluating Therapist Proficiency in MI Spirit and Skills

Recording client sessions is an especially powerful way to assess and strengthen MI skills. The Motivational Interviewing Treatment Integrity (MITI) code (Moyers et al., 2003) is a detailed tool for evaluating therapist proficiency in MI spirit and skills. It may be too exhaustive and resource intensive for the beginning MI practitioner, so we have developed a brief, easy-to-complete MI coding form to use while reviewing recorded sessions (Figure 5-6).

FIGURE 5-6: MI Coding Form

- Number of closed questions:
- Number of open questions:
- Number of simple reflections:
- Number of complex reflections:
- Change statements by client:
- Sustain statements by client:
- Therapist talk time (approx):

Targets:
Twice as many reflections as questions
At least 50% complex reflections
No more than 50% therapist talk time

MI "Spirit"	(low)				(high)
Partnership	1	2	3	4	5
Acceptance	1	2	3	4	5
Compassion	1	2	3	4	5
Evocation	1	2	3	4	5

The "coach" or observer listens to either a live or recorded session and on the coding sheet places checkmarks beside the appropriate category for the type of utterance made by the counsellor or the client. At the end of the interview, the observer adds up the checkmarks for each category to get a total number of open and closed questions, simple and complex reflections and client change statements. The observer then provides an overall rating of therapist talk time and rates the degree to which the counsellor demonstrated MI spirit—partnership, acceptance, compassion and evocation—in the session. The coding sheet can be completed by the therapist or by a clinical or peer supervisor.

The coding sheet can be used individually for a counsellor's own reflection and self-assessment, or in individual or group clinical supervision. It can also be adapted so the counsellor can gather more detailed feedback about his or her proficiency in MI skills. For example, the counsellor can include a section to note MI-consistent and MI-inconsistent behaviours and responses. Counsellors new to MI can use the coding sheet as a structured way to view demonstration videos online: it will help them recognize specific micro-skills and how they are used in practice (see the Resources section for links to MI videos). In the end, our clients are our best teachers, and regular practice and post-session reflection help to highlight areas of strength and areas for continued focus.

Conclusion

Adia's case example illustrates some of the pitfalls that occur when helping professionals use a highly directive or confrontational style. At the end of the addiction assessment (which Adia seemingly attended only out of duress), both Adia and her counsellor felt frustrated, discouraged and hopeless. Yet Adia has a wealth of personal resources that she has brought to bear on the problems and roadblocks in her life: she is surviving as a single parent; she manages to feed and house herself and her children; she is committed to finishing high school so she can have more choices in her life; she has tried—and by her own reports succeeded in—stopping her drug use in the past; and she is used to doing things on her own initiative. A motivational approach that elicited Adia's hopes, dreams, goals and strategies might have led to a more positive outcome in this treatment encounter. At the least, Adia would have felt heard, validated and understood—and therefore more inclined to trust that the counsellor had her best interests in mind.

The major objective in MI is to guide the client in the direction of change using a combination of core skills and specific strategies, practised with an underlying MI spirit. Just focusing on helping a client explore his or her ambivalence about changing can enhance motivation, and has the added benefit of communicating non-judgmental acceptance of where the person is at, building rapport and strengthening therapeutic alliance. Although there is no one approach that is likely to be the best or most appropriate intervention for every client, MI represents a useful and important evidence-based approach to addiction counselling.

Revisiting the self-assessment

Now that you have read the chapter, is there anything in your responses to the self-assessment questions posed at the beginning of this chapter that you would change? Take another look at the following client statements, and write down one or two sentences in response. Then compare your answers with the ones you formulated at the beginning of the chapter. What, if anything, is different? What implications does this have for your clinical practice?

1. Client: *It's easy for you to tell me all these things I have to do. When was the last time you had someone on your case all the time?*
Counsellor:
_____
_____

2. Client: *I've tried everything and nothing seems to help. What's the point?*
Counsellor:
_____
_____

Practice Tips

Miller and colleagues (2004) and Miller and Rollnick (2013) suggest overall guidelines for using MI core skills:

- Resist the "righting reflex" and practise listening to your client with unconditional acceptance and compassion. This is the essential starting point for MI, and is key to the spirit of the approach.
- Don't ask more than two questions in a row. Open-ended questions are followed up with reflective listening to convey understanding and empathy and to further the conversation. Asking a lot of questions conveys an expert, one-up position on the part of the counsellor, rather than the equal partnership—client and counsellor are both experts—that characterizes MI.
- Aim for a two-to-one ratio of reflections to questions. In other words, try to offer two reflections for every question asked. Remember that reflective listening is a complex skill that takes practice. It may be useful to set a small, incremental goal, such as committing to listening to a client carefully throughout the session and offering a single tentative reflection of what you have understood. Aim for more than 50 per cent complex (versus simple) reflections. Complex reflections are more evocative of clients' own goals, concerns and hopes. Again, formulating complex reflections takes practice. As clinicians become more adept at reflective listening, complex reflections become easier to frame and articulate in one-to-one interactions with clients.
- Aim to do less than 50 per cent of the talking in the conversation. The goal is to facilitate the client's own exploration of the problem or issue.
- Avoid "roadblocks" or counsellor behaviour that gets in the way of enhancing motivation for change. This includes giving advice or making suggestions without asking the client's permission, as well as warning or threatening the client.

Resources

Publications

Martino, S., Ball, S.A., Gallon, S.L., Hall, D., Garcia, M., Ceperich, S. et al. (2006). *Motivational Interviewing Assessment: Supervisory Tools for Enhancing Proficiency (MIA STEP)*. Salem, OR: Northwest Frontier Addiction Technology Transfer Center, Oregon Health and Science University. Retrieved from www.motivationalinterview.org/Documents//MIA-STEP.pdf

Matulich, B. (2010). How to Do Motivational Interviewing: A Guidebook for Beginners. San Diego, CA: Author.

Miller, W.R. & Rollnick, S. (2009). Ten things that motivational interviewing is not. *Behavioural and Cognitive Psychotherapy, 37*, 129–140.

Miller, W.R. & Rollnick, S. (2013). *Motivational Interviewing: Helping People Change* (3rd ed.). New York: Guilford Press.

Moyers, T.B., Martin, T., Manuel, J.K., Miller, W.R. & Ernst, D. (2010). *Revised Global Scales: Motivational Interviewing Treatment Integrity 3.1.1 (MITI 3.1.1)*. Retrieved from http://casaa.unm.edu/download/miti3_1.pdf

Rollnick, S., Miller, W.R. & Butler, C.C. (2008). *Motivational Interviewing in Health Care: Helping Patients Change Behavior*. New York: Guildford Press.

Rosengren, D.B. (2009). Building Motivational Interviewing Skills: A Practitioner Workbook. New York: Guilford Press.

Internet

Center on Alcoholism, Substance Abuse, and Addictions
    http://casaa.unm.edu
Motivational Interviewing
    www.motivationalinterview.net
Motivational Interviewing Network of Trainers
    www.motivationalinterviewing.org
Motivational interviewing videos on YouTube
    www.youtube.com/user/teachproject#p/u
    www.youtube.com/user/MerloLab#g/u

References

Draycott, S. & Dabbs, A. (1998). Cognitive dissonance: A theoretical grounding of motivational interviewing. *British Journal of Clinical Psychology, 37*, 355–364.

Gaume, J., Gmel, G., Faouzi, M. & Daeppen, J.B. (2009). Counselor skill influences outcomes of brief motivational interventions. *Journal of Substance Abuse Treatment, 37*, 151–159.

Herie, M. & Selby, P. (2007, April). Getting beyond "Now is not a good time to stop smoking": Increasing motivation to stop smoking. *Smoking Cessation Rounds, 1* (2).

Hettema, J., Steele, J. & Miller, W.R. (2005). Motivational interviewing. *Annual Review of Clinical Psychology, 1,* 91–111.

LaBrie, J.W., Lamb, T.F., Pedersen, E.R. & Quinlan, T. (2006). A group motivational interviewing intervention reduces drinking and alcohol-related consequences in adjudicated college students. *Journal of College Student Development, 47,* 267–280.

Lundahl, B. & Burke, B.L. (2009). The effectiveness and applicability of motivational interviewing: A practice-friendly review of four meta-analyses. *Journal of Clinical Psychology, 65,* 1232–1245.

Lundahl, B.W., Kunz, C., Brownell, C., Tollefson, D. & Burke, B.L. (2010). A meta-analysis of motivational interviewing: Twenty-five years of empirical studies. *Research on Social Work Practice, 20,* 137–160.

Martino, S., Ball, S.A., Gallon, S.L., Hall, D., Garcia, M., Ceperich, S. et al. (2006). *Motivational Interviewing Assessment: Supervisory Tools for Enhancing Proficiency (MIA STEP).* Salem, OR: Northwest Frontier Addiction Technology Transfer Center, Oregon Health and Science University. Retrieved from www.motivationalinterview.org/Documents//MIA-STEP.pdf

Martino, S., Carroll, K., Kostas, D., Perkins, J. & Rounsaville, B. (2002). Dual diagnosis motivational interviewing: A modification of motivational interviewing for substance-abusing patients with psychotic disorders. *Journal of Substance Abuse Treatment, 23,* 297–308.

Medley, A.R. & Powell, T. (2010). Motivational interviewing to promote self-awareness and engagement in rehabilitation following acquired brain injury: A conceptual review. *Neuropsychological Rehabilitation, 20,* 481–508.

Miller, W. (1999). Toward a theory of motivational interviewing. *Motivational Interviewing Newsletter: Updates, Education and Training, 6* (3), 2–4.

Miller, W.R. & Moyers, T.B. (2006). Eight stages in learning motivational interviewing. *Journal of Teaching in the Addictions, 5* (1), 3–17.

Miller, W.R. & Rollnick, S. (2002). *Motivational Interviewing: Preparing People for Change* (2nd ed.). New York: Guilford Press.

Miller, W.R. & Rollnick, S. (2009). Ten things that motivational interviewing is not. *Behavioural and Cognitive Psychotherapy, 37,* 129–140.

Miller, W.R. & Rollnick, S. (2010). What's new since MI-2? Presentation at the International Conference on Motivational Interviewing, Stockholm, Sweden. Retrieved from http://motivationalinterview.org/Documents/Miller-and-Rollnick-june6-pre-conference-workshop.pdf

Miller, W.R. & Rollnick, S. (2013). *Motivational Interviewing: Helping People Change* (3rd ed.). New York: Guilford Press.

Miller, W.R. & Rose, G.S. (2009). Toward a theory of motivational interviewing. *American Psychologist, 64,* 527–537.

Miller, W.R., Sorenson, J.L., Selzer, J.A. & Brigham, G.S. (2006). Disseminating evidence-based practices in substance abuse treatment: A review with suggestions. *Journal of Substance Abuse Treatment, 31*, 25–39.

Miller, W.R., Yahne, C.E., Moyers, T.B., Martinez, J. & Pirritano, M. (2004). A random-ized trial of methods to help clinicians learn motivational interviewing. *Journal of Consulting and Clinical Psychology, 72*, 1050–1062.

Moyers, T., Martin, T., Catley, D., Harris, K. & Ahluwalia, J.S. (2003). Assessing the integrity of motivational interviewing interventions: Reliability of the motivational interviewing skills code. *Behavioural and Cognitive Psychotherapy, 31*, 177–184.

Moyers, T.B., Martin, T., Houck, J.M., Christopher, P.J. & Tonigan, J.S. (2009). From in-session behaviors to drinking outcomes: A causal chain for motivational inter-viewing. *Journal of Consulting and Clinical Psychology, 77*, 1113–1124.

Naar-King, S. & Suarez, M. (2011). *Motivational Interviewing with Adolescents and Young Adults.* New York: Guilford Press.

Prochaska, J.O. & DiClemente, C.C. (1984). *The Transtheoretical Approach: Crossing Traditional Boundaries of Therapy.* Homewood, IL: Dow Jones/Irwin.

Prochaska, J.O. & Norcross, J.C. (2007). *Systems of Psychotherapy: A Transtheoretical Analysis* (6th ed.). Belmont, CA: Thompson Brooks/Cole.

Project MATCH Research Group. (1999). Summary of Project MATCH. *Addiction, 94,* 31–34.

Rogers, C.R. (1980). *A Way of Being.* New York: Houghton Mifflin.

Rollnick, S., Miller, W.R. & Butler, C.C. (2008). *Motivational Interviewing in Health Care: Helping Patients Change Behavior.* New York: Guilford Press.

Rosengren, D.B. (2009). *Building Motivational Interviewing Skills: A Practitioner Workbook.* New York: Guilford Press.

Vansteenkiste, M. & Sheldon, K.M. (2006). There's nothing more practical than a good theory: Integrating motivational interviewing and self-determination theory. *British Journal of Clinical Psychology, 45*, 63–82.

West, R. (2005). Time for a change: Putting the Transtheoretical (Stages of Change) model to rest. *Addiction, 100*, 1036–1039.

Williams, G.C., McGregor, H.A., Sharp, D., Levesque, C., Kouides, R.W., Ryan, R.M. & Deci, E.L. (2006). Testing a self-determination theory intervention for motivat-ing cessation: Supporting autonomy and competence in a clinical trial. *Health Psychology, 25*, 91–101.

Chapter 6

Neurobiology of Substance Use Disorders and Pharmacotherapy

Rachel A. Rabin and Tony P. George

Increasing evidence suggests that substance use disorders have a biological foundation and may be best understood as a chronic brain illness (McLellan et al., 2000). Multiple neurobiological processes are highly affected and altered when recreational drug use progresses to chronic use. Understanding substance use disorders within a neurobiological framework may be advantageous for developing effective and successful pharmacotherapies specifically tailored to treat people with these illnesses.

What Is a Substance Use Disorder?

Substance use disorders is an umbrella term that encompasses both substance abuse and substance dependence.[1] *Substance abuse* occurs when the drug is used in a manner that does not conform to social norms. The *Diagnostic and Statistical Manual of Mental Disorders* ([DSM-IV-TR] American Psychiatric Association [APA], 2000) defines substance abuse as the use of a psychoactive substance causing social and/or occupational impairment evidenced by one of the following clinical features, as captured in the mnemonic HELP (George, 2003):
- drug use in Hazardous situations
- neglecting External obligations
- Legal problems triggered by drug use
- interPersonal problems related to persistent drug use.

Substance dependence is a constellation of physiological adaptations that includes tolerance and withdrawal, as well as functional consequences from uncontrollable consumption. Such consequences include a persistent desire or unsuccessful attempts to reduce substance use; use in larger amounts than intended; impairment in important social, occupational or recreational activities; greater amount of time spent obtaining the substance; and continued use despite recurrent problems. The presence of three or more of these symptoms in one month warrants a diagnosis of substance dependence.

---

1 The DSM-5 was published in May 2013. The terms "abuse" and "dependence" have been eliminated and replaced with the terms "addiction" and substance "use" disorders (e.g., "alcohol use disorder" rather than "alcohol abuse" or "alcohol dependence").

This diagnosis can occur with or without physiological dependence, but physiological dependence alone is not sufficient for a diagnosis.

The most common licit and illicit substances of abuse or dependence include nicotine, alcohol, marijuana, opiates, cocaine, hallucinogens, stimulants, sedative-hypnotics, anxiolytics, anesthetics and inhalants (National Institute on Drug Abuse, 2009). However, hallucinogen dependence differs from substance dependence involving other classes of drugs in that it is not associated with the classic patterns of tolerance and withdrawal liability. The extent of hallucinogen tolerance appears to be minimal and a clear withdrawal syndrome has not yet been well established (APA, 2000; Kosten et al., 1987). While hallucinogens tend not to cause physiological dependence, chronic users may experience psychological dependence or "cravings" for hallucinogens (APA, 2000).

Drug craving is the desire for previously experienced effects of a psychoactive substance. This desire can become compelling and can increase in the presence of both internal and external cues, particularly with (perceived) substance availability. It is characterized by an increased likelihood of drug-seeking behaviours and drug-related thoughts (World Health Organization, 2004). Drug cravings can persist, or even return long after drug use has been discontinued, which may, in part, account for the typically high rate of relapse.

Opioid analgesic drugs are recommended for the management of severe pain. While psychological dependence is quite rare in people chronically treated with opioid analgesics, physical dependence can develop (Portenoy, 1990). Notably, only about two to six per cent of medical patients with no history of substance misuse abuse analgesics when they are medically administered, adhering to strict guidelines (Fields, 2007). It should be common practice for clinicians to screen for risk factors associated with addiction before starting patients on any opioid treatment plan.

Prevalence of Substance Use Disorders in Canada

Substance use is a growing problem in Canada. According to the 2004 Canadian Addiction Survey (Adlaf et al., 2005), the prevalence of psychoactive substance use has increased over the decade preceding the survey.

The study found that although most Canadians drink alcohol in moderation, approximately six per cent of past-year drinkers engaged in heavy drinking (five drinks or more in a single sitting for males, and four or more drinks for females) at least once a week, and 25.5 per cent reported heavy drinking at least once a month (Adlaf et al., 2005). A 2002 Statistics Canada survey revealed that 641,000 (2.6 per cent) of Canadians age 15 years and older (3.8 per cent males and 1.3 per cent females) reported symptoms consistent with alcohol dependence at some time during the 12 months prior to the survey (Tjepkema, 2004).

In the Statistics Canada survey, about 3.1 million people—13 per cent of the population—reported that they had used illicit drugs in the past year (Tjepkema, 2004). Almost half of people who used drugs (49 per cent) had done so at least monthly, and nine per cent acknowledged daily use. Furthermore, the number of Canadians dependent on illicit drugs in 2002 was reported to be 194,000 (0.8 per cent) (Tjepkema, 2004).

According to the Canadian Tobacco Use Monitoring Survey, 17 per cent of Canadians age 15 and older were current tobacco smokers in 2003, and 17 per cent were daily smokers (Health Canada, 2011).

Societal Costs and Burdens

Substance use disorders can cause significant social, emotional and economic disruption to the person, his or her family and society as a whole. These disorders affect the general population directly and indirectly in terms of health care, premature death, disability, law enforcement, loss of productivity and the costs associated with research and prevention. In 2002, 0.8 per cent of Canadian deaths resulted from illicit drug use, 16.6 per cent from tobacco use and just under two per cent from alcohol use (Rehm et al., 2006). The leading causes of death linked to illegal drug use were overdose, drug-related suicide and diseases such as hepatitis and HIV. The total annual cost of substance abuse in Canada reached $39.8 billion (see Rehm et al., 2006).

Neurobiology of Reward and Addiction

To understand substance use disorders within a neurobiological framework, practitioners need to recognize the underlying neurocircuitry of critical brain pathways, the mediating actions of endogenous neurotransmitters, and their effects at specific receptor sites.

Acute Effects of Drugs of Abuse

Mesolimbic dopamine system

One common feature of all drugs of abuse is their ability to either directly or indirectly increase brain levels of the neurotransmitter dopamine. Dopamine is associated with the euphoric and positive reinforcing effects of drugs of abuse, as well as with natural rewards elicited from food or sex, for example. Addictive drugs boost dopamine up to 100 times more than natural rewards, and for sustained periods (Di Chiara & Imperato, 1988; Volkow et al., 2009). This powerful effect strongly motivates some people to repeatedly engage in drug-taking behaviours.

While there are several dopamine systems in the brain, the one most often associated with addiction is the mesolimbic dopamine system (Koob & Bloom, 1988). The mesolimbic pathway originates in the ventral tegmental area (VTA) of the midbrain and innervates several structures of the limbic system, including the nucleus accumbens (NAc) (See Figure 6-1.) This circuit is involved in the conscious experience of the drug's effect, the user's cravings and the compulsion to continuously administer the drug (Cami & Farre, 2003).

FIGURE 6-1: Dopamine Mesolimbic ("Brain Reward") Pathways

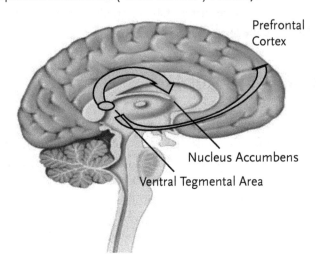

The reinforcing properties of addictive drugs depend on their ability to increase dopamine in the synapses made by the VTA neurons in the nucleus accumbens. Increased dopamine transmission in the NAc is responsible for the acute high experienced or the initial reinforcing effects of the drug. This can be conceptualized as *positive reinforcement* (Janhunen & Ahtee, 2007), given that a rewarding stimulus directly increases the probability that a response will recur.

Drugs of abuse can either directly or indirectly stimulate the "reward circuit" of the brain. For example, cocaine acts by blocking the removal of dopamine from the synaptic gap (the space between two neurons). Cocaine binds tightly at the dopamine transporter, forming a complex that prevents the transporter from fulfilling its reuptake function. Cocaine prevents dopamine from being reabsorbed by the neurons that released it and thus increases dopamine concentration in the synapse, exciting the nervous system for an extended period of time.

Like cocaine, amphetamines increase the concentration of dopamine in the synapse, but through a more complex process. Amphetamines are similar in structure to dopamine and therefore can move from outside the neuron into the cell via dopamine transporters or directly by diffusing through the neural membrane. Once inside, amphetamines force dopamine out of their storage vesicles and expel them into the synapse. Amphetamines appear to actually have multiple methods for enhancing dopamine transmission; they are also thought to behave like cocaine and inhibit synaptic dopamine reuptake.

In contrast, alcohol, nicotine, opiates and marijuana work indirectly by stimulating neurons that modulate dopamine cell firing. For example gamma-aminobutyric acid (GABA) neurons contain receptors that nicotine, opiate or cannabinoid receptors can act upon (Kreek et al., 2002).

While dopamine is the primary neurotransmitter involved in substance use disorders, GABA, norepinephrine, serotonin, acetylcholine, glutamate, endocannabinoids and other neurotransmitters are also implicated (Galanter & Kleber, 2008).

Endogenous opioid peptide systems

The endogenous opioid system is composed of receptors and their ligands (molecules that bind to a specific receptor). Originally thought to be involved only in mediating the effects of opiates, this system is now recognized as having a role in the behavioural and neurochemical effects of multiple drugs of abuse (Trigo et al., 2010).

Opioids exert their effects by binding to one of three opioid receptors: mu, delta or kappa. The mu opioid receptors, and to a lesser extent delta receptors, mediate positive reinforcement through dopamine release (Johnson & North, 1992) after being activated directly (e.g., with morphine) or indirectly (e.g., with alcohol, cannabinoids, nicotine) (Contet et al., 2004). Stimulation of these receptors leads to feelings of euphoria. They give a boost of pleasure in a way that also reduces the brain's perception of pain.

In contrast, kappa opioid receptor activation is not reinforcing; its activation can actually decrease dopamine. Stimulation of kappa opioid receptors can produce aversive responses, specifically dysphoria, hallucinations and malaise. In fact, blockade of these receptors has been shown to decrease substance intake by attenuating the negative emotional state associated with drug use (Walker & Koob, 2008).

Neuroadaptation

While increases in extracellular dopamine are acutely reinforcing, this increase in itself does not mediate the persistent behavioural consequences of substance use disorders. These disorders are thought to be the result of repeated stimulation of the mesolimbic pathway, which triggers reorganization in the brain's neurocircuitry. Long-lasting molecular and cellular plasticity can result in compromised neural mechanisms that mediate positive reinforcement, craving and relapse. These changes serve to motivate the user to continue to administer the drug (Koob & Le Moal, 2008). As people become more driven to administer the drug, the drive can also progress to a state of *negative reinforcement*, in which the removal of (or the subjective need to alleviate) the uncomfortable symptoms associated with withdrawal leads to drug re-administration.

Neuroplasticity refers to the brain's remarkable ability to change structurally or functionally in response to stimuli from the environment. It is the mechanism that underlies learning and memory. Drugs of abuse can modulate neuroplasticity, while neuroplasticity in the mesocorticolimbic reward pathway may drive the development of drug addiction (Everitt et al., 2008).

Neuroadaptation refers to the process whereby the brain attempts to compensate for the drug's effect so that it can attempt to function normally. Ironically, these alterations contribute to the development of dependence. Changes are long-lasting and not readily reversible (Hyman et al., 2006). Repetitive substance use corrupts the normal circuitry of the brain and triggers neurobiological changes associated with aberrations in the dopamine systems. Researchers have proposed that adaptations in these dopaminergic circuits make the addicted person more responsive to the increases in dopamine that are produced by drugs of abuse and less sensitive to the physiological increases in dopamine produced by natural reinforcers (Volkow et al., 2004). To the degree that a person is addicted, they require the extra dopamine that drugs provide.

Neuroadaptations have been documented not only for dopamine systems, but also for other neurotransmitters: glutamate, GABA, opiates, serotonin and various neuro-peptides. At a cellular level, chronic drug intake has been reported to alter the density of certain receptors in order to adapt to the strong imbalances of neurotransmitter levels. Neurons accomplish this by either reducing ("downregulating") or increasing ("upregu-lating") the number of receptors for a specific neurotransmitter. For example, chronic nicotine exposure can cause desensitization of nicotinic receptors in the brain, leading to an upregulation of such receptors. This is associated with increased dopamine respon-siveness within the VTA or other dopamine systems and may contribute to a heightened response, a phenomenon known as sensitization.

Sensitization refers to the phenomenon that occurs with repeated administration of a drug, which elicits escalating effects at a given dose. It may be best conceptualized as reverse tolerance. This response can persist for months after the last drug exposure (Robinson & Berridge, 1993). Moreover, sensitization is thought to mediate drug-, cue- and stress-induced relapse (Kalivas & Stewart, 1991). Interestingly, tolerance may develop to select drug effects, while sensitization develops to others, presumably reflect-ing the different properties of the affected circuits. The clinical implication of tolerance is that people with addiction require more and more of the substance to get the same clinical effect, or the same amount of the drug becomes less effective. With sensitization, the use of the drug over time leads to more pronounced clinical effects (e.g., cocaine-induced paranoid thinking).

Relapse is the resumption of drug-seeking or drug-taking behaviour after a period of abstinence to a level of intensity comparable to that attained before the initiation of abstinence. Chronic relapse is a significant problem and a core feature of drug addiction (Kleber, 2007). Relapse rates are estimated to be between 35 and 85 per cent and often occur within the first three to six months after cessation (George, 2011). Research has identified numerous risk factors that predict vulnerability to relapse, including genetic predisposition, stress and conditioned positive reinforcers, such as specific places or par-aphernalia. Given that substance dependence is a heterogeneous condition, predicting the exact time course from abstinence to relapse is difficult. Rates can vary as a function of severity of addiction, type of drug, genetics, gender, the presence of a comorbid disor-der and treatment compliance.

Enhanced understanding of the neurobiological processes implicated in addic-tion, such as neuroadaptation and neuroplasticity, may lead to pharmacotherapies and other treatment approaches that help improve rates of recovery.

Genetic Vulnerability Factors

We are entering an era where substance use disorders are increasingly recognized as chronic medical disorders, similar to hypertension, schizophrenia and diabetes (McLellan et al., 2000). Adopting such a perspective may help to move society away from regarding substance use disorders as behavioural weaknesses, and emphasize certain neurochemical and neurobiological vulnerabilities that predispose and perpetuate addictions. Hereditary factors have long been implicated in the development of these disorders (Gurling et al., 1985). In fact, research suggests an eight-fold increased risk of drug-related disorders among first-degree relatives of people with substance use disorders (George, 2003).

Genetic risk plays an important contributory role to the addiction process at the psychosocial and biological levels. Genetic variation may partially underlie complex personality and physiological traits, such as impulsivity, risk taking, behavioural inhibition and stress sensitivity, which may, in part, be responsible for the initiation of drug use, as well as the transition to compulsive use (Kreek et al., 2005). For example, novelty-seeking traits may lead a person to experiment with alcohol at an earlier age, and research has demonstrated a strong association between early onset of alcohol use and alcohol dependence (Sartor et al., 2009).

Genetic polymorphisms may also contribute to a person's predisposition to addiction. A polymorphism is a change in the sequence of DNA and occurs with fairly high frequency in the general population. Variants in the coding region of genes can alter enzyme activity and affect receptor function and neurotransmitter systems. These alterations can make a person more vulnerable to developing a substance use disorder, and can also reduce risk for addiction, making a person more resilient (Kreek et al., 2004).

Polymorphisms in genes coding for specific enzymes can result in altered drug metabolism. For example, CYP2A6 is the enzyme that metabolizes nicotine and is thought to play a role in nicotine dependence. Genetic variations in this gene have been linked with several different smoking behaviours and response to therapies (Thorgeirsson et al., 2010).

Specific polymorphisms for CYP2A6 code for reduced enzymatic activity; people who possess this variant tend to smoke fewer cigarettes per day, are less dependent on nicotine and may have an easier time quitting smoking compared to people with variants that code for normal activity.

Interestingly, a recent study showed that slow metabolizers are three times more likely to become addicted to tobacco than are normal nicotine metabolizers (O'Loughlin et al., 2004). This may seem counterintuitive, but investigators theorize that people with reduced enzymatic activity experience prolonged exposure to nicotine and enhanced rewarding effects, despite consuming fewer cigarettes (O'Loughlin et al., 2004).

This type of paradigm extends to other substances of abuse, as polymorphisms in genes coding for the enzymes CYP2D6 and ALDH1B/C have been implicated in opioid dependence and alcohol dependence, respectively (Kreek et al., 2004).

Certain polymorphisms in genetic coding can also lead to altered receptor function, and cause neurotransmitter systems to function aberrantly. Variants of the dopamine D2 receptor have been linked to heroin dependence (Vereczkei et al., 2009), and repeat polymorphisms in the cannabinoid receptor gene have been associated with cocaine, amphetamine and heroin abuse (Ballon et al., 2006; Comings et al., 1997).

Polymorphisms affecting dopamine neurotransmission have also been associated with heightened risk for substance use disorders (Forbes et al., 2009).

While genetic information remains stable over a person's lifetime, the way in which genes are regulated may be influenced by external factors through a process called epigenetics. Epigenetic mechanisms modify gene activity without changing the sequence of DNA. These processes can activate, increase or repress the expression of different genes and in essence act as a "switching mechanism." Recent evidence suggests that epigenetic mechanisms may, in part, mediate brain changes associated with repeated drug exposure. For example, chronic cocaine exposure is known to induce a distinct set of genes in the NAc, some of which remain elevated for days to weeks (McClung & Nestler, 2003). These modifications may be involved in regulating behavioural responses to drugs of abuse, including behavioural sensitivity, conditioned responses and relapse (Kumar et al., 2005), ultimately leading to the development and maintenance of addiction (McClung & Nestler, 2003).

Understanding basic principles of neuronal and behavioural alterations that occur with addiction will ultimately lead to the identification of new targets for treating substance use disorders and novel approaches for prevention.

Pharmacological Treatments

Understanding the cellular mechanisms, neural circuitry and neuroplasticity resulting from compulsive drug use has tremendous implications in the prevention and treatment of substance use disorders, and the development of medications. Broadly speaking, medication interventions can be classified as agonists, partial agonists or antagonists. Each of these is described below. Table 6-1 at the end of this section presents a complete summary of evidence-based pharmacological treatments.

Agonist Therapy

The agonist approach uses a similar drug to mimic certain aspects of the abused substance by stimulating a relevant receptor involved in the drug addiction (e.g., nicotinic or mu-opioid receptor). This type of therapy is often referred to as substitution or maintenance therapy. Using this approach, an addictive agent is replaced with one that has less addictive potential and a better safety profile due to its pharmacological characteristics.

Methadone

Methadone is an example of an agonist used to treat opioid dependence (Bao et al., 2009). The opioid-withdrawing brain cannot distinguish between methadone and the abused opioid (e.g., heroin, oxycodone, morphine), as both relieve withdrawal symptoms such as body aches, nausea, diarrhea, anxiety and elevated pulse. Methadone is readily absorbed and is long-lasting, with a half-life (the time required for half of the drug to be eliminated from the body) between 12 and 100 hours (Reisine & Pasternak, 1996). Methadone produces different euphoric effects from person to person, but it is effective in blocking craving and withdrawal for 24 to 36 hours (Scimeca et al., 2000). It is a successful maintenance therapy because it keeps people in treatment, reduces their use of injection drugs (and of thus acquiring or transmitting diseases) and reduces overdose risk. Methadone decreases opioid abuse more successfully than treatments that do not incorporate this therapy. Optimum duration of maintenance on methadone remains unclear, but outcomes are best with extended treatment (Kleber, 2007).

Nicotine replacement therapy

Nicotine replacement therapy (NRT) uses pure nicotine to treat nicotine or tobacco dependence. NRT takes several forms, including transdermal patch, gum, lozenge, vapour inhaler and sublingual tablet; and each form varies in its duration of action (George, 2011). While the more slowly absorbed vehicles (gum and patch) help reduce withdrawal symptoms, the more rapidly absorbed agents (inhaler and spray) treat both nicotine withdrawal and craving, and achieve better smoking cessation rates. NRTs deliver nicotine without the additional exposure to carcinogens and other aromatic hydrocarbons in cigarettes (Joseph et al., 1996).

Partial Agonists

While agonists are chemicals that bind to receptors and fully stimulate them to produce their effects, partial agonists work by both stimulating and blocking receptors. More specifically, these drugs primarily stimulate receptors at low doses, and block them at higher doses.

Varenicline

Varenicline is approved in Canada and the United States for the treatment of nicotine dependence. It acts as a partial agonist at the nicotinic acetylcholine receptor (nAChR), the same receptor on which nicotine itself acts. Research has demonstrated promising effects using this compound. One study found that after one year of abstinence, the odds of quitting with varenicline were 2.5 to three times greater than with placebo (Jorenby et al., 2006), making it the most effective treatment available for nicotine dependence.

Buprenorphine

Compared to methadone, buprenorphine is a relatively new treatment option for opioid dependence, with a higher safety profile and easier accessibility. Methadone patients generally require once-daily dosing, but many people on buprenorphine can be treated once every two or three days. Buprenorphine is a mu-opioid receptor partial agonist. It has very high affinity and low intrinsic activity at the mu-receptor and thus will displace opioid full agonists, such as abused opioids, from the receptor. Buprenorphine's long duration of action is due to its long half-life and slow dissociation from mu-opioid receptors. At increasing doses, buprenorphine has a ceiling effect. In other words, it reaches a maximum euphoric effect and subsequently does not continue to increase linearly with increasing doses of the drug; in fact, at higher doses, the antagonist effects of this drug become more prominent. Accordingly, these properties explain why overdose of buprenorphine is rare and why it is unlikely to cause respiratory depression, a major concern with full opioid agonists such as heroin and methadone. Furthermore, buprenorphine may be less sedating than full mu-opioid agonists while still decreasing cravings for other opioids and preventing opioid withdrawal. Having opioid-dependent patients comply with buprenorphine therapy remains a clinical issue (Boothby & Doering, 2007).

Antagonists

Like agonists, antagonists compete with the substance of abuse for the receptor binding sites. However, antagonists do not stimulate the receptor. Instead, the effects of the abused substance are blocked, thereby attenuating or eliminating the rewarding or reinforcing effects of the substance.

Naltrexone

Naltrexone is a mu-opioid receptor antagonist and is thought to reduce both cravings and euphoria related to alcohol consumption (O'Brien et al., 1996; O'Malley et al., 1992). Studies have demonstrated its effectiveness in decreasing alcohol consumption and increasing the time to relapse (Anton & Swift, 2003). Not only is naltrexone an approved treatment option for alcohol dependence; it has also been shown to be effective in treating opioid dependence (Roozen et al., 2006).

Disulfiram

In 1948, disulfiram was the first medication to be approved by the U.S. Food and Drug Administration for alcohol dependence. Disulfiram works by inhibiting aldehyde dehydrogenase, an enzyme involved in alcohol metabolism, which results in the buildup of the compound acetaldehyde. Acetaldehyde is a very toxic substance that causes many of the hangover symptoms heavy drinkers experience. In the normal metabolic

TABLE 6-1

Evidence-Based Pharmacotherapies for Substance Use Disorders and Their Characteristics

PHARMACOLOGIC TREATMENT	TARGETED SUBSTANCE USE DISORDER	ADMINISTRATION ROUTE	SITE OF ACTION	MECHANISM	SUBJECTIVE EXPERIENCE
Methadone	Opioid	Oral	Mu-opioid receptors	Full agonist	Relieves withdrawal symptoms
Buprenorphine	Opioid	Transdermal, oral	Mu-opioid receptors	Partial agonist	Relieves drug cravings, prevents euphoric high
Naltrexone	Opioid, alcohol	Injection	Mu-opioid receptors	Antagonist	Prevents euphoria, reduces craving and helps prevent relapse
Disulfiram	Alcohol, cocaine	Oral	Enzyme inhibitor – aldehyde dehydrogenase	Inhibits alcohol metabolism	Adverse reaction when combined with alcohol; anti-craving effect with cocaine
Acamprosate	Alcohol	Oral	Glutamate receptor	Antagonist	Reduces cravings and overall desire to drink alcohol; helps maintain abstinence
NRTs	Nicotine	Transdermal, oral, nasal	Nicotinic acetylcholine receptors	Full agonist	Suppress withdrawal symptoms
Bupropion	Nicotine	Oral	Dopamine transporters; nicotinic acetylcholine receptors	Antagonist	Eases withdrawal symptoms and cravings
Varenicline	Nicotine	Oral	Nicotinic acetylcholine receptors	Partial agonist	Reduces cravings and withdrawal symptoms

process, the body continues to oxidize acetaldehyde into acetic acid, which is harmless. Disulfiram interferes with this metabolic process by blocking this last conversion step. If alcohol is ingested when disulfiram is in the system, the concentration of blood acetaldehyde levels may be five to 10 times higher than that found with alcohol alone. This leads to a disulfiram-ethanol reaction and results in aversive symptoms such as nausea, headaches, flushing, warmness, vomiting, shortness of breath and blurred vision (Garbutt, 2009). Disulfiram is one of the few demonstrably effective interventions for alcohol dependence, both alone and as an adjunct to psychosocial methods. However, its success is highly correlated with compliance (Brewer, 2000) and is not effective if taken intermittently.

Conclusion

Substance use disorders clearly have a neurbiological basis. Adopting a neurobiological framework is critical given that pharmacotherapeutic interventions, in combination with behavioural treatments, may be our best method for treating people with these disorders. There is considerable enthusiasm in the scientific community about incorporating advances in neuroscience, imaging techniques and pharmaceutical technology not only in improving existing pharmacotherapies, but also in developing new potential agents. Such approaches hold great hope and promise for people with substance use disorders, their families and society as a whole.

Practice Tips

- Clinicians should understand the underlying neurocircuitry of the critical brain pathways, the mediating actions of endogenous neurotransmitters and their effects at specific receptor sites. Increasing evidence suggests that prolonged exposure to abusive substances can produce long-lasting changes in drug-reward circuitry, leading to sensitization and high relapse rates.
- Numerous neurotransmitter systems can be targeted for effective pharmacological treatment interventions. An example is the mu-opioid receptor, which is the target of methadone in opioid-dependence treatment.
- Explore whether withdrawal symptoms, both in the acute and subacute stages, should be treated with medication.
- Consider maintenance therapy as best practice for the treatment of opioid dependence, as well as most other substances.
- Consider a combination of pharmacotherapy, psychosocial intervention and continuous, close monitoring.

Resources

Publications

Cami, J. & Farre, M. (2003). Drug addiction. *New England Journal of Medicine, 349,* 975–986.

Kosten, T.R. & George, T.P. (2002). The neurobiology of opioid dependence: Implications for treatment. *Science & Practice Perspectives, 1,* 13–20.

Internet

Canadian Centre on Substance Abuse
   www.ccsa.ca/Eng/Pages/Home.aspx
National Institute on Drug Abuse
   www.nida.nih.gov/nidahome.html

References

Adlaf, E.M., Begin, P. & Sawka, E. (2005). *Canadian Survey (CAS): A National Survey of Canadians' Use of Alcohol and Other Drugs: Prevalence of Use and Related Harms: Detailed Report.* Ottawa: Canadian Centre on Substance Abuse.

American Psychiatric Association (APA). (2000). *Diagnostic and Statistical Manual of Mental Disorders* (text rev.). Washington, DC: Author.

Anton, R.F. & Swift, R.M. (2003). Current pharmacotherapies of alcoholism: A U.S. perspective. *American Journal on Addictions, 12* (Suppl. 1), 53–68.

Ballon, N., Leroy, S., Roy, C., Bourdel, M.C., Charles-Nicolas, A., Krebs, M.O. & Poirier, M.F. (2006). (AAT)n repeat in the cannabinoid receptor gene (CNR1): Association with cocaine addiction in an African-Caribbean population. *Pharmacogenomics, 6,* 126–130.

Bao, Y., Liu, Z., Epstein, D.H., Du, C., Shi, J. & Lu, L. (2009). A meta-analysis of retention in methadone maintenance by dose and dosing strategy. *American Journal of Drug and Alcohol Abuse, 35,* 28–33.

Boothby, L.A. & Doering, P.L. (2007). Buprenorphine for the treatment of opioid dependence. *American Journal of Health-System Pharmacy, 64,* 266–272.

Brewer, C., Meyers, R.J. & Johnsen J. (2000). Does disulfiram help to prevent relapse in alcohol abuse? *CNS Drugs, 14,* 329–341.

Cami, J. & Farre, M. (2003). Drug addiction. *New England Journal of Medicine, 349,* 975–986.

Comings, D.E., Muhleman, D., Gade, R., Johnson, P., Verde, R., Saucier, G. & MacMurray, J. (1997).Cannabinoid receptor gene (CNR1): Association with IV drug use. *Molecular Psychiatry, 2,* 161–168.

Contet, C., Kieffer, B.L. & Befort, K. (2004). Mu opioid receptor: A gateway to drug addiction. *Current Opinion in Neurobiology, 14*, 370–378.

Di Chiara, G. & Imperato, A. (1988). Drugs abused by humans preferentially increase synaptic dopamine concentrations in the mesolimbic system of freely moving rats. *Proceedings of the National Academy of Science, 85*, 5274–5278.

Everitt, B.J., Belin, D., Economidou, D., Pelloux, Y., Dalley, J.W. & Robbins, T.W. (2008). Neural mechanisms underlying the vulnerability to develop compulsive drug-seeking habits and addiction. *Philosophical Transactions of the Royal Society B: Biological Sciences, 363*, 3125–3135.

Fields, H.L. (2007). Should we be reluctant to prescribe opioids for chronic non-malignant pain? *Pain, 129*, 233–234.

Forbes, E.E., Brown, S.M., Kimak, M., Ferrell, R.E., Manuck, S.B. & Hariri, A.R. (2009). Genetic variation in components of dopamine neurotransmission impacts ventral striatal reactivity associated with impulsivity. *Molecular Psychiatry, 14*, 60–70.

Galanter, M. & Kleber, H.D. (Eds.). (2008). *The American Psychiatric Publishing Textbook of Substance Abuse Treatment* (4th ed.). Arlington, VA: American Psychiatric Publishing.

Garbutt, J.C. (2009). The state of pharmacotherapy for the treatment of alcohol dependence. *Journal of Substance Abuse Treatment, 36* (Suppl. 1), S15–23.

George, T.P. (2003). Biological basis of drug addiction. In J.C. Soares & S. Gershon (Eds.), *Handbook of Medical Psychiatry* (1st ed., pp. 581–594). New York: Marcel Dekker.

George, T.P. (2011). Nicotine and tobacco. In L. Goldman & A. Schafer (Eds.), *Cecil Textbook of Medicine* (24th ed., pp. 142–146). New York: Elsevier.

Gurling, H.M., Grant, S. & Dangl, J. (1985). The genetic and cultural transmission of alcohol use, alcoholism, cigarette smoking and coffee drinking: A review and an example using a log linear cultural transmission model. *British Journal of Addiction, 80*, 269–279.

Health Canada. (2011). *Canadian Tobacco Use Monitoring Survey (CTUMS) 2011*. Ottawa: Author. Retrieved from www.hc-sc.gc.ca/hc-ps/tobac-tabac/research-recherche/stat/ctums-esutc_2011-eng.php

Hyman, S.E., Malenka, R.C. & Nestler, E.J. (2006). Neural mechanisms of addiction: The role of reward-related learning and memory. *Annual Review of Neuroscience, 29*, 565–598.

Janhunen, S. & Ahtee, L. (2007). Differential nicotinic regulation of the nigrostriatal and mesolimbic dopaminergic pathways: Implications for drug development. *Neuroscience and Biobehavioral Reviews, 31*, 287–314.

Jorenby, D.E., Hays, J.T., Rigotti, N.A., Azoulay, S., Watsky, E.J., Williams, K.E. et al. (2006). Efficacy of varenicline, an alpha4beta2 nicotinic acetylcholine receptor partial agonist, vs placebo or sustained-release bupropion for smoking cessation: A randomized controlled trial. *JAMA, 296*, 56–63.

Johnson, S.W. & North, R.A. (1992). Opioids excite dopamine neurons by hyperpolarization of local interneurons. *Journal of Neuroscience, 12*, 483–488.

Joseph, A.M., Norman, S.M., Ferry, L.H., Prochazka, A.V., Westman, E.C., Steele, B.G. et al. (1996). The safety of transdermal nicotine as an aid to smoking cessation in patients with cardiac disease. *New England Journal of Medicine, 335,* 1792–1798.

Kalivas, P.W. & Stewart, J. (1991). Dopamine transmission in the initiation and expression of drug- and stress-induced sensitization of motor activity. *Brain Research Reviews, 16,* 223–244.

Kleber, H.D. (2007). Pharmacologic treatments for opioid dependence: Detoxification and maintenance options. *Dialogues in Clinical Neuroscience, 9,* 455–470.

Koob, G.F. & Bloom, F.E. (1988). Cellular and molecular mechanisms of drug dependence. *Science, 242,* 715–723.

Koob, G.F. & Le Moal, M. (2008). Addiction and the brain antireward system. *Annual Review of Psychology, 59,* 29–53.

Kosten, T.R., Rounsaville, B.J., Babor, T.F., Spitzer, R.L. & Williams, J.B. (1987). Substance-use disorders in DSM-III-R: Evidence for the dependence syndrome across different psychoactive substances. *British Journal of Psychiatry, 151,* 834–843.

Kreek, M.J., LaForge, K.S. & Butelman, E. (2002). Pharmacotherapy of addictions. *Nature Reviews Drug Discovery, 1,* 710–726.

Kreek, M.J., Nielsen, D.A., Butelman, E.R. & LaForge, K.S. (2005). Genetic influences on impulsivity, risk taking, stress responsivity and vulnerability to drug abuse and addiction. *Nature Neuroscience, 8,* 1450–1457.

Kreek, M.J., Nielsen, D.A. & LaForge, K.S. (2004). Genes associated with addiction: Alcoholism, opiate, and cocaine addiction. *Neuromolecular Medicine, 5,* 85–108.

Kumar, A., Choi, K.H., Renthal, W., Tsankova, N.M., Theobald, D.E., Truong, H.T. et al. (2005). Chromatin remodeling is a key mechanism underlying cocaine-induced plasticity in striatum. *Neuron, 48,* 303–314.

McClung, C.A. & Nestler, E.J. (2003). Regulation of gene expression and cocaine reward by CREB and ΔFosB. *Nature Neuroscience, 6,* 1208–1215.

McLellan, A.T., Lewis, D.C., O'Brien, C.P. & Kleber, H.D. (2000). Drug dependence, a chronic medical illness: Implications for treatment, insurance, and outcomes evaluation. *JAMA, 284,* 1689–1695.

National Institute on Drug Abuse (NIDA). (2009). *DrugFacts: Treatment Approaches for Drug Addiction.* Retrieved from www.drugabuse.gov/infofacts/treatmeth.html

O'Brien, T.P., Metallinos, D.L., Chen, H., Shin, M.K. & Tilghman, S.M. (1996). Complementation mapping of skeletal and central nervous system abnormalities in mice of the piebald deletion complex. *Genetics, 143,* 447–461.

O'Loughlin, J., Paradis, G., Kim, W., DiFranza, J., Meshefedjian, G., McMillan-Davey, E. et al. (2004). Genetically decreased *CYP2A6* and the risk of tobacco dependence: A prospective study of novice smokers. *Tobacco Control, 13,* 422–428.

O'Malley, S.S., Jaffe, A.J., Chang, G., Schottenfeld, R.S., Meyer, R.E. & Rounsaville, B. (1992). Naltrexone and coping skills therapy for alcohol dependence. *Archives of General Psychiatry, 49,* 881–887.

Portenoy, R.K. (1990). Chronic opioid therapy in nonmalignant pain. *Journal of Pain Symptom Management, 5* (Suppl. 1), 46–62.

Rehm, J., Baliunas, D., Brochu, S., Fischer, B., Gnam, W., Patra, J. et al. (2006). *The Costs of Substance Abuse in Canada 2002: Highlights.* Ottawa: Canadian Centre on Substance Abuse. Retrieved from www.ccsa.ca

Reisine, T. & Pasternak G. (1996). Opioid analgesics and antagonists. In A.G. Gilman, T.W. Rall, A.S. Nies & P. Taylor (Eds.), *Goodman and Gilman's The Pharmacological Basis of Therapeutics* (9th ed., pp. 521–555). New York: McGraw Hill.

Robinson, T.E. & Berridge, K.C. (1993). The neural basis of drug craving: An incentive-sensitization theory of addiction. *Brain Research, 18,* 247–291.

Roozen, H.G., de Waart, R., van der Windt, D.A., van den Brink, W., de Jong, C.A. & Kerkhof, A.J. (2006). A systematic review of the effectiveness of naltrexone in the maintenance treatment of opioid and alcohol dependence. *European Neuropsychopharmacology, 16,* 311–323.

Sartor, C.E., Lynskey, M.T., Bucholz, K.K., Madden, P.A.F., Martin, N.G. & Heath, A.C. (2009). Timing of first alcohol use and alcohol dependence: Evidence of common genetic influences. *Addiction, 104,* 1512–1518.

Scimeca, M.M., Savage, S.R., Portenoy, R. & Lowinson, J. (2000). Treatment of pain in methadone-maintained patients. *Mount Sinai Journal of Medicine, 67,* 412–422.

Thorgeirsson, T.E., Gudbjartsson, D.F., Surakka, I., Vink, J.M, Amin, N., Geller, F. et al. (2010). Sequence variants at CHRNB3-CHRNA6 and CYP2A6 affect smoking behaviour. *Nature Genetics, 42,* 448–453.

Tjepkema, M. (2004). Alcohol and illicit drug dependence. *Supplement to Health Reports, 15.* Statistics Canada Catalogue no. 82-003. Retrieved from www.statcan.gc.ca/pub/82-003-s/2004000/pdf/7447-eng.pdf

Trigo, J.M., Martin-Garcia, E., Berrendero, F., Robledo, P. & Maldonado, R. (2010). The endogenous opioid system: A common substrate in drug addiction. *Drug and Alcohol Dependence, 108,* 183–194.

Vereczkei, A., Sasvari-Szekely, M. & Barta, C. (2009). The role of genetic variants of the dopaminergic system in heroin dependence. *Neuropsychopharmacologia Hungarica, 11,* 95–101.

Volkow, N.D., Fowler, J.S., Wang, G.J., Bater, R. & Telang, F. (2009). Imaging dopamine's role in drug abuse and addiction. *Neuropharmacology, 56* (Suppl. 1), 3–8.

Volkow, N.D., Fowler, J.S., Wang, G.J. & Swanson, J.M. (2004). Dopamine in drug abuse and addiction: Results from imaging studies and treatment implications. *Molecular Psychiatry, 9,* 557–569.

Walker, B.M. & Koob, G.F. (2008). Pharmacological evidence for a motivational role of kappa-opioid systems in ethanol dependence. *Neuropsychopharmacology, 33,* 643–652.

World Health Organization. (2004). *Neuroscience of Psychoactive Substance Use and Dependence.* Geneva: Author.

Chapter 7

Physical Effects of Alcohol and Other Drugs

Meldon Kahan

Fifteen months ago, Paolo, a 45-year-old man, went to the emergency department of a community hospital presenting with severe anxiety. Three days before the emergency visit, he had abruptly stopped taking lorazepam and codeine because he was unable to renew his prescriptions. The emergency physician diagnosed benzodiazepine and opioid withdrawal, prescribed a small supply of both medications and referred Paolo to the nearby withdrawal management centre.

The centre then referred Paolo to a hospital-based addiction medicine service, where he was assessed by a therapist. Paolo told the therapist he had moved to the city on short notice because his elderly mother was ill and needed constant care. He reported feeling hopeless and depressed after a long-term relationship ended two years ago, and had had to quit a well-paying position as a conference organizer last year because he couldn't concentrate as a result of increased drug use. Paolo also reported physical and psychological symptoms of withdrawal, including achiness, nausea, insomnia and a marked worsening of anxiety. The therapist felt that Paolo was still in benzodiazepine and opioid withdrawal, despite the prescription he received in the emergency department. She also felt he had a mood and generalized anxiety disorder. She referred him to the service's addiction physician, who saw him a few days later.

Both the physician and the therapist continued to see Paolo over the next several months, and communicated regularly with each other over the phone. The physician initiated buprenorphine treatment for codeine dependence, and tapered the lorazepam to a much lower dose. The physician also initiated antidepressant treatment and connected Paolo with a family physician. The therapist provided ongoing solution-focused therapy, encouraging Paolo to get help caring for his mother, and to exercise regularly and attend Narcotics Anonymous meetings. She also taught him simple cognitive strategies for dealing with stress and cravings, and organized referrals to an inpatient addiction program and an outpatient cognitive-behavioural therapy program for anxiety.

One year later, Paolo reports that his mood and activity levels are much improved, and that he has enrolled in a new business course.

Substance use counsellors can play an important role in maintaining their clients' physical health. They are frequently called upon to explain the health risks of alcohol and other drugs, and to inform clients of ways to minimize these risks. They often communicate with the client's family physician and other health care providers. Counsellors may be the first professionals to become aware of signs and symptoms of impending illness in a client. This chapter summarizes the health effects of the major drugs of abuse, recognizing the role that counsellors can play in helping their clients cope with the physical effects of substance use.

Key Concepts

Tolerance

Psychoactive (mood- or consciousness-altering) drugs tend to have a diminished effect with repeated use, a phenomenon known as *tolerance*. Tolerance occurs when the nervous system adapts to regular drug use. For example, alcohol activates the GABA system, the system of neurons, receptors and neurotransmitters that inhibits the activity of the central nervous system (CNS). It also inhibits the NMDA system, which balances the GABA system by increasing CNS activity. These two actions combine to cause the CNS to slow down, resulting in sedation, the primary effect of alcohol. With repeated use, the CNS compensates by increasing the number and sensitivity of NMDA receptors on nerve cells. The NMDA system is thus able to overcome the sedating effects of alcohol, allowing a person who drinks heavily to act almost normally despite having consumed large amounts of alcohol.

Withdrawal

The nervous system requires days or weeks to adjust to the sudden cessation of drug use, causing a set of signs and symptoms known as *withdrawal*. For example, tolerance makes the NMDA system of people who drink heavily more active (see above), so when the person quits drinking, he or she experiences symptoms of an overactive nervous system. When tolerance develops, a balance is achieved between the sedative effect of alcohol and the increased activity of the NMDA activity in the brain. When alcohol is discontinued abruptly, the brain is left with the unopposed increased NMDA activity, leading to withdrawal symptoms. Withdrawal (like tolerance) is most common and severe with sedative and opioid use. While physical symptoms of withdrawal usually resolve in a week or two, people who use substances heavily over the long term may experience mood disturbances and craving for weeks or even months, due to semi-permanent changes in the nervous system.

Physical Dependence

Physical dependence refers to tolerance and withdrawal. It often accompanies psychological dependence, but the two are not the same. For example, people who are psychologically dependent on cocaine experience little or no physical withdrawal, and people taking daily doses of opioids for chronic pain often experience withdrawal if they abruptly stop the opioid, even if they are not psychologically dependent.

Dependence Liability

The ability of a drug to produce reinforcing states, such as pleasure or euphoria, is known as *dependence liability*. Drugs within the same class may vary in their dependence liability; for example, among opioids, heroin and oxycodone have a higher dependence liability than codeine. Dependence liability is influenced by pharmacological factors, such as how quickly the drug reaches the brain. Genetic, social and psychological factors are also important, and people vary widely in their response to particular drugs. For example, most people do not experience pleasant psychoactive effects when they take opioids for pain, but a few people do, placing them at higher risk for abuse and dependence.

Research suggests that drugs of abuse cause euphoria by increasing the release of the neurotransmitter dopamine in the "reward pathway," a bundle of nerves in the mid-portion of the brain. The reward pathway is closely tied to two other brain functions—memory and executive function: a person who is addicted to a drug experiences pleasure from taking it, remembers the pleasurable feeling and feels driven to acquire the drug to feel the pleasure again. The reward pathway's natural function is to be activated by non-drug activities, such as eating, sex and close contact. Drugs of abuse thus "hijack" a brain mechanism that promotes survival of our species.

Intoxication and Overdose

Intoxication refers to impaired functioning resulting from the immediate psychoactive and physical effects of a drug. Intoxication results in *overdose* when it threatens vital functions of the nervous system, such as respiration and heart rate. The severity of intoxication and overdose depends on the amount of drug used; the route of administration; the person's age, gender, tolerance and concurrent drug use; and environmental cues. The most dangerous overdoses occur when people use a mixture of opioids and sedatives, especially when they lack tolerance to these substances.

Pharmacotherapy

Medications can be used in numerous ways to treat substance dependence. In agonist substitution therapy, the prescribed drug is in the same class as the addicting drug, and is therefore able to relieve craving and withdrawal symptoms. Examples include methadone for heroin dependence and the nicotine patch for nicotine dependence. In anti-craving therapy, prescribed drugs modify the effects of neurotransmitters involved in drug craving and withdrawal. Naltrexone and acamprosate are two examples of drugs that reduce cravings for alcohol. Antagonist medication blocks the action of the addicting drug, thus reducing its reinforcing effect (as with naltrexone for opioid dependence). Finally, in aversive therapy, the medication induces unpleasant physical symptoms when the addicting drug is taken, for example, disulfiram used with alcohol.

Pharmacotherapy varies widely in effectiveness. Methadone is highly effective. Medications for alcohol and nicotine dependence are modestly effective, but are nonetheless important adjuncts to psychosocial treatment. No pharmacotherapy has yet proven effective for cocaine dependence.

Alcohol

Most adults in our society who drink alcohol do so moderately and without problems. However, excess alcohol use creates a huge burden of sickness, death and health care costs, outweighing the combined effects of all other drugs of abuse except tobacco (Single et al., 1999). The following is a discussion of some common alcohol-related problems.

Intoxication

The severity of intoxication is related to the amount and speed of consumption, gender, body size, tolerance, stomach contents and genetic variation in metabolism. Alcohol is metabolized by the liver at a rate of about one drink per hour. While consuming one or two drinks has a mild disinhibiting and relaxing effect, consuming four or more drinks in less than two hours typically causes increased sedation with impaired judgment, slurred speech, lack of co-ordination and slow response time. Intoxication also affects mood and behaviour, and may cause emotional lability, impulsivity, anger and depression. Ten or more drinks can cause coma and death from decreased breathing or choking on vomit.

The risks of acute alcohol intoxication are greatest among adolescents and older adults, and when alcohol is consumed along with other drugs, especially sedatives. Adolescents have little experience with the intoxicating effects of alcohol and are more likely to engage in risky behaviours, and older adults have less tolerance to alcohol.

Alcohol Withdrawal

People are at risk for alcohol withdrawal if they consume at least six drinks per day for more than a week. Withdrawal becomes more severe with larger amounts and longer duration of drinking and with increased age (Brower et al., 1994), although there are large individual variations.

Withdrawal begins between six and 24 hours after the person's last drink. Physical symptoms usually resolve within three to seven days, but some people have insomnia, anxiety and anxious or depressed mood for weeks afterward. Signs and symptoms of withdrawal include tremors, sweating, fast pulse, high blood pressure, vomiting and anxiety. Grand mal seizures can occur in the first two or three days of withdrawal. Other complications include irregular heartbeat, hallucinations and delirium tremens.

Delirium tremens (DTs) occurs after three to five days of severe, untreated withdrawal. People who are hospitalized due to a medical illness are at greatest risk for developing DTs. Symptoms include extreme confusion and disorientation, with vivid visual and auditory hallucinations and sometimes fever, sweating and tremor. Deaths can occur from electrolyte imbalance or an irregular heartbeat.

Patients experiencing alcohol withdrawal require a calm, supportive environment. Benzodiazepines are the treatment of choice for those who need medication; they are highly effective and very safe (Holbrook et al., 1999). Treatment can be facilitated by using the 10-item Clinical Institute Withdrawal Assessment (CIWA) Scale, which measures the severity of withdrawal (Devenyi & Harrison, 1985; Erstad & Cotugno, 1995; Holbrook et al., 1999). A nurse or other health care worker administers the scale every one to two hours. Patients are asked about symptoms of withdrawal (e.g., anxiety) and are observed for signs of withdrawal (e.g., tremor). They are given benzodiazepines when they score 10 or higher. Additional doses are usually not needed once the CIWA score is consistently less than 8.

The counsellor's role

Counsellors should ask all clients with alcohol problems about withdrawal symptoms. Clients sometimes mistakenly attribute withdrawal symptoms to anxiety. Withdrawal-induced anxiety occurs at a set time of day (typically morning or afternoon, 10 to 12 hours after the last drink), is usually accompanied by tremor and is quickly relieved by alcohol. Counsellors should urgently refer clients to a physician on-site or to the emergency department if the clients have clearly visible tremors when reaching for an object, or if they are walking unsteadily; sweating profusely; or are confused, disoriented or hallucinating. Referral is especially important if the person has had withdrawal seizures or delirium in the past; is elderly; lives alone; has serious medical problems, such as heart disease; or is dependent on other medications, such as benzodiazepines. People who report having had a seizure within the past day or two should also be referred for medical attention.

Detoxification options

Counsellors should consider referral to a withdrawal management service ("detox centre") if clients are intoxicated and might go into withdrawal some hours later, or if their withdrawal is mild and no longer requires medical attention. Staff at these centres are usually experienced at assessing withdrawal and know when a client requires urgent medical care. All withdrawal management services are affiliated with a nearby emergency department.

Planned outpatient medical detoxification is an option for people who don't require urgent treatment for withdrawal, but are having trouble abstaining from alcohol because of recurrent withdrawal symptoms in the morning. Counsellors can organize outpatient detoxification in consultation with a physician or nurse. Clients are advised to have their last drink the night before and attend the facility the next morning. At the facility, they are given a benzodiazepine medication every one to two hours, according to their CIWA score. They may be sent home or to a withdrawal management service after completing treatment. Outpatient detoxification should be undertaken as part of a comprehensive treatment plan, since by itself, detoxification is not likely to result in long-term abstinence.

Some substance use treatment facilities provide inpatient medical detoxification. This is usually an elective, pre-booked procedure, and is often followed by participation in a formal inpatient or outpatient program.

"Home detox" is useful for clients who are unable or unwilling to attend a treatment facility, medical clinic or withdrawal management service. Older clients in particular can benefit from home detoxification. The person should be assessed daily by a nurse or physician for the first two or three days. If benzodiazepines are required, a nurse or responsible family member should dispense them, with a physician available for urgent phone consultation if needed.

Cardiovascular Effects and Low-Risk Drinking Guidelines

Light drinkers tend to live longer than abstainers or heavy drinkers. Alcohol prevents clumping of platelets—tiny particles in the blood that form clots—and elevates levels of high-density lipoprotein, a type of cholesterol that protects against heart disease. As a result, alcohol prevents heart attacks and strokes. In women, the benefits of alcohol may be outweighed by an increased risk of breast cancer.

Canadian Centre on Substance Abuse low-risk guidelines recommend no more than 15 drinks per week for men and 10 per week for women (Butt et al., 2011). To reduce long-term health risks, the guidelines advise no more than two drinks a day most days for women or three drinks a day most days for men (Butt et al., 2011). A lower weekly amount is suggested for women because they tend to be smaller and have a lower volume of blood than men, along with other differences that will result in a higher blood alcohol level than in men for a given rate of alcohol consumption.

The cardiovascular benefits of alcohol apply mainly to older adults. While older adults who drink moderately may live longer on average, the mortality rate for young people increases directly with the amount consumed due to death from accidents, violence and suicide (Andreasson et al., 1988).

Most of the cardiovascular benefits of alcohol are obtained with less than one drink per day. At higher doses, alcohol can harm the cardiovascular system. Intoxication or withdrawal can trigger an irregular heartbeat, sometimes causing sudden death. Three drinks or more per day can raise blood pressure, causing strokes and other problems. Heavy alcohol use can damage the heart muscle, causing a condition known as cardiomyopathy. The weakened heart muscle is unable to pump blood efficiently, causing fatigue and shortness of breath.

Alcoholic Liver Disease

Alcoholic liver disease occurs in three stages. The first is called fatty liver, in which the liver accumulates fat and becomes enlarged. This stage is reversible with reduced drinking, and usually lacks observable symptoms. The second stage is alcoholic hepatitis, or inflammation of the liver. This stage may also have no symptoms, but sometimes people become seriously ill. They may develop jaundice, the signs of which are yellow skin, dark urine and whitish stools. They may also develop vomiting, fever and pain in the liver area (i.e., the right upper abdomen below the ribs).

Repeated or prolonged episodes of alcoholic hepatitis lead to the third stage, cirrhosis, in which large portions of the liver have died and been replaced by scar tissue. This damage is irreversible, even if alcohol use is stopped. Cirrhosis is a major cause of death in Canada. The risk of developing cirrhosis is between 10 and 20 per cent for men who consume six drinks per day for 10 to 20 years. Women face an equivalent risk if they have three drinks per day (Kahan & Wilson, 2002). Chronic daily drinking is worse for the liver than binge drinking.

With advanced cirrhosis, the liver cannot fully metabolize proteins, which creates the buildup of intermediate chemicals containing ammonia. These chemicals are toxic to the brain and may cause a condition called hepatic encephalopathy. In the early stages of encephalopathy, people are fatigued, forgetful and accident-prone. They may experience day-night reversal (sleeping during the day and being up at night). In the later stages, people become confused, drowsy and may sink into a coma.

Encephalopathy can be triggered by sedating drugs, infections, electrolyte disturbances, gastrointestinal bleeding and other causes. People with advanced cirrhosis should avoid sedatives such as benzodiazepines, avoid high-protein meals and report any new illness to their doctor right away. Encephalopathy is prevented and treated with a low-protein diet and laxatives, such as lactulose (which prevents the ammonia compounds from being absorbed). Sometimes hospitalization is required.

Cirrhosis may also cause death through internal bleeding. Blood normally flows from the intestines into the portal vein, which enters into the liver. The scar tissue in the cirrhotic liver may lead to increased pressure in the portal vein, causing it to back up into veins in the esophagus. These veins then become swollen and engorged, a condition called esophageal varices. Varices sometimes burst, causing profuse and often fatal bleeding into the gastrointestinal tract. Bleeding varices can be prevented with medications called beta blockers, which lower the blood pressure in the esophageal veins.

Ascites (pronounced "ah-sy-tees"), a condition in which the abdomen fills with fluid, is also due in part to obstructed blood flow. Ascites is often the first sign of severe cirrhosis and impending liver failure. Ascites is controlled with diuretics ("water pills") and a low-salt diet.

The mainstay of treatment is reduced drinking. Clients with alcoholic liver disease should be told that fatty liver and alcoholic hepatitis are reversible with abstinence or reduced drinking; the liver is one of few organs in the body with cells that can regenerate. While cirrhosis is not reversible, the liver can function normally even if large portions are permanently scarred. People with cirrhosis can often lead normal lives as long as they stop drinking completely. Reduced drinking strategies are not recommended for people with cirrhosis, since even moderate alcohol consumption may promote liver damage.

People with advanced cirrhosis sometimes require a liver transplant for survival. Most transplant programs will only place someone who is alcohol-dependent on their waiting list if the person has participated in a treatment program, has been abstinent for at least six months to two years and has strong social supports. The person's counsellor often has a key role in advocating for the client with transplant programs. Only 10 per cent of people who have undergone a transplant relapse to drinking (Maldonado & Keeffe, 1997).

Gastritis, Esophagitis and Pancreatitis

Gastritis is a common complication of heavy alcohol consumption. Alcohol causes irritation and erosion of the stomach lining, producing discomfort and pain in the upper abdominal area. Gastritis is potentially serious because it can result in internal bleeding, the symptoms of which are bloody or dark-brown vomit and bloody or black tarry stools. Gastritis often heals quickly with abstinence. A variety of medications promote healing by reducing the production of acid in the stomach.

Alcohol also causes inflammation in the esophagus (esophagitis). Symptoms of esophagitis include heartburn and vomiting. It can be prevented by reduced drinking, and is treated with medications that reduce acid production.

Inflammation of the pancreas (pancreatitis) causes severe abdominal pain and vomiting, often requiring hospitalization. The condition can become chronic, causing prolonged or recurrent abdominal pain. People with chronic pancreatitis may require frequent hospitalizations and surgery, and regular use of painkillers. Chronic pancreatitis does not always fully resolve, even with abstinence.

Trauma

Alcohol consumption is a major cause of trauma-related death and injury, including motor vehicle crashes, work-related injuries and violence (assaults and suicide). Even moderate alcohol consumption can impair driving ability (Lowenstein et al., 1990). Alcohol intoxication increases the risk of trauma by impairing judgment and co-ordination, slowing reaction time and causing impulsivity and emotional lability. Adolescents and young adults congregating in large groups are especially at risk for violence and accidents.

Cancer

Moderate alcohol consumption (two drinks per day) is associated with a modestly elevated risk of breast cancer, perhaps due to the effects of alcohol on estrogen metabolism (Bradley et al., 1998). Alcohol also acts as a carcinogen and co-carcinogen (i.e., it increases the effect of other carcinogens) for esophageal, colorectal, pancreatic and laryngeal cancers (Brown & Devesa, 2002).

Dementia

Heavy drinking is associated with a number of neurological disorders. One common and serious disorder is dementia, defined as a global decrease in cognitive functioning (Williams & Skinner, 1990). Alcoholic dementia differs from the most common form of dementia, Alzheimer's disease, in that it is potentially reversible with abstinence (although only some people recover and recovery may only be partial). The cognitive changes of alcoholic dementia may be subtle, such as decreased ability to think abstractly. Counsellors who suspect dementia should refer clients to a neurologist or psychologist for neuropsychological testing and possibly a brain (CT) scan. Clients should be advised of the diagnosis and of the potential for recovery with abstinence. Enlisting the aid and support of the client's family may be helpful.

Cerebellar Disease

Alcohol can damage the cerebellum, a part of the brain that controls balance and equilibrium. People with cerebellar disease have tremors of the hands and walk with a wide-based gait, as if they were on a moving ship. Sometimes they require a cane or walker to maintain their balance.

Peripheral Neuropathy

Alcohol may damage the nerves in the feet and legs, causing a condition known as peripheral neuropathy. People with this syndrome may experience decreased sensation and painful burning sensations in their feet.

Wernicke-Korsakoff Syndrome

People who drink heavily often eat poorly, and the metabolism of alcohol depletes the body's stores of the B vitamins. This can lead to a severe deficiency of vitamin B1 (thiamine), causing Wernicke-Korsakoff syndrome. In the Wernicke's phase of this syndrome, people become drowsy, and their walking and eye movements become unco-ordinated. Wernicke's is a medical emergency, requiring prompt administration of intravenous thiamine. If not treated in time, such people typically develop Korsakoff's syndrome, in which they exhibit marked impairment of short-term memory. People with Korsakoff's may not remember an event that occurred 10 minutes earlier. They rarely recover and frequently require institutionalization.

Blackouts

A blackout is a type of amnesia in which the person is unable to remember events that took place during the previous evening's drinking binge. People may on occasion behave in a bizarre or dangerous manner during a blackout.

Reproductive Effects

Drinking during pregnancy can cause fetal alcohol spectrum disorder (FASD), the features of which are delayed growth, cognitive impairment and sometimes facial abnormalities, such as short eye openings. Affected children may also have cognitive-behavioural problems such as hyperactivity, speech disorders and deficits in learning and memory. These problems can persist into adolescence and adulthood.

FASD varies widely in severity, depending on the amount and timing of maternal alcohol consumption and other factors. For example, a child may have only cognitive deficits with no facial abnormalities. A safe level of alcohol consumption during pregnancy has not been established and abstinence is the most prudent recommendation (Bradley et al., 1998; Eustace et al., 2003). Alcohol consumption in the first trimester of pregnancy is thought to be particularly dangerous. However, there is no evidence of harm from occasional drink during the first trimester, before the woman has discovered she is pregnant.

Alcohol use during pregnancy is associated with low-birthweight infants, hypertension in the mother and other problems. Other reproductive effects include erectile dysfunction in men, irregular menstrual cycles in women and infertility in both men and women.

Psychiatric Effects

Heavy drinking can induce depression. Alcohol-induced depression usually resolves within several weeks of abstinence, distinguishing it from a primary mood disorder (Freed, 1981). Heavy drinkers are at high risk for suicide, because of alcohol-induced depression and the impulsivity and lack of judgment associated with acute intoxication (Freed, 1981; Inskip et al., 1998). Heavy drinking can also induce or exacerbate anxiety disorders and psychosis (Soyka, 1994).

Laboratory Detection of Alcohol

One common abnormality that may be detected in people who drink heavily is an elevated level of the liver enzyme gamma-glutamyl transferase (GGT) (Mihas & Tavassoli, 1992). Another abnormality is an increase in the size of red blood cells, as measured by a test called mean cell volume (MCV). At least four drinks per day is usually needed to produce these elevations.

Blood tests such as GGT and MCV are not as sensitive as a clinical interview in detecting alcohol problems. However, periodic tests can be used to confirm clients' self-reports of reduced alcohol intake. With abstinence or reduced drinking, GGT usually returns to normal within two to four weeks, and MCV within three months.

Pharmacological Treatment of Alcohol Dependence

Medications for alcohol dependence can be a useful adjunct to psychosocial treatment. Naltrexone (ReVia) has been shown in several controlled trials to reduce the intensity and frequency of alcohol binges and cravings (Anton et al., 1999; Garbutt et al., 1999). Naltrexone diminishes the pleasurable and reinforcing effects of alcohol by blocking the action of endorphins, which are neurotransmitters that affect mood. Naltrexone cannot be used with people who take opioids regularly because it will trigger severe withdrawal.

Acamprosate has also been shown to be effective in treating alcohol dependence. It blocks the neurotransmitter glutamate, relieving craving and mood instability caused by prolonged alcohol withdrawal (Garbutt et al., 1999). Baclofen, ondansetron and topiramate can also help reduce craving (Johnson et al., 2000; Johnson et al., 2003).

Disulfiram is another drug that acts by inhibiting a liver enzyme that metabolizes alcohol, causing the buildup of a toxic metabolite called acetaldehyde (Garbutt et al., 1999; Wright & Moore, 1990). People who drink alcohol while on disulfiram may experience chest pain, headache, flushed face, vomiting and irregular heartbeat. The reaction is potentially fatal because blood pressure can drop precipitously and the heart can go into a dangerous rhythm. The person should not drink for at least seven days after taking disulfiram. Disulfiram is most effective in maintaining abstinence when it is dispensed under the supervision of a family member or pharmacist.

Nicotine

For a detailed discussion of working with clients who are dependent on nicotine, see Chapter 11.

Psychoactive Effects

Nicotine dependence is the most common substance use disorder. Nicotine is known as the "chameleon drug"; it acts as a sedative when the smoker is anxious and a stimulant when the smoker is fatigued (Brands et al., 2000). It reaches the brain within seconds, and the average smoker takes up to 200 puffs a day. This makes nicotine a very reinforcing drug with a high relapse rate.

Withdrawal

Nicotine withdrawal is characterized by fatigue, irritability, gastrointestinal upset and craving for cigarettes. While the acute withdrawal resolves in five days, craving can last for many months, and relapse rates are high. Smokers are likely to experience withdrawal when they quit if they need a cigarette within half an hour of waking, and if they smoke a pack a day or more.

Opioids

Opioids (also known as narcotics) act on endorphin receptors in the brain to produce pain relief and (in some people) euphoria. Heroin is the main illegal opioid; prescription opioids include oxycodone (OxyContin, OxyNEO), codeine (Tylenol 3), hydromorphone (Dilaudid) and morphine.

Overdose

Opioids in high doses suppress the brain centres that control breathing and heartbeat, with potentially fatal results. People are at greatest risk for opioid overdose if they don't use opioids every day and are not fully tolerant, or if they have also taken benzodiazepines or other sedating drugs. Signs of overdose include pinpoint pupils; slow, drawling speech; and "nodding off" (brief episodes of falling asleep). Even if the therapist is able to engage the person in conversation, the person could die once he or she is alone and falls asleep. Clients with these symptoms should be referred for immediate medical evaluation, and should not be left alone.

Withdrawal

Opioid withdrawal causes flu-like symptoms, such as muscle aches, sweating, chills and goosebumps, runny nose and eyes, nausea and diarrhea. Psychological symptoms include insomnia, anxiety, depression and strong cravings for opioids. Psychological symptoms usually cause considerably greater distress than physical symptoms. Withdrawal begins between six and 24 hours after the last use, depending on whether the opioid is short- or long-acting. Physical symptoms peak at two to three days and usually resolve within five to seven days. Insomnia, dysphoria and drug craving may persist for months.

Opioid withdrawal does not have medical complications, except during pregnancy (see below). However, opioid withdrawal is by no means harmless. It is associated with severe depression, and clients in withdrawal should be assessed for suicidal ideation. Also, people lose much of their tolerance after a few days of abstinence and are at risk for overdose if they relapse.

Opioid withdrawal can be treated with methadone or buprenorphine (see Chapter 12) or with clonidine, a non-narcotic drug that blocks the nervous impulses in the brain that cause withdrawal symptoms. Treatment of withdrawal by itself rarely results in long-term abstinence and should be combined with methadone or buprenorphine maintenance and psychosocial treatment.

Reproductive Effects

Pregnant women who are dependent on heroin have a high infant mortality rate, due to delayed growth of the fetus and premature labour. Opioid withdrawal during pregnancy can induce uterine contractions, causing miscarriage in the first trimester or premature labour during the third trimester. To avoid these risks, pregnant women dependent on opioids should, as a rule, be offered methadone or buprenorphine maintenance. Women who are dependent on heroin have better prenatal care, improved nutrition and substantially lower infant mortality rates when placed on methadone (Kaltenbach et al., 1998).

Infants born to mothers who are dependent on opioids are at risk for withdrawal, characterized by irritability, vomiting and poor feeding. Unrecognized neonatal withdrawal can cause seizures and death, so pregnant clients should be encouraged to disclose opioid use to their caregivers. Withdrawal is treated with small, tapering doses of morphine (Osborn et al., 2002).

Opioid Use and Chronic Pain

Addiction is not common among chronic pain patients on opioids. Most pain patients do not experience euphoria with opioid use, only pain relief. However, North America is witnessing a marked increase in prescription opioid misuse because physicians are prescribing opioids to many more patients and at higher doses. Examples of controlled-release opioids include Hydromorph Contin (hydromorphone), OxyContin (oxycodone) and Duragesic (transdermal fentanyl patch). Controlled release opioids have a greater risk of overdose and addiction than immediate-release opioids because they come in much higher dose formulations. Also, patients can alter the tablets to maximize their euphoric effect, by crushing the pills before swallowing them, snorting them or mixing them in water and then injecting the crushed pills. Newer formulations, such as OxyNEO, a reformulated OxyContin, are "tamper resistant"; that is, they work as well as their original formulations when swallowed, but are difficult to crush or inject.

Physical versus Psychological Dependence

Physical dependence refers to tolerance and withdrawal. Any patient who takes opioids daily for chronic pain may experience withdrawal if the opioids are suddenly discontinued. However, this does not mean the person is "addicted" or psychologically dependent on the opioids. The term *opioid dependence* (to imply addiction to opioids) has been replaced in the latest revision of the *Diagnostic and Statistical Manual of Mental Disorders* with the term *opioid use disorder* (American Psychiatric Association, 2013). A person who is physically but not psychologically dependent on opioids does not have an opioid use disorder.

Opioid Use Disorder in Patients with Chronic Pain

It can be difficult for counsellors and physicians to distinguish therapeutic opioid use from opioid dependence. Opioid use disorder should be suspected in pain patients who:
- have risk factors for misusing opioids. The major risk factor is a current or past history of addiction to alcohol, cocaine or other drugs. The more recent, severe or prolonged the addiction, the greater the person's risk of becoming addicted to opioids. Other risk factors are having an active mental disorder (e.g., depression or posttraumatic stress disorder) and being under age 40.
- take opioids far in excess of what would normally be required for their pain condition. Patients with lower back pain, fibromyalgia and other common pain conditions usually don't need opioids, and if they do, they respond to low doses.
- rapidly escalate their dose. Tolerance to the analgesic effects of opioids develops slowly, and patients are often able to remain on the same dose for months or years. However, tolerance to the euphoric effects of opioids develops within days, forcing patients addicted to the drug to increase their dose to achieve the same effect.

Eventually, they begin to experience distressing withdrawal symptoms at the end of a dosing interval, forcing them to take the opioid just for withdrawal relief.

- take the medication in a binge rather than scheduled pattern, to achieve the desired psychoactive effect or ward off withdrawal symptoms.
- display "aberrant drug-related behaviours," such as harassing the physician for script refills, acquiring opioids from other doctors or "the street," or crushing oral opioids for injection or snorting.
- experience severe and prolonged withdrawal if they run out. While any patient who regularly uses opioids may experience withdrawal if he or she abruptly stops the drug, those with opioid use disorder tend to experience frequent and distressing withdrawal with marked psychological symptoms. This is in part because they tend to use high doses in a binge pattern.

Laboratory Detection

Immunoassay and chromatography are the two main laboratory techniques used to detect opioids in urine. The immunoassay detects some opioids up to seven days after the last use. Immunoassay does not distinguish between different types of opioids. Chromatography only detects opioids for one or two days, but it can identify specific opioids.

Medical Treatment of Opioid Use Disorder

Patients with chronic pain who also have an opioid use disorder should be considered for methadone or buprenorphine treatment (see Chapter 12). Both these medications are opioids and can effectively relieve pain, withdrawal symptoms and craving.

Benzodiazepines

Benzodiazepines are among the most commonly prescribed drugs. Their main action is to diminish anxiety and induce sleep, but they are also used to treat alcohol withdrawal and prevent certain types of seizures. People become tolerant to the sleep-inducing effects of benzodiazepines, but do not develop significant tolerance to their anxiety-reducing effects. Most patients take the medication as prescribed, and benzodiazepine dependence is not common.

A number of benzodiazepines are available that differ in their duration of action and abuse liability. For example, diazepam (Valium) and chlordiazepoxide (Librium) are long-acting, while triazolam (Halcion) and alprazolam (Xanax) are short-acting. Diazepam, triazolam and lorazepam (Ativan) have higher abuse liabilities than oxazepam, chlordiazepoxide or clonazepam.

Intoxication and Overdose

Intoxication on large doses of benzodiazepines is clinically similar to alcohol intoxication. There is little risk of lethal overdose when benzodiazepines are used by themselves; however, an overdose involving benzodiazepines combined with alcohol or opioids is very dangerous.

Rebound Insomnia

Benzodiazepines suppress the deep and the rapid eye movement stages of the sleep cycle. When the drug is withdrawn suddenly, people experience sleep interrupted by vivid dreams. This "rebound insomnia" occurs after about three weeks of nightly use, and may take several weeks to resolve.

Other Effects

Benzodiazepine use increases the risk of motor vehicle accidents, and can cause falls and confusion in elderly people. Long-acting benzodiazepines, such as diazepam, flurazepam and chlordiazepoxide, are particularly hazardous for older adults.

Psychiatric Effects

Benzodiazepines can contribute to depression, particularly with high doses and in people with a pre-existing mood disorder. Benzodiazepines sometimes have a disinhibiting effect, especially among people with psychosis or certain personality disorders.

Laboratory Detection

Long-acting benzodiazepines such as diazepam can be detected for up to 20 days or longer with some immunoassay methods. Certain benzodiazepines such as clonazepam are difficult to detect on urine drug screens.

Withdrawal

Withdrawal symptoms begin one to two days after stopping short-acting benzodiazepines, and two to five days after stopping long-acting benzodiazepines. Withdrawal is more severe with high doses of short-acting benzodiazepines; with longer duration of use; and with people who are older or have concurrent anxiety, mood or substance use disorders. Withdrawal resolves within a few weeks for most people, but for some it may persist for months (Lader, 1994; Petursson, 1994; Pimlott & Kahan, 2000).

People who abruptly stop taking benzodiazepines are at risk for seizures, delirium and hallucinations if they have used large amounts for prolonged periods (50 mg or more of diazepam per day, or the equivalent dose of another benzodiazepine daily, for more than a few weeks). Those who suddenly stop therapeutic doses (30 mg or less of diazepam, or the equivalent dose of another benzodiazepine) tend to experience two groups of symptoms: anxiety-related symptoms (emotional lability, insomnia, agitation, irritability, poor concentration and panic attacks) and subtle neurological symptoms (distortions of visual and auditory stimuli, blurry vision, unsteadiness of gait, depersonalization or déjà vu sensations) (Busto et al., 1986).

The Decision to Taper

Patients who are dependent on high doses of benzodiazepines should be tapered off the drug, since the risks of continued use far outweigh the benefits. However, because therapeutic use does not generally result in severe social disruption or physical harm, and because withdrawal can be prolonged and difficult, the decision to taper a patient should be made only after a careful assessment of the risks and benefits. The risks, outlined above, include a possible increase in anxiety, depression and suicidal ideation. The benefits might not be apparent until tapering is well underway. People who are tapered off benzodiazepines frequently report feeling more alive, energetic and clear-headed. They may be better able to make important life decisions and obtain greater benefit from psychotherapy.

Approach to Tapering

People taking very high doses may need to be tapered in an inpatient setting. Those on therapeutic doses should be tapered slowly as outpatients over a period of several weeks or months (DuPont, 1990). It is medically easiest to taper the patient with the benzodiazepine he or she is taking, but people who find this difficult might have greater success if they are switched to another benzodiazepine. Tapering with long-acting agents such as diazepam or clonazepam may allow for a smoother withdrawal, although diazepam can be misused and is not a safe option for older adults or people with liver disease. Patients taking alprazolam or triazolam should be tapered with these agents, or with clonazepam. Use of adjunctive agents such as gabapentin or anxiolytic antidepressants may be helpful in difficult cases.

For physicians who are tapering patients, a weekly reduction of no more than 5 mg of diazepam (or equivalent) is suggested. The daily dispensing schedule (two, three or four times per day) should be kept the same until near the end. Clients should be advised not to miss doses or speed up the taper on their own because this will generate withdrawal symptoms and "detoxification fear." The taper should be slowed near the end, as people often find the last pill the most difficult to discontinue. The patient should have a say in the rate of the taper; there is usually no need to complete the taper in a set time period. Frequent pharmacy pickup might be necessary if the patient repeatedly runs out of pills.

A program of therapeutic support must be in place before tapering is attempted. Frequent follow-up visits should be organized, weekly if necessary. The client should be asked whether he or she feels any benefits of the tapering, as well as any withdrawal symptoms. Counsellors should watch for signs of depression and suicidal ideation during tapering.

Cannabis

Cannabis (marijuana and hashish) is the most commonly used illicit drug in Canada. It is usually smoked but may be taken orally. Cannabis causes relaxation and a feeling of well-being accompanied by mild hallucinogenic effects, such as distortion in the sense of time, difficulty with abstract thinking and concentration, and vivid visual and auditory perceptions. Effects last several hours. Cannabis intoxication can sometimes trigger panic attacks and an irregular heartbeat.

The overall risk of becoming dependent on cannabis is low compared with alcohol and other drugs. However, cannabis use and cannabis-related problems are very common among youth. In 2008, 17 per cent of a sample of Canadian adolescents between age 13 and 15 reported using cannabis in the past year (Hammond et al., 2011). In a prospective study of 2,500 youth using cannabis, 81 per cent of high-frequency cannabis users met one or more criteria for cannabis dependence (Nocon et al., 2006). The majority of cannabis users admitted to a substance use treatment program in Ontario were in high school and under 20 years old (Urbanoski et al., 2005).

Medical Uses

An oral synthetic form of cannabis is used to treat nausea caused by chemotherapy. Cannabis is being studied as an analgesic, muscle relaxant and appetite stimulant in the treatment of serious medical conditions such as multiple sclerosis and HIV, but to date there is little evidence to support its medical use for common pain conditions such as back pain (Gurley et al., 1998; Killestein et al., 2002; Watson et al., 2000). While cannabis may be more effective than placebo, it is significantly less effective than standard medications such as opioids (Furlan et al., 2011), and often causes disturbing cognitive and neurological side-effects (Honarmand et al., 2011; Martin-Sanchez, 2009). For therapeutic use, oral cannabis or cannabis inhaled through a vaporizer is preferred over smoked cannabis, because inhalation does not contain impurities (some of which are carcinogenic). Oral use is also preferred over smoking, as it does not cause the same rapid increase in blood level of cannabis, which puts the person at risk for intoxication and other side-effects.

Withdrawal

More than 40 per cent of daily or frequent cannabis smokers experience withdrawal symptoms on cessation of the drug: these symptoms may involve fatigue and weakness or anxiety and restlessness. The symptoms are often distressing enough to cause users to resume smoking (Hasin et al., 2008; Weisdorf, 2000). Daily cannabis users may also experience rebound anxiety and emotional volatility after stopping use. Further research is needed to determine the role of medications in relieving withdrawal symptoms.

Psychiatric Effects

Evidence suggests that cannabis can exacerbate depression (Rey et al., 2002), impair cognitive functioning (Solowij et al., 2002), induce psychosis (Basu et al., 1999), trigger schizophrenia in people who are predisposed (Hambrecht & Hafner, 2000) and worsen symptom control in people with schizophrenia (Caspari, 1999). Adolescents and people with primary psychiatric disorders appear to be particularly vulnerable to the psychiatric effects of cannabis (Johns, 2001; Rey et al., 2002). Frequent cannabis use in adolescents is also associated with adjustment problems, such as crime and other illicit drug use (Fergusson et al., 2002).

Health Effects

Epidemiological and pathological studies suggest that chronic cannabis use can cause or accelerate chronic obstructive lung disease (chronic bronchitis), and may be a risk factor for lung cancer, although it is difficult to control for confounding with tobacco use (Berthiller et al., 2008; Henry et al., 2003). Cannabis use during pregnancy has been associated with cognitive defects in children (Wong et al., 2011). It is also a risk factor for motor vehicle accidents (Mann et al., 2007).

Laboratory Detection

Regular use of cannabis is detected in the urine for 20 days or longer. Second-hand cannabis smoke is generally not detectable on urine drug screens.

Sedatives

Benzodiazepines have largely replaced earlier generations of prescription sedatives. Fiorinal is the only non-benzodiazepine sedative that is still commonly prescribed. It is a combination of ASA, codeine and a barbiturate known as butalbital. Most patients take Fiorinal in moderate doses to treat migraine headaches, but some patients become addicted.

Barbiturates can induce depression, and overdoses with these drugs are more dangerous than benzodiazepine overdoses. Patients who abruptly stop high doses (such as 10 tablets per day of Fiorinal) can develop a dangerous and potentially fatal withdrawal that can include seizures, psychosis, delirium and an irregular heartbeat. The treatment drug of choice is phenobarbital. Phenobarbital may be used as part of an outpatient tapering program for people who use sedatives moderately, or in an inpatient setting for those who use them heavily.

Solvents

Inhalation of solvents, such as gasoline or glue, produces intoxication similar to that of alcohol, with slurred speech, sedation and disinhibition. Distortions of vision and sense of time can also occur. Death can occur from suffocation or an irregular heartbeat.

Prolonged use of solvents can result in tolerance, withdrawal and dependence. The most serious medical consequence of solvent use is permanent brain damage, which is similar to alcohol-related brain damage but more severe and with a younger age of onset. As with alcohol, solvents damage the cerebellum (responsible for balance) and cerebrum (cognition and memory). Solvent use during pregnancy can cause premature birth and birth defects. Psychiatric effects of prolonged solvent use include depression, suicidal ideation and paranoia.

Cocaine

Cocaine causes a rapid buildup of several neurotransmitters in the brain, including dopamine (which causes euphoria) and epinephrine and norepinephrine (which stimulate the heart and nervous system). The euphoria usually lasts no more than 20 minutes with smoking and injection, but longer with oral or nasal use. The effects on the heart and nervous system last for hours. The first few uses of cocaine produce the most intense euphoria, with feelings of elation, boundless energy and confidence. With regular use, the person tends to experience a brief "rush" lasting seconds or minutes, followed by agitation and paranoia.

Cocaine can be injected into a vein, smoked, inhaled through the nose ("snorting") or taken orally. Nasal inhalation irritates the lining of the nose and creates a milder euphoria than injecting or smoking. Some people "binge" on cocaine, injecting or smoking it multiple times over several days, followed by days or weeks of abstinence.

"Crack" is made by mixing cocaine with baking soda, forming a small solid rock that makes a popping sound when heated. Heating releases pure cocaine vapour, which circulates through the lungs and reaches the brain within seconds. Crack reaches a wider market than cocaine powder because it is easy to use and can be sold in small $10 to $20 packets.

Withdrawal

People who have just finished a cocaine binge sleep deeply for one to two days. This is followed by one or more weeks of intense cravings for cocaine, depression, insomnia with nightmares, and feelings of emptiness and irritability. Whether these phases represent a true physiological withdrawal remains controversial.

Overdose

Cocaine overdose can cause seizures, severe hypertension, rapid heartbeat, fever and delirium, and eventually coma and death.

Cardiovascular Effects

Cocaine can trigger a marked rise in blood pressure, a rapid and irregular heartbeat, and spasms of the blood vessels (Warner, 1993). This can result in strokes, brain hemorrhages, heart attacks and ruptured aneurysms. While people with underlying hypertension or heart disease are at greatest risk, these complications have been reported to occur even in young, healthy adults taking small doses of cocaine. Combined cocaine and alcohol use creates a metabolite called cocaethylene, which appears to enhance cardiovascular toxicity (Pennings et al., 2002).

Reproductive Effects

Cocaine taken during pregnancy can cause the placenta to separate from the uterus, resulting in severe hemorrhage and the death of the fetus (Keller & Snyder-Keller, 2000). Cocaine can also trigger premature labour. Regular use of cocaine during pregnancy may cause delayed growth of the fetus, due to poor blood supply through the placenta. Often people who use cocaine receive inadequate prenatal and medical care (Kaltenbach & Finnegan, 1998).

Other Physical Effects

Grand mal seizures are very common among those who use cocaine, typically occurring within minutes of use. Like other stimulants, cocaine suppresses appetite, leading to marked weight loss (Warner, 1993).

Psychiatric Effects

Cocaine can have profound psychiatric effects. People who are acutely intoxicated on cocaine display a wide variety of psychiatric symptoms, including delusions, paranoia, hallucinations (especially tactile), delirium and severe anxiety. Paranoid delusional disorders and other types of psychoses have been linked with chronic cocaine use. Symptoms may persist for months after the person has stopped using cocaine, and antipsychotic medication is often required. Cocaine can induce severe depression, and people who use cocaine heavily are at high risk of suicide.

Concurrent cocaine and alcohol use increases the risk of depression, violence and suicide (Cornelius et al., 1998; Salloum et al., 1996).

Laboratory Detection

The metabolite of cocaine, benzoylecgonine, is detected in urine by immunoassay methods for three to seven days after use.

Methamphetamine

Methamphetamine is manufactured in clandestine labs using common household materials and ephedrine, an ingredient used in cold medicines. It acts in a somewhat similar manner to cocaine: it stimulates the release of dopamine and other neurotransmitters from the nerve terminals in the brain. Like cocaine, methamphetamine is a powder that can be taken orally, by snorting or smoking, or by injection.

Symptoms of methamphetamine intoxication are similar to symptoms of cocaine intoxication, except that they last hours rather than minutes. Regular methamphetamine use is associated with marked weight loss and dental problems. Injection use can lead to hepatitis C, HIV and other complications. Psychiatric complications, including paranoia and psychosis, can occur, similar to what can occur with cocaine addiction. People who are addicted to methamphetamine are at higher risk for violence and suicide, due to acute intoxication and chronic psychiatric effects.

Hallucinogens

Hallucinogenic drugs, such as LSD, mescaline and psilocybin, can cause intense hallucinations, as well as distortions in the sense of time, disorientation and confusion. These experiences are often perceived as pleasant, but occasionally they are frightening. The reaction usually resolves in one or two hours, but psychotic symptoms occasionally persist for protracted periods, even months, in rarer cases. Tolerance and withdrawal do not occur with hallucinogens.

In the weeks and months after stopping use, a small percentage of people may experience "flashbacks," in which they briefly relive past episodes of drug use. Though vivid and disturbing, flashbacks tend to last only minutes, and diminish in frequency and intensity over time.

Anabolic Steroids

Anabolic steroids are derived from the male sex hormone testosterone (Kahan & Wilson, 2002). They are used by athletes and bodybuilders to enhance performance and increase muscle bulk and by adolescent males to improve their appearance. Anabolic steroids are rarely prescribed by physicians; the drugs are acquired illicitly from veterinary sources. They are frequently taken in heavy doses followed by reduced dosing or abstinence ("cycling" or "stacking"). Steroids are taken orally or by injection. Long-term steroid use has serious health effects (Bolding et al., 2002; Parssinen & Seppala, 2002).

Dependence

Steroids can induce euphoria, perhaps through the release of endorphins in the central nervous system, and there have been case reports of steroid dependence. Abruptly stopping heavy steroid use can cause withdrawal, which is characterized by fatigue, depression and craving.

Psychiatric Effects

People who use steroids can develop symptoms of aggression ("steroid rage"), depression and suicidal ideation, hypomania and psychosis. Most symptoms resolve with abstinence, but depression may persist for months.

Health Effects

Steroids raise cholesterol levels and promote the formation of blood clots, resulting in heart attacks and strokes. Those who use steroids may be at higher risk for liver cancer. Women may experience irregular periods and masculinizing effects, such as acne, deepened voice and facial hair. Men can develop small testicles, low sperm count, decreased sex drive and enlarged breasts. Steroids can stop bone growth in adolescents. Needle sharing can cause viral hepatitis or HIV.

Other Drugs

The drugs described below are classified as hallucinogenic stimulants (MDMA), sedatives (GHB, flunitrazepam), and dissociative anesthetics (ketamine and PCP). Little is known about their long-term health effects. They are usually taken in oral form and their effects last for several hours. They are usually not detectable on standard urine drug screens.

MDMA ("Ecstasy")

The psychoactive effects of MDMA (3,4-methylenedioxymethamphetamine, commonly called "ecstasy") are due to the release of serotonin and dopamine in the brain. People who use ecstasy report feeling more sensual and affectionate, hence its other names "empathy" or "love drug." Tolerance develops quickly, but it does not appear to cause withdrawal.

The acute toxic effects of ecstasy are due to the release of serotonin. People who take antidepressants or other drugs that elevate serotonin are at greatest risk. Symptoms and signs include fever, sweating, fast pulse, muscle rigidity and twitching, seizures and jaw clenching. Some of the medical complications of ecstasy are due to the circumstances in which it is used—prolonged dancing in a hot room without adequate fluid replacement can lead to dehydration and electrolyte imbalances, which have potentially serious consequences (Gowing et al., 2002). Regular ecstasy use is also associated with depression (Verheyden et al., 2003), and case reports suggest that it can trigger psychosis (Vecellio et al., 2003).

Gamma Hydroxybutyrate

Gamma hydroxybutyrate (GHB) is a potent sedative, with effects similar to alcohol. There is a small margin between the intoxicating dose and the dose that can cause coma and death. Combining GHB with alcohol is particularly dangerous.

GHB causes dependence and withdrawal. The withdrawal syndrome is similar to that of alcohol, but longer (up to 15 days) and more severe (Bowles et al., 2001; Craig et al., 2000; Dyer et al., 2001). Symptoms include tremors, seizures, hallucinations, paranoia and delirium. Barbiturates such as phenobarbital are the treatment drug of choice.

Flunitrazepam

Flunitrazepam (Rohypnol) is a potent, short-acting benzodiazepine. Because it has pronounced sedative and amnesia effects, it has been used to commit sexual assault on unsuspecting strangers ("date rape"). Other sedating drugs have also been used for this purpose, including alcohol and GHB.

Ketamine

Ketamine (commonly known as "special K") is a dissociative anesthetic. Those who use the drug experience a dream-like state, with confusion and hallucinations, out-of-body sensations and a distorted sense of time. Ketamine use can lead to coma and decreased respiration, particularly if taken with alcohol or other sedatives. It can also have serious cardiovascular and neurological complications, such as irregular heartbeat and seizures.

Phencyclidine

Phencyclidine (PCP) is also a dissociative anesthetic. It is smoked or "snorted." It can cause disorientation; acute psychotic symptoms, including hallucinations and delusions; and violent behaviour. Like ketamine, it has serious medical complications, such as seizures.

Conclusion

Alcohol and other drug problems are associated with a wide variety of serious physical and psychiatric problems. Counsellors should inform their clients of these health risks, and be alert to the symptoms and signs of physical and psychiatric illness in clients. They should also encourage their clients' primary care physicians to assist with follow-up and relapse prevention.

Practice Tips

Clients often have a close, long-term relationship with their primary care provider, and the provider can play an important role in relapse prevention. Primary care providers should:

- regularly follow up and monitor the client, which includes taking a substance use history, and in some cases ordering blood tests and urine drug screens
- prescribe medications to reduce craving and promote abstinence as needed
- be cautious in prescribing potentially addicting drugs, such as opioids, stimulants and benzodiazepines
- treat medical complications of substance use
- monitor compliance with medications and other recommended treatments

- identify and address mental and physical disorders that can trigger relapse, such as chronic pain, anxiety or depression
- encourage active self-care and a healthy lifestyle (exercise, sleep, spending time with friends and family)
- encourage ongoing participation in self-help groups and outpatient follow-up.

Counsellors should:
- refer clients for medical care and actively encourage them to attend appointments. (Booking these appointments with the client from your office improves their show rates!)
- communicate regularly with their clients' primary care providers, and educate the providers about treatment of substance use problems
- ensure that treatment plans are co-ordinated, and that the goals and roles created for clients, counsellors, primary care providers and other care providers are appropriate and understood by all involved
- reinforce the merits of working together to find the best solutions to clients' problems related to addictive behaviour and to achieve and maintain goals of improved health and well-being.

References

American Psychiatric Association. (2013). *Diagnostic and Statistical Manual of Mental Disorders* (5th ed.). Washington, DC: Author.

Andreasson, S., Allbeck, P. & Romelsjo, A. (1988). Alcohol and mortality among young men: Longitudinal study of Swedish conscripts. *British Medical Journal, 296,* 1021–1025.

Anton, R.F., Moak, D.H., Waid, L.R., Latham, P.K., Malcolm, R.J. & Dias, J.K. (1999). Naltrexone and cognitive behavioral therapy for the treatment of outpatient alcoholics: Results of a placebo-controlled trial. *American Journal of Psychiatry, 156,* 1758–1764.

Basu, D., Malhotra, A., Bhagat, A. & Varma, V.K. (1999). Cannabis psychosis and acute schizophrenia. A case-control study from India. *European Addiction Research, 5* (2), 71–73.

Berthiller J., Straif, K., Boniol, M., Voirin, N., Benhaïm-Luzon, V., Ayoub, W.B. et al. (2008). Cannabis smoking and risk of lung cancer in men: A pooled analysis of three studies in Maghreb. *Journal of Thoracic Oncology, 3,* 1398–1403.

Bolding, G., Sherr, L. & Elford, J. (2002). Use of anabolic steroids and associated health risks among gay men attending London gyms. *Addiction, 97,* 195–203.

Bowles, T.M., Sommi, R.W. & Amiri, M. (2001). Successful management of prolonged gamma-hydroxybutyrate and alcohol withdrawal. *Pharmacotherapy, 21,* 254–257.

Bradley, K., Badrinath, S., Bush, K., Boyd-Wickizer, J. & Anawalt, B. (1998). Medical risks for women who drink alcohol. *Journal of General Internal Medicine, 13,* 627–639.

Brands, B., Kahan, M., Selby, P. & Wilson, L. (Eds.) (2000). *Management of Alcohol, Tobacco and Other Drug Problems: A Physician's Manual.* Toronto: Centre for Addiction and Mental Health.

Brower, K.J., Mudd, S., Blow, F.C., Young, J.P. & Hill, E.M. (1994). Severity and treatment of alcohol withdrawal in elderly versus younger patients. *Alcohol Clinical Experimental Research, 18,* 196–201.

Brown, L.M. & Devesa, S.S. (2002). Epidemiologic trends in esophageal and gastric cancer in the United States. *Surgical Oncology Clinics of North America, 11,* 235–256.

Busto, U., Sellers, E.M., Naranjo, C.A., Cappell, H., Sanchez-Craig, M. & Sykora, K. (1986). Withdrawal reaction after long-term therapeutic use of benzodiazepines. *New England Journal of Medicine, 315,* 854–859.

Butt, P., Beirness, D. & Stockwell, T. (2011). *Alcohol and Health in Canada: A Summary of Evidence and Guidelines for Low-Risk Drinking.* Ottawa: Canadian Centre on Substance Abuse.

Caspari, D. (1999). Cannabis and schizophrenia: Results of a follow-up study. *European Archives of Psychiatry and Clinical Neuroscience, 249,* 45–49.

Cornelius, J.R., Thase, M.E., Salloum, I.M., Cornelius, M.D., Black, A. & Mann, J.J. (1998). Cocaine use associated with increased suicidal behavior in depressed alcoholics. *Addictive Behaviors, 23,* 119–121.

Craig, K., Gomez, H.F., McManus, J.L. & Bania, T.C. (2000). Severe gamma-hydroxybutyrate withdrawal: A case report and literature review. *Journal of Emergency Medicine, 18,* 65–70.

Devenyi, P. & Harrison, M.L. (1985). Prevention of alcohol withdrawal seizures with oral diazepam loading. *Canadian Medical Association Journal, 132,* 798–800.

DuPont, R.L. (1990). A physician's guide to discontinuing benzodiazepine therapy. *Western Journal of Medicine, 152,* 600–603.

Dyer, J.E., Roth, B. & Hyma, B.A. (2001). Gamma-hydroxybutyrate withdrawal syndrome. *Annals of Emergency Medicine, 37,* 147–153.

Erstad, B.L. & Cotugno, C.L. (1995). Management of alcohol withdrawal. *American Journal of Health-System Pharmacy, 52,* 697–709.

Eustace, L.W., Kang, D.H. & Coombs, D. (2003). Fetal alcohol syndrome: A growing concern for health care professionals. *Journal of Obstetric, Gynecologic, and Neonatal Nursing, 32,* 215–221.

Fergusson, D.M., Horwood, L.J. & Swain-Campbell, N. (2002). Cannabis use and psychosocial adjustment in adolescence and young adulthood. *Addiction, 97,* 1123–1135.

Freed, E.X. (1981). Changes in weekly self-ratings of depression by hospitalized alcoholics. *Journal of Psychiatric Treatment and Evaluation, 3,* 451–454.

Furlan, A.D., Chaparro, L.E., Irvin, E. & Mailis-Gagnon, A. (2011). A comparison between enriched and non-enriched enrolment randomized withdrawal trials of opioids for chronic non-cancer pain. *Pain Research and Management, 16*, 337–351.

Garbutt, J.C., West, S.L., Carey, T.S., Lohr, K.N. & Crews, F.T. (1999). Pharmacological treatment of alcohol dependence: A review of the evidence. *Journal of the American Medical Association, 281*, 1318–1325.

Gowing, L.R., Henry-Edwards, S.M., Irvine, R.J. & Ali, R.L. (2002). The health effects of ecstasy: A literature review. *Drug and Alcohol Review, 21*, 53–63.

Gurley, R.J., Aranow, R. & Katz, M. (1998). Medicinal marijuana: A comprehensive review. *Journal of Psychoactive Drugs, 30*, 137–147.

Hambrecht, M. & Hafner, H. (2000). Cannabis, vulnerability, and the onset of schizophrenia: An epidemiological perspective. *Australian and New Zealand Journal of Psychiatry, 34*, 468–475.

Hammond, D., Ahmed, R., Yang, W.S., Brukhalter, R. & Leatherdale, S. (2011). Illicit substance use among Canadian youth: Trends between 2002 and 2008. *Canadian Journal of Public Health, 102*, 7–12.

Hasin, D.S., Keyes, K.M., Alderson, D., Wang, S., Aharonovich, E. & Grant, B.F. (2008). Cannabis withdrawal in the United States: Results from NESARC. *Journal of Clinical Psychiatry, 69*, 1354–1363.

Henry, J.A., Oldfield, W.L. & Kon, O.M. (2003). Comparing cannabis with tobacco. *British Medical Journal, 326*, 942–943.

Holbrook, A.M., Crowther, R., Lotter, A., Cheng, C. & King, D. (1999). Meta-analysis of benzodiazepine use in the treatment of acute alcohol withdrawal. *Canadian Medical Association Journal 160*, 649–655.

Honarmand, K., Tierney, M.C., O'Connor, P. & Feinstein, A.(2011.). Effects of cannabis on cognitive function in patients with multiple sclerosis. *Neurology, 76*, 1153–1160.

Inskip, H.M., Harris, E.C. & Barraclough, B. (1998). Lifetime risk of suicide for affective disorder, alcoholism and schizophrenia. *British Journal of Psychiatry, 172*, 35–37.

Johns, A. (2001). Psychiatric effects of cannabis. *British Journal of Psychiatry, 178*, 116–122.

Johnson, B.A., Ait-Daoud, N., Bowden, C.L., DiClemente, C.C., Roache, J.D., Lawson, K. et al. (2003). Oral topiramate for treatment of alcohol dependence: A randomised controlled trial. *The Lancet, 361*, 1677–1685.

Johnson, B.A., Roache, J.D., Javors, M.A., DiClemente, C.C., Cloninger, C.R., Prihoda, T.J. et al. (2000). Ondansetron for reduction of drinking among biologically predisposed alcoholic patients: A randomized controlled trial. *Journal of the American Medical Association, 284*, 963–971.

Kahan, M. & Wilson, L. (Eds.). (2002). *Management of Alcohol, Tobacco and Other Drug Problems: A Pocket Guide for Physicians and Nurses.* Toronto: Centre for Addiction and Mental Health.

Kaltenbach, K., Berghella, V. & Finnegan, L. (1998). Opioid dependence during pregnancy: Effects and management. *Obstetrics and Gynecology Clinics of North America, 25*, 139–151.

Kaltenbach, K. & Finnegan, L. (1998). Prevention and treatment issues for pregnant cocaine-dependent women and their infants. *Annals of the New York Academy of Sciences, 846*, 329–334.

Keller, R.W., Jr. & Snyder-Keller, A. (2000). Prenatal cocaine exposure. *Annals of the New York Academy of Sciences, 909*, 217–232.

Killestein, J., Hoogervorst, E.L., Reif, M., Kalkers, N.F., Van Loenen, A.C., Staats, P.G. et al. (2002). Safety, tolerability, and efficacy of orally administered cannabinoids in MS. *Neurology, 58*, 1404–1407.

Lader, M. (1994). Anxiolytic drugs: Dependence, addiction and abuse. *European Neuro-psychopharmacology, 4*, 85–91.

Lowenstein, S.R., Weissberg, M.P. & Terry, D. (1990). Alcohol intoxication, injuries, and dangerous behaviors—and the revolving emergency department door. *Journal of Trauma, 30*, 1252–1258.

Maldonado, J.R. & Keeffe, E.B. (1997). Liver transplantation for alcoholic liver disease: Selection and outcome. *Clinics in Liver Disease, 1*, 305–321.

Mann, R.E., Adlaf, E., Zhao, J., Stoduto, G., Ialomiteanu, A., Smart, R.G. & Asbridge, M. (2007). Cannabis use and self-reported collisions in a representative sample of adult drivers. *Journal of Safety Research, 38*, 669–674.

Martin-Sanchez, E. (2009.). Systematic review and meta-analysis of cannabis treatment for chronic pain. *Pain Medicine, 10*, 1353–1368.

Mihas, A.A. & Tavassoli, M. (1992). Laboratory markers of ethanol intake and abuse: A critical appraisal. *American Journal of Medical Sciences, 303*, 415–428.

Nocon, A., Wittchen, H.U., Pfister, H., Zimmermann, P. & Lieb, R. (2006). Dependence symptoms in young cannabis users? A prospective epidemiological study. *Journal of Psychiatric Research. 40*, 394–403.

Osborn, D.A., Cole, M.J. & Jeffery, H.E. (2002). Opiate treatment for opiate withdrawal in newborn infants. *Cochrane Database of Systematic Reviews, 2002* (3): CD002059.

Parssinen, M. & Seppala, T. (2002). Steroid use and long-term health risks in former athletes. *Sports Medicine, 32*, 83–94.

Pennings, E.J., Leccese, A.P. & Wolff, F.A. (2002). Effects of concurrent use of alcohol and cocaine. *Addiction, 97*, 773–783.

Petursson, H. (1994). The benzodiazepine withdrawal syndrome. *Addiction, 89*, 1455–1459.

Pimlott, N. & Kahan, M. (2000). Management of benzodiazepine dependence and withdrawal. In B. Brands (Ed.), *Management of Alcohol, Tobacco and Other Drug Problems: A Physician's Manual* (pp. 154–170). Toronto: Centre for Addiction and Mental Health.

Rey, J.M., Sawyer, M.G., Raphael, B., Patton, G.C., & Lynskey, M. (2002). Mental health of teenagers who use cannabis. Results of an Australian survey. *British Journal of Psychiatry, 180*, 216–221.

Salloum, I.M., Daley, D.C., Cornelius, J.R., Kirisci, L. & Thase, M.E. (1996). Disproportionate lethality in psychiatric patients with concurrent alcohol and cocaine abuse. *American Journal of Psychiatry, 153*, 953–955.

Single, E., Robson, L., Rehm, J. & Xie, X. (1999). Morbidity and mortality attributable to alcohol, tobacco, and illicit drug use in Canada. *American Journal of Public Health, 89,* 385–390.

Solowij, N., Stephens, R.S., Roffman, R.A., Babor, T., Kadden, R., Miller, M. et al. (2002). Cognitive functioning of long-term heavy cannabis users seeking treatment. *JAMA, 287,* 1123–1131.

Soyka, M. (1994). Alcohol dependence and schizophrenia: What are the interrelationships? *Alcohol and Alcoholism* (Suppl. 2), 473–478.

Urbanoski, K.A., Strike, C.J. & Rush, B.R. (2005). Individuals seeking treatment for cannabis-related problems in Ontario: Demographic and treatment profile. *European Addiction Research, 11,* 115–123.

Vecellio, M., Schopper, C. & Modestin, J. (2003). Neuropsychiatric consequences (atypical psychosis and complex-partial seizures) of ecstasy use: Possible evidence for toxicity-vulnerability predictors and implications for preventative and clinical care. *Journal of Psychopharmacology, 17,* 342–345.

Verheyden, S.L., Henry, J.A. & Curran, H.V. (2003). Acute, sub-acute and long-term subjective consequences of "ecstasy" (MDMA) consumption in 430 regular users. *Human Psychopharmacology, 18,* 507–517.

Warner, E.A. (1993). Cocaine abuse. *Annals of Internal Medicine, 119,* 226–335.

Watson, S.J., Benson, J.A., Jr. & Joy, J.E. (2000). Marijuana and medicine: Assessing the science base—A summary of the 1999 Institute of Medicine report. *Archives of General Psychiatry, 57,* 547–552.

Weisdorf, T. (2000). Cannabis. In B. Brands (Ed.), *Management of Alcohol, Tobacco and Other Drug Problems: A Physician's Manual* (pp. 203–208). Toronto: Centre for Addiction and Mental Health.

Williams, C.M. & Skinner, A.E.G. (1990). The cognitive effects of alcohol abuse: A controlled study. *British Journal of Addiction, 85,* 911–917.

Wong, S, Ordean, A. & Kahan, M. (2011). Substance use in pregnancy: A clinical practice guideline. *Journal of the Society of Obstetrics and Gynecology of Canada, 33,* 367–384.

Wright, C. & Moore, R.D. (1990). Disulfiram treatment of alcoholism. *American Journal of Medicine, 188,* 647–655.

SECTION 2

CLINICAL INTERVENTIONS

Chapter 8

Screening and Assessment Practices

Linda Sibley

Scarlett is a 24-year-old woman who has been experiencing periods of sadness since she was 14. She sometimes drinks to feel better. She has always felt different from other women her age and is not interested in dating. After a childhood car accident left her unconscious for several hours, she began to have difficulties at school. She managed to graduate from high school, but continued to have trouble focusing on things.

Scarlett was caught for underage drinking several times but has had no legal problems. She has been moderately active socially and has a few close friends. Over the years, she has seen her family doctor for various concerns and tells her family that she feels "down and stressed out." Her doctor has prescribed antidepressants, which she takes inconsistently, a fact that concerns her parents. Scarlett says the medication "isn't going to help anyway."

Over the years, her family has set up appointments for her with counsellors, but she then drops out, saying the counsellors "don't understand me." Her family has never had the opportunity to be involved in a case conference with her family physician or counsellors to find out more about why these sessions aren't helping.

The family is concerned because since returning home after graduation from college, Scarlett has been out a lot at night drinking with friends. There is a lot of tension and conflict at home around her behaviour. Unbeknownst to her family, Scarlett has been experimenting with drugs since graduating from college. Her family has been urging her to search for full-time work and move out of the house, which has left Scarlett feeling unsupported, misunderstood and unable to follow through. Her parents have now held a family meeting with Scarlett and told her that they want her to make an appointment with the local addiction centre. They have given her an ultimatum, and she has agreed to follow through.

Screening and assessment are the foundation of good clinical practice in the treatment of substance use problems and other health care concerns. These two vital first steps determine clients' needs and preferences, their motivation for change, and the barriers and supports around achieving their personal goals.

The purpose of screening is to determine whether there is evidence of a problem. If the screening is positive, assessment follows, which allows the interviewer to determine the extent of the problem and how it has affected other areas of the person's life. In essence, an assessment involves gathering detailed information about the problem. These clinical activities help the interviewer and the client decide what next steps to consider and what the treatment plan might be.

The process of screening and assessment is sometimes quite fluid and difficult to define in practice. If the counsellor's role is to conduct both screening and assessment, the process may be seamless within a session, as well as from session to session. The transition from screening to assessment may even be imperceptible to the client, though there is a continuum, in that information acquired in determining the possibility of a problem can then be used to evaluate the nature and extent of the problem (Centre for Addiction and Mental Health [CAMH], 2006). The counsellor should explain these distinct phases to the client, so he or she knows what to expect.

Although this chapter focuses primarily on screening and assessing substance use problems, it is difficult to discuss these issues without also addressing mental health concerns and behavioural addictions (see Chapters 16 and 20). This chapter describes the properties and processes of screening and assessment and how information gathering in the screening phase leads to better outcomes in assessment and, ultimately, in the treatment planning phase. We discuss some current screening and assessment measures, but focus on the overarching principles of screening and assessment and the importance of these processes to the client and the clinician, as well as to the larger health care and social services system. Shared protocols in these two important phases create a common language between clinicians and sectors: we explore the role this connection plays in community development and strengthening the treatment system's capacity to serve the public.

Screening

It is important to screen for substance use concerns early in the counselling process. If the person doing the screening does not have the resources to provide a more comprehensive assessment or treatment, the client may need to be linked to other clinicians or agencies that can provide these services. A proper screening allows the interviewer (a health care provider, counsellor or therapist) to identify at the outset of the therapeutic relationship all or as many of the clinical issues the client brings to counselling as possible.

A "positive" screen for a specific issue (e.g., alcohol use problem, trauma) warrants further examination and a thorough discussion about choices to be made, opportunities for change and the relationship of this issue to other circumstances in the person's life.

Screening Procedures

Screening may be conducted over the phone or face to face. Virtual Internet screening protocols between agencies and institutions are implemented when clinical information can be securely transmitted. Some clinical websites have self-referral forms and self-tests that people can complete. The Ontario Telemedicine Network allows for video conferencing with client consent and also administers screening and assessment procedures.[1]

Screening in community-based addiction settings is done to determine whether the client is in the right place to receive the services delivered in that setting. If the client needs to be referred to a more appropriate setting, the screening process will help determine that need and be able to legitimize the referral so the reason for the referral can be explained in concrete terms to the client and family. Specialized or residential services may be required, which involve moving or referring clients to other programs, agencies or organizations. Unlike in an emergency department, wait times in community-based agencies are most often determined chronologically by order of contact or by date of physical attendance in a clinical setting, rather than by chronicity or acuity of symptoms.

The distress and urgency felt by people with substance use issues and the myths about motivation fuel the expectation that treatment providers should make an immediate referral to *treatment,* which unfortunately is still mostly understood as "residential programming." The public often misunderstands the importance of screening and assessment and wants to "get on with treatment," especially in urgent situations, for example, where regaining custody of children from child welfare or getting back to work are foremost in the client's mind. However, the screening process may uncover significant barriers that may impede the person's progress or ability to achieve his or her goals, and therefore is an important process that cannot be overlooked.

Because the addiction treatment system is under-resourced, wait-lists are common. Screening determines whether there is any evidence of substance use first and foremost, and next, whether there is any evidence of concerns about or consequences of use.

In some cases, screening will determine that the client has already made changes and that the current course of action is sufficient, in which case referrals to aftercare or other supports will be made.

Crises and practical concerns

Although seeking treatment for substance use problems is not always precipitated by a crisis, some event or set of circumstances has often occurred to draw attention to these problems. Clients themselves may have come to some realization that a problem exists, or someone close to them may have identified concerns about use or its consequences. It is not uncommon for legal, relationship or employment problems to be identified as the catalyst for change. Whatever reasons are identified, screening procedures and tools allow clinicians to systematically determine that a problem actually exists, as well as to

---

1 For more information about screening and assessment through the Ontario Telemedicine Network, visit www.otn.ca.

examine the source of the person's motivation for change and need for formalized external treatment or supports.

Historically, when clients present and report substance use problems, treatment professionals have rushed to provide solutions, for example, recommending abstinence when that goal may be premature, inappropriate or not helpful at the time. Screening protocols are needed to determine the problem and identify other immediate crises, health or mental health concerns, or other barriers to participating in the screening process.

Clients often have very practical concerns that, while they are not necessarily the purpose of the visit, must also be given priority. These concerns may include:

- shelter and housing
- food
- physical health care
- interpersonal crises.

To address these concerns, the clinician may take direct action or connect the client with relevant community resources. Supporting the client through any crisis is important in itself and helps build an ongoing connection (Skinner, 2005).

Clients may self-refer or be referred by another professional because of other unmet needs or critical situations related to issues such as withdrawal symptoms, overdose, violence, trauma, loss or legal problems that could or should interrupt the screening and assessment process.

Screening Practices by Setting

Screening determines whether substance use problems exist or have in the past, addresses the concerns the client identifies as the reason for coming for treatment, and explores any crises that may have precipitated the visit. Screening also allows the interviewer to explore whether the client is in a position to examine next steps.

In hospital emergency departments, triage determines which patient will be seen immediately and which patients will wait. Wait times may not be determined chronologically, and more serious health care problems will take precedence. Patients provide information about the acuity and severity of their symptoms or injuries and details of the situation (unless of course they aren't conscious or capable), which helps health care providers decide who should be seen first.

Injuries related to substance use may involve observable signs and symptoms, such as obvious intoxication or the distinct odour of alcohol or inhalants, or physical events attributed to specific drugs, such as cardiac incidents related to stimulant use. If the client is unconscious or incoherent, a toxicology screen is performed, which involves drawing blood to determine or confirm the presence of substances. Through triage processes, the patient's needs are identified and decisions are made about the next natural step in the process. Using a decision tree, these next steps might include doing X-rays and blood work or questioning the patient or the person accompanying the patient. The source and nature of the symptoms or injury and the context and circumstances may affect how quickly the patient will be seen and whether a referral to his or her family physician will be made.

Telehealth Ontario also triages clients. Registered nurses ask the caller screening questions and follow decision trees to make clinical decisions, recommendations and referrals. (Similar protocols are used with people calling or using Webchat through ConnexOntario.) The substance use, mental health and problem gambling referral agents follow protocols to help callers get to the next steps, whether those steps involve seeking emergency medical assistance, checking appointment availability across the province or virtually booking an appointment with a problem gambling treatment centre. Referrals are often made to addiction programs if a substance use problem is identified. For residential withdrawal management services, callers are screened primarily for evidence of intoxication (current or recent) or for symptoms of withdrawal to determine their eligibility. In terms of the continuum of care, this screening procedure is very similar to that of a hospital emergency department, where symptoms are quickly screened (triaged) to determine whether the person's level of need should be upgraded to requiring emergency medical services. Clients who do not require medical intervention to facilitate withdrawal or prevent life-threatening medical complications will be admitted to the residential or community withdrawal management service if beds are available. This is similar to the triaging that happens in the emergency department to consider medical complications that can exist during substance withdrawal.[2]

Screening and Assessment: Two Steps in Identifying Addiction-related Problems

Screening is conducted not only to determine where the client is at, but also to give the client positive teaching and feedback. It is the first step in the decisional algorithm described below.

If a screening for alcohol problems determines that there is no problem, the interviewer gives the person information about safe drinking limits and reinforces the person's healthy behaviours. The interviewer could also use this as an opportunity to explore why the person does not use alcohol: in some cases of abstinence, the person is actually an ex-user.

If there is no problem but the person has a family history of addiction or has had previous problems, the interviewer should provide relevant information in the session (e.g., about safe drinking guidelines, drinking and driving) and make a note to ask the client screening questions regularly if he or she is to return for follow-up.

If the risk of alcohol problems is low, with mild consequences, the interviewer should give advice and information (e.g., direct the client to an online tool to evaluate drinking;[3] suggest a book or brief counselling.)

---

2 For a fuller description of Ontario's withdrawal management service continuum and for other service definitions, visit www. connexontario.ca.
3 One example of an online tool people can use to evaluate their drinking is www.alcoholhelpcenter.net.

If the risk is moderate, the interviewer might recommend brief outpatient treatment and a more in-depth assessment.

If the problem appears to be severe, the client will qualify for the second step—a more in-depth assessment to determine eligibility and fit for more intensive treatment for addiction-related problems. (See Babor et al., 1989, Alcohol Use Disorders Identification Test [AUDIT] algorithm for levels.)

Screening for addiction problems needs to be a capacity in *all* health care and social service settings, while comprehensive assessment falls under the purview of specialized addiction treatment settings. The role of a decisional algorithm is to provide decision rules to make this process work effectively.

Assessment processes and tools engage the client further in a dialogue about clinical concerns and the impact of substances. Assessment tools allow the clinician to systematically explore each area of the client's life and his or her personal circumstances. The assessment process should encourage both client and clinician to examine together the biopsychosocial implications of substance use. In this process, the client participates fully in identifying and prioritizing issues and deciding what to do about each issue. The client retains full control over the pace of the examination, the steps to take and the timing for decisions about change. Should the client be less experienced in this process, the clinician can assist through education and teach the client how to identify issues, determine how important change is right now and develop a strategy for change. The clinician benefits by observing the knowledge level and experience the client has in identifying concerns and motivation for change. Through this exploration of issues and concerns, the clinician will be able to assess how much education will be required and which motivational interviewing strategies will be most effective. The clinician can then assist the client as much or as little as required in identifying issues and concerns, as well as in making the choices required to accomplish goals.

Standardized screening and assessment practices have greatly improved. Ontario has been using standardized assessment tools for more than a decade, and common screening tools are being shared in many regions of the province. Screening and assessment protocols may cross over communities, creating a more cohesive system for the client who needs this continuity of care.

Many communities and regions have developed shared screening protocols in addiction and mental health settings. In addiction settings, clinicians screen for mental health issues, and clinicians in mental health settings screen for addiction issues (CAMH, 2006). These shared protocols are referred to as "universal screening protocols."

The screening and assessment phases of care are quite distinct from one another in theory and practice, and require different tools. Role clarity is essential: interviewers should know when they are providing screening services and how this differs from assessment services.

Screening and assessment services may be offered in a single setting and with a single interviewer, or they may be offered by a series of staff in a program or agency. The client might attend a group interview for screening and be assessed individually, or may undergo an individual assessment first, followed by a group. The demand for service, the size of the community and the type of agency will determine these processes.

In some communities, one program or agency may screen and another will complete the assessment. Practitioners in primary care settings, other health care providers, school guidance counsellors and corrections professionals may screen clients and refer them to a specific addiction or mental health agency for assessment.

The specific tools used for screening and assessment may vary depending on the agency and the sector of health care or social services.

Screening and Assessment as Interpersonal Processes

Even more important than using the best screening and assessment tools is engaging and connecting with the client during the process. It is for this reason that some have argued that services should use their most skilled counsellors to do this part of the work. One evidence-based approach for screening and assessment is motivational interviewing (Miller & Rollnick, 2013). This approach has been shown to enhance client engagement in providing personal information and helping clients move forward with decisions and actions. Motivational interviewing is grounded in building empathic connection through empathic listening skills. For more about motivational interviewing, see Chapter 5.

The Stages of Change model provides another valuable framework for engaging clients who qualify for treatment but are ambivalent or not ready for change (Prochaska et al., 1995). This approach helps counsellors understand the client's perspective on change.

Even when faced with compelling reasons for change, some people have great difficulty accepting the need for change or identifying a desire for change. It is common for people with substance use problems to be referred by someone else (e.g., family, employers, doctors) without themselves recognizing the need for change. Clients who have been referred by others may be able to describe the stress they are experiencing, but may not link their substance use to other issues, such as marital conflict or workplace problems that led to disciplinary action resulting in the referral. Historically, these clients were said to be "in denial" of the "truth." By applying the stages of change paradigm, clinicians have come to understand that the client is not in denial, but rather, is in a different stage of understanding the issues and simply does not see what others see. Clients who present in this manner are considered to be in the precontemplation stage (DiClemente, 2003).

Typically, the family member or other referral source is less ambivalent about the client's need for change, and this disparity may have already been a source of discord. Careful screening and assessment avoid falling into the trap of premature referral to treatment, which is usually unsuccessful. Empathically engaging the client—sometimes even in the initial phone call—is critical.

Figure 8-1 illustrates the Stages of Change model (Prochaska et al., 1995). The clinician's task varies depending on what stage the client is at. Traditionally, clinicians have presumed that the client is in the action stage. The Stages of Change model allows the clinician to determine the client's stage of change and make a response appropriate to that stage.

FIGURE 8-1: The Stages of Change Model

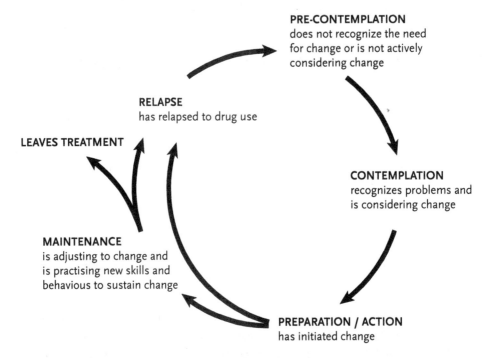

PRE-CONTEMPLATION
does not recognize the need for change or is not actively considering change

RELAPSE
has relapsed to drug use

LEAVES TREATMENT

CONTEMPLATION
recognizes problems and is considering change

MAINTENANCE
is adjusting to change and is practising new skills and behaviours to sustain change

PREPARATION / ACTION
has initiated change

Scarlett's parents identified the issues they were concerned about, and were pushing for action. Scarlett agreed to make an appointment at an addiction agency because of her parents' ultimatum. She will likely attend the appointment not having made any decisions about whether she wants to cut down on her drinking, and without being aware of the relationship between her not getting a job and her substance use. Scarlett does not see what others around her see, and she does not identify her behaviours as problematic. This indicates that Scarlett is in the precontemplation stage of change.

Although Scarlett's family may feel the right to be concerned, Scarlett may not be drinking and partying any more than do her friends. If the family confronts Scarlett about her drinking, she will be unable to hear the family's concern or objectively assess for herself whether her drinking is a problem. If Scarlett makes an appointment at the local addiction centre to placate her parents, she may procrastinate by booking it for a few weeks away, then deciding not to attend the appointment, and then waiting to re-book.

Common Screening Questions

Remember that the purpose of screening is not to determine the degree of the problem, but to determine whether a problem exists and whether a comprehensive assessment is needed. Each substance use or behaviour-related problem can be screened with a few basic questions. This is a good opportunity not only to ask these questions, but also to educate clients about healthy behaviours or about the need to examine more risky ones.

Not every screening protocol involves implementing tools or measures right away. For example, health care workers and people working in primary care or social services can ask basic questions about alcohol consumption to determine whether referral to an addiction centre might be needed. A series of well-placed questions in a conversation can elicit important information and be less intimidating for clients who are nervous about formal testing measures.

Basic questions should be used in a "universal" way; this means that the clinician asks the same questions of every client in a standardized interview or with a questionnaire. Simple questions can be dispersed throughout an interview. The clinician should normalize use (rather than using judgmental language implying that the client's substance use is abnormal). The clinician should also explain to the client why questions are being asked and what will happen with the information. Clients should know that they can speak freely and ask questions. Referrals to virtual sources of information or self-tests may be a good idea, as some clients want to educate themselves. If clinicians in primary care or community care settings can ask only one question, such as "Have you had more than five drinks on any one occasion over the last three months?" (for a man) or "Have you had more than four drinks?" (for a woman), and the client answers "no," further questions are not needed (Fleming et al., 1997).

Examples of basic questions about alcohol use might include:
- How often do you have a drink containing alcohol?
- How many drinks containing alcohol do you have on a typical day when you are drinking?
- Are there times when you drink more than this?
- What negative consequences have resulted from your use of alcohol? (CAMH, 2008)

These types of questions inform the clinician about the client's patterns and frequency of drinking. They also provide a sense of the person's alcohol tolerance, and a quick but silent guess about the person's weight will determine how intoxicated he or she should be with a given amount of alcohol. (Smaller men and women should feel more intoxicated and have a higher blood alcohol level.)

A more comprehensive screening would address tobacco use, specific types of substance use and addictive behaviours such as gambling, sex and Internet use.[4]

Affirmative answers to basic screening questions mean the interviewer should then use a formal screening tool and steer the conversation in that direction. The

[4] For sample screening questions about prescription and over-the-counter drug use, and use of illegal drugs, inhalants and tobacco, see *Substance Use, Concurrent Disorders and Gambling Problems in Ontario: A Guide for Helping Professionals* (CAMH, 2008), p. 19. For questions about gambling, see p. 49.

clinician should keep in mind that the client may have also already shared that he or she is not at all concerned about substance use or its long-term effects.

Some people share more information in a conversation than through a questionnaire or test. Computerized tests may appeal to any client: don't assume that only youth and young adults will prefer to use a computer. Most often in practice, a combination of computer, questionnaire and conversation is used.

Best Practice in Screening for Substance Use and Mental Health Disorders (Health Canada, 2002) suggests the following three screening questions, which should be investigated further if the person responds "yes" to one or more of them:

- Have you ever had any problems related to your use of alcohol or other drugs?
- Has a relative or friend, or a doctor or other health worker, been concerned about your drinking or other drug use, or suggested you cut down?
- Have you ever said to another person, "I don't have a problem" (with alcohol or other drugs) when, around the same time, you wondered whether you did have a problem? (Health Canada, 2002)

It is a good idea to practise asking these questions in an objective way that is non-judgmental and does not imply how much is "too much."

Returning to the case study of Scarlett, screening for the appropriateness of the referral will need to consider the following issues:

- Scarlett's stage of change
- evidence that there is some past or current concern about her substance use
- whether the referral is mandated (e.g., by probation, child welfare, physician)
- whether Scarlett is starting at the right place on the continuum of care. Is she in withdrawal from substances? Medically or mentally fragile?
- any previous experiences with the treatment system, including assessments or seeking assistance for substance use problems.

Scarlett's responses to the following questions will shape next steps in booking an appointment:

- How can I help you?
- How did you hear about our program?
- Are you currently using substances?
- Do you have substance use concerns or feel you have a problem?
- Do you feel you need assistance?
- Are you having any other concerns you wish to share?
- Is your family doctor aware of your decision to make an appointment?

The goal will be to get Scarlett to physically attend or commit to checking out the information virtually and then to call back. In most settings, screening activities include eliciting routine demographic information. Screening also asks about other issues; for example, in the case of Scarlett:

- What does Scarlett want? What are her intentions?

- What prompted Scarlett to attend this appointment (i.e., has there been a crisis? Are her basic needs for food, shelter and safety being met)?

Many agencies in Ontario offer education or information sessions about programs and choices available to people like Scarlett. Scarlett might be directed to ConnexOntario to learn about treatment options in her community, or to a social media site to learn from other people's experiences and stories.[5] Scarlett should be assured about her right to choose for herself and to decide what to do independent of her family. If she attends an initial session, she should be praised for going, given that it was her parents' concern, not her own, that motivated making an appointment. It may be helpful to explain that the session provides an opportunity for Scarlett to explore her substance use with no expectation that she acknowledge that a problem exists or commit to change. Scarlett may get information that can generate insights into improving her health and wellness. At this point, there is no clear indication that there is a substance use problem or that there is anything else of concern for Scarlett.

Admission and discharge criteria

Across jurisdictions, it is important to know admission and discharge criteria. In 2000, Ontario's admission and discharge criteria were created to assist with clinical decision making related to where to start with a client in screening, and how to progress in assessment to make treatment planning decisions. The admission and discharge criteria can be found in Appendix A of the *Admission and Discharge Criteria and Assessment Tools Clinical Manual: Helping Clients Navigate Addiction Treatment in Ontario Using the Admission and Discharge Criteria and Standardized Tools* (Cross & Sibley, 2010).

Initial screening and problem identification activities allow practitioners to identify the need for withdrawal and stabilization services, medical and psychiatric services or residential supports. These are important first steps in determining how to support clients as they begin to consider behaviour change. Practitioners need to rule out any physical health or safety issues or environmental concerns that may interfere with next steps to ensure the client is stable enough to act on referrals and invest in the treatment plan. Figure 8-2 presents a decision tree from Ontario's admission and discharge criteria (Cross & Sibley, 2010), outlining the systematic thinking that guides priority setting with clients.

---

5 One social media site where people share their experiences and stories is www.its-possible.ca.

FIGURE 8-2: Admission Decision Tree

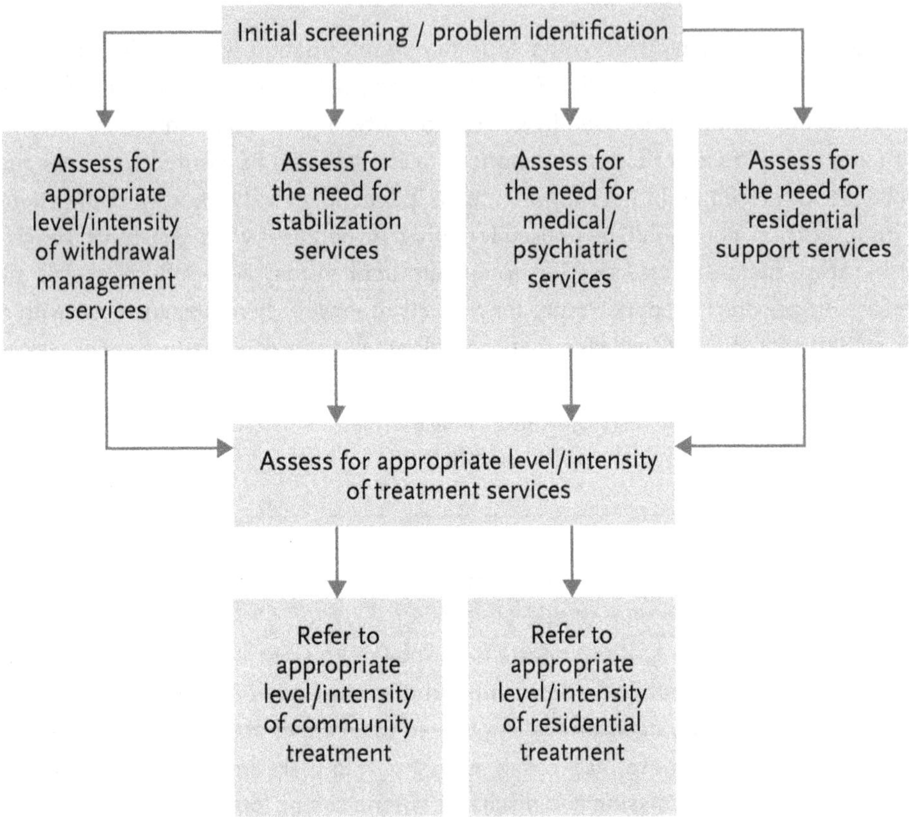

```
                    ┌──────────────────────────────────────────┐
                    │  Initial screening / problem identification │
                    └──────────────────────────────────────────┘
        │               │                  │                    │
        ▼               ▼                  ▼                    ▼
  ┌───────────┐  ┌───────────┐      ┌───────────┐        ┌───────────┐
  │ Assess for │  │ Assess for │      │ Assess for │        │ Assess for │
  │appropriate │  │the need for│      │the need for│        │the need for│
  │level/      │  │stabilization│     │medical/    │        │residential │
  │intensity   │  │services    │      │psychiatric │        │support     │
  │of withdrawal│ │            │      │services    │        │services    │
  │management  │  │            │      │            │        │            │
  │services    │  │            │      │            │        │            │
  └───────────┘  └───────────┘      └───────────┘        └───────────┘
        │               │                  │                    │
        │               ▼                  ▼                    │
        │      ┌─────────────────────────────────────┐         │
        └─────▶│ Assess for appropriate level/intensity│◀────────┘
               │       of treatment services          │
               └─────────────────────────────────────┘
                      │                    │
                      ▼                    ▼
               ┌───────────┐        ┌───────────┐
               │ Refer to   │        │ Refer to   │
               │appropriate │        │appropriate │
               │level/      │        │level/      │
               │intensity   │        │intensity   │
               │of community│        │of residential│
               │treatment   │        │treatment   │
               └───────────┘        └───────────┘
```

Source: Cross & Sibley (2010).

Benefits of Standardized Screening and Assessment

Routine consistent screening and assessment ensure that the same kind of information is elicited from each client, providing useful data from which to determine program needs and funding requirements to enhance clinical practice.

When a client is reassessed, either during or after treatment, any change in the client's scores can yield useful information about the client's progress. If a client leaves treatment and re-enters, screening and assessment results can be compared over time to determine whether improvement or deterioration has occurred.

Sharing consistent screening and assessment tools also makes it easier to communicate results to other clinicians. Using standardized measures across the service system creates a common language to improve understanding and ensure that referrals are more effective. These measures also reduce duplication of screening activities and assessments.

In Ontario, standardized assessment tools measure factors associated with the seven categories of client strengths and needs outlined below. These seven Admission and Discharge Criteria and Assessment Tools (ADAT) criteria are used as the basis for admission, treatment planning, referral and discharge decisions (Cross & Sibley, 2010). They closely resemble the six dimensions described by the American Society of Addiction Medicine.[6]

The seven ADAT criteria (Cross & Sibley, 2010) used in assessment are:

1. **Acute intoxication and withdrawal needs:** How intoxicated does the client get and which withdrawal symptoms are evident, if any?

2. **Emotional/behavioural needs:** Are there unmet or ongoing needs that can influence the treatment plan?

3. **Medical/psychiatric needs:** Are there unmet or ongoing needs that can influence the treatment plan?

4. **Treatment readiness:** How ready does the client appear to be to be able to make changes, and in which areas? A stage-based approach should be used to prepare the client using motivational interviewing techniques and respecting client choice.

5. **Recovery environment:** Is there evidence of support in the client's home environment? Does the client require stabilization services or other supports?

6. **Relapse potential:** Is there risk of relapse, and how much support might be required to achieve stated goals?

7. **Barriers and resources:** Are there personal, situational or environmental barriers that could be a detriment to the success of the stated treatment plan or behaviour change goals? (pp. 22–23)

When examining each of these strengths and needs criteria, the clinician can work with the client to prioritize needs and determine referrals to addiction-related services or non-addiction supports and services. Assessment tools should map onto these seven areas. The Global Appraisal of Individual Needs (GAIN) created by Dennis (2010) at Chestnut Health Systems is an example of a suite of tools that work with criteria like Ontario's seven areas of strengths and needs. Chestnut Health's tools move from screening (GAIN-Short Screener) to quick or more involved assessment tools (GAIN-Quick or GAIN-Intensive). The GAIN tools are designed to assess the criteria outlined in the *Diagnostic and Statistical Manual of Mental Disorders* (American Psychiatric Association, 2000), with algorithms embedded in the computerized version of the tool to match client answers to treatment plan suggestions. GAIN tools are used across the United States and meet state or federal legislation requirements.

In Canada, the GAIN-Intensive is used in Quebec as the standardized measure for substance use problems, and is also being adopted by other Canadian provinces.

---

6 For the six dimensions of client strengths and needs identified by the American Society of Addiction Medicine, visit www.asam.org/publications/patient-placement-criteria.

Screening for Addictions and Co-occurring Problems

Screening tools are not meant to replace a clinician's judgment. However, they can provide a preliminary indication of whether a client has a substance use and/or mental health problem. Some tools (dimensional tools) measure the quantity or frequency of a parameter such as substance use, while others map onto diagnostic criteria and indicate whether a mental health or substance use disorder is likely to be present. After asking a few questions, the clinician can then introduce the idea of using an objective measure called a screening tool to gather more details about the client's use and determine next steps (chosen by the client).

Psychometric criteria used to evaluate screening tools are discussed in *Review of Diagnostic Screening Instruments for Alcohol and Other Drug Use and Other Psychiatric Disorders* (Dawe et al., 2002), published by Australia's Commonwealth Department of Health and Ageing.

CAGE-AID

The CAGE Questionnaire Adapted to Include Drugs (CAGE-AID) is widely used in health care and addiction and mental health settings to screen for substance use problems.

The following four questions screen for thoughts about cutting down consumption, annoyance at others suggesting you have a problem, guilt associated with use and whether use occurs the next day to offset withdrawal symptoms.

1. Have you felt you ought to **C**ut down on your drinking or drug use?
2. Have people **A**nnoyed you by criticizing your drinking or drug use?
3. Have you felt bad or **G**uilty about your drinking or drug use?
4. Have you ever had a drink or used drugs first thing in the morning to steady your nerves or to get rid of a hangover (**E**ye-opener)?

A score of two or more "yes" answers indicates a positive CAGE and further evaluation is indicated.

Source: Brown, R.L. & Rounds, L.A. (1995). Conjoint screening questionnaires for alcohol and drug abuse. *Wisconsin Medical Journal, 94*, 135–140. Reprinted with permission.

Screening for Barriers and Co-occurring Issues

In addition to screening to determine whether a referral for a substance use assessment is required, the clinician also screens for barriers or complexities that might impede the client's recovery or require specialized approaches or skills. Research shows that different populations within the addiction treatment system experience specific issues that can create barriers if they are not included in universal screening protocols. Such protocols have been developed for a range of problems that co-occur with addiction (e.g., trauma, acquired brain injury, gender identity issues), challenging clinicians to be comprehensive and client-centred. While addiction remains the focus of screening, other problem areas may need to be explored as well.

Screening protocols exist for problems other than psychoactive substance use:

- **Problem gambling:** universal screening in health and social settings uses the Canadian Problem Gambling Index (Ferris & Wynne, 2001).
- **Trauma:** screening questions and tools can be used with recent newcomers from war-torn countries or soldiers returning from combat. Rather than trying to elicit information or details about trauma, the clinician should adopt a trauma-informed approach, recognizing the possibility of trauma in the person's life and addressing it—not necessarily with direct questions, but with an approach that considers safety, choice and empowerment of the client. (See Chapter 17 for more information about trauma.)
- **Acquired brain injury:** screening determines whether there is evidence of brain injury or cognitive damage from substance use that will impair insight or prevent the person from being able to participate fully in a substance use treatment program. Given the high rates of violence resulting in brain injury among people who are homeless, clinicians working with this population should screen every client. (See Chapter 18 for more information about acquired brain injury.)
- **Gender identity and sexual orientation issues:** screening tools include the Asking the Right Questions interviewing approach (Barbara et al., 2007). Clinicians should work this approach into all clinical interactions. (See Chapter 25 on sexual orientation and gender identity.)
- **Health concerns or complications:** ADAT's health screening form can help determine whether referral to a medical practitioner or hospital is needed (Cross & Sibley, 2010). It is not uncommon for people with substance use problems to have serious health and dental problems or complications that become obvious during screening or assessment, requiring the process to be postponed until the client is medically stabilized.
- **Violence against women:** the Ontario Woman Abuse Screening Project universally screens women entering many community services across the province.[7]
- **Concurrent disorders:** screening can be done using the GAIN-SS, which is a CAMH-modified universal screening tool used by many mental health organizations to screen

---

7 For more information about the Ontario Woman Abuse Screening Project, visit www.womanabusescreening.ca.

for substance use and gambling problems, and by many addiction agencies to screen for mental health concerns, including eating disorders. An undetected co-occurring problem can result in clients being bounced between the substance use and mental health systems, making frequent visits to the emergency department or being hospitalized. (See Chapter 16 for more information about concurrent disorders.)

Culture and Diversity

Evidence-based practice indicates that all agencies, institutions and practitioners should be able to deal effectively and empathically with anyone who comes through the door.

Agencies supported by government funding that serve the public are required to serve anyone who needs assistance. Thus it is not a matter of choice that practitioners learn about cultures in their community, but a moral imperative. Many professional development opportunities exist to expand this knowledge, and agencies should develop policy statements and strategic plans that reflect the value of culture and diversity and serving everyone in the community. Some agencies state these ideals but do little to implement them in actual practice.

Practitioners involved in screening and assessment must be well informed about available culture-based services and how to refer to them.

Considerations for Trauma-informed Work

Because of the high prevalence of trauma among people with substance use and mental health problems, clinicians should consider the possibility of a trauma history before or during screening and assessment. According to the Women, Co-occurring Disorders and Violence Study, more than 91 per cent of study participants reported a history of physical abuse, and 90 per cent reported sexual abuse (Jean Tweed Centre, 2013). Other populations for high risk of trauma include Aboriginal people who were in residential schools, people referred by child welfare to addiction services, military personnel, police officers, firefighters, paramedics, 911 call centre staff, people who work with trauma survivors, and witnesses of crime, natural disaster and family loss. Clinicians who work with these people need training about the relationship between trauma and substance use problems. Knowing about local programs and services that provide trauma treatment is critical to treatment planning.

Traumatic experiences may interfere with the client's ability to trust the clinician. Clinicians who observe guardedness in the client should consider the possibility of trauma and try to promote safety in the interview by being supportive and gentle, rather than trying to "break through" evasiveness that might look like resistance or denial. Questions should be asked in a way that does not retraumatize the client.[8]

---

8 For more information about working with clients who have trauma histories, see *Bridging Responses: A Front-Line Worker's Guide to Supporting Women Who Have Post-Traumatic Stress* (Haskell, 2001). The information does not apply exclusively to female clients.

Considerations for LGBTQ Communities

Issues around sexual orientation and gender identity do not necessarily make people more susceptible to substance use or mental health problems. However, stress or uncertainty in these areas may relate to the client's substance use, or to suicidal or self-harming behaviour (CAMH, 2012).

Screening questions can be used to determine whether issues around gender and sexual orientation are linked to substance use problems. If the screening reveals concerns, the assessment can explore them with specific questions or the clinician can use tools from the Asking the Right Questions manual (Barbara et al., 2007).

Screening questions can include asking how the client identifies in terms of gender identity and sexual orientation, and whether the client has a partner and how that partner identifies (demographic questions asked at intake may already request this information). Traditionally, clinicians have not explicitly asked about clients' sexual orientation and gender identity, and have assumed heterosexuality. But being in a heterosexual relationship does not mean a person identifies as heterosexual. Asking these questions can also be useful in determining the client's need for information about harm reduction and access to harm reduction supplies, and education about safer sex practices.

Interviewers who assume a client's heterosexuality send a message that they do not accept other identities and orientations. This bias can discourage clients from sharing important information. The interviewer should refer to an "intimate partner" or "significant other" as opposed to boyfriend, girlfriend, husband or wife. (Practitioners may erroneously assume the opposite gender when the client says "I am married" or "I have a spouse.")

Clinicians must also be careful not to pathologize or imply a pathological connection between clients' mental health and substance use concerns and their gender identity or sexual orientation. Appropriate signage can open discussion, just as displaying rainbow flags, stickers or symbols can open doors for clients so they know the environment is safe. The language used in the context of triage, screening or assessment must also create safety. The word "straight" has another meaning in the addiction field, so clinicians should not talk about "getting straight" because this language may be misunderstood.

Issues of sexual orientation and gender identity may be particularly sensitive among particular populations and cultures, such as youth. Interviewers should be discreet when speaking with families or other community members. Even seemingly benign inferences about a client's sexuality could make clients susceptible to bullying and other forms of discrimination. The interviewer should be aware of safety planning and other support services, and discuss possible referrals for the client as needed.

Clients Who Are Intoxicated

Clients may arrive for appointments under the influence of substances. Policies need to be in place to guide staff in these situations. When clients book an appointment, they need to be told that they must not arrive intoxicated. This will be difficult for clients who use daily, who are under stress or who are dependent on the substance and risk withdrawal. A solid understanding of harm reduction activities and techniques is very important in this work. Some drug use is more obvious than others: some substances have no odour and sometimes a client may not appear to be intoxicated.

In most clinical outpatient settings, clients who are obviously intoxicated will not be screened or assessed. However, the client could be referred to community or residential withdrawal management programs or to primary care (walk-in or urgent care centres) or emergency departments when warranted medically.

If the client is at risk to self or others, the clinician should follow agency protocols about risk assessment, referral and safety planning.[9]

If a client shows up for the appointment intoxicated, it is important to arrange safe transportation home. The clinician should ask about dependents and their whereabouts (i.e., underage children in child care, schools or at home) and safety in order to determine how to proceed. If the client has driven to the appointment, the clinician must explain that his or her keys will be taken away and alternative transportation arranged for the person's own safety and that of the public. If the person refuses to surrender the keys or leaves, the clinician must call 911. Intoxicated clients who arrive at the appointment on foot or by bicycle can also be a danger to themselves or others. The clinician must follow protocols established in the agency's policies and procedures.

Clients with Acquired Brain Injury or Fetal Alcohol Spectrum Disorder

Clients with an acquired brain injury (ABI) may have difficulty with concentration, memory, judgment and task initiation and completion; they may experience headaches or outbursts; and they may not be able to live independently. These are issues that are also common among people with substance use problems. The clinician must screen to determine whether the client's difficulties are related to an old or recent acquired brain injury (ABI).[10]

People referred to addiction treatment may have other diagnoses, such as fetal alcohol spectrum disorder (FASD), or they may have experienced accidents or injuries. Therefore, it is important to screen for other diagnoses and ask about past or recent accidents, injuries or violence. (See Chapter 18 for more information about ABI and FASD.)

---

9 Refer to the admission and discharge criteria in Appendix A of *Admission and Discharge Criteria and Assessment Tools Clinical Manual: Helping Clients Navigate Addiction Treatment in Ontario Using the Admission and Discharge Criteria and Standardized Tools* (Cross & Sibley, 2010).
10 One commonly used ABI screening tool is the HELPS. It is available at https://www.hnfs.com/va/static/rmh/4_helps_tbi.pdf.

Prolonged use of inhalants and non-beverage alcohol (e.g., mouthwash, rubbing alcohol) can cause cognitive damage. Clients with a history of using these substances need medical attention to determine the effects on brain functioning.

As with spinal injuries, a correlation exists between ABI and substance use problems. Some clients acquired the brain injury while under the influence of alcohol or other drugs.[11] In the recovery process, they may re-engage with substances. Some clients use substances to cope with feelings of aggression or anger.

The following are populations that may warrant screening for ABI or for evidence of cognitive damage caused by substance use problems:

- clients who have had sports injuries causing concussion (e.g., ice skating, soccer, snowboarding, skiing)
- clients who have played contact sports with or without helmets
- victims of recent violence (e.g., clients living with violence in shelters, abusive home environments)
- war veterans who may have sustained a head injury from an explosion (trauma may also trigger substance use)
- inmates in correctional settings or released into the community.

The following basic screening questions can help determine the presence of an ABI:

- Do you have a diagnosis of an acquired brain injury?
- Do you suspect you may have had a brain injury?
- How long has it been since your first brain injury?
- Have you ever lost consciousness or had a concussion?
- How long was your loss of consciousness?
- How many concussions have you had?

Assessment

When screening suggests that a substance use problem might exist, an assessment is an important next step. The assessment provides more detailed information and scores that can help the clinician and client understand the severity of the problem and its impact on the client's life (e.g., health, relationships, employment).

The interviewer should share the results of the screening tools or protocols with the client and gather the client's impressions about the results using motivational interviewing techniques. Asking open-ended questions about scores and for the client's interpretations and feelings about the results yields important information about the stages of change and the client's decision-making process.

The assessment should be conducted using a standardized process or tool that has been tested scientifically. Some assessment tools are interview protocols such as the Ontario Common Assessment of Need, in which questions are asked consistently with

---

11 For more about the signs and symptoms of traumatic brain injury, see www.brainline.org/content/2008/07/signs-and-symptoms.html.

each client but do not necessarily result in a single score. Other assessment tools yield scores that are interpreted with the client to determine next steps.

The interviewer must get permission from the client to proceed with the assessment. The interviewer should be able to describe the tools and process, what will be measured, how long it will take and what results might be apparent. At each step, the interviewer gathers evidence and information about the issue and checks in with the client for permission to continue. This is experienced as a mutual exploration of each step and of each outcome or result. It is important for the interviewer to remain silent periodically during the assessment and to observe the client's body language and facial expressions and watch for signs of stress or discomfort in order to create a successful assessment experience.

The interviewer must give the client the opportunity to ask questions during the assessment. Some assessment tools are self-administered in groups or via computer and others are administered individually by an interviewer.

Assessment Tools and Protocols

The Addiction Severity Index (ASI), AUDIT, Substance Abuse Subtle Screening Inventory (SASSI) and ADAT are well-known assessment tools used in Ontario. ADAT has been used for more than a decade and was developed to assess clients' strengths and needs, which all assessment tools should identify because strengths-based assessment leads to strengths-based treatment planning. This approach allows treatment providers to understand and prioritize the client's concerns and goals and build a solid foundation starting with what the client feels most confident about. In contrast, a problem-based approach focuses on areas in which the client is least skilled, and may arouse in the client fear of relapse and other concerns about substance use. Examining strengths and needs is a positive approach to treatment planning in which previous successes are highlighted to motivate the client in working toward the changes he or she is now considering.

The assessment should be performed with the understanding that the client's current stage of change may influence his or her understanding of the results, and that the feedback may move the client to the next stage of change (DiClemente, 2003). Research shows that this personalized feedback can influence decision making (Emmen et al., 2011).

A thorough assessment yields the following information:
- quantity and frequency of substance use
- historical onset and evolution of use
- which substances lead to the use of others and what substances the client prefers
- substances the client has tried and disliked, quit attempts, periods of abstinence
- goals the client has set and met
- treatment experiences and outcomes
- connection between substance use and life areas, including physical health, withdrawal effects and symptoms, legal status, relationships, employment or school, mental health, financial status

- the client's expectations for the future, decisions the client has made about substance use
- the client's recovery environment and supports.

> Scarlett is still in the precontemplative stage of change, so the interviewer will gather information that can be developed into feedback to share with Scarlett to help her reduce the amount and frequency of her alcohol use. The interviewer suspects that Scarlett's drinking may be related to being closeted as a lesbian or having gender identity issues and that Scarlett drinks to cope. Based on the screening and conversations, the interviewer senses that Scarlett's family has no idea that she is worrying about her sexuality and has in fact struggled with this since adolescence, when her drinking began. Scarlett reports no current relationships or intimate partners and diverts the conversation when asked about this part of her life. The interviewer considers how to approach this conversation after the assessment. The assessment will focus on Scarlett's substance use and its relationship to her mental health.

Motivational Dynamics in Screening and Assessment

Strong evidence suggests that the process of screening and assessing for substance use concerns can either motivate or de-motivate clients, affecting their likelihood of staying in treatment. Motivational interviewing has been shown to enhance the assessment process (Miller & Rollnick, 2013). While some assessment tools do not allow the clinician to deviate from the script, motivational interviewing techniques can be applied after assessment, with the clinician asking for comments and feedback and then using reflection skills to enhance motivation and learning. Enhancing motivation using information from the assessment is critical to moving the client into the next stage of change. (See Chapter 5 for more about motivational interviewing.)

When the assessment process or tool allows for reflection or motivational interviewing techniques, the interviewer can stop to reflect on the client's body language or other non-verbal messages and probe for deeper meaning using motivational interviewing techniques.

Treatment Planning

This section examines the seven areas of need identified by ADAT (Cross & Sibley, 2010) to determine appropriate next steps and referrals for Scarlett:

1. **Acute intoxication and withdrawal needs:** Scarlett drinks more on the weekends but is not a daily drinker. Although she may benefit from learning about lower-risk alcohol consumption and blood alcohol levels to reduce risky behaviour such as impaired driving, no referrals are warranted at this time. Scarlett may benefit from harm reduction strategies.

2. **Emotional and behavioural needs:** Although Scarlett may benefit from supportive counselling and cognitive-behavioural therapy to increase her coping skills, she does not have major concerns about emotional or behavioural issues at this time. As Scarlett opens up to her counsellor and becomes more engaged in the therapeutic relationship, such issues may emerge, at which time referrals could be made.

3. **Medical and psychiatric needs:** The clinician should refer Scarlett for a general physical exam and tests to rule out brain injury from her car accident. She should also be referred for brain functioning tests.

4. **Treatment readiness:** Scarlett does not believe she needs treatment for her drinking. She is in the precontemplative stage of change. She may need education and information about safer drinking choices and referrals for supportive counselling.

5. **Recovery environment:** Despite some conflict with her parents around their concern about her drinking and unemployment, Scarlett generally has a supportive home environment.

6. **Relapse potential:** Scarlett is likely to continue her weekend binges with friends. She may agree to participate in education sessions to prevent legal problems such as an impaired driving charge. Should Scarlett wish to cut down on her drinking, the clinician can discuss techniques and strategies to help her.

7. **Barriers and resources:** Scarlett has some financial barriers, but she has social and family supports, financial support through her parents and a university degree. With some counselling supports and education, Scarlett will likely meet her goals.

Motivational interviewing techniques can be used to discuss Scarlett's high-risk binge drinking, and harm reduction techniques should be recommended. Treatment goals will need to be based on Scarlett's preferences and should address the coming-out process if Scarlett decides to come out to her parents and friends. A referral to an LGBTQ service may be a good idea. Scarlett may benefit from specific information about how to avoid legal problems related to drinking and driving. Learning harm reduction techniques and getting advice and information about blood alcohol levels, for example, through a remedial measures program, may be helpful. If Scarlett screens positive for an ABI, referral for further assessment and treatment will be necessary. If screening or assessment identifies a mood disorder, treatment planning and referrals must address this issue. Once a therapeutic relationship has been established with Scarlett and she feels more trust with her counsellor, other information may surface that may result in other referrals for Scarlett, if she agrees to them.

Community Development through Shared Protocols

Health Canada recommends that all people seeking help from mental health services be routinely screened for co-occurring substance use problems, and that all people seeking help from substance use services be screened for co-occurring mental health problems. This helps to ensure that people will be welcomed wherever or however they enter the system (the "no wrong door" approach), and will have seamless and timely access to services (CAMH, 2006).

Many communities are adopting co-ordinated access agreements across child and family services and mental health and addiction sectors. These agreements or integrated service delivery systems allow for easier access for the community with one phone number to call and, in some cases, multiple access centres across a region or community. Shared screening tools and processes open the doors for these co-ordinated service delivery options.

Shared screening protocols are an excellent vehicle for cross-sector collaboration and training. Increased access points are good for the community that needs them, and cross-sector collaborations allow for increased skill sets across clinical networks. New partnerships and other shared service delivery options become possible as staff work more closely together to decrease the fail points in the system. Funders have an expectation of collaboration and integrated service delivery to increase the efficiencies and effectiveness in health care and social services.

Clients and their families should not have to access multiple agencies for screening and assessment for each concern; accordingly, staff in agencies that serve people with mental health and addiction issues should be able to educate clients about all the choices available.

Conclusion

Screening and assessment should be viewed as ongoing processes, rather than as discrete single events that occur only at intake or at the start of a new treatment relationship. Addiction problems can be quite complex, and it often takes time for a clear understanding to emerge. Clients with addiction problems are a diverse group, with clinical features that can change or emerge over time. Clinicians can best help clients if they have comprehensive information, and screening represents the first step in this process.

Over the next decade, ongoing changes in the health care system will focus on integrated service delivery, co-ordinated access and opportunities for cross-training. Counsellors who work outside of the specialized addiction services sector but who see clients with addiction problems should learn screening skills, be knowledgeable about the addiction services sector and train to administer standardized tools.

Many clinical settings will implement assessment groups or will use groups for screening and assessment to reduce wait times and free up time for new groups to ensure timely interventions.

The availability of online self-tests will increase, giving people greater access to information about their risk addiction problems, and the potential for self-change. Mobile applications will also grow as more and more consumers rely on hand-held devices. Applications already exist with which people can determine themselves whether they have a Facebook addiction, for example.

People who prefer online advice or counselling to face-to-face meetings will have access to a growing number of counsellors with expertise in online addiction, including online gambling, gaming or other online behaviour issues.

Counsellors will need to be able to incorporate computerized screening and assessment tools into their daily work, and to be able to incorporate this information into the client's electronic health record and data collection systems.

New types of behavioural or process addictions related to social media, gaming and online gambling are emerging and share some of the features of addiction to substances, such as loss of control and continued use despite adverse consequences. (See Chapter 20 about process addictions). The same criteria for screening and assessing alcohol or other drug problems can be applied to these process addictions.

Practice Tips

- Ensure that the environment is welcoming to clients, their families and significant others, and other visitors, from the moment they place a phone call or drop by to the time they come to an appointment. First contact is a very influential time for engaging the client, whether it be virtual, via telephone or in person.
- Be on time and do not keep clients waiting. Waiting can increase clients' feelings of nervousness and vulnerability.
- Ensure that the area you are working in affords privacy to clients and that they are as comfortable as possible during the assessment.
- Explain to clients that confidentiality is strictly upheld, except when disclosure is required by law: these legal limitations should be explained.
- Screen all clients in non-specialized settings for addiction and related problems. All non-specialized agencies should have protocols for screening, responding to and referring clients with addiction-related issues.
- Offer clients who have screened positive for addiction problems a comprehensive assessment to determine the nature of the problem and explore their options. Make the assessment process client-centred and responsive to clients' issues and concerns, recognizing that the *how* of assessment may be more important than the *what* of assessment. Motivational interviewing skills provide an evidence-based way of accomplishing this: if you are not trained in motivational interviewing, make a point of doing so because it is central to clinical practice.
- Use clinical findings as an opportunity to give feedback to clients about the nature of their problems and about opportunities for getting help.

- Develop your ability to move easily through assessment tools and protocols by engaging in practice sessions with colleagues, observing others who have more experience, doing dry runs to practise explaining things out loud, and becoming familiar with the paperwork and other procedures your protocol requires. It is important that clients feel you are confident administering the tools and that the interview flows well. If you are new to the tool itself or the process of assessment, explain to clients that you are on a learning curve and are interested in their feedback.
- Familiarize yourself with the CCSA core competencies of the Canadian Centre on Substance Abuse (CCSA), specifically those relating to screening and assessment skills. They can be found on the CCSA website (CCSA, 2010).
- Explain the importance of standardized assessment, outlining the benefits to clients and their treatment plan. Ensure that clients understand that assessment is an important part of the process and that the information it yields will help them understand the impact of substance use on their lives.
- Ensure that a policy or guideline is in place at your agency or private practice regarding the use of social media and virtual contact . These policies should describe how technology should be used to maintain contact with the client.
- Write down details of the next visit for clients, including all contact information and the date and time of the next visit if you are referring someone in crisis. With clients' permission, you might also e-mail them the information for the next visit. This may be helpful in maintaining contact with clients.

Resources

Publications

Center for Substance Abuse Treatment. (2007). *Screening, Assessment, and Treatment Planning for Persons with Co-occurring Disorders*. Rockville, MD: Substance Abuse and Mental Health Services Administration. Retrieved from http://store.samhsa.gov

Centre for Addiction and Mental Health (CAMH). (2006). *Navigating Screening Options for Concurrent Disorders*. Toronto: Author.

Croton, G. (2007). *Screening for and Assessment of Co-occurring Substance Use and Mental Health Disorders by Alcohol & Other Drug and Mental Health Services*. Victoria, Australia: Victorian Dual Diagnosis Initiative Advisory Group. Retrieved from www.nada.org.au/media/14706/vddi_screening.pdf

Health Canada. (2002). General issues in screening. *Best Practice in Screening for Substance Use and Mental Health.* Ottawa: Author. Retrieved from www.hc-sc.gc.ca/ hc-ps/pubs/adp-apd/bp_disorder-mp_concomitants/screening-depistage-eng.php

References

American Psychiatric Association. (2000). *Diagnostic and Statistical Manual of Mental Disorders* (4th ed., text rev.). Washington, DC: Author.

Babor, T.F., de la Fuente, J.R., Saunders, J. & Grant, M. (1989). *AUDIT—The Alcohol Use Disorders Identification Test: Guidelines for Use in Primary Health Care.* Geneva: World Health Organization.

Barbara, A.M., Chaim, G. & Doctor, F. (2007). *Asking the Right Questions 2: Talking with Clients about Sexual Orientation and Gender Identity in Mental Health, Counselling and Addiction Settings.* Toronto: Centre for Addiction and Mental Health.

Canadian Centre on Substance Abuse (CCSA). (2010). *Competencies for Canada's Substance Abuse Workforce.* Ottawa: Author. Retrieved from www.ccsa.ca/eng/ priorities/workforce/competencies

Centre for Addiction and Mental Health (CAMH). (2006). *Navigating Screening Options for Concurrent Disorders.* Toronto: Author.

Centre for Addiction and Mental Health (CAMH). (2008). *Substance Use, Concurrent Disorders and Gambling Problems in Ontario: A Guide for Helping Professionals.* Toronto: Author.

Centre for Addiction and Mental Health (CAMH). (2012). Substance use: Issues to consider for the lesbian, gay, bisexual, transgendered, transsexual, two-spirit, intersex and queer communities. Retrieved from www.camh.ca/en/hospital/about_camh/ health_equity/Pages/substance_use_lgbtttiq.aspx

Cross, S. & Sibley, L.B. (2010). *Admission and Discharge Criteria and Assessment Tools Clinical Manual: Helping Clients Navigate Addiction Treatment in Ontario Using the Admission and Discharge Criteria and Standardized Tools.* Toronto: Centre for Addiction and Mental Health. Retrieved from https://knowledgex.camh.net/ amhspecialists/Screening_Assessment/assessment/adat/Documents/ adat_tools_criteria_manual.pdf

Dawe, S., Loxton, N.J., Hides, L., Kavanagh, D.J. & Mattick, R.P. (2002). *Review of Diagnostic Screening Instruments for Alcohol and Other Drug Use and Other Psychiatric Disorders* (2nd ed.). Canberra, Australia: Commonwealth Department of Health and Ageing. Retrieved from www.health.gov.au

Dennis, M.L. (2010). Global Appraisal of Individual Needs (GAIN): A Standardized Biopsychosocial Assessment Tool. Bloomington, IL: Chestnut Health Systems.

DiClemente, C.C. (2003). *Addiction and Change: How Addictions Develop and Addicted People Recover.* New York: Guilford Press.

Emmen, M.J., Schippers, G.M., Bleijenberg, G. & Wollersheim, H. (2011). The Drinker's Check-up: A brief motivational intervention for early-stage problem drinkers. In W.M. Cox & E. Klinger (Eds.), *Handbook of Motivational Counseling: Goal-Based Approaches to Assessment and Intervention with Addiction and Other Problems* (pp. 505–530). Chichester, United Kingdom: John Wiley & Sons.

Ferris, J. & Wynne, H. (2001). *The Canadian Problem Gambling Index: Final Report.* Ottawa: Canadian Centre on Substance Abuse.

Fleming, M.F., Barry, K.L., Manwell, L.B., Johnson, K. & London, R. (1997). Brief physician advice for problem alcohol drinkers: A randomized controlled trial in community-based primary care practices. *JAMA, 277,* 1039–1045.

Haskell, L. (2001). *Bridging Responses: A Front-Line Worker's Guide to Supporting Women Who Have Post-Traumatic Stress.* Toronto: Centre for Addiction and Mental Health.

Health Canada. (2002). General issues in screening. *Best Practice in Screening for Substance Use and Mental Health.* Ottawa: Author. Retrieved from www.hc-sc.gc.ca/hc-ps/pubs/adp-apd/bp_disorder-mp_concomitants/screening-depistage-eng.php

Jean Tweed Treatment Centre. (2013). *Trauma Matters: Guidelines for Trauma-Informed Practices in Women's Substance Use Services.* Toronto: Author. Retrieved from www.jeantweed.com

Miller, W.R. & Rollnick, S. (2013). *Motivational Interviewing: Helping People Change* (3rd ed.) New York: Guilford Press.

Prochaska, J., Norcross, J. & DiClemente, C. (1995). *Changing for Good: A Revolutionary Six Stage Program for Overcoming Bad Habits and Making Your Life Positively Forward.* New York: Avon Books.

Skinner, W. (2005). Identifying, assessing and treating concurrent disorders: The client-counsellor relationship. In W.J.W. Skinner (Ed.), *Treating Concurrent Disorders: A Guide for Counsellors* (pp. 17–28). Toronto: Centre for Addiction and Mental Health. Retrieved from http://knowledgex.camh.net/amhspecialists/Screening_Assessment/screening/Pages/engaging_client.aspx

Chapter 9

Brief Interventions for At-Risk Drinking

John A. Cunningham and David C. Hodgins

Eric is 27 years old and operates a front-end loader for a road construction company. He works long hours to capitalize on good weather and often goes out with "the boys" after work to have a few beers and wind down. If he were to count drinks, Eric would find that he drinks four to six beers each time and, on weekends, he drinks about double this amount. Eric doesn't focus much on his alcohol consumption and sees his drinking as pretty typical of men his age. Although he is not particularly concerned about his drinking, his girlfriend is often upset that he comes home late and then falls asleep in front of the television. She has often been embarrassed when he is loud and obviously intoxicated at social events, the latest being her sister's wedding. Eric knows that he frequently drives home with blood alcohol above the legal limit, but feels that he is a good driver nonetheless. He also has been getting to work late on some mornings after he has had a few more drinks than usual.

Eric's situation is a common one. His alcohol use is starting to affect different areas of his life, and he has an increased risk of developing health concerns down the road. Yet Eric's risky drinking is not that severe, and extended treatment (whether inpatient or extended outpatient) may not be warranted. The reality is that many people with the types of at-risk drinking Eric is experiencing may never even seek help (Cunningham & Breslin, 2004). For some, their risky drinking will get worse; others may "mature out" of their at-risk drinking and either not drink at all in later life or drink moderately (Dawson et al., 2005). Eric's situation illustrates how the severity of alcohol concerns occurs on a continuum. His drinking is well above low-risk guidelines for safe drinking, but still well below the severity of drinking sometimes seen in treatment settings. The challenge is to decide on the type of help that might best be suited for Eric.

But why is help warranted for people like Eric? First, the costs to society are substantially greater from people engaged in at-risk drinking than from people with severe alcohol use disorder, simply because there are so many more of them (Stockwell et al., 2004). Second, there is great value in secondary prevention—helping people before their risky drinking gets too severe. Not everyone receiving an intervention will go on to develop severe alcohol use disorder. However, if many people can be helped for less than it would cost to provide treatment for a few people with more serious alcohol concerns, then these secondary prevention efforts make good health services sense. Finally, and most important, people like Eric would benefit from help. Many people who drink above low-risk levels recognize this need and say they would be interested in help to deal with their alcohol concerns, particularly if the services provided are in a format that matches their lower severity of alcohol use problems.

This chapter describes brief interventions designed to help people who drink at risky levels. These interventions come in various forms and have been applied in different settings—from outpatient addiction services through primary care health settings, and including various self-help approaches (e.g., books, Internet-based interventions). We review these interventions and give concrete examples of how they might help someone like Eric. In the Resources section, we provide links to freely accessible tools for use in brief interventions.

Definitions

Before reviewing brief interventions, it is worthwhile to define what is meant by "at-risk drinking." This is an intentionally vague term that covers the range of drinkers, from those who drink beyond recommended levels to those who have recognizable consequences associated with their drinking (and might even display mild forms of alcohol use disorder). We use the term because it is often difficult to define the exact severity of problems of participants in the research we have reviewed. An excellent quote by Heather (1989) on brief interventions in community settings is as applicable today as it was two decades ago:

> Evidence shows that brief interventions are effective and should be used for individuals who are not actively seeking help at specialist agencies. This justification is, again, independent of level of seriousness, although most recipients of community-based interventions will obviously have problems of a less severe variety. Moreover, when potential clients are not actively seeking help, then the cost-effectiveness kind of argument does become relevant and it is ethically legitimate to ask what is the least expensive way of reaching the greatest number of smokers or excessive drinkers, etc. (p. 366)

Outpatient Addiction Settings

In reviews of the research evidence supporting the effectiveness of different treatment approaches, brief interventions are ranked highest (Miller et al., 2003). Brief interventions generally have a similar format, whether they are offered in an outpatient or primary care setting. The content of most brief interventions follows the model captured in the acronym FRAMES, as outlined by Miller and Rollnick (1991):

- provide **F**eedback about the person's drinking
- stress personal **R**esponsibility for change
- provide clear **A**dvice to cut down on drinking
- provide a **M**enu of options for reducing drinking
- use an **E**mpathic approach in interacting with the client
- support **S**elf-efficacy by enhancing beliefs about ability to change.

In an outpatient setting, the prototypical example of a brief intervention is the Drinker's Check-Up (Miller et al., 1988). In this two-session intervention, the first session involves assessing the client's alcohol use and its consequences. In the second session, the information from the assessment is provided as feedback to the client, who is encouraged to set goals regarding alcohol consumption. This basic structure can be reduced to a 20-minute session or expanded to several sessions, with goal-setting exercises and other cognitive-behavioural tools to help meet these goals.

Common to all these interventions is the therapist's style. The therapist orientation is motivational (the Empathic component of the FRAMES acronym) and clear advice is provided non-judgmentally. Clients are encouraged to verbalize their own treatment goals in order to promote "buy-in" for changing alcohol consumption. Miller (2000) discusses the role of this empathic style of therapist interaction as a key ingredient in brief interventions—the factor that can spark a fire that can lead to large changes. (See Chapter 5 on motivational interviewing.)

Primary Care Settings

Primary health care would seem to be an ideal setting for brief interventions. Most people access primary health care services each year, and many of the health concerns they voice are directly or indirectly related to high levels of alcohol consumption. Extensive research has demonstrated the efficacy of brief interventions in primary care settings for at-risk alcohol use (Kaner et al., 2007), and substantial knowledge translation work has promoted the use of brief interventions in this setting. However, these efforts have met with only limited success, as brief interventions are still rarely implemented and are not regarded by many primary health care workers as a necessary part of their everyday practice. Reasons for this lack of adoption are myriad but appear to revolve around four factors—lack of training, lack of time, skepticism regarding effectiveness and concerns about patients' willingness to discuss their alcohol consumption. Ongoing efforts continue to address these concerns, and it is hoped that brief interventions will eventually be adopted widely as part of primary health care.

Brief interventions used in primary health care settings are very similar to those employed in outpatient addiction settings. Essentially, the primary health care worker asks questions about the patient's alcohol use. Those patients whose drinking is risky are then advised in an empathic way about ways to cut down on their drinking. Follow-up by the health care worker is sometimes offered or, when necessary, patients with more severe concerns are referred to a specialized addiction treatment. Brief interventions in primary health care settings generally take no more than 10 minutes. The intervention can be delivered by a physician, nurse or other health care professional (or a combination of both, e.g., a nurse conducts the assessment and the physician provides the intervention). The next section describes initiatives that are using self-administered electronic screeners in primary health care in an effort to promote brief interventions in this setting.

Brief Interventions People Can Use on Their Own

Brief interventions can be self-administered by people whose drinking levels might put them at risk of experiencing problems and who are interested in dealing with their alcohol concerns by themselves. The basic components, assessment followed by feedback, are the type of tools that can readily be translated into a self-help format. Since most people who drink at risky levels do not seek help, and many are interested in dealing with drinking concerns on their own, it makes sense to provide brief intervention tools people can use without having to seek clinical treatment.

Self-administered tools come in a variety of lengths and formats. Originally, these tools were provided in books (or booklets), and the person was essentially guided through the same sorts of exercises that would most commonly be used in an outpatient treatment setting (e.g., assessment, goal setting, relapse prevention). This format has been evaluated and shown to have some efficacy when used on its own (Apodaca & Miller, 2003). An added advantage has been associated with pairing a self-help book with a brief telephone contact or personalized assessment feedback summary (Sanchez-Craig et al., 1996).

More recent years have seen self-help tools translated into web-based formats (Cunningham et al., 2011). Not everyone (e.g., people with language or literacy barriers) has equal access to the Internet. However, for others, the Internet can help them overcome barriers to treatment, such as lack of services in geographically remote communities and concerns about privacy (Cunningham et al., 2006). Several versions of Internet interventions are available free of charge, two of which are listed in the Resources section.

The most common type of brief Internet intervention consists of a brief set of questions followed by a personalized feedback report that summarizes the person's drinking and provides an assessment of the severity of the drinking. Common in these personalized feedback reports are normative comparisons in which the person's drinking is compared to that of others of the same age and sex in the general population. This type of normative feedback is thought to motivate people to reduce their drinking, as many heavy drinkers are often surprised by how much more they drink than others. The sidebar opposite provides examples of personalized feedback that one of these free Internet interventions, the Check Your Drinking screener, might give to Eric, who was introduced in this chapter's opening case scenario.

Personalized feedback from the Check Your Drinking screener

Eric might receive this feedback:

You reported consuming 34 drinks per week. This is more than 95 per cent of Canadian men your age.

You reported drinking on about 100 per cent of days in the last year.

Based on your weekly drinking, you reported that you drank a total of 1,768 drinks in the last year.

You reported having 12 drinks on your heaviest drinking day.

If a drink usually costs you about $3.50, you spent approximately $6,188 in the last year, depending on where you drank (at home, in a bar, etc.).

You consumed about 400 calories from alcohol on days that you drank (one drink has about 100 calories).

You had enough alcohol in the last year to add roughly 51 pounds or 23 kilograms to your weight.

You reported consuming five or more drinks on one occasion more than once per week. This is more often than 96 per cent of Canadian men your age.

Your AUDIT score (a World Health Organization alcohol severity scale) is 14, which places your drinking in the range of a harmful drinker.

Based on your weight, it takes you two hours for the alcohol from one drink to leave your system and seven hours for four drinks.

Based on your weight, if you have 10 drinks, it will take about 18 hours until there is no alcohol in your system.

Last year you spent about 3,203 hours under the influence of alcohol.

Try the program at www.CheckYourDrinking.net to see the graphical feedback provided.

Other web-based interventions provide an array of cognitive-behavioural and relapse prevention tools commonly seen in treatment settings (e.g., drinking diaries, goal-setting tools, strategies for dealing with high-risk situations). In addition, some websites offer online support groups, where people can discuss concerns with others who are trying to reduce their drinking. As with self-help books, these online help centres can provide an extensive set of materials. In this sense, they are not brief interventions. However, from the perspective of the therapist or other front-line worker who is looking for tools to help people who drink above low-risk levels, these resources are brief because they can be recommended by the therapist and used quickly by the person without having to contact the therapist again. (Or perhaps some sort of a hybrid arrangement could be made, where the therapist periodically monitors or connects with the person if he or she runs into difficulties.)

Brief Interventions as Public Health Initiatives

A final type of brief intervention involves the translation of brief intervention materials into formats that are useful for public health initiatives. These tools might best be thought of as "ultra-brief" interventions. The bare bones of a brief intervention (a short assessment plus feedback) are offered in a self-test format in a pamphlet or other type of handout. These materials are then distributed widely as part of an educational campaign. The intent is to get people to think about their drinking and seek help if they feel the need. Some evidence reveals that these ultra-brief interventions can have a small impact on people's alcohol consumption by reducing their weekly consumption by about two drinks (Cunningham et al., 2008). These reductions are relatively minor but relevant when considered from a public health perspective: large numbers of people can be reached at low cost, and the materials can be provided to everyone rather than to just those who seek help. From a clinical perspective, these types of educational materials are useful because they can be distributed in different non-specialist health care settings and may encourage people to seek help when they would not normally do so.

Special Populations, Settings and Issues

Brief interventions have been offered in a variety of settings and for specific populations and issues. A few of the more common examples are described here.

Emergency Rooms and Hospitals

Alcohol is a contributing factor to many accidents and other physical health concerns. Thus, it is not a surprise that many people who engage in risky drinking can be found in emergency room settings, as well as in other general hospital clinics and wards. A lively area of research is attempting to validate the use of brief interventions in these settings, with the majority of work being conducted in emergency rooms (where wait times could potentially be used for other purposes, such as providing a brief intervention). While the research is not uniformly positive, there is promise that the provision of brief interventions in these settings is helpful (Bernstein et al., 2009).

University and College

The post-secondary years are often a time of experimentation and exploration, and risky drinking is generally most common at this developmental age. Unfortunately, students engaged in risky drinking can cause themselves and others a great deal of harm in both the short term and long term. Considerable resources have been devoted to developing and evaluating brief interventions in university and college settings. Whether the interventions are tailored specifically for this population or simply applied using the tools developed in other general population settings, evidence suggests they are helpful for students who are at risk of experiencing alcohol-related problems (Moreira et al., 2009).

Illicit Drugs and Tobacco

The use of other drugs in conjunction with risky drinking is common, particularly the combination of cigarette smoking and risky drinking. An extensive evidence base demonstrates the efficacy of brief interventions to help with smoking cessation (2008 PHS Guideline Update Panel, Liaisons, and Staff, 2008). Unfortunately, much less research has been done on the efficacy of brief interventions for other drug concerns. However, some initiatives are under way to adapt the brief intervention models for at-risk drinking and smoking to other drug concerns (Madras et al., 2009). However, the caveat, at least at present, is that only limited evidence exists that these interventions will work. (The flip side is that there is no real evidence indicating they will not work.)

Concurrent Alcohol and Mental Health Concerns

While there is little research in this area, brief interventions may have an important role to play in treatment for at-risk drinking among people with concurrent mental health concerns. The challenge is that addiction and mental health services are often provided as separate clinical services. To prevent the client with both mental health and addiction issues from falling between the cracks or being shuttled back and forth between specialty settings, some form of intervention for alcohol concerns needs to be provided within specialized mental health settings (just as mental health concerns should be addressed in addiction settings). Arguably, brief interventions could serve this role because they can be incorporated into other services without too much disruption or specialized training. However we *are* considering the use of brief interventions for people who engage in at-risk drinking and who have concurrent mental health concerns.

Conclusion

In some ways, brief interventions are the great equalizer because they can be administered to most populations in many settings. This is one of the main strengths of brief interventions. Most people with at-risk alcohol consumption do not show up in traditional addiction treatment settings. Brief interventions are the distillation of the key elements of addiction treatment, packaged in a way that makes them portable and usable in a variety of settings. More extended treatment in a specialized addiction agency would likely be more helpful for people who engage in risky drinking. However, if they will not come to this type of treatment (or will not stay once they get there), we would argue that is it better to provide them with something brief that we know can help rather than nothing at all.

The reality is that most people like Eric, whose story opened this chapter, are unlikely to show up in a specialized addiction treatment setting. If Eric were to seek treatment, it would likely be related to an impaired driving charge or pressure from his girlfriend, and then a brief intervention might be the best intervention. Special attention would need to be given to the motivational aspects of the intervention, as Eric may be ambivalent about change. Alcohol is probably still a "friend," but one with negative consequences.

More likely, Eric will not show up in addiction treatment, but he could be encouraged to reconsider his alcohol use in other settings. A primary health care setting is probably the most likely place where Eric's drinking could be addressed. Or, if Eric has an injury, then perhaps some sort of intervention could be conducted in an emergency room. Unfortunately, brief interventions are still rarely provided in primary care and hospital health care settings in Canada. It is hoped that this lack of service provision can be addressed soon, as there is much opportunity to help people with alcohol concerns in these settings.

Finally, Eric or his girlfriend might notice a pamphlet on drinking while filling a prescription at the pharmacy, or they might do a quick web search on drinking. Accessing an Internet-based intervention could serve as a step toward helping Eric deal with his alcohol concerns.

Practice Tips

Brief intervention materials are easily accessible to the general population and health care providers through bookstores and online. Even if these interventions do not lead to reduced drinking, they may increase a person's readiness to seek specialized treatment.

Online and print-based materials can be helpful for therapists who work with people presenting for other mental or physical health concerns where alcohol may play a role. Therapists can:
- provide evidence-based advice on reducing risky alcohol use
- address sensitive issues in a non-threatening and non-judgmental way
- "extend" therapy by monitoring a client's use of educational resources.
- (for other health care providers) routinely inquire about alcohol use and provide public health materials in waiting rooms.

Resources

Publications

Centre for Addiction and Mental Health & St. Joseph's Health Centre, Toronto. (2010). *Primary Care Addiction Toolkit*. Toronto: Author. Retrieved from http://knowledgex.camh.net/primary_care/toolkits/addiction_toolkit/Pages/default.aspx

National Institute on Alcohol Abuse and Alcoholism. (2005). *Helping Patients Who Drink Too Much: A Clinician's Guide*. Bethesda, MD: Author. Retrieved from http://pubs.niaaa.nih.gov/publications/Practitioner/CliniciansGuide2005/guide.pdf

Internet
Alcohol Help Center
   www.alcoholhelpcenter.net
Check Your Drinking
   www.CheckYourDrinking.net

References

2008 PHS Guideline Update Panel, Liaisons, and Staff. (2008). Treating tobacco use and dependence: 2008 update. U.S. Public Health Service Clinical Practice Guideline executive summary. *Respiratory Care, 53*, 1217–1222.

Apodaca, T.R. & Miller, W.R. (2003). A meta-analysis of the effectiveness of bibliotherapy for alcohol problems. *Journal of Clinical Psychology, 59*, 289–304.

Bernstein, E., Bernstein, J.A., Stein, J.B. & Saitz, R. (2009). SBIRT in emergency care settings: Are we ready to take it to scale? *Academic Emergency Medicine, 16*, 1072–1077.

Cunningham, J.A. & Breslin, F.C. (2004). Only one in three people with alcohol abuse or dependence ever seek treatment. *Addictive Behaviors, 29*, 221–223.

Cunningham, J.A., Kypri, K. & McCambridge, J. (2011). The use of emerging technologies in alcohol treatment. *Alcohol Research & Health, 33*, 320–326.

Cunningham, J.A., Neighbors, C., Wild, C. & Humphreys, K. (2008). Ultra-brief intervention for problem drinkers: Research protocol. *BMC Public Health, 8*, 298.

Cunningham, J.A., Selby, P.L., Kypri, K. & Humphreys, K.N. (2006). Access to the Internet among drinkers, smokers and illicit drug users: Is it a barrier to the provision of interventions on the World Wide Web? *Medical Informatics and the Internet in Medicine, 31*, 53–58.

Dawson, D.A., Grant, B.F., Stinson, F.S., Chou, P.S., Huang, B. & Ruan, W.J. (2005). Recovery from DSM–IV alcohol dependence: United States, 2001–2002. *Addiction, 100*, 281–292.

Heather, N. (1989). Psychology and brief interventions. *British Journal of Addiction, 84*, 357–370.

Kaner, E.F., Beyer, F., Dickinson, H.O., Pienaar, E., Campbell, F., Schlesinger, C. et al. (2007). Effectiveness of brief alcohol interventions in primary care populations. *Cochrane Database of Systematic Reviews,* (2), CD004148. doi: 10.1002/14651858. CD004148.pub3

Madras, B.K., Compton, W.M., Avula, D., Stegbauer, T., Stein, J.B. & Clark, H.W. (2009). Screening, brief interventions, referral to treatment (SBIRT) for illicit drug and alcohol use at multiple healthcare sites: Comparison at intake and 6 months later. *Drug and Alcohol Dependence, 99*, 280–295.

Miller, W.R. (2000). Rediscovering fire: Small interventions, large effects. *Psychology of Addictive Behaviors, 14*, 6–18.

Miller, W.R. & Rollnick, S. (1991). *Motivational Interviewing: Preparing People to Change Addictive Behavior.* New York: Guilford Press.

Miller, W.R., Sovereign, R.G. & Krege, B. (1988). Motivational interviewing with problem drinkers: II. The Drinker's Check-up as a preventive intervention. *Behavioural Psychotherapy, 16*, 251–268.

Miller, W.R., Wilbourne, P.L. & Hettema, J.E. (2003). What works? A summary of alcohol treatment outcome literature. In R.K. Hester & W.R. Miller (Eds.), *Handbook of*

Alcoholism Treatment Approaches: Effective Alternatives (3rd ed., pp. 13–63). Boston: Allyn & Bacon.

Moreira, M.T., Smith, L.A. & Foxcroft, D. (2009). Social norms interventions to reduce alcohol misuse in university or college students. *Cochrane Database of Systematic Reviews*, (3), CD006748. doi: 10.1002/14651858.CD006748.pub2

Sanchez-Craig, M., Davila, R. & Cooper, G. (1996). A self-help approach for high-risk drinking: Effect of an initial assessment. *Journal of Consulting and Clinical Psychology, 64*, 694–700.

Stockwell, T., Toumbourou, J.W., Letcher, P., Smart, D., Sanson, A. & Bond, L. (2004). Risk and protection factors for different intensities of adolescent substance use: When does the prevention paradox apply? *Drug and Alcohol Review, 23*, 67–77.

Chapter 10

Relapse Prevention

Marilyn Herie and Lyn Watkin-Merek

> George is a 22-year-old male who works sporadically at his family's restaurant with his mother and stepfather. He left school midway through Grade 11, and still lives with his parents. There is considerable conflict in the home about George not finding a job or supporting himself. About 10 months ago, the police were called when an argument George was having with his mother escalated and he threatened to kill her.
>
> George reported using marijuana regularly and drinking six beers on the day of his arrest. He stated that he typically drinks five or six beers "to get a buzz," and that while under the influence he "feels good." He also admitted that he uses marijuana to "calm down," but that it sometimes makes him feel paranoid. George attended outpatient treatment as a condition of probation, but began drinking and using cannabis again after a few weeks.
>
> George's family believes drugs are the source of all of his problems and wants to make sure he stops using alcohol and cannabis. His probation officer has also warned him that he needs to maintain abstinence or he will be in breach of his probation. George, on the other hand, does not regard his alcohol or cannabis use as problematic in the least—he thinks his family and probation officer are putting unreasonable pressure on him about his substance use.
>
> The other day George met up with some friends after working a shift in the restaurant. He was feeling stressed and angry at his mother's "nagging" and set out to get as drunk as possible. He remembers having an argument with another customer in a bar, which turned physical. He doesn't recall who threw the first punch, but when the police were called, he knew he was in serious trouble because of his probation.

The pattern of substance use described in this case scenario is common. Although it has contributed to George's interpersonal, work and legal problems, he is ambivalent about the benefits—or need—for long-term abstinence. George was able to stop using alcohol and cannabis while he was in treatment and for a few weeks afterwards, but his commitment to abstinence wavered as time passed. His family and his probation officer thought that once he completed treatment he would be "cured." Instead, about a month and a half after he completed an outpatient program, he went back to regular alcohol and cannabis use. It was not until George was forced to enter treatment a second time and began seriously working toward recovery that he was able to learn how to maintain abstinence in the longer term.

The chronic, relapsing nature of alcohol and other drug problems has been recognized since the early 1970s (Hunt et al., 1971). In the late 1970s and early 1980s, researchers began to focus on factors that affect the process of relapse (Litman et al., 1979, 1984; Wilson, 1980) and on the development of "relapse prevention" treatment strategies (Annis, 1986; Marlatt & Gordon, 1985). Despite advances in substance use treatment, relapse prevention continues to be a major issue (Hendershot et al., 2008). Research on the effectiveness of well-established treatment approaches (e.g., cognitive-behavioural therapy, dialectical behaviour therapy, interpersonal psychotherapy, 12-step facilitation therapy, motivational enhancement therapy) points to their effectiveness in reducing or eliminating substance use during the months following treatment, but also shows that most people will return to pre-treatment behaviour patterns within the first year (Project MATCH Research Group, 1997; Witkiewitz & Marlatt, 2007).

Relapse prevention treatments and strategies cannot reasonably be expected to prevent all recurring substance use episodes; instead, these strategies help people make small steps toward change. This fits with the current conceptualization of addiction as a chronic relapsing disorder or as a chronic disease, with many similar features as other chronic diseases, such as type 2 diabetes, cardiovascular disease and cancer (McLellan et al., 2000; White et al., 2003).

Relapse essentially means failure to maintain behavioural change, rather than failure to initiate it. Treatment approaches based on social learning theory (later termed social cognitive theory), specifically Bandura's theory of self-efficacy, hold that the strategies that are effective in initiating a change in health behaviour (including substance use) may be ineffective at maintaining that change over time and avoiding relapse (Bandura, 1986, 2004). Definitions of relapse have evolved over time from a binary "all or nothing" approach (where relapse is said to occur at the time of first drink or drug use) to consider the nuances of quantity and frequency measures, lifestyle changes and iterative progress in the direction of change (Maisto & Connors, 2006). From this standpoint, relapse and relapse prevention are better understood as continuous processes as opposed to discrete events.

This chapter examines the nature of relapse, along with some key questions: What is relapse? How do we define it? Are there problems with the term "relapse" itself? We then briefly outline a theoretical framework that attempts to explain relapse processes (Witkiewitz & Marlatt, 2007), as well as key biological, psychological, social, structural and spiritual factors that may affect relapse. In addition, highlights from the structured relapse prevention manual-based approach (Herie & Watkin-Merek, 2006) provide some key clinical tools for helping prevent relapse. Finally, we explore some of the research and practice implications for relapse prevention with diverse client populations.

Toward a Definition of Relapse

Although changing substance use behaviour is difficult, maintaining change is even more challenging (Connors & Maisto, 2006); that perhaps is the essence of the problem of relapse in addiction treatment.

Addiction research and treatment have been guided in the past by binary thinking, where "alcoholism" can be compared to pregnancy: "Either you have it or you don't, and there is nothing in between" (Miller, 1996, p. 15). This overly simplistic conceptualization of a complex problem has also been applied to treatment outcomes, judging them as either successful (abstinent) or relapsed (non-abstinent). But if treatment success were always to be judged on abstinence alone, almost all people who complete treatment would be considered "treatment failures" at some point in time.

Miller (1996) points out that the concept of relapse can in itself be harmful in its implicit imposition of a value judgment:

> Backsliding is an old synonym for sin, and few would fail to grasp which side of the relapse dichotomy is judged the more desirable. "Relapsed" has a connotation of failure, weakness and shame, of having fallen from a state of grace. Such overtones are likely to compromise self-regard and add needless affective meaning to what is a rather common behavioral event. (p. 25)

Roozen and Van de Wetering (2007) argue that the term "relapse prevention" should be changed to "relapse management" to better capture the neurobiological reality of addiction as a chronic condition. More recently, Marjot (2010) suggested changing the focus altogether, away from relapse and toward attachment (in this case, to substances of abuse and addiction). Defining relapse—once thought to be straightforward—has proven to be more complex.

Categorizing substance use treatment outcomes as either abstinent or non-abstinent ignores the behavioural changes that may occur post-treatment. For example, people may change the number of drinks they consume, the number of drinking days and the frequency of binge use. They may also change their use of other drugs, including prescription and over-the-counter drugs and tobacco, or they make improvements in social functioning or relationships.

Ideally, a definition of relapse should consider multiple factors. Miller (1996) identified the following factors:

- threshold (the amount of substance use)
- window (the period of time judged)
- reset (the period of abstinence required before a person can be considered to have relapsed)
- polydrugs (the types of substance use that constitute a relapse)
- consequences (behaviours and consequences associated with substance use required before a person can be considered to have relapsed)
- verification (self-report or collateral reports).

Asking a client whether he or she had a relapse can be interpreted in many ways: Did you drink (at all)? Did you drink above a certain threshold? Or, did you drink more than the limit you had set for yourself? Did you use drugs other than alcohol that were not identified as treatment targets? Was your alcohol use accompanied by any negative or harmful consequences? It is also important to consider whether self-reported alcohol use is corroborated by collateral information or biological measures.

That there is no single empirically or theoretically ideal combination of these factors highlights the inherent ambiguity in the term "relapse," and presents a major challenge in understanding and applying relapse prevention research findings (Bradizza et al., 2006). To confuse the issue even further, some studies distinguish between a "lapse" (an initial setback), a "relapse" (a return to pre-treatment substance use) and a "prolapse" (recovering from a relapse by making positive behaviour changes) (Witkiewitz & Marlatt, 2007). Other studies apply quantitative measures to differentiate lapses from relapses; for example, drinking at a level of 50 per cent or more constitutes relapse and less than 50 per cent constitutes a lapse. On the other hand, in harm reduction models, a lapse might be defined as any harmful consequences related to alcohol or other drug use, such as conflict with a partner or missing work (Witkiewitz & Marlatt, 2007).

Even if researchers and clinicians could develop and widely agree on a standard definition, the criteria for determining whether relapse occurs might vary across different substances. For example, any use of crack cocaine or injection drugs might constitute relapse, whereas having a single beer or a single cigarette might be considered a lapse (McKay et al., 2006). In the absence of a standard definition, McKay and colleagues (2006) proposed the following definition as a way to include the diversity of research findings on relapse and relapse prevention:

> We have labeled any alcohol or drug use in a given period after an intake or
> baseline assessment as a "relapse." With this definition, relapse is indicated
> by frequency measures of use that are greater than 0 for a given period
> (e.g., % days of heavy drinking > 0) or biological markers of use . . . as well
> as by assessments of specific episodes of use (e.g., a first smoking "lapse"
> after a quit date). (p. 110)

This definition can be useful as a way to capture the plethora of research on relapse prevention, but may be less applicable to clinical settings where a nuanced understanding of post-treatment substance use is more relevant to a client's experiences and processes of recovery.

Connors and Maisto (2006) suggest that "in its most basic form, relapse is the resumption of problematic behavior" (p. 107). Witkiewitz and Marlatt (2007) propose a definition of relapse that reflects the pragmatism of harm reduction: "Alcohol treatment outcomes may be characterized by the severity of alcohol-related problems, not the specific quantity or frequency of drinking" (p. 734). In summary, a client-centred definition of relapse should pay attention to three factors: (1) the person's progress toward treatment goals, including substance use, psychosocial or other goals; (2) the personal and social consequences related to alcohol or other drug use; and (3) the person's return to the problematic behaviour (i.e., substance use).

Theoretical Development: Marlatt's Relapse Prevention Model

The work of Alan Marlatt has been enormously influential in addiction treatment and research. His original cognitive-behavioural model of relapse is perhaps the best known and tested in the addiction field, and has been elaborated on and extended in recent years (Maisto & Connors, 2006). In his original conceptualization, Marlatt provided a cognitive-behavioural framework with testable hypotheses and practical strategies for working with relapse (Marlatt & Gordon, 1985). This section summarizes the framework as Marlatt first described it, followed by an overview of the ways in which Marlatt's original theory has been modified and expanded in recent years.

Marlatt conceptualizes relapse as a two-stage process, where the precipitants of substance use are distinct from the factors that prolong or sustain such use over time. Marlatt's research with people who experienced relapse led him to believe that relapse occurs as a result of a person's lack of coping skills to successfully avoid drinking or using other drugs in certain challenging situations (Marlatt & Gordon, 1980). Marlatt developed eight relapse determinants, also known as risk situations:

- unpleasant emotions
- physical discomfort
- pleasant emotions
- tests of personal control
- urges and temptations
- conflict with others
- social pressure to use
- pleasant times with others.

Marlatt's approach to relapse prevention treatment focuses on providing coping skills training for the risk situations that are particular to each client. His taxonomy of risk situations is clinically useful in that it gives the therapist a "handle" on how to work with clients to prevent or discuss relapse. Relapse is therefore addressed:

> in a pragmatic manner as an error, a lapse, a slip or temporary setback, and not an inevitable collapse on the road to recovery. Teaching people about high risk situations and how to cope with them more effectively is the essence of relapse prevention. (Marlatt, 1996, p. 47)

For example, in the case of George that opens this chapter, the risk situation—being in a bar—was exacerbated by unpleasant emotions (feeling stressed), conflict with others (George's mother) and social pressure to use (partying with friends who were also drinking). Helping George to recognize the situations and triggers that put him at risk is the first step in preventing relapse.

Instruments to assess risk across these domains were developed by Annis and Martin (Inventory of Drug-Taking Situations [IDTS], 1985a; Drug-Taking Confidence Questionnaire [DTCQ], 1985b), as well as by the Project MATCH Research Group (1997). The relevance of these relapse precipitants is such that they are still commonly used as questionnaire items in research trials (ElGeili & Bashir, 2005; Levy, 2008; Ramo & Brown, 2008; Zywiak et al., 2006).

However, Marlatt's original model (Marlatt, 1996; Marlatt & Gordon, 1980) has some shortcomings. Relapse precipitants can be multidimensional and interact in complex ways. Structural factors, such as substandard housing, limited occupational opportunities, poor access to health care and poverty can also affect behavioural change, as can motivation and ambivalence. Failure to cope may be evidence of a deficit in coping skills, but not necessarily. Furthermore, the negative experience of a relapse can solidify a person's intention to change. Finally, neurobiological factors in addiction and craving can have a considerable impact on craving and relapse risk. Marlatt's taxonomy may not sufficiently capture the "magic" of the substance, and (more importantly) a landmark study designed to test this taxonomy—the Relapse Replication and Extension Project (Lowman et al., 1996)—failed to support the predictive validity of these categories of risk situations. There was a call for a reconceptualization of the theory to include both interpersonal and intrapersonal relapse determinants, as well as a greater emphasis on cravings (Marlatt & Witkiewitz, 2005).

These critiques have been addressed in recent years as the model has been extended to encompass the temporal relationships among cognitive, behavioural, affective and biological processes affecting relapse (Witkiewitz & Marlatt, 2004, 2007). Hunter-Reel and colleagues (2009) proposed a further extension to the model to incorporate the mediating effects of social and structural factors on cognition, affect, behaviour and biology.

In this extended version of Marlatt's original model, relapse is viewed as a dynamic process, where slight or seemingly insignificant changes or events may trigger a downward spiral of craving, negative affect and decreased self-efficacy:

> The sheer disaster of a relapse crisis after an individual has been maintaining abstinence has bewildered patients, researchers and clinicians for years. The symbolism of "falling from the wagon" provides an illustration of the sudden, devastating experience of the chronic return to previous levels of abuse. This experience is often followed by the harsh realization that getting back on the wagon will not be as effortless as the fall from it. (Witkiewitz & Marlatt, 2007, pp. 728–729)

A contemporary understanding of relapse means considering the interplay of numerous factors. These include high-risk situations (as outlined above), within which are nested what Baker and colleagues (2004) have termed *tonic* processes (primarily stable) and *phasic* processes (primarily fluctuating) that are somewhat overlapping. Tonic processes relate to underlying levels of risk, and include distal risks, such as family history or number of addiction symptoms, as well as cognitive processes (i.e., cravings, self-efficacy, expectancies and motivation) and physical withdrawal. Phasic processes represent dynamic precipitants to relapse, and can also include cognitions and withdrawal, as well as coping behaviour, affect, substance use and perceived effects (reinforcement) (Witkiewitz & Marlatt, 2004). This framework has some research support and captures the complex and dynamic interplay of factors that may predict vulnerability to relapse (see Witkiewitz & Marlatt, 2007, for a review).

In the most recent iteration of the theory behind relapse, Witkiewitz and Marlatt (2007) propose catastrophe theory as a potentially helpful way to model and test these complex, non-linear processes. Catastrophe theory studies how sudden, discontinuous changes (like relapse) can result from slight changes in a system (which in this case would include biological, psychological and social systems). Although preliminary empirical support for modelling the theory appears promising, more research is needed to establish whether catastrophe theory can provide an even more robust explanation for the processes of relapse and recovery (McKay et al., 2006).

Key Factors in Relapse: A Biopsychosocial (and Structural/Spiritual) Perspective

The biopsychosocial perspective on addiction holds that addiction is the result of interacting biological, psychological and social factors (Griffiths, 2005; Maisto & Connors, 2006); this can be extended to include structural and spiritual factors (Herie & Skinner, 2010). This section reviews the evidence base for relapse risk factors in each of these domains, with implications for practice.

Biological Factors

The effects of substance use on the brain have been well known for decades (Leshner, 1997). Recent research on the neurobiology of addiction suggests that long-term or permanent changes in brain structures, particularly in the brain's executive functioning and reward systems, are a result of repeated drug administration (National Institute on Drug Abuse, 2010). For example, people with cocaine use disorder experience neuroadaptations that affect learning and memory function, which in turn influences treatment outcomes (i.e., leading to a greater likelihood of relapse) (Fox et al., 2009).

Research also supports the possibility that sex-related hormones affect relapse risk: in one study, high progesterone levels in women, characteristic of the midluteal phase (the days following ovulation), were associated with lower stress-induced and cocaine cue–induced cravings, compared to women with low or moderate progesterone levels (Sinha et al., 2007). In other words, fluctuating hormone levels in women who are menstruating may contribute to the intensity of cravings or cue sensitivity.

Some of the most recent work on biological factors in relapse has focused on genetic risks. Emerging evidence points to the likelihood that distal relapse risks are largely influenced by genetic factors, and genetic variations may even influence subjective experiences of drug cravings (Hendershot et al., 2008). For example, a recent study found that a particular genotype predicted post-treatment alcohol relapse and time to relapse (Wojnar et al., 2009). However, the literature on possible linkages between specific genetic markers and treatment outcomes is still very new and more research is needed.

Advances in technology, such as the ecological momentary assessment (EMA), have made it possible to gather "real-time" subjective data on relapse occurrences, and to compare these data to biological or genetic characteristics of study participants. EMA technology provides individuals with an electronic device they can always carry with them to record cravings and substance use episodes. Although still in an early stage, these methodological advances in relapse research hold some promise in comparing distal with proximal factors to increase our understanding of relapse processes and interactions (McKay et al., 2006).

Psychological Factors

A number of personality variables may be associated with relapse risk. These include negative cognitive style, feelings of inadequacy, ineffective coping, rigid personality style and external locus of control (Chatterjee & Chattopadhyay, 2005; Gordon et al., 2006). Assessing for these factors at intake can help with treatment planning and identifying supports during and after treatment.

Another potential risk factor for relapse is anxiety sensitivity. This term refers to a person's fear of anxiety symptoms, and can be measured through a standardized scale. Early smoking relapse has been shown to be strongly associated with anxiety sensitivity in adult smokers (Zvolensky et al., 2007), where people with higher anxiety sensitivity scores relapsed significantly sooner than those with lower scores.

Social learning theory posits that self-efficacy, a person's expectancy or belief in his or her ability to act in a certain way, is predictive of future behaviour. Research supports linkages between the ability to maintain abstinence and perceived self-efficacy as a predictor of lapse and relapse (Gordon et al., 2006; Gwaltney et al., 2005), although measures of self-efficacy may be compromised by self-report biases, such as impression management or deception (Demmel et al., 2006). Motivation likely also plays a role, with a strong association between high levels of motivation and short- and long-term abstinence (Schröter et al., 2006). A continuous assessment of self-efficacy and motivation may provide valuable feedback about treatment effectiveness and relapse risk.

Social Factors

Social factors can both increase risk of relapse and protect against it (Hunter-Reel et al., 2009). For example, the number of people in a person's social network and the person's attachment to a circle of social supports are protective factors. Similarly, higher levels of general and alcohol-specific support within the network and specific behaviours of network members predict drinking outcomes (Hunter-Reel et al., 2009; VanDeMark, 2007). Even attending a self-help group is related to positive outcomes in the short term (Mueller et al., 2007). Living alone and being single are risk factors that may be as—or more—important as coping skills in relation to relapse (Walter et al., 2006). Experience of chronic life stressors (e.g., in military settings) predicts post-treatment substance use, as does drug availability (Tate et al., 2006).

Less well known are the mechanisms by which these factors influence alcohol or other drug use behaviour, but it is likely that they interact with intrapersonal (psychological and biological) factors in complex ways (Hunter-Reel et al., 2009). These findings reinforce the importance of helping clients build robust social supports and networks that are supportive of client goals during and after treatment.

Social-Structural and Spiritual Factors

There is growing awareness that social-structural and spiritual factors, traditionally under-acknowledged in addiction research, are also key to understanding relapse. Stahler and colleagues (2010) found a link between neighbourhood factors, such as crime rates, and keeping outpatient treatment appointments at 30 days post-discharge, as well as increased risk of rehospitalization within one year. Other predictors include level of education, living independently, lack of continuing substance use treatment (Xie et al., 2005) and substance availability (Tate et al., 2006). Access to safe, stable housing, high-quality health care (including mental health services) and meaningful activities and opportunities cannot be underestimated in working with clients on sustaining their treatment progress and goals.

Some evidence suggests that spiritual factors may be related to treatment outcomes. For example, Sterling and colleagues (2007) investigated the association between self-reported spiritual growth during inpatient alcohol treatment and relapse and found that post-treatment alcohol use was associated with decreased spirituality. Associations between client self-reports of the importance of spirituality at admission and treatment and within-treatment craving and relapse (in combination with self-efficacy and depression) support the notion that practitioners need to pay attention to this area (Gordon et al., 2006). Engaging in prayer, relying on a "higher power" and finding a deeper meaning to one's life can be important complements to more main-stream treatment approaches (Davis & O'Neill, 2005; Harris et al., 2005).

In addition to traditional 12-step approaches to treatment that have an overarch-ing spiritual component (Wilson, 1962), research and treatment that apply Buddhist practices to relapse prevention, such as mindfulness meditation and mindfulness-based cognitive therapy, have been gaining in popularity over the past decade (Breslin et al., 2002; Marlatt, 2002; Vallejo & Hortensia, 2009; Witkiewitz et al., 2005; Zgierska et al., 2008). For example, people can use mindfulness to monitor their urges and cravings, and apply the Buddhist value of "non-attachment" to let go of cravings to use substances. The first randomized-controlled trial comparing mindfulness-based relapse prevention (MBRP) to treatment as usual found that people in the MBRP group had significantly lower rates of substance use, greater decreases in cravings and increases in acceptance and "acting with awareness" in the four-month post-intervention period (Bowen at al., 2009). However, these results are preliminary and more research is needed (Zgierska et al., 2009). As research support for the efficacy of mindfulness-based approaches to relapse prevention grows, this promising practice is likely to continue to find its way into mainstream addiction treatment programs.

Structured Relapse Prevention: A Manual-Based Approach

The structured relapse prevention treatment intervention (SRP) is a counselling approach for people with moderate to severe levels of alcohol or other drug addiction (Annis et al., 1996; Herie & Watkin-Merek, 2006). The treatment blends cognitive-behavioural therapy (CBT) with a motivational approach, and is based on Marlatt's relapse prevention model (Marlatt, 1996; Marlatt & Gordon, 1985). The therapy sessions address substance use triggers and provide structured coping skills training, and have also been adapted for people with concurrent mental health and addiction problems. SRP falls into the category of cognitive-behavioural coping skills approaches that are strongly rooted in social learning theory. A robust evidence base lends support for this type of intervention as a best practice in addiction treatment (Rohsenow & Monti, 2001; Roozen & Van de Wetering, 2007).

SRP is used in outpatient addiction treatment centres throughout Ontario—both with individuals and groups—and in residential treatment centres to help prepare clients for their return to the community, and as part of aftercare programs. Many adaptations have been made to the model originally outlined in the manual, based on the popula-tions served and sociocultural and linguistic considerations, as well as on counsellor preferences (Herie & Watkin-Merek, 2006). These iterations of SRP tend to conform to a basic two-phase approach, in which initiation-of-change strategies, such as avoidance and reliance on the support of others, are gradually complemented or replaced by more internalized coping strategies.

Overview of Structured Relapse Prevention Counselling

SRP counselling incorporates motivational interviewing strategies (Miller & Rollnick, 2002) to help clients commit to making changes to their substance use. Of course, some clients may not progress through these various components in a linear fashion due to motivational or other setbacks.

SRP comprises five components that can be delivered sequentially or in an ad hoc fashion, depending on the client's needs and readiness to change. In component 1, all clients at intake to SRP counselling are assessed for quantity and frequency of substance use, psychosocial resources and issues and any co-occurring problem areas, such as mental health or medical concerns. In component 2, clients are provided with individualized feedback of the assessment results during one or more motivational interviewing sessions. Clients who are willing to change their substance use will collaborate with their counsellor to develop an individually tailored treatment plan and set a treatment goal as part of component 3.

If clients are willing and able to commit to outpatient treatment, they progress through SRP components 4 and 5, delivered in either group or individual sessions. Component 4 focuses on helping clients initiate changes to their substance use (stabilization), and component 5 helps clients make the transition to maintenance strategies.

Each component of the treatment process is described in greater detail below, beginning with a discussion of the type of client for whom this treatment approach is likely to be most effective.

Component 1: Assessment

Carrying out an initial assessment is not unique to SRP—any addiction treatment program should begin this way. While various evidence-based brief screening and assessment tools exist (e.g., see Health Canada, 2007; Herie & Watkin-Merek, 2006), one assessment instrument in particular is important in preparing clients for SRP counselling: the Inventory of Drug-Taking Situations ([IDTS], Annis & Martin, 1985a; Turner et al., 1997). This tool helps to reveal the specific risk areas unique to each client, providing counsellors with a "road map" for areas to target in relapse prevention planning and coping skills training.

The IDTS-8 is an eight-item assessment and treatment planning tool adapted from the longer (50-item) version that gives a situational analysis of a client's substance use. The frequency of the client's past drinking or other drug use is assessed, following the classification system developed by Marlatt and Gordon (1985), across the eight risk areas discussed earlier in this chapter (unpleasant emotions, physical discomfort, pleasant emotions, tests of personal control, urges and temptations, conflict with others, social pressure to use and pleasant times with others). Figure 10-1 shows the questionnaire, which is relatively quick and easy for clients to complete on their own.

FIGURE 10-1: Inventory of Drug-Taking Situations (IDTS-8)

Inventory of Drug-Taking Situations (IDTS-8)

Name: _____ Date: _____

(check one box)
Is this your PRIMARY substance of abuse?   ☐
or
your SECONDARY substance of abuse?   ☐

IDENTIFYING CAUSES

The first step in trying to change your substance use habits and patterns is to identify the reasons that led to your use of alcohol or other drugs. Below are eight typical causes ("trigger situations").

Think of your drinking or other drug use **over the past year**, and circle any that apply to you.

1. *unpleasant emotions* (e.g., when I was angry, frustrated, bored, sad or anxious)

2. *physical discomfort* (e.g., when I was feeling ill or in pain)

3. *pleasant emotions* (e.g., when I was enjoying myself or just feeling happy)

4. *testing personal control* (e.g., when I started to believe I could handle alcohol or drugs)

5. *urges and temptations* (e.g., when I walked by a pub or saw something that reminded me of drinking or drug use)

6. *conflict with others* (e.g., when I had an argument or was not getting along with someone)

7. *social pressures* (e.g., when someone offered alcohol or drugs)

8. *pleasant times with others* (e.g., when I was out with friends or at a party).

   In terms of how often I drink or use drugs in each of the above situations, I would rank the "trigger situations" that I have circled above as follows:

   1st (most frequent): _____

   2nd (in frequency): _____

   3rd (in frequency): _____

(Depending on time available at this session, the next exercise might be a take-home assignment.)

AREAS OF RISK

Think about your drinking or other substance use in the last 12 months in each of the following situations. If you NEVER drank heavily or used other drugs in that situation, you would circle "0." If you ALMOST ALWAYS drank heavily or used other drugs in that situation, you would circle "100%." If your answer falls somewhere in between, place an **X** along the line so that it shows about how close to 0% or 100% you think is appropriate. In the example below, the **X** shows that the person drank heavily or used other drugs a little less than half the time in a particular risk situation.

EXAMPLE

In the last 12 months I drank heavily or used other substances:

| 0% | 25% | **X** 50% | 75% | 100% | = | 48% |

Never   Almost always

In the last 12 months I drank heavily or used other substances when I was experiencing:

1. *Unpleasant emotions*

| 0% | 25% | 50% | 75% | 100% | = | % |

Never   Almost always

2. *Physical discomfort*

| 0% | 25% | 50% | 75% | 100% | = | % |

Never   Almost always

3. *Pleasant emotions*

| 0% | 25% | 50% | 75% | 100% | = | % |

Never   Almost always

4. *Testing personal control*

| 0% | 25% | 50% | 75% | 100% | = | % |

Never   Almost always

5. *Urges and temptations*

| 0% | 25% | 50% | 75% | 100% | = | % |

Never   Almost always

6. *Conflict with others*

| 0% | 25% | 50% | 75% | 100% | = | % |

Never   Almost always

7. *Social pressures*

| 0% | 25% | 50% | 75% | 100% | = | % |

Never   Almost always

8. *Pleasant times with others*

| 0% | 25% | 50% | 75% | 100% | = | % |

Never   Almost always

Adapted from H.M. Annis & G. Martin (1985). *Inventory of Drug-Taking Situations* (4th ed.). Toronto: Addiction Research Foundation.

Component 2: Motivational interviewing

Motivational interviewing is a client-centred, collaborative approach that is highly respectful of clients' autonomy (Miller & Rollnick, 2002). The spirit, processes and strategies of motivational interviewing are discussed in greater detail in Chapter 5, but in brief, the approach is designed to help build clients' commitment and readiness for change. In SRP, one or more motivational interviewing sessions, delivered individually or in groups, can help engage clients who are reluctant to enter treatment or make changes to their substance use. The number of sessions devoted to motivational interviewing should be informed by the clients' needs and readiness, as well as by existing resources. A motivational style is also infused throughout SRP counselling sessions, since clients' motivation tends to fluctuate throughout treatment. Enhancing motivation is key to treatment success, as motivation has been associated with short- and long-term abstinence (Schröter et al., 2006).

Component 3: Individual treatment planning

Treatment planning is one of the most important components of SRP counselling. We have found the following strategies to be helpful in encouraging client collaboration in developing a treatment plan: goal setting and self-monitoring, identifying problem drinking or other drug use situations, identifying coping strengths and weaknesses and contracting for treatment. Each strategy is described in more detail below.

Goal setting and self-monitoring can be useful ways to facilitate client participation in the treatment planning process. Clients use self-monitoring forms to note their substance use goal each week—including their level of confidence in achieving this goal—and keep a daily record of any substance use, the circumstances surrounding that use, risky situations encountered and coping strategies used. Clients then discuss the self-monitoring with their counsellor during subsequent treatment sessions.

A fundamental part of planning for SRP treatment involves agreeing on the client's most problematic drinking or other drug use situations. The IDTS, which is given at assessment, provides this information in a systematic way based on the types of situations that triggered substance use over the past year. After discussing the IDTS results and the daily monitoring, clients are asked to rank the three most problematic triggers to substance use that they want to work on in treatment, and to give specific examples of past drinking or other drug use experiences for each situation. This exercise allows clients to analyze past situations in detail in order to identify what they might do differently in similar situations in the future. In addition, because the maintenance phase of SRP counselling focuses on planned exposure to high-risk situations for substance use (see below), it is important that both client and counsellor have a detailed overview of past drinking or other drug use scenarios.

The strengths, supports and coping responses already available to a client are invaluable in preventing relapse, and form the groundwork for developing successful homework assignments. The client must become more aware of his or her strengths and learn to use them effectively. Coping responses that the client may have used successfully in other areas may be quite effective, with only minor alterations, in addressing problematic drinking or other drug use situations. At this point in treatment planning, the clinician's task is to establish the client's existing repertoire of general coping behaviours, personal strengths and environmental resources. The process of reviewing the client's repertoire should provide a better appreciation of the possibilities open to the client, and should allow the client to focus on his or her strengths and successes rather than failures.

Coping skills training is of key importance in SRP counselling, with a comprehensive array of exercises and homework assignments spread across treatment sessions. The client selects priority areas for coping skills development from a list of topics, and these are addressed during group or individual sessions or provided as homework assignments. For example, during the early weeks of treatment, clients often choose to work on coping with cravings, managing stress or increasing social support. Later treatment sessions might address money issues, anger management or sexual relationships and dating.

Finally, the client is informed of the program's orientation and attendance requirements, the limits of client confidentiality and expectations for participation in planning and doing homework. Other possible treatment options are also presented. The client is then asked to decide whether he or she wishes to work toward change in substance use by entering SRP counselling. Clinicians may choose to use a treatment contract to formalize the client's commitment to enter treatment.

Component 4: Initiation counselling

The "heart" of SRP counselling is divided into two major phases: *initiation* (Component 4) and *maintenance* (Component 5). The initiation phase focuses on counselling strategies suitable for clients who are still struggling to quit or change their substance use, or those who are newly abstinent.

This initiation phase incorporates the substance use triggers identified by the client in the treatment plan. The focus is on helping clients anticipate substance use triggers for the coming week, and identify and commit to alternative coping strategies that don't involve drinking or other drug use. Clients must begin to identify and plan for high-risk situations in advance, so they can prepare alternative coping strategies.

Clients are encouraged to use coping plans that are known to be powerful strategies in initiating short-term behavioural change. These strategies include avoiding risky situations (e.g., drug use settings and drug-using friends), taking medications to help with cravings (e.g., nicotine replacement) or seeking out social support (e.g., from reliable friends or family members). Figure 10-2 shows the Weekly Plan (initiation phase) form that clients complete to guide them in anticipating substance use triggers and using relatively safe initiation strategies, such as avoidance and social support, to cope.

FIGURE 10-2: Weekly Plan (Initiation Phase) Form

NAME: _____ SUBSTANCE: _____ DATE: _____

SRP WEEKLY PLAN — INITIATION PHASE

The early weeks of changing your alcohol or other drug use can be a challenging time. We call this early period of behaviour change the "Initiation Phase," which can last for anywhere from one month to much longer. Research has shown that "initiating" a change in your behaviour is easier and more effective when you use some of the following powerful strategies.

- Think about what you have to lose if you don't change. What are the factors "pushing" you to change your drinking or drug use at this time?
- Think about situations that could arise and present a risk for you. Plan ahead of time what you will do so that you aren't caught off guard.
- Avoid risky places and friends who use alcohol or other drugs.
- Involve your spouse, another family member, or a trusted friend or sponsor.
- During the first couple of weeks of changing your drinking or other drug use, living in a supportive environment can be especially helpful.
- If you want to stop drinking, consider discussing the use of alcohol-sensitizing or anti-craving medication (e.g., Antabuse®, Temposil® or naltrexone) with your doctor. These drugs can be a big help in getting you over those difficult first few weeks.
- Set a goal for your drinking or other drug use—make a commitment to yourself.

Below is some space for you to think about what you would like to accomplish in the coming week and how you will do so.

GOAL: _____

Confidence in achieving this goal: ☐ 0% ☐ 20% ☐ 40% ☐ 60% ☐ 80% ☐ 100%

Describe **two substance use triggers** that are likely to arise over the coming week: Indicate the following: Where will you be? What time of day? Who, if anyone, will be present? What will you be doing, thinking, feeling?	For each of the two triggers, describe **several coping strategies** that you will be prepared to use: You may want to use some of the strategies listed above, or plan other ways of coping that will work for you.

Component 5: Maintenance counselling

This final component of SRP counselling focuses on strategies suitable for clients in the maintenance stage of change; that is, helping clients who have achieved relative stability with respect to substance use goals using initiation strategies, but who now need the tools and skills to maintain change over the longer term.

Although it can be argued that the term "relapse prevention" should be restricted to clients in the maintenance stage of change, in practice, clients do not progress from an exclusive use of initiation strategies (Component 4) to maintenance strategies (Component 5). Instead, they tend to combine both action and maintenance strategies throughout treatment, increasingly coming to rely on maintenance strategies toward the end of treatment. The distinction between initiation and maintenance strategies is emphasized so that clients are aware of which strategies they are using. The objective is to encourage clients to rely less on initiation strategies and to gain confidence in using maintenance strategies before treatment ends. This last phase of treatment involves four steps: (1) graduated real-life exposure to a client's high-risk situations for substance use; (2) homework tasks within each type of risk situation; (3) slow reduction of the client's reliance on initiation strategies, including reliance on pharmacological agents; and (4) homework tasks that promote self-attribution of control.

The Weekly plan form used to help clients learn and practise these maintenance strategies is shown in Figure 10-3. Several differences from the Weekly plan for initiation-phase sessions (Figure 10-2) should be noted. While clients in the initiation phase are asked to focus on anticipating drug use triggers that are likely to arise naturally over the coming week, clients in the maintenance stage are also asked to actually plan on entering self-identified high-risk situations.

Homework assignments must be designed to help clients experience success and begin to build confidence (self-efficacy) in their ability to cope in high-risk situations. Multiple homework assignments (i.e., three or more) should be agreed upon at each treatment session so the client quickly learns that a high-risk situation does not automatically imply a relapse. These assignments should draw on a wide variety of the client's coping strengths and resources. As the client's confidence grows, he or she moves up the hierarchy to more difficult situations. At this later stage, a slip or lapse is unlikely to be the major setback it might have been early in treatment because the client has already begun a "snowball effect" in the growth of self-efficacy. By the end of treatment, the client should take most of the responsibility for designing his or her own homework assignments.

In summary, clients who are in the action stage or initiation phase are encouraged to use avoidance (e.g., avoid drug use settings, drug-using friends), social support (e.g., a reliable friend or family member) and perhaps a protective or anti-craving medication. Clients in the maintenance stage, however, are expected to use a greater variety of coping alternatives that will make them more self-reliant. Consistent with research on the relationship of coping repertoire to outcome (Curry & Marlatt, 1985; Moser, 1993; Van Osch et al., 2008) and the superiority of many active coping strategies compared with

FIGURE 10-3: Weekly Plan (Maintenance Phase) Form

NAME: _____ SUBSTANCE: _____ DATE: _____

SRP WEEKLY PLAN—MAINTENANCE PHASE

Congratulations! You've successfully made some changes in your drinking or other drug use. The next step is to maintain those changes and prevent relapse. Research has shown that two of the most powerful strategies for maintaining behaviour change are to:

1. take stock of all of the high-risk situations that you are likely to encounter as a natural part of your lifestyle, and
2. gradually enter these situations, starting with a lower risk and working your way up.

The idea behind planning to enter situations in which you might be tempted to drink or use other drugs is that, if these situations are likely to arise at some point, it's better for you to be in control of where and when they do. The following are more tips for maintaining behaviour change.

- Experience each risk situation a few times before moving on to the next one.
- Make sure that you take the credit for success! For example, in the initiation phase of change, we encouraged you to seek the support of others. Now that you are learning to maintain change, it's important for you to know that you can "do it on your own" if you have to.
- Make sure that the situation you plan to enter is challenging, but not too challenging.
- If you are having difficulty with entering high-risk situations, you may be moving too quickly. Take your time! You can always go back to using some of the initiation strategies (like avoiding people, places and things, or relying on the support of others) until you feel more confident.

Two powerful strategies to help maintain changes in your drinking or other drug use are setting a goal and planning to enter risk situations. Below is space for you to plan what you would like to accomplish in the coming week.

GOAL: _____

Confidence in achieving this goal: ☐ 0% ☐ 20% ☐ 40% ☐ 60% ☐ 80% ☐ 100%

HOMEWORK ASSIGNMENT
Planned Exposure to a Substance Use Trigger

Describe triggering situation: _____
_____
_____

Planned experience:
When? _____
Where? _____
Who present? _____

Coping plan (be specific, describe exactly what you will say and do, what you will be thinking, etc.):
_____
_____
_____

OUTCOME REPORT

Did you attempt this assignment? ☐ No ☐ Yes
Were you successful? ☐ No ☐ Yes
Comment: _____
_____
_____

Did you use? ☐ No ☐ Yes   If Yes, how much?
_____

What, if anything, might you try doing differently next time?
_____
_____
_____

simple avoidance (Moos & Moos, 2007; Moser, 1993; Shiffman, 1985), clients in the maintenance stage are encouraged to develop a broad repertoire of coping alternatives that includes active as well as avoidant cognitive and behavioural coping responses.

Summary of the SRP approach

Although SRP counselling has been presented as a highly structured, ordered sequence of five counselling components, in practice, a dynamic interplay occurs between counselling components and a client's readiness to change. The components are designed to enhance client readiness to change, and client stage of change affects the choice of counselling components. While some clients may proceed in a linear fashion through the stages of change and counselling components, others may not. For example, an action-stage client who experiences a lapse to substance use while receiving initiation-stage counselling may need earlier counselling components, such as continued assessment and motivational interviewing. Similarly, a preparation-stage client may experience uncertainty regarding the decision to change when faced with signing an individual treatment contract. If this occurs, further exploration of the costs and benefits of change through motivational interviewing is required. Thus, the SRP treatment model takes into account clients' readiness to change—the SRP components can be individually tailored to fit clients' ongoing needs.

The purpose of treatment is to increase self-efficacy across all areas of perceived risk, since self-efficacy has been linked with relapse onset (Gwaltney et al., 2005). If the client fails to show improved confidence in coping with a particular risk situation, further work in this area should be considered before the client is discharged from treatment. The clinician must consider possible reasons why the client has not developed confidence in the identified area. For example, has the client successfully performed homework assignments involving entry into high-risk situations? If so, what self-inferences is the client drawing from those experiences? Such an inquiry by the clinician should uncover the reason for the client's lack of confidence in relation to the particular risk area and identify any further work that needs to be done before the client completes treatment.

Relapse Prevention with Diverse Client Populations

In any treatment intervention, the needs of diverse client populations need to be considered and treatment strategies tailored accordingly. Although this is a major concern in the treatment of substance use problems, little research has been done with many special populations and marginalized groups. This section highlights key considerations from existing research and clinical practice implications of relapse prevention counselling, taking into account gender, age (youth and older adults), ethnocultural factors, sexual diversity and concurrent mental health disorders. Note that there is great heterogeneity within these broad categories, so it is a challenge to extrapolate research and practice considerations to all clients. The points outlined in this section can act as signposts for issues to be aware of; however, clinical practice should always be informed by the unique needs and issues of each individual client.

Gender

In a review of research findings on relapse and gender, Walitzer and Dearing (2006) found that studies of alcohol relapse have revealed various factors, including negative mood, childhood trauma (especially sexual abuse), alcohol-related self-efficacy and poorer coping, to be associated with greater likelihood of relapse; however, these factors are not moderated by gender. Among men and women who are addicted to substances other than alcohol, women have been shown to be less prone to relapse than men. Marriage also affects relapse risk differently for men and women, possibly because of partner differences. For example, women with alcohol use disorder are more likely to have partners who are heavy drinkers, thus increasing their relapse risk. On the other hand, marriage is a protective factor for men with alcohol problems.

Research has also shown that men tend to report more negative social influences, greater exposure to substances and poorer coping skills than women (Walton et al., 2001). Women may be at higher risk for relapse following negative emotions or personal conflict, while men report positive experiences (pleasant times with others or pleasant emotions) as particular relapse risks (Walitzer & Dearing, 2006).

In general, women tend to report better coping mechanisms than men (Walton et al., 2001). Women also tend to see their substance use as secondary to more general problems, such as anxiety and depression. As a result, women use medical and psychiatric services more frequently than men and perceive these services as more effective (Osorio et al., 2002).

Youth

Few relapse prevention models focus on youth, although rates of post-treatment relapse (the overall percentage of youth who are not able to maintain their substance use goals) and time to relapse (the average time after treatment ends before a relapse occurs) appear similar for both adults and youth (Chung & Maisto, 2006). Youth-specific treatment approaches are important, given that young people face different developmental processes and challenges. Some research has explored ways of adapting treatment models to better fit the needs of younger clients.

Relapse prevention for young people needs to focus on issues of youth-parent relationships and peer group membership, as these are central to the lives and experiences of younger clients. Illicit substance use by youth is strongly related to parental support, as well as parental awareness and monitoring of the whereabouts and activities of their child (Miller & Plant, 2003). Peer influences, delinquency and re-offending behaviour are also strongly associated with youth substance use (Roget et al., 1998). In some cases, relapse prevention may need to include liaison with the juvenile justice system, or a contract with a specific substance use treatment provider.

Clinicians need to make feedback personally relevant to young clients, and avoid confrontation. Confrontation, with its authoritarian overtones, is especially likely to trigger a rebellious response and is unlikely to promote a therapeutic alliance. In addition, clinicians need to encourage young clients to actively prepare for relapse and to practise coping strategies. First Contact is a brief, four-session intervention adapted especially for youth (Breslin et al., 1999). This manual-based approach combines elements of cognitive-behavioural and motivational interviewing approaches, and includes brief screening tools, personalized feedback and exercises to identify and plan for high-risk situations. Given that many young people with addiction issues also experience other co-occurring problems, a treatment approach like First Contact can be a good way to engage them in a process for changing their substance use and enhance their motivation before addressing other specialized or long-term needs. Groups are the most widespread modality used with youth, due to the influence that pro-social peers have on one another and the greater opportunity for social skills training and development (Mason & Hawkins, 2009).

An important component of relapse prevention strategies with youth is the development of a behavioural contract, in this case a "relapse contract." This contract is created by all parties involved and might include family rules, school or job requirements, probation requirements, treatment attendance, urinalysis, social supports and relapse consequences. Any relapse episodes need to focus on what can be learned, as "learning by doing" is important in this stage of life.

Older Adults

Most research exploring relapse has focused across the adult age range rather than specifically on older adults. However, a few differences in treatment outcomes for older adults have been noted (Barrick & Connors, 2002). For example, high-risk situations among older adults tend to involve intrapersonal issues more frequently than among younger adults (Barrick & Connors, 2002). In addition, several age-specific issues have been found to be relevant to relapse prevention in older adults. Negative emotional states related to anxiety, interpersonal conflict, depression, loneliness, loss and social isolation constitute the highest-risk situations. Retirement, the death of a partner or child and the stressors of aging represent a risky time for alcohol or other drug use. Cognitive impairments associated with aging, no matter what the etiology, need to be assessed and taken into consideration in relapse planning for older adults (Barrick & Connors, 2002).

Schonfeld and colleagues (2000) evaluated a 16-week relapse prevention program called Get Smart and found that cognitive-behavioural programs that focus on identifying high-risk situations, coping skills and relapse plans worked well with older clients who have significant medical, social and substance use problems.

Ethnocultural Factors

Many treatment programs have difficulty attracting and retaining clients from diverse ethnocultural communities. Language, treatment philosophies and methods, clinician demographics and lack of agency knowledge or awareness of cross-cultural counselling implications create systemic barriers for many clients. Other factors, such as settlement experience, norms and values around substance use, or experiences of marginalization and discrimination, can also present significant barriers to treatment access and engagement.

Increasingly, the literature indicates that clinicians need to develop competence in working with clients from diverse racial, cultural, ethnic and religious backgrounds (Srivastava, 2007; Straussner, 2002). Ethnocultural competence, defined as "the ability of a clinician to function effectively in the context of ethnocultural differences" (Straussner, 2002, p. 35) is a critical skill in applying relapse prevention strategies and techniques.

It is important to recognize that "talk therapy" may not be normative in many cultures; some clients may find it difficult to share personal issues with a clinician from a culture they do not know well. Group treatment may make it difficult for members of some ethnocultural groups to disclose personal information, necessitating individual counselling in some cases. However, relapse prevention treatment targeted at individual clients may not be a good fit for people whose culture values family and community over "rugged individualism." Mainstream western culture has a more individualistic and personal growth world view than many other cultures that have collective and different experiences of history, values and social and family structures (Blume & de la Cruz, 2005). In some cases, family counselling might be a more appropriate way to address substance use and relapse.

Although some research has been carried out on substance use patterns and issues in different cultural groups, caution needs to be exercised in drawing particular clinical implications from this work, given the heterogeneity of ethnocultural groups. In addition, more research is needed to help develop relapse prevention approaches specific to different populations.

Indigenous Populations

Little research exists regarding relapse prevention applications for indigenous populations. One study exploring predictors of relapse among a sample of American Indian women found that negative messages about alcohol or other drug use in childhood and high self-efficacy were significant protective factors, and alcohol craving, conflict with others and social networks where alcohol was used were risk factors (Chong & Lopez, 2008). These relapse precipitants and protective factors are not dissimilar to those identified among general treatment populations (e.g., Gordon et al., 2006; Witkiewitz & Marlatt, 2007). Again, however, these research findings should be interpreted with caution, and may not be applicable to specific clients in specific First Nations communities.

Because of the great diversity among and within indigenous populations, it is impossible to generalize about traditional or non-traditional beliefs or preferences. Many clients may choose traditional healing approaches or teachings as a path to healing and recovery, while others may prefer mainstream approaches. Still others may find a combination of traditional and non-traditional approaches to be most suitable.

Aboriginal clients may face geographical barriers to accessing treatment. In rural or remote communities, access to treatment resources can be limited. Furthermore, health and recovery from substance use should be considered within the broader context of colonialism and historical (and current) oppression, as well as the impacts of intergenerational trauma. These issues are addressed in more detail in Chapter 24.

Sexual Diversity

There is very limited research about relapse prevention specific to lesbian, gay, bisexual, transsexual or transgendered people. However, as with all counsellor-client interactions, mutual respect, unconditional positive regard and attentiveness to the client's issues and goals should be paramount. Clients from sexually diverse groups often have issues relating to discrimination (homophobia, biphobia, transphobia), coming out, openness about sexual orientation or gender identity, family issues, involvement in the community and body image (Barbara et al., 2002). See Chapter 25 for specific suggestions on how to be intentionally inclusive with these client populations.

Concurrent Mental Health Disorders

Increasing recognition of the high co-prevalence rates of substance use and mental illness means that clinicians need to routinely screen for the presence of a concurrent disorder. (This is discussed in more detail in Chapter 16.) Ignoring or not properly recognizing concurrent disorders can affect clients' ability to recover successfully. Herie and colleagues (2006) identify various negative effects, including:

- premature dropout from treatment
- higher risk of relapse
- risk of harmful interactions between drugs of abuse and psychiatric medications
- misinterpretation of symptoms (e.g., are they signs of a mental health problem, the effects of substance use or signs of withdrawal from substances?)
- likelihood of needing more expensive services in future.

Various factors have made it difficult for agencies and health care settings to respond adequately to the needs of people with concurrent disorders: lack of specialist knowledge and skills in addiction, mental health or both; limited access to specialist diagnostic and other treatment services and providers; agency exclusion criteria; problem complexity; and fragmented treatment systems. Nevertheless, people with concurrent disorders are often best served where they present and, at the very least, within the context of an integrated treatment program or system (Health Canada, 2002).

To better empower clients in fostering a more helpful mindset about managing relapses, it is useful to normalize the idea that relapses occur in both substance use and mental health domains, and then attempt to help clients identify personalized "early warning signs" that their mental health is deteriorating. For example, indications of depression might include wanting to withdraw socially, beginning to lose interest in activities previously enjoyed and experiencing an increase in negative or pessimistic thinking.

Once the client becomes aware of these early warning signs, or red flags, encourage the client to develop strategies for coping and intervening early on in the cycle. Such interventions might include relaying symptoms to a caregiver and implementing personal coping strategies, such as using good self-care strategies and seeking social support, with the overall goal of circumventing a full relapse. Relapse prevention goals might include:

- working on a substance use goal of abstinence or reduction
- having slips less often, and having shorter-lasting slips should they occur within an abstinence-based goal
- using less of the problem substance (if used at all), and having fewer negative consequences associated with substance use
- recognizing the impact of substance use on mental health
- learning and recognizing early warning signs for mental health relapse
- developing and using an action recovery plan that can be implemented and practised in the real world, in between SRP sessions, which aims to support the maintenance of change.

People with severe mental illness may be more sensitive to the effects of alcohol and other drugs due to increased biological vulnerability, and therefore may experience more negative consequences from relatively small amounts of substance use. Thus, moderate use (e.g., two beers three times per week, or $20 worth of crack cocaine used once every few weeks) in someone with schizophrenia may result in negative consequences (such as increased psychotic symptoms) or dramatically increase the risk of more severe substance use. A key message when working with clients with serious and persistent mental illness is that the quantity of the substance use may be less important than the consequences. This is especially true in light of possible interactions between non-prescribed or illicit substances or alcohol and psychiatric medications.

A number of modifications may be helpful in running relapse prevention groups with clients who have concurrent disorders. These include implementing shorter group duration; using fewer clinical tools per treatment session; modifying clinical tools to incorporate concurrent disorder–specific treatment goals (e.g., taking prescribed medications, coping with the symptoms of mental illness or the side-effects of prescribed medications); taking more time in the group to process discussion around access to services and navigating the mental health and addiction treatment system; and making homework tools easier and simpler to complete (Herie et al., 2006).

Revisiting the Case Study

In the case study that opened this chapter, George does not really see his substance use as problematic: the drugs help him to relax and escape life's stresses and problems, but he is unhappy with the negative consequences he has been experiencing. Even if George were able to abstain completely from alcohol and cannabis in the short term, he would be left without the important (and effective) coping tools these drugs provide, ultimately leading him back into the same patterns of use.

An integrated motivational/cognitive-behavioural intervention like SRP could help George to explore the costs and benefits of his drug use, enhance his motivation for change and self-efficacy, identify situations where he is at higher risk of using and help him develop new, more effective coping skills. Other interventions, such as assessing for a possible concurrent disorder and providing occupational therapy, might be useful complements to relapse prevention treatment for George. A holistic approach would also consider the impacts of his relationship with his mother and stepfather, and his long-term hopes and goals.

Conclusion

This chapter has highlighted a number of clinical issues and considerations in addressing relapse to substance use. Treatment approaches must be considered against a backdrop of evolving research findings and theory, including recent research on the neurobiological factors, and extensions to theoretical models. These advances will likely affect—and perhaps challenge—mainstream approaches in the years to come. At this time, cognitive-behavioural treatments informed by social learning theory, such as the SRP model, demonstrate robust empirical support and can be used effectively with a variety of clinical populations. It is critical to ensure that relapse prevention strategies are tailored to the unique needs of clients and that the particular issues of diverse populations are considered. Relapse prevention is just one part of a more complex set of clinical considerations, but it can constitute an entry point and beginning of positive change and recovery.

Practice Tips

- Expect relapse: it is a normal result of the chronic nature of addictive disorders. Relapse should be considered in the context of clients' overall progress toward treatment goals, as well as the psychosocial impacts of substance use.
- Ensure that a dynamic model of relapse accounts for the complex interactions among and between biological, psychological, social, structural and spiritual factors in the client's life.
- Consider cognitive-behavioural therapy and motivational interviewing, informed by social learning theory, as relapse prevention interventions.
- Focus maintenance strategies on building self-efficacy in real-life risk situations. The coping strategies that help a person to initiate behavioural change differ from those needed to maintain change.
- Include identifying and analyzing risk situations (e.g., relapse triggers and consequences) in relapse risk assessments, as well as cognitive and behavioural alternatives to substance use.
- Use relapse planning, in which clients anticipate upcoming risk situations and identify possible coping strategies, when clients are both initiating and maintaining change.
- Tailor and adapt treatment interventions to fit the diverse needs of the client populations you serve.

Resources

Publications

Herie, M. & Watkin-Merek, L. (1997). *Structured Relapse Prevention: An Outpatient Approach to Group Treatment* (Video). Toronto: Addiction Research Foundation.

Herie, M. & Watkin-Merek, L. (2006). *Structured Relapse Prevention: An Outpatient Counselling Approach* (2nd ed.). Toronto: Centre for Addiction and Mental Health.

Substance Abuse and Mental Health Services Administration. (2010, October 14). *The N-SSATS Report: Clinical or Therapeutic Approaches Used by Substance Abuse Treatment Facilities.* Rockville, MD: Author. Retrieved from www.oas.samhsa.gov/2k10/238/238 ClinicalAp2k10Web.pdf

Internet

Addictive Behaviors Research Center, University of Washington
http://depts.washington.edu/abrc/

Alan Marlatt lecture on mindfulness-based relapse prevention
www.youtube.com/watch?v=3ri2YB0ApIg

Alcohol Help Center
www.alcoholhelpcenter.net/Default.aspx

Centre for Addiction and Mental Health. (2006). Overview of structured relapse prevention. Retrieved from http://knowledgex.camh.net/amhspecialists/specialized_treatment/relapse_prevention/srp/Pages/default.aspx

Mindfulness-Based Relapse Prevention
www.mindfulrp.com

References

Annis, H.M. (1986). A relapse prevention model for treatment of alcoholics. In W.R. Miller & N. Heather (Eds.), *Treating Addictive Behaviors: Processes of Change* (pp. 407–421). New York: Plenum.

Annis, H.M., Herie, M. & Watkin-Merek, L. (1996). *Structured Relapse Prevention*. Toronto: Addiction Research Foundation.

Annis, H.M. & Martin, G. (1985a). *Inventory of Drug-Taking Situations (IDTS-50)*. Toronto: Addiction Research Foundation.

Annis, H.M. & Martin, G. (1985b). *Drug-Taking Confidence Questionnaire (DTCQ-50)*. Toronto: Addiction Research Foundation.

Baker, T.B., Piper, M.E., McCarthy, D.E., Majeskie, M.R. & Fiore, M.C. (2004). Addiction motivation reformulated: An affective processing model of negative reinforcement. *Psychological Review, 111*, 33–51.

Bandura, A. (1986). *Social Foundations of Thought and Action*. Englewood Cliffs, NJ: Prentice Hall.

Bandura, A. (2004). Health promotion by social cognitive means. *Health Education & Behavior, 31*, 143–164.

Barbara, A.M., Chaim, G. & Doctor, F. (2002). *Asking the Right Questions: Talking about Sexual Orientation and Gender Identity during Assessment for Drug and Alcohol Concerns*. Toronto: Centre for Addiction and Mental Health.

Barrick, C. & Connors, G.J. (2002). Relapse prevention and maintaining abstinence in older adults with alcohol-use disorders. *Drugs & Aging, 19*, 583–594.

Blume, A.W. & de la Cruz, G.B. (2005). Relapse prevention among diverse populations. In G.A. Marlatt & D.M. Donavan (Eds.), *Relapse Prevention Maintenance Strategies in the Treatment of Addictive Behaviors* (2nd ed., pp. 45–64). New York: Guilford Press.

Bowen, S., Chawla, N., Collins, S.E., Witkiewitz, K., Hsu, S., Grow, J. et al. (2009). Mindfulness-based relapse prevention for substance use disorders: A pilot efficacy trial. *Substance Abuse, 30*, 295–305.

Bradizza, C.M., Stasiewicz, P.R. & Paas, N.D. (2006). Relapse to alcohol and drug use among individuals diagnosed with co-occurring mental health and substance use disorders: A review. *Clinical Psychology Review, 26*, 162–178.

Breslin, C., Sdao-Jarvie, K., Tupker, E. & Pearlman, S. (1999). *First Contact: A Brief Treatment for Young Substance Users.* Toronto: Centre for Addiction and Mental Health.

Breslin, F.C., Zack, M. & McMain, S. (2002). An information-processing analysis of mindfulness: Implications for relapse prevention in the treatment of substance abuse. *Clinical Psychology: Science and Practice, 9*, 275–299.

Chatterjee, U. & Chattopadhyay, P.K. (2005). Relapse prevention in drug abuse: Personality determinants. *Social Science International, 21* (1), 56–62.

Chong, J. & Lopez, D. (2008). Predictors of relapse for American Indian women after substance abuse treatment. *American Indian and Alaska Native Mental Health Research, 14* (3), 24–48.

Chung, T. & Maisto, S.A. (2006). Relapse to alcohol and other drug use in treated adolescents: Review and reconsideration of relapse as a change point in clinical course. *Clinical Psychology Review, 26*, 149–161.

Connors, G.J. & Maisto, S.A. (2006). Relapse in the addictive behaviors. *Clinical Psychology Review, 26*, 107–108.

Curry, S.G. & Marlatt, G.A. (1985). Unaided quitters' strategies for coping with temptations to smoke. In S. Shiffman & T.A. Wills (Eds.), *Coping and Substance Use* (pp. 243–265). New York: Academic Press.

Davis, K.E. & O'Neill, S.J. (2005). A focus group analysis of relapse prevention strategies for persons with substance use and mental disorders. *Psychiatric Services, 56*, 1288–1291.

Demmel, R., Nicolai, J. & Jenko, D.M. (2006). Self-efficacy and alcohol relapse: Concurrent validity of confidence measures, self-other discrepancies and prediction of treatment outcome. *Journal of Studies on Alcohol, 67*, 637–641.

ElGeili, E.S.S. & Bashir, T.Z. (2005). Precipitants of relapse among heroin addicts. *Addictive Disorders and Their Treatment, 4*, 29–38.

Fox, H.C., Jackson, E.D. & Sinha, R. (2009). Elevated cortisol and learning and memory deficits in cocaine dependent individuals: Relationship to relapse outcomes. *Psychoneuroendocrinology, 34*, 1198–1207.

Gordon, S.M., Sterling, R., Siatkowski, C., Raively, K., Weinstein, S. & Hill, P.C. (2006). Inpatient desire to drink as a predictor of relapse to alcohol use following treatment. *American Journal on Addictions, 15*, 242–245.

Griffiths, M. (2005). A "components" model of addiction within a biopsychosocial framework. *Journal of Substance Use, 10*, 191–197.

Gwaltney, C.J., Shiffman, S., Balabanis, M.H. & Paty, J.A. (2005). Dynamic self-efficacy and outcome expectancies: Prediction of smoking lapse and relapse. *Journal of Abnormal Psychology, 114*, 661–675.

Harris, M., Fallot, R.D. & Bereley, R.W. (2005). Qualitative interviews on substance abuse relapse and prevention among female trauma survivors. *Psychiatric Services, 56*, 1292–1296.

Health Canada. (2002). *Best Practices: Concurrent Mental Health and Substance Use Disorders*. Ottawa: Author. Retrieved from www.hc-sc.gc.ca/ahc-asc/pubs/drugs-drogues/bp_disorder-mp_concomitants/index_e.html

Health Canada. (2007). *Best Practice in Screening for Substance Use and Mental Health Disorders*. Retrieved from www.hc-sc.gc.ca/hc-ps/pubs/adp-apd/bp_disorder-mp_concomitants/screening-depistage-eng.php

Hendershot, C.S., Marlatt, G.A. & George, W.H. (2008). Relapse prevention and the maintenance of optimal health. In S.A. Shumaker, J.K. Ockene & K.A. Riekert (Eds.), *Handbook of Health Behaviour Change* (pp. 127–149). New York: Springer.

Herie, M. & Skinner, W. (2010). *Substance Abuse in Canada*. Don Mills, ON: Oxford University Press.

Herie, M., Tsanos, A. & Watkin-Merek, L. (2006). Adapting the SRP approach. In M. Herie & L. Watkin-Merek (Eds.), *Structured Relapse Prevention: An Outpatient Counselling Approach* (2nd ed., pp. 123–133). Toronto: Centre for Addiction and Mental Health.

Herie, M. & Watkin-Merek, L. (2006). *Structured Relapse Prevention: An Outpatient Counselling Approach* (2nd ed.). Toronto: Centre for Addiction and Mental Health.

Hunt, W.A., Barnett, L.W. & Brach, L.G. (1971). Relapse rates in addiction programs. *Journal of Clinical Psychology, 27*, 455–456.

Hunter-Reel, D., McCrady, B. & Hildebrandt, T. (2009). Emphasizing interpersonal factors: An extension of the Witkiewitz and Marlatt relapse model. *Addiction, 104*, 1281–1290.

Leshner, A.I. (1997). Addiction is a brain disease, and it matters. *Science, 278* (5335), 45–47.

Levy, M.S. (2008). Listening to our clients: The prevention of relapse. *Journal of Psychoactive Drugs, 20*, 167–172.

Litman, G.K., Eiser, J.R., Rawson, N.S.B. & Oppenheim, A.N. (1979). Differences in relapse precipitants and coping behaviors between alcohol relapsers and survivors. *Behaviour Research and Therapy, 17*, 89–94.

Litman, G.K., Stapleton, J., Oppenheim, A.N., Peleg, M. & Jackson, P. (1984). The relationship between coping behaviors, their effectiveness and alcoholism relapse and survival. *British Journal of Addiction, 79*, 283–291.

Lowman, C., Allen, J., Stout, R.L. & the Relapse Research Group. (1996). Replication and extension of Marlatt's taxonomy of relapse precipitants: Overview of procedures and results. *Addiction, 91* (Suppl.), 51–71.

Maisto, S.A. & Connors, G.J. (2006). Relapse in the addictive behaviors: Integration and future directions. *Clinical Psychology Review, 26*, 229–231.

Marjot, D. (2010). It's reunion, not relapse. *Addiction, 105*, 374–375.

Marlatt, G.A. (1996). Taxonomy of high risk situations for alcohol relapse: Evolution and development of a cognitive-behavioral model. *Addiction, 91* (Suppl.), 37–49.

Marlatt, G.A. (2002). Buddhist philosophy and the treatment of addictive behavior. *Cognitive and Behavioral Practice, 9*, 44–50.

Marlatt, G.A. & Gordon, J.R. (1980). Determinants of relapse: Implications for the maintenance of behavior change. In P. Davidson & S. Davidson (Eds.), *Behavioral Medicine: Changing Health Lifestyles* (pp. 71–127). New York: Brunner/Mazel.

Marlatt, G.A. & Gordon, J.R. (1985). *Relapse Prevention: Maintenance Strategies in the Treatment of Addictive Behaviors.* New York: Guilford Press.

Marlatt, G.A. & Witkiewitz, K. (2005). Relapse prevention for alcohol and drug problems. In G.A. Marlatt & D.M. Donovan (Eds.), *Relapse Prevention: Maintenance Strategies in the Treatment of Addictive Behaviors* (2nd ed., pp. 1–43). New York: Guilford Press.

Mason, W.A. & Hawkins, J.D. (2009). Adolescent risk and protective factors: Psychosocial. In R.K. Ries, S.C. Miller, D.A. Fiellin & R. Saitz (Eds.), *Principles of Addiction Medicine* (4th ed., pp. 1383–1390). Philadelphia: Lippincott, Williams & Wilkins.

McKay, J.R., Franklin, T.R., Patapis, N. & Lynch, K.G. (2006). Conceptual, methodological and analytical issues in the study of relapse. *Clinical Psychology Review, 26*, 109–127.

McLellan, A.T., Lewis, D.C., O'Brien, C.P. & Kleber, H.D. (2000). Drug dependence, a chronic medical illness: Implications for treatment, insurance, and outcomes evaluation. *JAMA, 284*, 1689–1695.

Miller, P. & Plant, M. (2003). The family, peer influences and substance use: Findings from a study of U.K. teenagers. *Journal of Substance Use, 8*, 19–26.

Miller, W.R. (1996). What is a relapse? Fifty ways to leave the wagon. *Addiction, 91* (Suppl.), 15–27.

Miller, W.R. & Rollnick, S. (2002). *Motivational Interviewing* (2nd ed.). New York: Guilford Press.

Moos, R.H. & Moos, B.S. (2007). Treated and untreated alcohol-use disorders: Course and predictors of remission and relapse. *Evaluation Review, 31*, 564–584.

Moser, A.E. (1993). Situational antecedents, self-efficacy and coping in relapse crisis outcome: A prospective study of treated alcoholics. Unpublished doctoral dissertation, York University, Toronto.

Mueller, S.E., Petitjean, S., Boening, J. & Wiesbeck, G.A. (2007). The impact of self-help group attendance on relapse rates after alcohol detoxification in a controlled study. *Alcohol and Alcoholism, 42*, 108–112.

National Institute on Drug Abuse. (2010). *Drugs, Brains and Behavior: The Science of Addiction.* Bethesda, MD: U.S. Department of Health and Human Services. Retrieved from http://drugabuse.gov/scienceofaddiction/sciofaddiction.pdf

Osorio, R., McCusker, M. & Salazar, C. (2002). Evaluation of a women-only service for substance misusers. *Journal of Substance Use, 7,* 41–49.

Project MATCH Research Group. (1997). Matching alcoholism treatments to client heterogeneity: Project MATCH posttreatment drinking outcomes. *Journal of Studies on Alcohol, 58,* 7–29.

Ramo, D.E. & Brown, S.A. (2008). Classes of substance abuse relapse situations: A comparison of adolescents and adults. *Psychology of Addictive Behaviors, 22,* 372–379.

Roget, N.A., Fisher, G.L. & Johnson, M.L. (1998). A protocol for reducing juvenile recidivism through relapse prevention. *Journal of Addictions and Offender Counselling, 19,* 33–43.

Rohsenow, D.J. & Monti, P.M. (2001). Relapse among cocaine abusers: Theoretical, methodological and treatment considerations. In F.M. Tims, C.G. Leukefeld & J.J. Platt (Eds.), *Relapse and Recovery in Addictions* (pp. 355–378). Newhaven, CT: Yale University Press.

Roozen, H.G. & Van de Wetering, B.J.M. (2007). Neuropsychiatric insights in clinical practice: From relapse prevention toward relapse management. *American Journal on Addictions, 16,* 530–531.

Schonfeld, L., Dupree, L.W., Dickson-Fuhrmann, E., McKean Royer, C., McDermott, C.H., Rosansky, J.S. et al. (2000). Cognitive-behavioural treatment of older veterans with substance abuse problems. *Journal of Geriatric Psychiatry Neurology, 13,* 124–129.

Schröter, M., Collins, S.E., Frittrang, T., Buchkremer, G. & Batra, A. (2006). Randomized controlled trial of relapse prevention and a standard behavioral intervention with adult smokers. *Addictive Behaviors, 31,* 1259–1264.

Shiffman, S. (1985). Preventing relapse in ex-smokers: A self-management approach. In G.A. Marlatt & J.R. Gordon (Eds.), *Relapse Prevention* (pp. 472–520). New York: Guilford Press.

Sinha, R., Fox, H., Hong, K.I., Sofuoglu, M., Morgan, P.T. & Bergquist, K.T. (2007). Sex steroid hormones, stress response, and drug craving in cocaine-dependent women: Implications for relapse susceptibility. *Experimental and Clinical Psychopharmacology, 15,* 445–452.

Srivastava, R. (2007). *The Healthcare Professional's Guide to Clinical Cultural Competence.* Toronto: Mosby/Elsevier.

Stahler, G.J., Mennis, J., Cotlar, R. & Baron, D.A. (2010). The influence of neighborhood environment on treatment continuity and rehospitalization in dually diagnosed patients discharged from acute inpatient care. *American Journal of Psychiatry, 166,* 1207–1208.

Sterling, R.C., Weinstein, S., Losardo, D., Raively, K., Hill, P., Petrone, A. & Gottheil, E. (2007). A retrospective case control study of alcohol relapse and spiritual growth. *American Journal on Addictions, 16* (1), 56–61.

Straussner, S.L. (2002). Ethnic cultures and substance abuse. *Counselor: The Magazine for Addiction Professionals, 3* (6), 34–38.

Tate, S.R., Brown, S.A., Glasner, S.V., Unrod, M. & McQuaid, J.R. (2006). Chronic life stress, acute stress events, and substance availability in relapse. *Addiction Research & Theory, 14*, 303–322.

Turner, N.E., Annis, H.M. & Sklar, S.M. (1997). Measurement of antecedents to drug and alcohol use: Psychometric properties of the Inventory of Drug-Taking Situations (IDTS). *Behaviour Research and Therapy, 35*, 465–483.

Vallejo, Z. & Hortensia, A. (2009). Adaptation of mindfulness-based stress reduction program for addiction relapse prevention. *Humanistic Psychologist, 37*, 192–206.

VanDeMark, N.R. (2007). Policy on reintegration of women with histories of substance abuse: A mixed methods study of predictors of relapse and facilitators of recovery. *Substance Abuse Treatment, Prevention, and Policy, 2*. doi: 10.1186/1747-597X-2-28

Van Osch, L., Lechner, L., Reubsaet, A., Wigger, S. & de Vries, H. (2008). Relapse prevention in a national smoking cessation contest: Effects of coping planning. *British Journal of Health Psychology, 13*, 525–535.

Walitzer, K.S. & Dearing, R.L. (2006). Gender differences in alcohol and substance use relapse. *Clinical Psychology Review, 26* (2), 128–148.

Walter, M., Gerhard, U., Duersteler-MacFarland, K.M., Weijers, H.G., Boening, J. & Wiesbeck, G.A. (2006). Social factors but not stress-coping styles predict relapse in detoxified alcoholics. *Neuropsychobiology, 54*, 100–106.

Walton, M.A., Blow, F.C. & Booth, B.M. (2001). Diversity in relapse prevention needs: Gender and race comparisons among substance abuse treatment patients. *American Journal of Drug and Alcohol Abuse, 27*, 225–240.

White, W., Boyle, M. & Loveland, D. (2003). Addiction as chronic disease: From rhetoric to clinical application. *Alcoholism Treatment Quarterly, 20*, 107–130.

Wilson, B. (1962). *The AA Service Manual Combined with Twelve Concepts for World Services* (1999–2000 ed.). Alcoholics Anonymous World Services.

Wilson, G.T. (1980). Cognitive factors in lifestyle changes: A social learning perspective. In P.O. Davidson & S.M. Davidson (Eds.), *Behavioral Medicine: Changing Health Lifestyles* (pp. 3–37). New York: Brunner/Mazel.

Witkiewitz, K. & Marlatt, G.A. (2004). Relapse prevention for alcohol and drug problems: That was Zen, this is Tao. *American Psychologist, 59*, 224–235.

Witkiewitz, K. & Marlatt, G.A. (2007). Modeling the complexity of post-treatment drinking: It's a rocky road to relapse. *Clinical Psychology Review, 27*, 724–738.

Witkiewitz, K., Marlatt, G.A. & Walker, D. (2005). Mindfulness-based relapse prevention for alcohol and substance use disorders. *Journal of Cognitive Psychotherapy, 19*, 211–228.

Wojnar, M., Brower, K.J., Strobbe, S., Ilgen, M., Matsumoto, H., Nowosad, I. et al. (2009). Association between Val66Met brain-derived neurotrophic factor (BDNF) gene polymorphism and post-treatment relapse in alcohol dependence. *Alcoholism Clinical and Experimental Research, 33*, 693–702.

Xie, H., McHugo, G.J., Fox, M.B. & Drake, R.E. (2005). Substance abuse relapse in a ten-year prospective follow-up of clients with mental and substance use disorders. *Psychiatric Services, 56*, 1282–1287.

Zgierska, A., Rabago, D., Chawla, N., Kushner, K., Koehler, R. & Marlatt, A. (2009). Mindfulness meditation for substance use disorders: A systematic review. *Substance Abuse, 30*, 266–294.

Zgierska, A., Rabago, D., Zuelsdorff, M., Coe, C., Miller, M. & Fleming, M. (2008). Mindfulness medication for relapse prevention: A feasibility pilot study. *Journal of Addiction Medicine, 2*, 165–173.

Zvolensky, M.J., Bernstein, A., Cardenas, S.J., Colotla, V.A., Marshall, E.C. & Feldner, M.T. (2007). Anxiety sensitivity and early relapse to smoking: A test among Mexican daily, low-level smokers. *Nicotine and Tobacco Research, 9*, 483–491.

Zywiak, W.H., Stout, R.L., Longabaugh, R., Dyck, I., Connors, G.J. & Maisto, S.A. (2006). Relapse-onset factors in Project MATCH: The Relapse Questionnaire. *Journal of Substance Abuse Treatment, 31*, 341–345.

Chapter 11

Tobacco Interventions for People with Alcohol and Other Drug Problems

Peter Selby, Megan Barker and Marilyn Herie

Raisa began using substances at a very early age. She grew up in a small town in northern Ontario with her mother, who has bipolar disorder, and her stepfather, who drank heavily and was often unemployed. Her stepfather began sexually abusing Raisa when she was 11 years old. Around the same time she began smoking. To cope with the ongoing abuse, Raisa started drinking at age 12 and started experimenting with other drugs by age 15. She eventually dropped out of school and ran away from home to Toronto in order to escape her abusive stepfather.

Raisa is now 35 years old, homeless and addicted to alcohol, opioids and crack cocaine. She often smokes up to 70 cigarettes a day. She is being treated as an inpatient at a local mental health and addiction centre as a consequence of a recent suicide attempt. The centre is a smoke-free environment, and Raisa is finding it very difficult to get through the day without smoking many cigarettes because she can only go outside for a cigarette three times a day. Even with these breaks incorporated into her schedule, Raisa has been caught smoking in her room and seems frustrated, angry, anxious and restless.

Raisa is one of many people for whom tobacco was the first drug of addiction. More importantly, tobacco use is often the last to be addressed, yet has the highest risk of morbidity and mortality. It is clear that being given limited designated times to smoke does not work for Raisa. She is likely experiencing nicotine withdrawal, leading her to smoke in her room despite the rules on the unit. This is also jeopardizing her treatment—she has been warned that if she continues to smoke on the unit she will be discharged.

The issue of tobacco use among people with mental health and substance use problems is not new or unique; yet comprehensive, evidence-based, integrated cessation or withdrawal management interventions are not uniformly available for clients who smoke. Raisa's tobacco addiction is as much of a concern as the other substance use and mental health issues that led her into treatment. Tobacco is the primary cause of preventable death in the developed world. It continues to remain Ontario's number one drug problem, accounting for 42 per cent of drug-related costs to the economy, 59 per cent of drug-related hospital days and 86 per cent of all drug-related deaths (Rehm et al., 2006). Among people entering addiction treatment, smoking prevalence remains disproportionately high, ranging between 49 and 98 per cent (Schroeder, 2009). In a review of the addiction treatment literature, Guydish and colleagues (2011) found that people who smoke and who also have other addictions smoke more heavily, are less successful in their attempts to quit smoking and are more likely to die from tobacco-related causes than from all other substance-related causes combined. In addition, tobacco is the leading cause of death among people with addiction and/or mental health problems (Hurt et al., 1996). These findings suggest that although clinicians in addiction treatment settings may be helping clients reduce the risks associated with using other substances, failing to address clients' tobacco use means overlooking their area of potentially highest risk. Tobacco cessation warrants a significant systematized response from addiction treatment programs.

Although the benefits of smoking cessation are well known, substance use treatment programs often overlook the opportunity to motivate and counsel clients to quit. Treatment providers frequently believe that it is unrealistic to counsel clients to address tobacco use at the same time as dealing with another substance use problem. They know that quitting smoking can, for most clients, be even more difficult than giving up the substance for which they are seeking treatment (Kozlowski et al., 1989; Ziedonis et al., 2007). However, a significant number of clients in substance use treatment are willing to accept treatment for tobacco use (Joseph et al., 2004; Prochaska et al., 2007; Schroeder & Morris, 2010), and substance use counsellors may be ideally situated to offer this treatment. Furthermore, addressing smoking may help to improve the success of substance use treatment (Kohn et al., 2003; Prochaska, 2010).

In this chapter, we examine the rationale and importance of integrating tobacco cessation interventions with other substance use treatment. We discuss the evidence for intervening with this population and describe a humanistic framework for addressing tobacco use. Our goal is to help counsellors motivate and counsel their clients to quit smoking and engage in relapse prevention. We encourage behaviour change among counsellors themselves so they will increasingly see smoking cessation treatment in addiction settings as a standard of care and a duty of practice, akin to that for any other substance use problem (Torrijos & Glantz, 2006).

Health Effects of Tobacco Use

The negative health effects of tobacco use are multi-layered and appear not to spare any major organ system. Cigarettes remain the only legally available consumer product that will kill at least 50 per cent of the people who use them as intended by the manufacturer (Peto et al., 1996). Tobacco use kills an estimated 37,000 Canadians annually (Rehm et al., 2006) and accounts for more deaths than alcohol, illicit drugs, HIV, hepatitis C, suicide, murder and motor vehicle accidents combined (Jha & Chaloupka, 1999; Makomaski Illing & Kaiserman, 1999). Smoking is responsible for the death of approximately six million people each year (World Health Organization, 2011). Unless we encourage and help people to quit, 500 million people alive today will die in the 21st century from tobacco use (Jha et al., 2006).

The costs of tobacco use are unprecedented. In 2002, Canadians spent 17 billion dollars in health care and economic costs, of which 43 per cent accounted for substance use and misuse costs (Rehm et al., 2006). Moreover, 3.8 million hospital days were attributed to substance use and misuse, the majority of which were a consequence of smoking (Rehm et al., 2006).

The health effects of smoking and environmental tobacco smoke exposure have been described over most of the last century (Bartecchi et al., 1995; Repace, 2006; Wald & Hackshaw, 1996) (see Table 11-1). However, many people who smoke remain unaware of all the risks of using tobacco (Cunningham et al., 2007). Smoke from cigarettes contains about 7,000 chemicals, of which at least 69 cause cancer, including carbon monoxide, hydrogen cyanide, polyaromatic hydrocarbons such as benzene, pesticides and tobacco-specific nitrosamines (U.S. Department of Health and Human Services, 2010). The increased health risks are seen in all people who smoke and in people who do not smoke but are exposed to environmental tobacco smoke. There is no safe level of cigarette smoking or exposure to environmental tobacco smoke. Moreover, there is a consistent association between the amount of smoke exposure and the risk of mortality. Since cigarettes are the most frequently used tobacco product, cigarette smoke is the leading cause of tobacco-related mortality (Centers for Disease Control and Prevention, 2008). While smokeless tobacco does not appear to carry the same risk for lung cancer and chronic obstructive pulmonary disease associated with smoking, the risks for oral diseases and cancers are significant (Critchley & Unal, 2003).

Although the most well-known health effects of smoking are lung cancer and emphysema, tobacco use is attributed to a myriad of chronic medical conditions. Table 11-1 presents a more comprehensive list of the adverse effects associated with tobacco use. We currently face a chronic disease epidemic. As our population continues to age and the burden of chronic disease is further realized, the need for strategies to address tobacco dependence becomes more compelling.

TABLE 11-1

Health Effects of Smoking and Environmental Tobacco Smoke Exposure

CANCER
• lung (85 per cent of lung cancers occur in smokers; one in 20 smokers will develop lung cancer) • mouth, tongue, larynx and pharynx, stomach and bladder
CARDIOVASCULAR DISEASE
• heart attacks (smoking accounts for 40 to 45 per cent of heart attacks in people under age 65) • strokes • peripheral vascular disease
LUNG DISEASE
• chronic obstructive pulmonary disease (COPD) or emphysema (85 per cent of cases are due to smoking; one in seven smokers who smoke one pack per day for 20 years will develop COPD) • higher risk for pneumonia • worsening of asthma
DISEASES OF THE MOUTH
• gingivitis • tooth loss • bad breath
EFFECTS IN WOMEN
• osteoporosis • breast cancer (controversial) • adverse health effects in pregnancy for mother and fetus
EFFECTS ON SKIN
• skin wrinkles (smoking ages skin by 15 to 20 years)
MISCELLANEOUS
• burns • poor wound and fracture healing • gastro-esophageal reflux disease or acid reflux • deafness • age-related blindness (number one cause of blindness in Canada) • dementia

Sources: Bartecchi et al., 1994, 1995; MacKenzie et al., 1994; West & Shiffman, 2007.

Additive Health Effects of Combined Tobacco and Other Substance Use

The burden of chronic disease and other health effects is disproportionately higher in people with substance use disorders who use tobacco. A landmark study of mortality in people with alcohol addiction found that 50 per cent died from tobacco-related causes and 34 per cent from alcohol-related causes (Hurt et al., 1996). Many of the health effects seen in substance-using populations may be due to the amount smoked and the duration of smoke exposure. Additionally, the literature suggests that people may benefit from quitting both drugs concurrently (Patkar, Lundy et al., 2002; Patkar, Sterling et al., 2002).

Cigarette Smoking Is Highly Addictive

In the past, it was argued that because nicotine does not cause intoxication and impairment, smoking was simply a bad habit, not a true addiction (Herie & Skinner, 2010; Robinson & Pritchard, 1992). Today, the addictive nature of nicotine in tobacco is no longer in question. Studies of both animals and humans have shown that nicotine causes dopamine release in the same regions of the brain as other drugs of abuse (Balfour, 2002). Inhaled smoke delivers nicotine to the brain within 20 seconds, making it highly addictive (Rose et al., 1999) and comparable to opioids, alcohol and cocaine (Jarvis, 2004; Stolerman & Jarvis, 1995).

   The *Diagnostic and Statistical Manual of Mental Disorders* (DSM-IV-TR) lacked a diagnosis for "nicotine abuse" as there was for "substance abuse" (American Psychiatric Association [APA], 2000). The only diagnostic category for tobacco use disorders was "nicotine dependence," with "nicotine withdrawal" as a symptom. The DSM-5, released in May 2013, combines substance abuse and dependence into one disorder (APA, 2010). Under the revision, "nicotine dependence" is referred to as "nicotine use disorder"— many people who currently smoke did not meet DSM-IV-TR criteria for nicotine dependence, but were nevertheless physically dependent on nicotine, as evidenced by withdrawal and tolerance (Moolchan et al., 2002). Combining substance abuse and dependence helps legitimize nicotine use as a substance use disorder, and allows for classification of levels of severity.

   Fifty-seven per cent of people who smoke daily report having their first cigarette within the first 30 minutes of waking (Canadian Tobacco Use Monitoring Survey, 2010). The only other substance so widely used upon waking is caffeine. Most people in substance use treatment who smoke feel it is harder to quit smoking than to quit the drug for which they are seeking treatment (Kozlowski et al., 1989; Ziedonis et al., 2007). This begs the question: which drug is the client's true "drug of choice"?

More tobacco facts

Cigarette design

Cigarettes consist of a tobacco column made from shredded tobacco leaf, reconstituted tobacco (other parts of the tobacco plant that have been crushed, made into sheets and shredded) and puff tobacco (loose-leaf tobacco that has been freeze-dried with ammonia and Freon to double its volume). Although Canadian cigarettes do not contain additives, or reconstituted or puff tobacco, they are not safer than American cigarettes.

The light and mild deception

So-called light or mild cigarettes are created by making ventilation holes in the filter either mechanically or with lasers. Smokers compensate to get the nicotine they desire by using a combination of strategies: they increase the volume or number of puffs per cigarette or block the ventilation holes (National Cancer Institute, 2001). Moreover, since the late 1970s, the nicotine content of Canadian cigarettes has been increasing steadily (Rickert, 2000). Although the light and mild descriptors are no longer allowed in Canada, colour coding on cigarette packaging still perpetuates the deception.

Tobacco use in Aboriginal populations

The commercial use of tobacco by Canada's Aboriginal population has contributed to devastating health effects and societal repercussions. Recent data indicates that 59 per cent of Aboriginal people in Canada smoke, and that they can begin smoking as early as age 7 or 8 (Herie & Skinner, 2010). The prevalence of smoking among the Aboriginal population is about three to four times that of the general Canadian population.

For many First Nations communities, tobacco is a ceremonial and spiritual plant. The ceremonial use of tobacco typically involves burning it or using it in a smudge, but not inhaling the smoke (Bartecchi et al., 1995; Vidal, 1997). This tobacco may be used in different contexts depending on the particular community's customs and beliefs. Traditional tobacco has been used as a sacred medicine to treat various physical ailments and purify the mind and body (Health Canada, 2003).

Although the tobacco plant is sacred among some First Nations, it is not revered by all groups or by the Inuit (Von Gernet, 2000). However, more than 70 per cent of Inuit people smoke and Inuit women have the highest rates of lung cancer compared with other populations on a global scale (Herie & Skinner, 2010)

The Métis population also has a higher smoking rate than the general Canadian population. In 2006, 31 per cent of Métis adults smoked daily, down from 37 per cent in 2001 (Janz et al., 2009). Additionally, 61 per cent of Métis adults were non-smokers in 2006, compared with 54 per cent in 2001 (Janz et al., 2009).

Is Tobacco a Gateway Drug?

Although most people who smoke do not go on to develop other substance use problems, smoking is often the first drug of use for most people who later develop alcohol or other drug problems. In a review of adolescent mental health and addiction problems, it was found that early onset of smoking—before age 13—predicted later mental health and substance use disorders (Upadhyaya et al., 2002).

In a prospective study that followed 684 adolescents age 14 to 18 until age 24, lifetime history of smoking, especially in those who smoked daily, significantly increased the chances of future alcohol, cannabis or other illicit drug and polysubstance use in young adulthood (Lewinsohn et al., 1999). Remaining abstinent from smoking for a 12-month period was associated with a lower risk of future alcohol use disorders.

In susceptible individuals, it appears that smoking may be a gateway drug. More than 80 per cent of youth with substance use disorders use tobacco concurrently, become highly dependent and continue using tobacco through adulthood (Myers & MacPherson, 2004; Upadhyaya et al., 2003). Efforts to discourage youth from smoking or to help them quit could also help to prevent other addictions (Ellickson et al., 2001).

Prevalence of Smoking and Association with Other Substance Use

In Canada, the prevalence of smoking in the general population is 16.7 per cent (Reid et al., 2012). Here, and in other developed countries, smoking is more prevalent among people who have lower education, lower social class, blue-collar occupations, psychiatric illness and/or alcohol and other drug problems (Bergen & Caporaso, 1999; Kumra & Markoff, 2000; Minian et al., 2008). In substance use treatment populations, the prevalence of smoking may be as high as 85 to 90 per cent (Sullivan & Covey, 2002) and is often also high among treatment providers.

In terms of alcohol use and smoking, a large U.S. general population study found that the incidence of smoking increases with the amount of alcohol consumed (Dawson, 2000). Smoking was found in 22.5 per cent of lifetime alcohol abstainers, 27.6 per cent of non-abstainers, 53 per cent of heavy drinkers and 55.5 per cent of people with a diagnosis of either alcohol abuse or addiction in the past year.

Another U.S. population-based study found that 71 per cent of people who used illicit drugs also smoked (Richter et al., 2002). The study showed that the likelihood of smoking increased with the number of drugs used. Those who reported using more than one drug were 2.4 times more likely to smoke than those who used only one drug. Also in the United States, a study of 452 injection drug users found that 91 per cent smoked (Clarke et al., 2001). This association between substance use and smoking has been observed in an Australian study (Degenhardt & Hall, 2001).

The reasons for the association between substance use and smoking are complex. Research tells us that substance use corresponds with increased smoking. In laboratory studies, the administration of opioids, alcohol, cocaine, caffeine or amphetamine increased the amount of tobacco participants smoked (Spiga et al., 1998). Conversely, smoking can also increase cravings for other substances. In cocaine users, exposure to tobacco in the presence of cocaine cues leads to more intense cravings for cocaine (Epstein et al., 2010; Reid et al., 1998). Schoedel and Tyndale (2003) demonstrated that when people drink they may be able to smoke many more cigarettes, and when they smoke, they may be able to drink more. This is because alcohol and nicotine reciprocally enhance drug metabolism and elimination.

This complex association suggests that quitting smoking may be difficult for people who are actively drinking. However, the current literature on alcohol treatment and concurrent smoking indicates that "concurrent tobacco dependence treatment does not jeopardize alcohol and non-nicotine drug outcomes" (Kalman et al., 2010, p. 6). As a general guideline, people can and should attempt to quit both substances together, assuming they are ready to do so.

Client Readiness to Address Smoking

Studies show that many clients are ready to attempt smoking cessation while they are in substance use treatment. In a study of 207 clients admitted to an inpatient alcohol and other drug treatment program, 23.7 per cent were willing to attempt smoking cessation (Saxon et al., 1997). Ten per cent had abstained from smoking at six-week follow-up. Clients attending methadone maintenance clinics have shown similar rates of willingness to attempt smoking cessation (Richter et al., 2001). About 13 per cent of clients undergoing alcohol and other drug treatment have quit smoking without formal help at 12-month follow-up (Kohn et al., 2003).

In a study of 1,007 young adults who smoke, those with an active alcohol problem in the preceding year were 60 per cent less likely to quit smoking than those who did not have an alcohol problem. However, if the alcohol problem was inactive, the person was as likely to quit smoking as someone without an alcohol problem (Breslau et al., 1996). Moreover, a study of 100 smokers attending a tobacco dependence clinic showed that those entering tobacco treatment who had a history of recent illicit drug use were less likely to be successful in tobacco cessation treatment (Stapleton et al., 2009). Investigators noted that initially illicit drug users appeared to be as motivated to quit smoking as non–illicit drug users. However, continued use of illicit drugs undermined their quit process. These findings strengthen the notion that active illicit drug use appears to have a significant effect on the success of attempting to stop smoking. Protocols that focus on concurrent treatment may be the most effective approach in cases of active illicit drug use.

Although only 25 per cent of clients may be willing to quit smoking while they undergo treatment for other substance use, many are willing to explore the issue (Bernstein & Stoduto, 1999; Campbell et al., 1998; Schroeder & Morris, 2010).

Furthermore, if tobacco use is not addressed during treatment for other substance use problems, there is a possibility that clients who currently do not smoke may initiate or relapse to smoking. In Kohn and colleagues' (2003) study of a substance use treatment program where smoking was not addressed, about 12 per cent of clients either started to smoke or relapsed to smoking.

Relationship between Smoking Cessation and Other Substance Use Treatment Outcomes

Effect of Quitting Smoking on Recovery from Alcohol and Other Drug Problems

Several studies have shown that quitting smoking during substance use treatment can increase rates of abstinence from alcohol and other drugs (Bobo et al., 1987; Joseph et al., 2004; Kohn et al., 2003; Lemon et al., 2003). Kohn and colleagues (2003) measured the effect of smoking on substance use treatment prognosis in terms of the number of days clients were abstinent. The longest period of abstinence occurred with clients who quit smoking after they began treatment (311 days) and with those who did not smoke when they began treatment (295 days). The shortest period of abstinence was found among clients who continued to smoke (258 days) or who started or resumed smoking (247 days) (Kohn et al., 2003). Quitting smoking during treatment for drugs other than alcohol has also been shown to reduce drug cravings (Campbell et al., 1995; Lemon et al., 2003).

Clients in substance use treatment may be more motivated and confident about changing their use of substances other than tobacco, and seeking to address smoking may affect treatment retention. Stotts and colleagues (2003) found that clients who chose to change only their alcohol use were more likely to stay in treatment than clients who chose to change their smoking and drinking concurrently. However, the study did not determine why clients who chose to quit both alcohol and tobacco were more likely to leave treatment prematurely. These results should be interpreted with caution because the study examined only a small sample of clients, who may not be representative of general addiction treatment populations. In addition, clients with polysubstance use and more complex problems may be more likely to drop out of treatment, regardless of their smoking status or tobacco use goals (Dutra et al., 2008).

Other studies show that counselling clients to quit smoking during substance use treatment does not interfere with treatment success. Prochaska and colleagues (2004) conducted a meta-analysis of randomized controlled trials to evaluate tobacco dependence treatment for people with concurrent substance use. They found that clients who received tobacco dependence treatment were 25 per cent more likely to achieve long-term abstinence from alcohol and illicit drugs. These findings suggest that clinical treatment of tobacco dependence does not interfere with other addiction treatment and may actually enhance treatment outcomes (Prochaska, 2010).

Clients in substance use treatment may also have underlying comorbid conditions that could affect treatment delivery. For example, depression can interfere with a person's ability to quit smoking (Kenford et al., 2002; Lerman et al., 2002; Patten et al., 2001). The risk of major depression can be seven times higher in those with a history of major depression who attempt to quit smoking (Glassman et al., 2001). In a Canadian study of 161 men and women in early recovery from alcohol problems, Currie and colleagues (2001) found that clients were more likely to use cigarettes to manage depression. Identifying and treating concurrent disorders is an essential component of developing effective treatment plans for clients with substance use and other issues. (Treatment approaches for concurrent disorders are discussed in Chapter 16.)

In general, addressing smoking in clients with alcohol and other drug problems is safe and beneficial. A prospective study led by Kohn and colleagues (2003) evaluated the impact of smoking status on treatment outcomes for clients seeking treatment for alcohol and illicit drugs. At 12-month follow-up, clients who had quit smoking during treatment were more likely to have remained abstinent from alcohol and illicit drugs. The evidence suggests that clients in substance use treatment who are ready to quit smoking should receive intensive smoking cessation treatment. However, if a client is having difficulty coping with the physical and emotional impact of quitting smoking, it may be prudent for the counsellor to discuss delaying the quit attempt until the client feels more stable.

Effects of Alcohol and Other Drug Use on Quitting Smoking

Drinking affects the ability to quit smoking and is also a risk factor for relapse to smoking. This may be due to the association of drinking with smoking, the loss of inhibition caused by alcohol, the environment in which both may be consumed or some other unknown factor.

In studies assessing the effects of substance use on smoking cessation, past sub-stance use history did not affect the ability to quit or remain abstinent from smoking (Abrams et al., 2003; Humfleet et al., 1999). However, even low to moderate alcohol use at any time predicted relapse to smoking. Marijuana use did not predict relapse to smoking.

Kalman and colleagues (2002) found that the ability to quit smoking appears to be related to the length of time the person has abstained from alcohol. People who had been abstinent for a long time did not differ from the general population in their ability to quit smoking, which was between 20 to 30 per cent of those who quit in the action stage.

Such findings suggest that abstinence from substances increases the chances of quitting smoking. Conversely, it also appears that quitting smoking can increase the chances of abstinence from other substances.

Methadone Maintenance and Smoking Cessation

The prevalence of smoking among clients in methadone maintenance therapy is as high as 90 per cent (Clarke et al., 2001). Methadone dose increases are known to increase cravings for nicotine and the intensity of nicotine withdrawal (Nahvi et al., 2006; Schmitz et al., 1994; Story & Stark, 1991). Moreover, smoking may serve as a positive reinforcement for methadone due to the long-term association between opi-oids and nicotine in these clients (Elkader et al., 2009; McCool & Richter, 2003; Spiga et al., 1998). Another factor that helps to explain the high rates of tobacco use in this population is the presence of concurrent depression (Elkader et al., 2009).

In a study that explored the relationship between smoking and methadone, 168 clients enrolled in two methadone programs stated that using illicit drugs was a trigger to smoke, but that smoking was not a trigger to use illicit drugs (Stein & Anderson, 2003). They did not report using cigarettes as a means to cope with urges to use drugs, and thought that quitting smoking at the same time as quitting other drugs was appro-priate. However, Frosch and colleagues (2000) found that intensity of smoking was related to use of illicit opioids and cocaine during methadone treatment. These findings suggest that smoking may not trigger illicit opioid use, but that heavier smoking may be associated with increased likelihood to use opioids and cocaine. Further research in this area is warranted before we can generalize the results to this population.

Although people who use illicit opioids perceive quitting smoking to be harder than quitting opioid use (Frosch et al., 2000), many people in methadone maintenance treatment have the motivation to quit smoking and are interested in receiving tobacco dependence treatment (Frosch et al., 1998; Shadel et al., 2005). In a cross-sectional study that assessed the level of motivation to quit smoking among outpatients enrolled in four urban methadone maintenance clinics, results showed that close to 50 per cent had contemplated quitting, and an additional 22 per cent were preparing to quit (Nahvi et al., 2006). Moreover, clients who receive integrated methadone maintenance therapy and smoking cessation treatment are more likely to quit both substances (Lemon et al., 2003). In a recent review of the literature assessing the efficacy of tobacco dependence treatment for people receiving methadone maintenance therapy, Okoli and colleagues (2010) found that tobacco dependence treatment did not increase or worsen substance use, and that most interventions resulted in reduced smoking. These findings suggest that even people with more severe and complex substance use problems can quit smoking when cessation interventions are offered as part of an integrated, holistic substance use treatment approach.

Goals of Tobacco Dependence Treatment

The overall goal of smoking cessation treatment is no different than that of any other addiction treatment. The most important step is to engage clients in the process to improve their health and engage in a life of recovery without tobacco. A general approach to treatment should emphasize client autonomy and goal setting by evoking the client's own reasons for change. Evidence suggests that counsellors should jointly negotiate substance use—including tobacco—goals at treatment entry, and integrate stage-based cessation interventions into addiction treatment programs (2008 PHS Guideline Update Panel, Liaisons, and Staff, 2008; Bernstein & Stoduto, 1999; Campbell et al., 1998). This requires a systematic approach that involves consistently screening for smoking status, assessing for readiness, advising and helping clients to stop smoking (and working to enhance motivation for those who are not ready to change) and helping prevent relapse for those who have already quit. This process of screening and assessment, offering advice and motivational enhancement, and developing relapse prevention strategies collaboratively with clients is in line with general addiction treatment approaches and interventions.

Implementing Cessation Treatment in Addiction Treatment Settings

A 2011 survey of 223 addiction treatment programs in Canada found that 54 per cent of all programs provided clients with at least some assistance to quit smoking (Currie et al., 2003). Outpatient programs (65 per cent) were more likely to offer services than residential programs (44 per cent). However, in most programs, smoking cessation services were offered on an individual ad hoc basis based on client request, and only 10 per cent had formal smoking cessation services. Twelve per cent were contemplating the addition of formal cessation services. All programs offered smoking cessation as an optional part of treatment. Currently, the most common format is sequential treatment of alcohol or other drug use, followed by tobacco dependence treatment. However, it should be noted that this study simply provided an environmental scan of the situation in Canada and not necessarily a recommendation of best practices for this client population.

Treating tobacco dependence in clients with other substance use problems has historically been neglected in addiction treatment settings. Barriers have included lack of funding, agency mandates that exclude tobacco cessation, and lack of knowledge and skills. The three most common myths are that people in substance use treatment are not motivated to quit smoking, that they will relapse to other drug use if they attempt to quit, and that they are unable to quit (Campbell et al., 1995; Teater & Hammond, 2009; Ziedonis et al., 2007). Many counsellors feel that clients should not try to take on too much at once or that requiring clients to quit smoking will prevent them from attending treatment for their other substance use problems (Ziedonis et al., 2006). The smoking status of the counsellor is another barrier (practitioners who smoke are less likely to offer tobacco dependence treatment), although many clients do not think it affects the counsellor's ability to be an effective clinician (Bernstein & Stoduto, 1999; Ziedonis et al., 2007). In addition, clinicians may not address tobacco use because it does not visibly impair the user and its effects become evident only in the long term (Bartecchi et al., 1995).

However, long-term health is not the only reason to focus on tobacco dependence concurrently with other substance use treatment: people in nicotine withdrawal may smoke other smokers' cigarette butts, putting themselves at risk for communicable diseases such as tuberculosis (Aloot et al., 1993), or they may commit crimes to obtain cigarettes (DiFranza & Coleman, 2001).

Addiction counsellors are uniquely situated to intervene because they are knowledgeable about principles of recovery, are seen as credible sources for treating addiction and often have long-term therapeutic relationships with their clients (Currie et al., 2003; McFall et al., 2005). Moreover, while addiction counsellors may hesitate to ask clients about their smoking or to advise them to quit (Friend & Levy, 2004), they are in fact experts in behavioural change strategies that could be used to help clients quit smoking (Schroeder & Morris, 2010). By simply applying the knowledge and skills they already use on a daily basis to the context of smoking cessation, counsellors can have a profound effect on the health and well-being of their clients.

Strategies to help overcome some of the barriers to smoking cessation treatment include policy changes at the treatment system and agency levels, staff training with ongoing coaching and support, and access to counselling and medical services to help both staff and clients stop smoking (Bernstein & Stoduto, 1999; Campbell et al., 1998; Knudsen et al., 2010; Teater & Hammond, 2009).

Program and Systemic Changes

Smoking is socially infectious; the smell and sight of smoking are triggers for many smokers trying to quit. To reduce triggers, addiction treatment programs need to create an environment conducive to recovery, and provide management support for smoke-free policies and options for clients. Nutrition and exercise, if not part of the treatment program, are essential to help clients prevent weight gain after they have stopped smoking. Exercise also has the additional benefit of improving mood.

Staff should not be allowed to smoke with clients; ideally, they would be offered help to overcome their own addiction to tobacco. Management can also help arrange treatment for staff members interested in quitting smoking through on-site programs or employee assistance programs (Moher et al., 2003). Currently, many jurisdictions have free telephone quit lines and web-based resources to help people stop smoking. Management can also ensure they budget for smoking cessation medications, since many staff may not be able to afford them on their income, or their employee benefits program may be inadequate. Integrating smoking cessation into the values and mission of the treatment agency is also important.

Smoke-Free Policies

Smoke-free policies and indoor spaces help people quit smoking (Stephens et al., 2001). Fortunately, policies and bylaws that protect people from environmental tobacco smoke are now more commonplace, and many buildings are smoke free. Many addiction treatment facilities do not permit smoking indoors, but clients are free to smoke outside. More progressive facilities do not permit smoking anywhere on the property and require clients who smoke to participate in a cessation program. At a minimum, tobacco-use policies should address where smoking is permitted on the property, whether tobacco products are allowed on inpatient units and ways of responding to clients who do not follow the policy. These policies should also include interventions to address smoking by clients and staff, and should establish appropriate boundaries about staff smoking with clients and clients' tobacco use during breaks in treatment sessions.

Implementing smoke-free policies in addiction treatment settings can be a challenge, as counsellors do not always feel equipped to provide tobacco cessation treatment and support. Moreover, some clients regard smoke-free policies as unnecessarily punitive, or view tobacco use as a coping strategy they use while they try to reduce or quit other substances. A multi-pronged approach to organizational change—including support from management and administration, staff training, clear communication and a menu of treatment options for clients and staff—is key to successfully implementing and rolling out smoke-free policies in addiction treatment settings.

The Addressing Tobacco through Organizational Change (ATTOC) model is one example of a comprehensive approach to smoke-free policy implementation (Ziedonis et al., 2007). The model's primary goal was to address tobacco in addiction treatment settings by providing staff training, offering treatment for staff and clients, and supporting the organization in preparing for change. Willamette Family Treatment Services (WFTS), the largest treatment centre in Oregon, decided to implement smoke-free grounds for staff and created designated smoking areas for client use. Initially, staff and clients were resistant to the policy, and were concerned that the "right to smoke" would be truncated (Ziedonis et al., 2007). To address this issue, WFTS formed a leadership committee focused on tobacco that included staff from every clinical program. This inclusive committee facilitated staff training, provided resources and smoking cessation medication to staff and clients, and kept the organization informed of the policy's implementation by maintaining open communication. WFTS reported that the ATTOC model not only facilitated a gradual shift in the centre's tobacco culture; it also made the transition to being smoke free as seamless as possible (Ziedonis et al., 2007). Using a model such as ATTOC that supports organizational change makes the implementation of smoke-free policies less of a challenge.

In Canada, the Centre for Addiction and Mental Health (CAMH) became a smoke-free facility in 2005, prohibiting smoking inside all buildings and within nine metres of all entrances. The policy also introduced a nicotine replacement therapy order sheet, order sets and medical directives, and prohibited client smoking rooms. In 2011, CAMH extended the smoke-free policy to include no smoking of any kind by clients, family members, staff, volunteers or any visitors to CAMH's main facilities, except in designated areas.

The policy's implementation strategy has focused on three dimensions: clients, staff and the community (CAMH, 2011, internal corporate communication). Clients are offered cessation counselling and medications, recreational programming and other supports, as well as education about the policy. Staff members are offered training and resources on the policy, and support is offered for those interested in quitting. The community has provided extra receptacles for cigarette butts and has implemented provisions for cleaning up extra litter on surrounding public property. Consultation and open communication are another important part of the policy and allow staff to voice their concerns, suggestions and support of the policy at any time. Despite anticipated challenges with implementation and enforcement, the transition to a smoke-free CAMH has been steady (CAMH, 2011, internal corporate communication).

Staff Training

There is evidence that counsellor training about smoking cessation coupled with client education significantly changes clients' attitudes and readiness to quit smoking as part of their treatment plan (Knudsen & Studts, 2010; Perine & Schare, 1999). Staff attitudes are likely to change with a comprehensive approach that includes policy change and staff education (Campbell et al., 1998; Teater & Hammond, 2009).

Clinicians are often hesitant to engage clients in smoking cessation interventions because they feel they lack the skills and training (Sarna et al., 2000; Twardella & Brenner, 2005; Vogt et al., 2005). Evidence-based training programs designed to enhance clinician knowledge and skills in delivering tobacco cessation interventions can help instil confidence.

In Canada, an initiative that has become the benchmark for intensive cessation counselling is the TEACH project (Training Enhancement in Applied Cessation Counselling and Health). Funded by the Ontario Ministry of Health and Long-Term Care as part of the Smoke-Free Ontario Strategy, TEACH is a knowledge translation project that offers Canada's only university-accredited certificate program in tobacco dependence treatment (Herie et al., 2011). TEACH recently conducted a rigorous program evaluation to determine the program's impact on practitioner behaviour and treatment capacity in Ontario. Post-training evaluations reported that in each curriculum area covered by the TEACH program, practitioners had set concrete goals to incorporate their new knowledge and skills into clinical practice (Herie et al., 2011). Additionally, at six-month follow-up, more than half of TEACH trained practitioners (55.4%) reported having offered intensive individual tobacco dependence treatment sessions to clients (Herie et al., 2011). These encouraging results suggest that the program is having an impact on clinicians' daily practice.

Components of Clinical Intervention

The components of an evidence-based brief clinical intervention are collectively known as the "Five A" model: Ask, Advise, Assess, Assist and Arrange (2008 PHS Guideline, 2008). This model can be used with all populations, including pregnant women, adolescents, smokers with medical comorbidities, older smokers, smokers with mental illness and other addictions and members of racial and ethnic minority groups. Regardless of the population, it is important to ensure that every client is asked about tobacco use and offered an appropriate clinical intervention.

1. Ask

All substance use treatment clients should be screened for tobacco use and their interest in quitting (2008 PHS Guideline, 2008). Counsellors should record the types of tobacco products used, along with the quantity and frequency of use. The level of nicotine dependence can be measured using the Fagerström Test for Nicotine Dependence (Heatherton et al., 1991) or the Cigarette Dependence Scale (Etter et al., 2003). These tests guide the use of nicotine replacement therapy. For people who smoke less than 10 cigarettes per day or who smoke occasionally, behavioural treatment and advice may suffice. For people who are heavily dependent, intensive counselling and medications may be necessary. Those who have quit should be congratulated and supported in maintaining their cessation while in treatment and during aftercare. They should also be advised to avoid environmental tobacco smoke.

Explore relevant aspects of the client's history

A careful psychiatric history should be obtained whenever possible, with special attention to depression, anxiety, eating disorders, psychotic disorders and bipolar disorders. These conditions are associated with higher prevalence of smoking and difficulty quitting (El-Guebaly et al., 2002). A person on psychiatric medications should not stop smoking abruptly without first consulting a doctor or pharmacist to make sure the medication dose does not need to be adjusted. Exploring past quit attempts helps counsellors understand the person's level of dependence, psychological and social strengths, successful behaviours and strategies used in past quit attempts and relapse triggers. Since it often takes four to 11 attempts to stop smoking completely, educating clients about smoking cessation as a process rather than an event helps build hope in those who have tried but not yet succeeded in quitting, and who may experience a sense of failure.

Clients with a history of major depression should be evaluated with a depression rating scale such as the Patient Health Questionnaire (PHQ-9) (Spitzer et al., 1999) or the Beck Depression Inventory (Beck & Steer, 1987). If a client is currently depressed, it is important to treat the depression while or before the client attempts to quit smoking. For a client who is not currently depressed, it is important to monitor depressive symptoms while the person is attempting to quit smoking.

Ask also about medical symptoms. People who smoke are more likely to report respiratory, cardiovascular, gastrointestinal, and nose and throat problems.

2. Advise

All clients should be advised to quit smoking due to its detrimental health effects (2008 PHS Guideline, 2008). Some clients may resent being advised to quit when they are seeking treatment for other substance use problems. Therefore, sensitivity to the client's readiness is important. In some areas, practitioners prefer to give the advice only after they have assessed the client's readiness to hear the information.

3. Assess

Assessing the client's readiness to quit as measured by a composite scale of importance and confidence could help in tailoring treatment. A stage-matched intervention may have some benefit and should be employed. For the purposes of smoking cessation, the stages of change are defined as follows:

- **precontemplation:** not ready to quit smoking in the next six months
- **contemplation:** ready to quit in the next six months but not the next month
- **preparation:** ready to quit within the next month
- **action:** has quit smoking, but for less than six months
- **maintenance:** has quit smoking for more than six months
- **relapse or treatment failure:** smoking at least one cigarette per day for seven consecutive days or smoking one or more cigarettes on one or more days in a two-week period (Hughes, Keely et al., 2003) is considered a relapse or failure of the intervention. Smoking less than either of those amounts should be considered a lapse or slip. Note that 97 per cent of lapses become full-blown relapses, and helping clients refrain from lapsing even once is optimal (McEwen et al., 2006).

Clients who resume smoking should be reassessed for their willingness to try again, since many are still interested in addressing their tobacco use. Remember that change typically follows a non-linear pattern. People are susceptible to both intra-therapeutic and extra-therapeutic factors that can move them in either direction along the continuum of change.

4. Assist

There is a strong relationship between the intensity of counselling and smoking cessation. Treatment may be delivered in groups or individually. Each session should be longer than 10 minutes (ideally 30 to 60 minutes). At least four sessions with an aftercare component are recommended. Treatment should involve problem solving and intra-treatment and extra-treatment social support.

The addition of cognitive-behavioural therapy to address depression in clients with a history of alcohol addiction has been shown to increase treatment attendance and short-term success in quitting smoking (Patten et al., 2001).

All clients should be encouraged to use pharmacotherapy unless there is a medical contraindication. Counsellors can encourage clients to discuss the issue with their family doctor or pharmacist.

Motivational techniques, such as exploring the pros and cons of changing, should be used with all clients. In the preparation phase (i.e., if the client is ready to quit in the next 30 days), clients should be encouraged to set a target quit date. It is also important in this phase to discuss strategies clients can use to cope with withdrawal, cravings and cues; extra-therapeutic social support is recommended. To increase the odds of quitting, living space and vehicles should be smoke free (2008 PHS Guideline, 2008; Stephens et al., 2001). Harm reduction strategies include smoking outdoors and gradually reducing the number of cigarettes smoked per day but not switching to light or ultra-light cigarettes, since people tend to compensate for the lower level of nicotine by taking more puffs or inhaling more deeply (Kozlowski et al., 1998).

For people who are unwilling to quit, motivational interviewing techniques to explore and resolve their ambivalence and resistance are recommended. (For more about motivational interviewing, see Chapter 5.)

Another effective strategy to help clients initiate behaviour change is the Behavior Change Roadmap: The 4 Point Plan. It guides clients through four crucial steps that can end destructive behaviours, such as smoking, and leads them to adopt healthier lifestyles. The four steps are: Strategize, Take Action, Optimize and Prevent Relapse. The *My Change Plan* workbook (Nicotine Dependence Service, 2011) outlines the steps of the 4 Point Plan and is an excellent tool for clinicians to use when developing a quit plan with clients.[1]

---

1 The *My Change Plan* workbook is available for free download on the TEACH website at www.nicotinedependenceclinic.com/English/teach/resources/Assessment%20Tools/My%20Change%20Plan%20Booklet.pdf.

Use of pharmacotherapy

In all the clinical trials conducted to date, pharmacotherapy approximately doubles the chances of quitting and sustaining the quit (2008 PHS Guideline, 2008; Hughes, Keely et al., 2003; Nides, 2008; Silagy et al., 2002; Stead et al., 2008). Nicotine replacement therapy (nicotine patch, gum, inhaler, lozenge or mouth spray) and bupropion SR (Zyban) all produce similar long-term abstinence rates. Varenicline (Champix) has been shown in some studies to be significantly more efficacious than NRT or bupropion monotherapy (Keating et al., 2006; Oncken et al., 2006; Tonstad et al., 2006). For more details about how to prescribe first-line smoking cessation medications and their potential side-effects, refer to the Pharmacotherapy for Smoking Cessation web link in the "Resources" section of this chapter.

Nicotine replacement therapy

Nicotine replacement therapy (NRT) can be used by anyone who smokes more than 10 cigarettes per day. It is available in several forms over the counter. NRTs currently available in Canada are nicotine gum, patch, inhaler, lozenge and mouth spray. NRT replaces some of the nicotine a smoker would typically acquire from a smoking a cigarette. It is a safer delivery system of nicotine because it does not contain the thousands of chemicals and carcinogens found in cigarette smoke (Ontario Medical Association, 2008). The nicotine delivered through NRT is absorbed by the body at a much slower rate, thus true addiction to NRT is rare (Hughes, 2008). This makes NRTs a viable option for clients who are looking to reduce consumption or sustain their quit.

One study found that clients with past alcohol problems were likely to respond favourably to NRT, continuing with a sustained quit at six-month follow-up (Hughes, Novy et al., 2003). The recommended duration of treatment varies from seven to 52 weeks of medication and should be tailored to each client. Some clients may find it difficult to stop nicotine gum, but it is safer than smoking (Hurt et al., 1995), and clients can be helped to stop use without risking relapse to smoking.

Bupropion

Prescription medications can also be recommended for clients interested in quitting. Bupropion SR, also referred to as Zyban, is classified as an antidepressant, but is also prescribed in smoking cessation. Bupropion SR may be the best choice for clients with a history of depression due to its antidepressant effects and its ability to be combined safely with other common antidepressants (DeBattista et al., 2003; Kennedy et al., 2002). It is also the least expensive oral medication officially indicated for smoking cessation (Selby, 2007). Bupropion is contraindicated for clients with predispositions to seizures, eating disorders, uncontrolled bipolar disorder and pregnant women. Bupropion may be safely combined with NRT and is associated with higher six-month abstinence rates than either medication alone.

Varenicline

Varenicline, also referred to as Champix, has the highest quit rate of existing therapies available to clients (Keating et al., 2006; Oncken et al., 2006; Tonstad et al., 2006). This partial agonist acts by binding to nicotinic acetylcholine receptors in the brain, and stimulates dopamine levels to a lesser degree than would be elicited by a cigarette (Nides, 2008). This reduces the withdrawal and cravings a person would normally experience when trying to quit. The most recent Cochrane review found that "varenicline increased the chances of successful long-term smoking cessation between two- and threefold compared with pharmacologically unassisted quit attempts" (Cahill et al., 2008, p. 2). Although varenicline has not been approved for use in combination with other pharmacotherapies for smoking cessation, these combinations are being investigated (Ebbert, Burke et al., 2009; Ebbert, Croghan et al., 2009).

The varenicline package insert contains a black box warning label about post-marketing reports of neuropsychiatric side-effects, including suicidal and homicidal ideation, in people taking varenicline (Coe, 2012). Williams and colleagues (2011) examined these reports and concluded that "despite case reports of serious neuropsychiatric symptoms in patients taking varenicline, including changes in behaviour and mood, causality has not been established" (p. 1). Similarly, Cerimele and Durango (2012) examined published reports describing the use of varenicline in clients with schizophrenia. They found that of the 260 clients with schizophrenia who received varenicline, five per cent experienced the onset or worsening of psychiatric symptoms, and no clients experienced suicidal ideation or behaviours (Cerimele & Durango, 2012). These analyses provide encouraging support for varenicline as an effective smoking cessation medication that can be used safely with neuropsychiatric populations.

A meta-analysis by Singh and colleagues (2011) suggested that varenicline may be associated with a small increased risk of adverse cardiovascular events. Prochaska and Hilton (2012) conducted a similar meta-analysis that included more trials (22 versus 14) and did not include events reported after 30 days of medication discontinuation. They found no relationship between varenicline use and increased cardiovascular serious adverse events. The summary estimate for the risk difference was 0.27 per cent, which was not found to be clinically or statistically significant. Therefore, current data does not support a causal link between varenicline and cardiovascular events.

Nortriptyline and clonidine

Second-line medications such as nortriptyline, an antidepressant, and clonidine, an antihypertensive, can be prescribed, but are not officially indicated for smoking cessation (Selby, 2007). Although these pharmacotherapies have evidence of efficacy, their risks and potential side-effects make them less desirable than the first-line medications discussed earlier.

Best practices in pharmacotherapy

The Canadian Action Network for the Advancement, Dissemination and Adoption of Practice-Informed Tobacco Treatment (CAN-ADAPTT) clinical practice guideline states that it is best practice to tailor smoking cessation pharmacotherapy to each person's clinical needs and preferences (CAN-ADAPTT, 2011). Thus, the choice of medication, dosage and duration of use is highly dependent on individual differences and contraindications. It is also recommended that pharmacological interventions be combined with psychosocial interventions for optimal effectiveness in helping clients quit smoking (CAN-ADAPTT, 2011).

Alternative therapies and treatments

There is no scientific evidence suggesting that acupuncture and laser therapy are effective in smoking cessation (2008 PHS Guideline, 2008; Lancaster et al., 2000). Any efficacy that has been demonstrated in anecdotal cases may have resulted from positive expectancies. The effectiveness of hypnosis is still uncertain, as research in this area has not been very robust. However, it is recommended that hypnosis not be used as an evidence-based approach because there are many other well-established approaches to cessation (2008 PHS Guideline, 2008).

A potential new treatment option for tobacco dependence that is currently being researched is transcranial magnetic stimulation (TMS). TMS is a non-invasive therapeutic approach used to excite neurons in the brain. Neurons achieve excitation by weak electric currents induced in brain tissue by rapidly changing magnetic fields. As a result, brain activity can be modified without a surgical procedure or external electrodes (Brody & Cook, 2011). TMS provides clinical researchers with a tool to map out brain functioning and has shown promising results in the treatment of depression (Slotema et al., 2010). Delivering TMS to the prefrontal cortex has been shown to reduce cravings for cigarettes, alcohol, illicit drugs and food (Fecteau et al., 2010), and in some cases, has been shown to reduce intake (Barr et al., 2008; Feil & Zangen, 2010).

Cytisine is another treatment being explored for use in tobacco dependence treatment. Like varenicline, cytisine is a partial agonist that binds to the nicotinic receptors in the brain, and acts to reduce cravings and make cigarettes less satisfying if a lapse occurs (Etter et al., 2008; Tutka & Zatoński, 2006). West and colleagues (2011) assessed the efficacy and safety of cytisine compared with placebo in a single-centre study. The results showed that participants in the cytisine group achieved a sustained abstinence rate of 8.4 per cent compared with 2.4 per cent in the placebo group, suggesting that cytisine can be effective for smoking cessation. It is also a low-cost treatment, available for $15 for a course of treatment in Poland, and $6 in Russia (Tutka & Zatoński, 2006). Cytisine is currently not marketed on a global scale.

Another treatment undergoing research for tobacco dependence treatment is the nicotine vaccine. The major intended use of the vaccine is to prevent relapse after users dependent on the drug achieve abstinence (Hall & Gartner, 2011). The vaccine acts by inducing the body to manufacture nicotine antibodies. These antibodies bind to nicotine in the blood and prevent it from reaching the brain (Cornuz et al., 2008). It is hypothesized that these antibodies will diminish the positive effects associated with nicotine in the first few months of treatment when clients are likely to relapse. The most advanced vaccine candidate, NicVAX, failed to demonstrate efficacy in phase III clinical trials, although earlier phases revealed a correlation between the vaccine and higher abstinence rates in participants with higher immunity to nicotine (Fahim et al., 2011). Despite these results, research continues to advance and will focus on improving vaccine effectiveness and combining the vaccine with other pharmacological interventions.

5. Arrange

Periodic follow-up is recommended for clients who are not ready to quit. For those who have quit, follow-up sessions are advised during the first week of quitting to explore slips, negative mood and other predictors of relapse. Thereafter, the frequency and duration of follow-ups can be decided based on individual preferences and staff availability.

Measures of Success

Success can be measured in several ways. First, standard measures look at biochemically verified reports, such as exhaled carbon monoxide levels of less than 10 ppm or urinary or salivary cotinine (a metabolite or byproduct of nicotine, thus a biomarker for exposure to tobacco). Another way to measure success is to use self-reports of continuous abstinence (not even a single puff of a cigarette) six months after the quit date, while other studies also look at quit rates at one year as a measure of success. Since clients enter substance use treatment at different stages of change with respect to quitting smoking, it is more realistic to monitor changes in readiness rather than only smoking cessation rates. Thus, an effective tobacco intervention program moves clients in the precontemplation stage into contemplation and so on. This is not dissimilar to measuring success in addressing other substance use: small incremental changes in a positive direction, treatment engagement and retention, enhanced commitment and motivation to change, and reducing harms represent tangible and important treatment gains.

Revisiting the Case Study

After about a week into her inpatient stay, Raisa began using NRT because she hated the constant withdrawal and cravings from only being allowed to smoke three times per day. To her surprise, she found that the nicotine patch, in combination with the breakthrough medications (gum and lozenge) she was given, helped her cravings. Raisa decided to attend a new smoking cessation group on the unit. The confidence she gained from the group and her use of the medications made her determined to quit smoking along with her other drug use. Raisa recognized that her recovery was not going to be easy, but she told herself that if she could be smoke free—a goal that she never in her wildest dreams imagined accomplishing—then she could do anything.

Conclusion

Clients like Raisa want and need to be offered evidence-based clinical approaches to smoking cessation in addiction treatment settings. First, health care practitioners should ask clients about their smoking and determine their level of interest in quitting. This conversation should be followed up with an assessment of the client's psychiatric history. In the case of Raisa, the sexual abuse she experienced as a child coincided with the initiation of her tobacco use. This would be an issue worth exploring with Raisa because it could play a role in triggering relapse and might be a barrier to particular quit strategies.

Second, health care practitioners should advise clients about the harms associated with smoking, bearing in mind clients' sensitivity to their readiness to quit. If the client is ready to proceed through treatment, it is important to assist him or her in the process. A client like Raisa, regardless of readiness to quit, should be encouraged to use pharmacotherapy to deal with nicotine withdrawal while in a smoke-free environment. Counselling, cognitive-behavioural therapy, motivational interviewing and pharmacotherapy are all evidence-based approaches that counsellors can use to help their clients with tobacco cessation. Finally, it is vital to arrange follow-up with clients to track their progress, determine predictors of relapse and help them sustain their quit.

Tobacco is a potential gateway drug that prematurely kills about 50 per cent of regular users. Ten thousand people worldwide are killed daily from an addiction that, until recently, has been underrecognized in the addiction field. Given the serious health consequences of tobacco use, every counsellor needs to intervene. Although many clients have difficulty quitting smoking, with appropriate interventions, they can be helped to address their tobacco use. The "Five A" model for smoking cessation provides an approach that focuses on the client, matching treatment to his or her individual stage of change.

Clients who wish to address their smoking can do so without jeopardizing their recovery from substance use problems. Smoking cessation may even help them in their recovery from other substance use problems, and protect against relapse (Sullivan & Covey, 2002).

Practice Tips

- Identify every client who uses tobacco and offer at least a brief intervention at each clinical visit. This should be the standard of care and duty of practice of all health care professionals.
- Treat tobacco dependence concurrently with other substance use treatment.
- Make quitting smoking a recommended treatment goal in addiction treatment settings because abstinence from substances increases the chances of quitting smoking. Moreover, quitting smoking can also increase the chances of abstinence from other substances.
- Emphasize client autonomy and goal setting as a general approach to treatment by evoking the client's own reasons for change.
- Combine psychosocial techniques with pharmacotherapy for optimal tobacco dependence treatment.
- Consider applying the "Five A" model (Ask, Advise, Assess, Assist and Arrange) as an evidence-based brief clinical intervention with any population.
- Encourage all clients to use pharmacotherapy unless there is a medical contraindication. Pharmacotherapy approximately doubles the chances of quitting and sustaining the quit.

Resources

Publications

2008 PHS Guideline Update Panel, Liaisons, and Staff. (2008). *Clinical Practice Guideline: Treating Tobacco Use and Dependence: 2008 Update.* Rockville, MD: Department of Health and Human Services. Retrieved from www.ahrq.gov/clinic/tobacco/treating_tobacco_use08.pdf

Els, C., Kunyk, D. & Selby, P. (2012). *Disease Interrupted: Tobacco Reduction and Cessation.* Charleston, SC: CreateSpace.

Ontario Medical Association. (2008). Rethinking stop smoking medications: Treatment myths and realities. *Ontario Medical Review, 75* (1), 22–34.

TEACH Project. (n.d.). Pharmacotherapy for smoking cessation. Retrieved from https://www.nicotinedependenceclinic.com/English/teach/resources/Visual%20Aids/Pharmacotherapy%20for%20smoking%20cessation.pdf

Ziedonis, D.M., Guydish, J., Williams, J., Steinberg, M. & Foulds, J. (2006). Barriers and solutions to addressing tobacco dependence in addiction treatment programs. *Alcohol Research and Health, 29,* 228–235.

Internet

CAN-ADAPTT (Canadian Action Network for the Advancement, Dissemination and
Adoption of Practice-Informed Tobacco Treatment)
www.can-adaptt.net

Canadian Council for Tobacco Control
www.cctc.ca

Nicotine Dependence Service (Centre for Addiction and Mental Health)
www.nicotinedependenceclinic.com

Ontario Tobacco Research Unit
www.otru.org

Smokers' Helpline
www.smokershelpline.ca

You Can Make It Happen
http://youcanmakeithappen.ca

References

2008 PHS Guideline Update Panel, Liaisons, and Staff. (2008). *Clinical Practice Guideline: Treating Tobacco Use and Dependence: 2008 Update.* Rockville, MD: Department of Health and Human Services. Retrieved from www.ahrq.gov/clinic/ tobacco/treating_tobacco_use08.pdf

Abrams, D.B., Niaura, R., Brown, R.A., Emmons, K.M., Goldstein, M.G. & Monti, P.M. (2003). *The Tobacco Dependence Treatment Handbook: A Guide to Best Practices.* New York: Guilford Press.

Aloot, C.B., Vredevoe, D.L. & Brecht, M.L. (1993). Evaluation of high-risk smoking practices used by the homeless. *Cancer Nursing, 16,* 123–130.

American Psychiatric Association (APA). (2000). *Diagnostic and Statistical Manual of Mental Disorders* (text rev.). Washington, DC: Author.

American Psychiatric Association (APA). (2010). DSM-5 development. R 31: Tobacco use disorder. Retrieved from www.dsm5.org/ProposedRevisions/Pages/ proposedrevision.aspx?rid=459

Balfour, D.J.K. (2002). The neurobiology of tobacco dependence: A commentary. *Respiration, 69,* 7–11.

Barr, M.S., Fitzgerald, P.B., Farzan, F., George, T.P. & Daskalakis, Z.J. (2008). Transcranial magnetic stimulation to understand the pathophysiology and treatment of substance use disorders. *Current Drug Abuse Reviews, 1,* 328–339.

Bartecchi, C.E., MacKenzie, T.D. & Schrier, R.W. (1994). The human costs of tobacco use. *New England Journal of Medicine, 330,* 907–912.

Bartecchi, C.E., MacKenzie, T.D. & Schrier, R.W. (1995, May). The global tobacco epidemic. *Scientific American, 272,* 44–51.

Beck, A. & Steer, R.A. (1987). *Manual for the Revised Beck Depression Inventory*. San Antonio, TX: Psychological Corp.

Bergen, A.W. & Caporaso, N. (1999). Cigarette smoking. *Journal of the National Cancer Institute, 91*, 1365–1375.

Bernstein, S.M. & Stoduto, G. (1999). Adding a choice-based program for tobacco smoking to an abstinence-based addiction treatment program. *Journal of Substance Abuse Treatment, 17*, 167–173.

Bobo, J.K., Gilchrist, L.D., Schilling, R.F.D., Noach, B. & Schinke, S.P. (1987). Cigarette smoking cessation attempts by recovering alcoholics. *Addictive Behaviors, 12*, 209–215.

Breslau, N., Peterson, E., Schultz, L., Andreski, P. & Chilcoat, H. (1996). Are smokers with alcohol disorders less likely to quit? *American Journal of Public Health, 86*, 985–990.

Brody A.L. & Cook, I.A. (2011). Manipulation of cigarette craving with transcranial magnetic stimulation. *Biological Psychiatry, 70*, 702–703.

Cahill, K., Stead, L.F. & Lancaster, T. (2008). Nicotine receptor partial agonists for smoking cessation. *Cochrane Database of Systematic Reviews, 3*, CD006103.

Campbell, B.K., Krumenacker, J. & Stark, M.J. (1998). Smoking cessation for clients in chemical dependence treatment. A demonstration project. *Journal of Substance Abuse Treatment, 15*, 313–318.

Campbell, B.K., Wander, N., Stark, M.J. & Holbert, T. (1995). Treating cigarette smoking in drug-abusing clients. *Journal of Substance Abuse Treatment, 12*, 89–94.

Canadian Action Network for the Advancement, Dissemination and Adoption of Practice-Informed Tobacco Treatment (CAN-ADAPTT). (2011). *Canadian Smoking Cessation Clinical Practice Guideline*. Toronto: Centre for Addiction and Mental Health. Retrieved from https://www.nicotinedependenceclinic.com/English/CANADAPTT/Guideline/Introduction.aspx

Canadian Tobacco Use Monitoring Survey. (2010). CTUMS 2010 Wave 1 survey results. Ottawa: Health Canada. Retrieved from www.hc-sc.gc.ca

Centers for Disease Control and Prevention. (2008). Smoking-attributable mortality, years of potential life lost, and productivity losses—United States, 2000–2004. *Morbidity and Mortality Weekly Report, 57*, 1226–1228.

Cerimele, J.M. & Durango, A. (2012). Does varenicline worsen psychiatric symptoms in patients with schizophrenia or schizoaffective disorder? A review of published studies. *Journal of Clinical Psychiatry, 73*, 1039–1047.

Clarke, J.G., Stein, M.D., McGarry, K.A. & Gogineni, A. (2001). Interest in smoking cessation among injection drug users. *American Journal of Addiction, 10*, 159–166.

Coe, J. (2012). Varenicline. In C. Els, D. Kunyk & P. Selby (Eds.), *Disease Interrupted: Tobacco Reduction and Cessation* (pp. 163–169). Charleston, SC: CreateSpace.

Cornuz, J.S., Zwhalen, S., Jungi, W.F., Osterwalder, J., Klingler, K., Van Melle, G. & Cerny, T. (2008). A vaccine against nicotine for smoking cessation: A randomized controlled trial. *PLOS ONE, 3*, 2547.

Critchley, J.A. & Unal, B. (2003). Health effects associated with smokeless tobacco: A systematic review. *Thorax, 58*, 435–443.

Cunningham, J.A., Selby, P.L. & Faulkner, G. (2007). Increasing perceived choice about change in smokers: Implications. *Addictive Behaviors, 32*, 1907–1912.

Currie, S.R., Hodgins, D.C., el-Guebaly, N. & Campbell, W. (2001). Influence of depression and gender on smoking expectancies and temptations in alcoholics in early recovery. *Journal of Substance Abuse, 13*, 443–458.

Currie, S.R., Nesbitt, K., Wood, C. & Lawson, A. (2003). Survey of smoking cessation services in Canadian addiction programs. *Journal of Substance Abuse Treatment, 24*, 59–65.

Dawson, D.A. (2000). Drinking as a risk factor for sustained smoking. *Drug and Alcohol Dependence, 59*, 235–249.

DeBattista, C., Solvason, H.B., Poirier, J., Kendrick, E. & Schatzberg, A.F. (2003). A prospective trial of bupropion SR augmentation of partial and non-responders to serotonergic antidepressants. *Journal of Clinical Psychopharmacology, 23*, 27–30.

Degenhardt, L. & Hall, W. (2001). The relationship between tobacco use, substance-use disorders and mental health: Results from the National Survey of Mental Health and Well-Being. *Nicotine and Tobacco Research, 3*, 225–234.

DiFranza, J.R. & Coleman, M. (2001). Sources of tobacco for youths in communities with strong enforcement of youth access laws. *Tobacco Control, 10*, 323–328.

Dutra, L., Stathopoulou, G., Basden, S.L., Leyro, T.M., Powers, M.B. & Otto, M.W. (2008). A meta-analytic review of psychosocial interventions for substance use disorders. *American Journal of Psychiatry, 165*, 179–187.

Ebbert, J.O., Burke, M.V., Hays, J.T., Hurt, R.D. (2009). Combination treatment with varenicline and nicotine replacement therapy. *Nicotine & Tobacco Research, 11*, 572–576.

Ebbert J.O., Croghan, I.T., Sood, A., Schroeder, D.R., Hays, J.T. & Hurt, R.D. (2009). Varenicline and bupropion sustained-release combination therapy for smoking cessation. *Nicotine & Tobacco Research, 11*, 234–239.

El-Guebaly, N., Cathcart, J., Currie, S., Brown, D. & Gloster, S. (2002). Smoking cessation approaches for persons with mental illness or addictive disorders. *Psychiatric Services, 53*, 1166–1170.

Elkader, A.K., Brands, B., Selby, P. & Sproule, B.A. (2009). Methadone-nicotine interactions in methadone maintenance treatment patients. *Journal of Clinical Psychopharmacology, 29*, 231–238.

Ellickson, P.L., Tucker, J.S. & Klein, D.J. (2001). High-risk behaviors associated with early smoking: Results from a 5-year follow-up. *Journal of Adolescent Health, 28*, 465–473.

Epstein, D.H., Marrone, G.F., Heishman, S.J., Schmittner, J. & Preston, K.L. (2010). Tobacco, cocaine, and heroin: Craving and use during daily life. *Addictive Behaviors, 35*, 318–324.

Etter, J.F., Le Houezec, J. & Perneger, T.V. (2003). A self-administered question-naire to measure dependence on cigarettes: The cigarette dependence scale. *Neuropsychopharmacology, 28*, 359–370.

Etter, J.F., Lukas, R.J., Benowitz, N.L., West, R. & Dresler, C.M. (2008). Cytisine for smoking cessation: A research agenda. *Drug & Alcohol Dependence, 92*, 3–8.

Fahim, R.E., Kessler, P.D., Fuller, S.A. & Kalnik, M.W. (2011). Nicotine vaccines. *CNS & Neurological Disorders—Drug Targets, 10*, 905–915.

Fecteau, S., Fregni, F., Boggio, P.S., Camprodon, J.A. & Pascual-Leone, A. (2010). Neuromodulation of decision-making in the addictive brain. *Substance Use & Misuse, 45*, 1766–1786.

Feil, J. & Zangen, A. (2010). Brain stimulation in the study and treatment of addiction. *Neuroscience & Biobehavioral Reviews, 34*, 559–574.

Friend, K.B. & Levy, D.T. (2004). Adoption of tobacco treatment interventions by sub-stance-abuse-treatment clinicians. *Drugs: Education, Prevention and Policy, 11*, 1–20.

Frosch, D.L., Shoptaw, S., Jarvik, M.E., Rawson, R.A. & Ling, W. (1998). Interest in smoking cessation among methadone maintained outpatients. *Journal of Addictive Disorders, 17* (2), 9–19.

Frosch, D.L., Shoptaw, S., Nahom, D. & Jarvik, M.E. (2000). Associations between tobacco smoking and illicit drug use among methadone-maintained opiate-dependent individuals. *Experimental and Clinical Psychopharmacology, 8*, 97–103.

Glassman, A.H., Covey, L.S., Stetner, F. & Rivelli, S. (2001). Smoking cessation and the course of major depression: A follow-up study. *The Lancet, 357*, 1929–1932.

Guydish, J., Passalacqua, E., Tajima, B., Chan, M., Chun, J. & Bostrom, A. (2011). Smoking prevalence in addiction treatment: A review. *Nicotine & Tobacco Research, 13*, 401–411.

Hall, W. & Gartner, C. (2011). Ethical and policy issues in using vaccines to treat and prevent cocaine and nicotine dependence. *Current Opinion in Psychiatry, 24*, 191–196.

Health Canada (2003). *Building and Sustaining Partnerships: A Resource Guide to Address Non-traditional Tobacco Use*. Ottawa: Author. Retrieved from www.hc-sc.gc.ca

Heatherton, T.F., Kozlowski, L.T., Frecker, R.C. & Fagerström, K.O. (1991). The Fagerström Test for Nicotine Dependence: A revision of the Fagerström Tolerance Questionnaire. *British Journal of Addiction, 86*, 1119–1127.

Herie, M., Connolly, H., Voci, S., Dragonetti, R. & Selby, P. (2011). Changing practi-tioner behavior and building capacity in tobacco cessation treatment: The TEACH Project. *Patient Education and Counselling, 86*, 49–56.

Herie, M. & Skinner, W. (2010). *Substance Abuse in Canada*. Toronto: Oxford University Press.

Hughes, J. (2008). Significance of off-label use of NRT. *Addiction, 103*, 1704–1705.

Hughes, J.R., Keely, J.P., Niaura, R.S., Ossip-Klein, D.J., Richmond, R.L. & Swan, G.E. (2003). Measures of abstinence in clinical trials: Issues and recommendations. *Nicotine & Tobacco Research, 5*, 13–25.

Hughes, J.R., Novy, P., Hatsukami, D.K., Jensen, J. & Callas, P.W. (2003). Efficacy of nicotine patch in smokers with a history of alcoholism. *Alcoholism: Clinical and Experimental Research, 27,* 946–954.

Humfleet, G., Munoz, R., Sees, K., Reus, V. & Hall, S. (1999). History of alcohol or drug problems, current use of alcohol or marijuana, and success in quitting smoking. *Addictive Behaviors, 24,* 149–154.

Hurt, R.D., Offord, K.P., Croghan, I.T., Gomez-Dahl, L., Kottke, T.E., Morse, R.M. & Melton, L.J. (1996). Mortality following inpatient addictions treatment: Role of tobacco use in a community-based cohort. *Journal of the American Medical Association, 275,* 1097–1103.

Hurt, R.D., Offord, K.P., Lauger, G.G., Marusic, Z., Fagerström, K.O., Enright, P.L. & Scanlon, P.D. (1995). Cessation of long-term nicotine gum use—a prospective, randomized trial. *Addiction, 90,* 407–413.

Janz, T., Seto, J. & Turner, A. (2009). *Aboriginal Peoples Survey, 2006: An Overview of the Health of the Métis Population.* Ottawa: Statistics Canada.

Jarvis, M.J. (2004). ABC of smoking cessation: Why people smoke. *British Medical Journal, 328,* 277–279.

Jha, P. & Chaloupka, F. (1999). *Curbing the Epidemic: Governments and the Economics of Tobacco Control.* Washington, DC: World Bank.

Jha, P., Chaloupka, F.J., Corrao, M. & Jacob, B. (2006). Reducing the burden of smoking world-wide: Effectiveness of interventions and their coverage. *Drug and Alcohol Review, 25,* 597–609.

Joseph, A.M., Willenbring, M.L., Nugent, S.M. & Nelson, D.B. (2004). A randomized trial of concurrent versus delayed smoking intervention for patients in alcohol dependence treatment. *Journal of Studies on Alcohol, 65,* 681–691.

Kalman, D., Kim, S., DiGirolamo, G., Smelson, S. & Ziedonis, D. (2010). Addressing tobacco use disorder in smokers in early remission from alcohol dependence: The case for integrating smoking cessation services in substance use disorder treatment programs. *Clinical Psychology Review, 30,* 12–24.

Kalman, D., Tirch, D., Penk, W. & Denison, H. (2002). An investigation of predictors of nicotine abstinence in a smoking cessation treatment study of smokers with a past history of alcohol dependence. *Psychology of Addictive Behaviors, 16,* 346–349.

Keating, G.M. & Siddiqui, M.A. (2006). Varenicline: A review of its use as an aid to smoking cessation therapy. *CNS Drugs, 20,* 945–960.

Kenford, S.L., Smith, S.S., Wetter, D.W., Jorenby, D.E., Fiore, M.C. & Baker, T.B. (2002). Predicting relapse back to smoking: Contrasting affective and physical models of dependence. *Journal of Consulting and Clinical Psychology, 70,* 216–227.

Kennedy, S.H., McCann, S.M., Masellis, M., McIntyre, R.S., Raskin, J., McKay, G. & Baker, G.B. (2002). Combining bupropion SR with venlafaxine, paroxetine, or fluoxetine: A preliminary report on pharmacokinetic, therapeutic, and sexual dysfunction effects. *Journal of Clinical Psychiatry, 63,* 181–186.

Knudsen, H.K. & Studts, J.L. (2010). The implementation of tobacco-related brief interventions in substance abuse treatment: A national study of counselors. *Journal of Substance Abuse Treatment, 38*, 212–219.

Knudsen, H.K., Studts, J.L., Boyd, S. & Roman, P.M. (2010). Structural and cultural barriers to the adoption of smoking cessation services in addiction treatment organizations. *Journal of Addictive Diseases, 29*, 294–305.

Kohn, C.S., Tsoh, J.Y. & Weisner, C.M. (2003). Changes in smoking status among substance abusers: Baseline characteristics and abstinence from alcohol and drugs at 12-month follow-up. *Drug and Alcohol Dependence, 69*, 61–71.

Kozlowski, L.T., Goldberg, M.E., Yost, B.A., White, E.L., Sweeney, C.T. & Pillitteri, J.L. (1998). Smokers' misperceptions of light and ultra-light cigarettes may keep them smoking. *American Journal of Preventive Medicine, 15*, 9–16.

Kozlowski, L.T., Wilkinson, D.A., Skinner, W., Kent, C., Franklin, T. & Pope, M. (1989). Comparing tobacco cigarette dependence with other drug dependencies: Greater or equal "difficulty quitting" and "urges to use," but less "pleasure" from cigarettes. *JAMA, 261*, 898–901.

Kumra, V. & Markoff, B.A. (2000). Who's smoking now? The epidemiology of tobacco use in the United States and abroad. *Clinics in Chest Medicine, 21*, vii–9.

Lancaster, T., Stead, L., Silagy, C. & Sowden, A. (2000). Effectiveness of interventions to help people stop smoking: Findings from the Cochrane Library. *British Medical Journal, 321*, 355–358.

Lemon, S.C., Friedmann, P.D. & Stein, M.D. (2003). The impact of smoking cessation on drug abuse treatment outcome. *Addictive Behaviors, 28*, 1323–1331.

Lerman, C., Roth, D., Kaufmann, V., Audrain, J., Hawk, L., Liu, A., Epstein, L. (2002). Mediating mechanisms for the impact of bupropion in smoking cessation treatment. *Drug and Alcohol Dependence, 67*, 219–223.

Lewinsohn, P.M., Rohde, P. & Brown, R.A. (1999). Level of current and past adolescent cigarette smoking as predictors of future substance use disorders in young adulthood. *Addiction, 94*, 913–921.

MacKenzie, T.D., Bartecchi, C.E. & Schrier, R.W. (1994). The human costs of tobacco use. *New England Journal of Medicine, 330*, 975–980.

Makomaski Illing, E.M. & Kaiserman, M.J. (1999). Mortality attributable to tobacco use in Canada and its regions, 1994 and 1996. *Chronic Diseases in Canada, 20*, 111–117.

McCool, R.M. & Richter, K.P. (2003). Why do so many drug users smoke? *Journal of Substance Abuse Treatment, 25*, 43–49.

McEwen, A., Hajek, P., McRobbie, H. & West, R. (2006). *Manual of Smoking Cessation: A Guide for Counsellors and Practitioners.* Malden, MA: Blackwell.

McFall, M., Saxon, A.J., Thompson, C.E., Yoshimoto, D., Malte, C., Straits-Troster, K. & Steele, B. (2005). Improving the rates of quitting smoking for veterans with posttraumatic stress disorder. *American Journal of Psychiatry, 162*, 1311–1319.

Minian, N., Schwartz, R., Garcia, J., Selby, P. & McDonald, P. (2008). *A Model for Assessing Gaps in Smoking Cessation Systems and Services in a Local Public Health Unit.* Toronto: Ontario Tobacco Research Unit.

Moher, M., Hey, K. & Lancaster, T. (2003). Workplace interventions for smoking cessation. *Cochrane Database of Systemic Reviews,* (2), CD003440.

Moolchan, E.T., Radzius, A., Epstein, D.H., Uhl, G., Gorelick, D.A., Cadet, J.L. & Henningfield, J.E. (2002). The Fagerström Test for Nicotine Dependence and the Diagnostic Interview Schedule: Do they diagnose the same smokers? *Addictive Behaviors, 27,* 101–113.

Myers, M.G. & MacPherson, L. (2004). Smoking cessation efforts among substance abusing adolescents. *Drug and Alcohol Dependence, 73,* 209–213.

Nahvi, S., Richter, K., Li, X., Modali, L. & Arnsten, J. (2006). Cigarette smoking and interest in quitting in methadone maintenance patients. *Addictive Behaviors, 31,* 2127–2134.

National Cancer Institute. (2001). *Risks Associated with Smoking Cigarettes with Low Machine-Measured Yields of Tar and Nicotine.* Bethesda, MD: Author.

Nicotine Dependence Service. (2011). *My Change Plan: Workbook for Making Healthy Changes.* Toronto: Centre for Addiction and Mental Health. Retrieved from https://www.nicotinedependenceclinic.com/English/teach/resources/Assessment%20Tools/My%20Change%20Plan%20Booklet.pdf

Nides, M. (2008). Update on pharmacologic options for smoking cessation treatment. *American Journal of Medicine, 121* (Suppl. 4), 20–31.

Okoli, C.T.C., Khara, M., Procyshyn, R.M., Johnson, J.L., Barr, A.M. & Greaves, L. (2010). Smoking cessation interventions among individuals in methadone maintenance: A brief review. *Journal of Substance Abuse Treatment, 38,* 191–199.

Oncken, C., Gonzales, D., Nides, M., Rennard, S., Watsky, E., Billing, C.B. et al. (2006). Efficacy and safety of the novel selective nicotine acetylcholine receptor partial agonist, varenicline, for smoking cessation. *Archives of Internal Medicine, 166,* 1571–1577.

Ontario Medical Association. (2008). Rethinking stop smoking medications: Treatment myths and realities. *Ontario Medical Review, 75* (1), 22–34.

Patkar, A.A., Lundy, A., Leone, F.T., Weinstein, S.P., Gottheil, E. & Steinberg, M. (2002). Tobacco and alcohol use and medical symptoms among cocaine dependent patients. *Substance Abuse, 23,* 105–114.

Patkar, A.A., Sterling, R.C., Leone, F.T., Lundy, A. & Weinstein, S.P. (2002). Relationship between tobacco smoking and medical symptoms among cocaine-, alcohol-, and opiate-dependent patients. *American Journal of Addiction, 11,* 209–218.

Patten, C.A., Gillin, J.C., Golshan, S., Wolter, T.D., Rapaport, M. & Kelsoe, J. (2001). Relationship of mood disturbance to cigarette smoking status among 252 patients with a current mood disorder. *Journal of Clinical Psychiatry, 62,* 319–324.

Perine, J.L. & Schare, M.L. (1999). Effect of counselor and client education in nicotine addiction on smoking in substance abusers. *Addictive Behaviors, 24,* 443–447.

Peto, R., Lopez, A.D., Boreham, J., Thun, M., Heath, C., Jr. & Doll, R. (1996). Mortality from smoking worldwide. *British Medical Bulletin, 52* (1), 12–21.

Prochaska, J.J. (2010). Failure to treat tobacco use in mental health and addiction treatment settings: A form of harm reduction? *Drug and Alcohol Dependence, 110,* 177–182.

Prochaska, J.J., Delucchi, K. & Hall, S.M. (2004). A meta-analysis of smoking cessation interventions with individuals in substance abuse treatment or recovery. *Journal of Consulting and Clinical Psychology, 72,* 1144–1156.

Prochaska, J.J. & Hilton, J.F. (2012). Risk of cardiovascular serious adverse events associated with varenicline use for tobacco cessation: Systematic review and meta-analysis. *British Medical Journal, 344,* e2856. doi: 10.1136/bmj.e2856

Prochaska, J.J., Rossi, J.S., Redding, C.A., Rosen, A.B., Tsoh, J.Y., Humfleet, G.L. & Hall, S.M. (2007). Depressed smokers and stage of change: Implications for treatment interventions. *Drug and Alcohol Dependence, 76,* 143–151.

Rehm, J., Gnam, W., Popova, S., Baliunas, D., Brochu, S., Fischer, B. et al. (2006). The costs of alcohol, illegal drugs, and tobacco in Canada, 2002. *Journal of Studies on Alcohol and Drugs, 68,* 886–895.

Reid, J.L., Hammond, D., Burkhalter, R. & Ahmed, R. (2012). *Tobacco Use in Canada: Patterns and Trends* (2012 edition). Waterloo, ON: Propel Centre for Population Health Impact, University of Waterloo.

Reid, M.S., Mickalian, J.D., Delucchi, K.L., Hall, S.M. & Berger, S.P. (1998). An acute dose of nicotine enhances cue-induced cocaine craving. *Drug and Alcohol Dependence, 49,* 95–104.

Repace, J.L. (2006). Exposure to secondhand smoke. In W.R. Ott, A.C. Steineman & L.A. Wallace (Eds.), *Exposure Analysis* (pp. 201–236). Boca Raton, FL: CRC Press.

Richter, K.P., Ahluwalia, H.K., Mosier, M.C., Nazir, N. & Ahluwalia, J.S. (2002). A population-based study of cigarette smoking among illicit drug users in the United States. *Addiction, 97,* 861–869.

Richter, K.P., Gibson, C.A., Ahluwalia, J.S. & Schmelzle, K.H. (2001). Tobacco use and quit attempts among methadone maintenance clients. *American Journal of Public Health, 91,* 296–299.

Rickert, W. (2000). Today's cigarettes: Steps toward reducing the health impact. In R.G. Ferrence, J. Slade, R. Room & M. Pope (Eds.), *Nicotine and Public Health* (pp. 135–158). Washington, DC: American Public Health Association.

Robinson, J.H. & Pritchard, W.S. (1992). The role of nicotine in tobacco use. *Psychopharmacology (Berl), 108,* 397–407.

Rose, J.E., Behm, F.M., Westman, E.C. & Coleman, R.E. (1999). Arterial nicotine kinetics during cigarette smoking and intravenous nicotine administration: Implications for addiction. *Drug and Alcohol Dependence, 56,* 99–107.

Sarna, L.P., Brown, J.K., Lillington, L., Rose, M., Wewers, M.E. & Brecht, M.L. (2000). Tobacco interventions by oncology nurses in clinical practice: Report from a national survey. *Cancer, 89,* 881–889.

Saxon, A.J., McGuffin, R. & Walker, R.D. (1997). An open trial of transdermal nicotine replacement therapy for smoking cessation among alcohol- and drug-dependent inpatients. *Journal of Substance Abuse Treatment, 14,* 333–337.

Schmitz, J.M., Grabowski, J. & Rhoades, H. (1994). The effects of high and low doses of methadone on cigarette smoking. *Drug and Alcohol Dependence, 34*, 237–242.

Schoedel, K.A. & Tyndale, R.F. (2003). Induction of nicotine-metabolizing CYP2B1 by ethanol and ethanol-metabolizing CYP2E1 by nicotine: Summary and implications. *Biochimica et Biophysica Acta, 1619*, 283–290.

Schroeder, S.A. (2009). A 51-year-old woman with bipolar disorder who wants to quit smoking. *Journal of the American Medical Association, 301*, 522–531.

Schroeder, S.A. & Morris, C.D. (2010). Confronting a neglected epidemic: Tobacco cessation for persons with mental illness and substance abuse problems. *Annual Review of Public Health, 31*, 297–314.

Selby, P. (2007). Smoking cessation. In J. Gray (Ed.), *Therapeutic Choices* (5th ed., pp. 146–157). Ottawa: Canadian Pharmacists Association.

Shadel, W.G., Stein, M.D., Anderson, B.J., Herman, D.S., Bishop, S., Lassor, J.A. & Niaura, R. (2005). Correlates of motivation to quit smoking in methadone-maintained smokers enrolled in a smoking cessation trial. *Addictive Behaviors, 30*, 295–300.

Silagy, C., Lancaster, T., Stead, L., Mant, D. & Fowler, G. (2002). Nicotine replacement therapy for smoking cessation. *Cochrane Database of Systemic Reviews*, (4), CD000146.

Singh S., Loke, Y.K., Spangler, J.G. & Furberg, C.D. (2011). Risk of serious adverse cardiovascular events associated with varenicline: A systematic review and meta-analysis. *Canadian Medical Association Journal, 183*, 1359–1366. doi: 10.1503/cmaj.110218

Slotema, C.W., Blom, J.D., Hoek, H.W. & Sommer, I.E. (2010). Should we expand the toolbox of psychiatric treatment methods to include repetitive transcranial magnetic stimulation (rTMS)? A meta-analysis of the efficacy of rTMS in psychiatric disorders. *Journal of Clinical Psychiatry, 71*, 873–884.

Spiga, R., Schmitz, J. & Day, J., II. (1998). Effects of nicotine on methadone self-administration in humans. *Drug and Alcohol Dependence, 50*, 157–165.

Spitzer R., Kroenke, K. & Williams, J. (1999). Validation and utility of a self-report version of PRIME-MD: The PHQ Primary Care Study. *JAMA, 282*, 1737–1744.

Stapleton, J.A., Keaney, F. & Sutherland, G. (2009). Illicit drug use as a predictor of smoking cessation treatment outcome. *Nicotine & Tobacco Research, 11*, 685–689.

Stead, L.F., Perera, R., Bullen, C., Mant, D. & Lancaster, T. (2008). Nicotine replacement therapy for smoking cessation (Review). *The Cochrane Library, 3*, 1–160.

Stein, M.D. & Anderson, B.J. (2003). Nicotine and drug interaction expectancies among methadone maintained cigarette smokers. *Journal of Substance Abuse Treatment, 24*, 357–361.

Stephens, T., Pederson, L.L., Koval, J.J. & Macnab, J. (2001). Comprehensive tobacco control policies and the smoking behaviour of Canadian adults. *Tobacco Control, 10*, 317–322.

Stolerman, I.P. & Jarvis, M.J. (1995). The scientific case that nicotine is addictive. *Psychopharmacology (Berl), 117*, 2–10, 14–20.

Story, J. & Stark, M.J. (1991). Treating cigarette smoking in methadone maintenance clients. *Journal of Psychoactive Drugs, 23,* 203–215.

Stotts, A.L., Schmitz, J.M. & Grabowski, J. (2003). Concurrent treatment for alcohol and tobacco dependence: Are patients ready to quit both? *Drug and Alcohol Dependence, 69,* 1–7.

Sullivan, M.A. & Covey, L.S. (2002). Current perspectives on smoking cessation among substance abusers. *Current Psychiatry Reports, 4,* 388–396.

TEACH Project. (2012). *Training Enhancement in Applied Cessation Counseling and Health.* Retrieved from www.teachproject.ca/resources.htm

Teater, B. & Hammond, G.C. (2009). The protected addiction: Exploring staff beliefs toward integrating tobacco dependence in substance abuse treatment services. *Journal of Alcohol and Drug Education, 53* (2), 52–70.

Tonstad, S., Tonnesen, P., Hajek, P., Williams, K.E., Billing, C.B. & Reeves, K.R. (2006). Effect of maintenance therapy with varenicline on smoking cessation: A randomized controlled trial. *JAMA, 296,* 64–71.

Torrijos, R.M. & Glantz, S.A. (2006). The U.S. Public Health Service "treating tobacco use and dependence clinical practice guidelines" as a legal standard of care. *Tobacco Control, 15,* 447–451.

Tutka, P. & Zatoński, W. (2006). Cytisine for the treatment of nicotine addiction: From molecule to therapeutic efficacy. *Pharmacological Reports, 58,* 777–798.

Twardella, D. & Brenner, H. (2005). Lack of training as a central barrier to the promotion of smoking cessation: A survey among general practitioners in Germany. *European Journal of Public Health, 15,* 140–145.

Upadhyaya, H.P., Brady, K.T., Wharton, M. & Liao, J. (2003). Psychiatric disorders and cigarette smoking among child and adolescent psychiatry inpatients. *American Journal on Addictions, 12,* 144–152.

Upadhyaya, H.P., Deas, D., Brady, K.T. & Kruesi, M. (2002). Cigarette smoking and psychiatric comorbidity in children and adolescents. *Journal of the American Academy of Child and Adolescent Psychiatry, 41,* 1294–1305.

U.S. Department of Health and Human Services. (2010). *How Tobacco Smoke Causes Disease: The Biology and Behavioral Basis for Smoking-Attributable Disease. A Report of the Surgeon General.* Atlanta, GA: U.S. Department of Health and Human Services, Centers for Disease Control and Prevention, National Center for Chronic Disease Prevention and Health Promotion, Office on Smoking and Health. Retrieved from www.surgeongeneral.gov/library/reports/tobaccosmoke/full_report.pdf

Vidal, C. (1997). Historical background on tobacco. Retrieved from www.niichro.com/Tobacco/Tobac1.html

Vogt, F., Hall, S. & Marteau, T.M. (2005). General practitioners' and family physicians' negative beliefs and attitudes towards discussing smoking cessation with patients: A systematic review. *Addiction, 100,* 1423–1431.

Von Gernet, A. (2000). Origins of nicotine use and the global diffusion of tobacco. In R.G. Ferrence, J. Slade, R. Room & M. Pope (Eds.), *Nicotine and Public Health* (pp. 3–15). Washington, DC: American Public Health Association.

Wald, N.J. & Hackshaw, A.K. (1996). Cigarette smoking: An epidemiological overview. *British Medical Bulletin, 52* (1), 3–11.

West, R. & Shiffman, S. (2007). *Fast Facts: Smoking Cessation.* Abingdon, United Kingdom: Health Press.

West, R., Zatonski, W., Cedzynska, M., Lewandowska, D., Pazik, J., Aveyard, P. & Stapleton, J. (2011). Placebo-controlled trial of cytisine for smoking cessation. *New England Journal of Medicine, 365,* 1193–1200.

Williams, J.M., Steinberg, M.B., Steinberg, M.L., Gandhi, K.K., Ulpe, R. & Foulds, J. (2011). Varenicline for tobacco dependence: Panacea or plight? *Expert Opinion Pharmacotherapy, 12,* 1799–1812.

World Health Organization. (2011). *World No Tobacco Day: The WHO Framework Convention on Tobacco Control.* Retrieved from http://whqlibdoc.who.int/hq/2011/ WHO_NMH_TFI_11.1_eng.pdf

Ziedonis, D.M., Guydish, J., Williams, J., Steinberg, M. & Foulds, J. (2006). Barriers and solutions to addressing tobacco dependence in addiction treatment programs. *Alcohol Research and Health, 29,* 228–235.

Ziedonis, D.M., Zammarelli, L., Seward, G., Oliver, K., Guydish, J., Hobart, M. & Meltzer, B. (2007). Addressing tobacco use through organizational change: A case study of an addiction treatment organization. *Journal of Psychoactive Drugs, 39,* 451–459.

Chapter 12

Opioid Addiction

Rosanra Yoon

> Mingyu is a 38-year-old woman who has been attending structured relapse pre-
> vention sessions for an alcohol use disorder. She is on a sick leave from her job
> as a paralegal assistant. She has a history of depression and anxiety, as well as
> a history of heroin use in her 20s. Last year, Mingyu was hit by a car while cross-
> ing the street, which resulted in a fractured collar bone and chronic back pain.
>
> During one of her sessions, Mingyu is extremely agitated and anxious. She
> tells the counsellor that her doctor refuses to continue to prescribe the opioid
> pain medications she has been taking daily. She has run out of her pills and
> is extremely upset by the withdrawal symptoms and increased pain. Feeling
> desperate, she went to a walk-in clinic yesterday to get her pain addressed.
> She is craving a drink but knows she shouldn't drink and feels she cannot
> cope with having no pain medication. Her plan is to borrow some oxycodone
> and morphine from her friend; Mingyu feels guilty about doing this but feels
> there is no other way. She also tells the counsellor that another friend is on
> methadone and that she might take a sip or two of her friend's methadone if
> things become really bad.

Engaging and supporting people who have opioid dependence in a collaborative partnership is essential to reducing the personal, social and health-related harms associated
with opioid addiction. Of key importance for clinicians is developing a foundational
understanding of the nature of opioids, conducting routine assessment and screening
and knowing about treatment options. This chapter provides an overview of opioid addiction, pharmacological and psychosocial support interventions and considerations for
special populations, such as women and people with high-risk opioid use.

It is estimated that more than 15 million people worldwide use illicit opioids—
about 11 million of whom use heroin (World Health Organization [WHO], 2009).
Because of the high prevalence of heroin use, its illicit status and its addictive potential,
much of the clinical literature has addressed this drug specifically.

However, in recent years, Canada, the United States and other developed countries have experienced a rise in illicit use of prescription opioids (Compton & Volkow,
2006; Hayden et al., 2005). In Canada, between 321,000 and 914,000 people used

prescription opioids for non-medical reasons in 2003. Among people engaged in illicit opioid use, about 72,000 were using either heroin, prescription opioids, or both. The majority engaged in illicit use of prescription opioid medications (Popova et al., 2009).

The harms associated with opioid addiction are significant: it can lead to reduced quality of life, the loss of meaningful relationships and activities and adverse physical and mental health sequelae. Of concern are the risks associated with intravenous administration, such as hepatitis C and HIV, and mortality from accidental overdoses, violence and suicide. People with opioid addiction do not fit one homogenous profile with one clear-cut presenting issue. Many may misuse other substances and medications in addition to having concurrent mental health and physical health problems that need to be addressed in a comprehensive manner (Noel et al., 2006). They may also require assistance with housing, and with legal, child welfare and vocational issues. Assessing the urgency of these issues and taking appropriate action are required. The most effective approaches address these issues in an integrated manner, co-ordinating services and collaborating with members of the client's circle of care.

Medication-assisted therapy, using methadone and buprenorphine, for example, in conjunction with psychosocial interventions is recommended as a best practice for people with opioid addiction (National Institute for Health and Clinical Excellence, 2007; WHO, 2009). However, despite this recommendation, only an estimated 26 per cent of people with opioid addiction in Canada were receiving methadone maintenance therapy in 2003 (Popova et al., 2006). Most are not in any type of treatment, putting them at the highest risk of poor health outcomes and accidental overdose. Stigma and misconceptions around opioid addiction, and around medications such as methadone and buprenorphine used to treat it, are often barriers to seeking help and engaging in treatment. The lack of availability of medication-assisted therapy is also an issue, especially in smaller communities.

Opioids: An Overview

The term *opioid* refers collectively to substances derived from the poppy plant, such as opium, morphine and codeine, as well as semi-synthetic (e.g., heroin) and synthetic forms (e.g., methadone). Opioids are psychoactive in that they bind to receptors in the brain and central and peripheral nervous system. They relieve pain and cause sedation, as well as reducing gastrointestinal motility (movement of the large and small intestines) (Kahan et al, 2006; National Institute for Health and Clinical Excellence [NICE], 2007). Due to their pain-relieving qualities, opioids have been used for many years for analgesia, while poppy derivatives such as opium have been used for many centuries.

Opioid addiction is a chronic and relapsing condition frequently marked by periods of stability and relapse. As such, a long-term approach to recovery and engagement at different points along the recovery journey is essential for best outcomes and treatment retention.

Appropriate prescribing of opioids for pain management is an important and effective intervention for managing acute pain. However, since some people are at higher risk for developing opioid addiction, it is important to conduct a comprehensive assessment of risk factors before initiating prescription opioid pain management (Kahan et al., 2006). People with a family or personal history of substance use problems are at higher risk of opioid misuse and addiction (Walwyn et al., 2010).

People who use opioids daily for weeks or months start to develop long-lasting changes in the function and structure of certain brain areas involved in learning, memory, decision making, mood and response to stress. These changes leave people vulnerable to relapsing to opioid use for months, sometimes even years, after they have stopped taking opioids.

Tolerance (needing more and more of the substance to achieve the same effect) to the euphoric, psychological effects of opioids develops quickly compared to tolerance to the pain-relieving qualities. People with opioid addiction commonly need to increase the amounts taken to continue to feel euphoria and to avoid withdrawal symptoms.

Drug tolerance in and of itself does not necessarily mean a person is addicted to the drug. Physiological tolerance to opioids can be lost in as little as a few consecutive days of abstinence. This is extremely important for the person engaged in treatment or cessation to understand because resuming the usual opioid dose after quitting for a few days poses a high risk of accidental overdose and death. This quick loss of tolerance is the primary cause of accidental death among people after they have completed a withdrawal management program, a prolonged jail stay or a 21-day treatment program. Clinicians must inform clients of this risk and advise them on how to deal with it when they are engaged in treatment or achieving a period of abstinence.

Types of Opioids

Heroin

Derived from the opium poppy, heroin is a semi-synthetic opiate and is the most commonly misused opioid worldwide (WHO, 2009). Although it can be snorted or smoked, the greatest risks associated with heroin use are often related to intravenous use that carries high risks associated with HIV and hepatitis C transmission through sharing injection equipment (e.g., needles, spoons, cottons). Other adverse consequences of intravenous use are skin infections, collapsed veins, potentially fatal bacterial infections of the heart valves and the high risk of overdose. Asking clients how they administer heroin, providing information about harm reduction strategies and connecting clients to primary health care services to address their physical health needs are essential ways to reduce the harms related to intravenous drug use.

Prescription Opioids

Non-medical use of prescription opioids—either alone or in combination with heroin or other substances—is a growing trend and is now more prevalent than heroin use in Canada (Fischer et al., 2008; Popova et al., 2009). Examples of prescription opioids include oxycodone, codeine, morphine, hydromorphone and fentanyl.

Modes of administration

Many types of oral prescription opioids exist, ranging from short-acting to sustained-release formulations in varying doses. These drugs can be taken in different ways, that is, by varying routes of administration. Ingesting opioids orally tends to be the least risky mode of administration, as oral intake slows down the rate of absorption. Crushing or chewing tablets is a frequent practice because it causes more euphoria by increasing the rate of oral absorption. Tablets may also be crushed and snorted intra-nasally for faster absorption. Intravenous administration of opioids has the fastest absorption rate: people may crush tablets to dilute in liquid or extract the opioid from transdermal patch preparations.

Misuse of the fentanyl contained in long-acting transdermal patches, which are intended to be applied to the skin for slow release of the opioid medication over time and replaced every two or three days, carries significant risks. Transdermal patches pose potentially fatal risks when people inject the medication into a vein, replacing a slow, sustained-release method with a fast-acting route, as intravenous fentanyl use is very dangerous. Sometimes people take the opioid by other risky routes, such as through the rectum. Obtaining prescription opioids by purchasing them from illicit sources, or from friends or family members, can also be dangerous because users may be unaware of safe doses.

The therapist should ask not only about how much of a drug a client is taking, but also about the route of administration. Knowing whether a client is crushing and snorting, chewing tablets or crushing and dissolving tablets for intravenous administration is important to assess for high-risk routes of use. Using a harm reduction approach, clinicians should support clients in using safer routes (e.g., oral versus intravenous) and safe techniques and supplies, providing them with information to help make less risky choices.

Patterns of Problematic Opioid Use

Problematic opioid use can appear as either opioid misuse or opioid addiction. Opioid misuse involves repeated use of the drug in ways other than intended or prescribed despite negative consequences to the person. Opioid addiction is marked by features that include:

- compulsive use and preoccupation with taking opioids
- continued use despite worsening personal circumstances and negative consequences from use

- tolerance—needing to take more and more of the substance to achieve the same effect
- withdrawal symptoms when opioid use stops
- loss of control over use
- cravings.

Note that physiological dependence alone is not a sign of opioid misuse or addiction. Key aspects in addition to physiological dependence are increasing loss of control over use and compulsive use despite harms directly caused by use. People can become physically dependent on opioids with long-term use, even when taking the drugs as prescribed, but dependence does not necessarily imply addiction (Kahan et al., 2006).

Behavioural signs and patterns of both opioid misuse and addiction include:
- running out of prescriptions early, escalating the dose, "losing" prescriptions, forging prescriptions, breaking the law to obtain opioids
- drawing on multiple sources of opioids (family, friends, diverted sources from the street market; prescriptions from multiple providers—ER, family MD, pain specialist, walk-in clinics)
- showing a decline in personal functioning (e.g., school or work performance suffers, social isolation, relationship problems, physical illnesses)
- experiencing withdrawal symptoms
- showing increasing tolerance
- altering the mechanism of delivery (crushing pills, altering patches, taking oral or transdermal preparations intravenously).

Assessment and Engagement

Problematic Opioid Use

Assessment

A detailed and comprehensive biopsychosocial assessment of illicit substance use is extremely important and should cover the following areas:
- substance use history—current and past, looking at patterns of use, duration of use, routes and periods of abstinence or stability from all substances, including opioids
- history of past drug treatment experiences
- medical and mental health history, including history of chronic pain
- current medications and treatments
- family history of addiction
- legal problems, drinking while under the influence charges
- a partner or roommate who uses drugs
- children and their care
- pregnancy
- current family doctors, specialists, services

- housing
- finances
- family and social supports
- self-concept and coping patterns
- resilience and strengths.

People who are addicted to opioids have a high prevalence of co-occurring depression and anxiety, which are usually untreated. Women in particular may have high rates of concurrent mental health problems, histories of physical or sexual abuse and related unresolved trauma, lower social and economic status and unhealthy relationship dynamics that may include domestic violence (Jones & Fiellin, 2007).

Historically, women have been under-represented in treatment. Moreover, few treatment programs have addressed the specific needs of women who often take on care-giving roles in child rearing or who may experience gender-related social stigma related to substance use.

Using a trauma-informed lens in the assessment and being sensitive to the woman's current experience is important to develop rapport and establish a collaborative therapeutic relationship that supports the woman's goals for recovery.

A comprehensive assessment and screening of mental health and coping can provide an opportunity to connect the person to mental health treatment while he or she is in opioid addiction treatment (Wild et al., 2005). Ideally, clients with complex problems receive integrated and co-ordinated care from practitioners who work collaboratively, using a comprehensive biopsychosocial approach to treatment and change management.

Engagement

The clinician's own values, beliefs, attitudes and level of evidence-based knowledge of opioid addiction and treatment options play a significant role in engaging the person in treatment options. A respectful, open and non-judgmental approach that is collaborative and that honours the client's autonomy and choice is the most important foundation in engaging and working with people who have opioid addiction. It is also essential to provide accurate information about treatment options, holistically assess the person's needs and work together with the person's circle of care. Motivational strategies have been demonstrated to be effective with this population (Miller & Rollnick, 2002).

Illicit opioid use and treatment such as methadone maintenance therapy are highly stigmatized. Clinicians must be sensitive to stigma and engage clients in a dialogue of their experience of opioid addiction in terms of their conceptualization and understanding of why they use opioids, their goals for recovery and how they perceive treatment.

Many people with problematic opioid use may not see themselves as "addicts." A collaborative discussion about how their use has become problematic, their lived experience of opioids over time and what they identify as their needs and goals to achieve wellness is more beneficial than a polarizing discussion about whether or not the person has an addiction. Dispelling myths and providing information on the risks and harms of opioid use help to normalize the person's experience and self-perception.

Clinicians should explain the various treatment options and evidence for their effectiveness. Treatment options must be discussed in a non-coercive manner that allows the client to make a decision based on the best available evidence and his or her own preference for treatment. By participating in their own treatment planning, clients can feel a greater sense of personal choice and control over the process, and be more engaged and committed to treatment (Zeldman et al., 2004).

In addition to connecting the person to treatment and services, it is equally important, if not more so, to work collaboratively as a team with the person's existing circle of care providers and supports, such as family, family doctor, specialists and other services. This team approach should be discussed together with the client; the client is the central member of this team and needs to understand why involvement with all members of the circle of care and support is important. For many people with problematic prescription opioid use, the worry that their current prescriber may suddenly discontinue prescribing is a common and legitimate fear that needs to be discussed collaboratively with them, allowing them to make a choice. This dialogue may afford the opportunity for the clinician to support the person engaging in treatment, as well as being a liaison and advocate for the person's recovery.

Chronic Pain and Problematic Opioid Use

Assessment

It is very important to conduct a comprehensive assessment for people who report chronic pain and opioid use. The assessment should cover all the elements of a thorough addiction assessment described earlier, as well as a history of the person's chronic pain issues (Kahan et al., 2006).

Engagement

Clinicians play an important role in engaging the person with chronic pain and illicit opioid use by discussing the role of opioids in the client's overall coping, balancing the pros and cons of the opioid use and finding out how the client relates the opioid use to pain issues. The client should know that the risk of opioid addiction is highest among people with a history of substance use problems and appreciate that adequate pain treatment should not come at the expense of developing opioid addiction as a sequelae. Clinicians can provide further information about chronic pain management.

The client should be encouraged to have a candid and transparent dialogue with his or her physician or pain specialist to evaluate current pain management in light of the adverse risk of developing problematic opioid use.

Opioid Intoxication

People with opioid intoxication usually present as sedated, with slurred speech, decreased breathing rate and slowing physical and mental abilities (Kahan & Marsh, 2000).

Assessment

Clinicians need to be keenly aware of the signs and symptoms of opioid intoxication and intervene quickly by assessing the level of sedation and connecting the person for immediate medical assessment. Many other factors could be contributing to the sedation, such as having used other sedating substances or having an underlying medical condition.

Signs and symptoms of opioid intoxication include:
- drowsiness
- pinpoint pupils
- slurred speech
- slowed mental and physical abilities
- poor balance (Kahan & Marsh, 2000).

Engagement

Effective intervention starts with ensuring the safety of people who are intoxicated and supporting their decision making. They may be anxious or agitated and may experience mood fluctuations; they need support and validation of their experience, and clear, simple options for managing their intoxication. If the person is not easily roused and has slowed breathing, clinicians should ensure the person is quickly assessed by a medical practitioner or call for emergency services.

Opioid Withdrawal

People going through opioid withdrawal can experience serious distress and physical discomfort. For the most commonly misused opioids, withdrawal symptoms start to peak two or three days after the last use. Acute physical symptoms improve after five to seven days from last use; however, the psychological symptoms of intense cravings, anxiety and low mood, as well as subacute physical symptoms, may last for weeks, even months. The persistence of these symptoms is a factor in relapse risk.

Assessment

Clinicians should routinely assess the person's coping and mood following withdrawal, as support and further counselling are needed after withdrawal from opioids. People at this stage are at higher risk of impulsive self-harm behaviours such as suicide (Kahan & Marsh, 2000). Clinicians must assess mental status and develop a safety plan. Most people in opioid withdrawal can safely come off opioids in non-medical withdrawal management settings or on their own. Those with complex medical problems or concurrent mental health problems that may worsen during withdrawal should seek medically supervised medical withdrawal management.

Signs and symptoms of opioid withdrawal include:
- anxiety
- mood changes
- agitation
- watery eyes
- runny nose
- goosebumps or chills
- diarrhea
- stomach cramps
- nausea/vomiting
- insomnia
- irritability
- muscle aches
- sweating
- fever
- increased sensation of pain
- opioid cravings.

Engagement

Validating the client's experience and demonstrating empathy and emotional support are particularly important, given the unpleasant and distressing process of withdrawal. Comfort measures such as low lighting, adequate hydration and rest are important considerations.

Clinicians need to know about available services for withdrawal management in the client's area in order to offer support and connect the person to services in a timely manner.

Treatment

Opioid Addiction

A continuum of service should be offered that is comprehensive and integrated.

Best outcomes are achieved with psychosocial interventions combined with pharmacotherapy. Opioid addiction is a chronic and relapsing condition, so a long-term treatment approach is needed (Scherbaum & Specka, 2008). Engaging the client in meaningful treatment throughout the recovery journey is essential. Improving quality of life is key.

Treatment goals include:

- reducing or stopping opioid use
- reducing current and future harms associated with opioid use
- improving the quality of life and well-being of the person
- setting medium- and longer-term goals.

Medication-assisted therapy

Pharmacological treatment using methadone or buprenorphine in combination with psychosocial intervention has been found to be very effective, with only 20 to 30 per cent of people experiencing relapse or treatment failure (Maremmani & Gerra, 2010; NICE, 2007).

Methadone

Methadone has very good outcomes for people who are addicted to opioids, as evidenced by rates of treatment retention and improvements in psychosocial well-being and quality of life (Mattick et al., 2003). Methadone is a long-acting agonist opioid that, at the right dose, allows the person to feel comfortable and remain free of withdrawal symptoms for 24 hours. This is in contrast to heroin and illicitly used prescription opioids, which have a short period of action (four to six hours), leading to numerous episodes of withdrawal throughout the day, which then leads to the development of tolerance and a pattern of dependence (Kahan & Marsh, 2000).

People can access methadone maintenance therapy by connecting with a methadone provider or clinic. Methadone is dispensed as a liquid mixed with juice that is taken daily. Until a period of stability is achieved, as evidence by improved psychosocial functioning and abstinence from opioids, the person is given his or her dose daily at a pharmacy, and is observed taking it. With increasing stability, take-home doses of methadone are provided. Methadone is a potent long-acting medication that requires the person to take on responsibilities to ensure safe storage and handling of take-home doses. Clinicians should discuss the importance of not giving away or selling doses, not missing doses and communicating with the prescriber any changes to the person's health or response to methadone.

It is important to advise clients on methadone maintenance therapy to avoid sedating substances such as alcohol and benzodiazepines to minimize the chance of interactions that can lead to overdose.

Buprenorphine

Buprenorphine is a partial opioid agonist at lower doses and an opioid antagonist at higher doses. It is available as a sublingual oral tablet for medication-assisted therapy. Buprenorphine is taken once daily and, like methadone, eliminates withdrawal symptoms for 24 hours when taken at the right dose. Taking buprenorphine is safer than taking methadone because the risk of overdose is much lower due to buprenorphine's high affinity to receptors; in other words, if additional opioids are taken, buprenorphine acts like an agonist by displacing other opioids (Handford et al., 2011).

Withdrawal management

Withdrawal management should not be a stand-alone intervention because it has poor outcomes when it is not paired with other psychosocial or ongoing treatment options such as substitution therapy. Most people in withdrawal management only relapse within six months. As such, withdrawal management alone is not the best approach for treatment success (WHO, 2009).

Opioid withdrawal management can be done on an outpatient basis, using buprenorphine or methadone with medical supervision and psychosocial supports, or without medical supervision in a non-medical withdrawal management facility with psychosocial support and intervention. As mentioned earlier, inpatient medical withdrawal management is recommended for people with concurrent mental health or medical issues that may become exacerbated in the context of withdrawal.

Physical symptoms of opioid withdrawal such as upset stomach, nausea and diarrhea can be alleviated with over-the-counter preparations and comfort measures, such as applying warmth (e.g., a hot water bottle) to relieve muscle aches.

Relapse prevention

Gaining the skills and support needed for relapse prevention is very important to sustain improvements and abstinence from opioids in recovery. Clinicians should discuss and collaboratively work with the client on the following areas throughout all phases of the recovery journey:
- coping with cravings
- avoiding triggers
- adaptive coping skills
- self-care
- physical and mental well-being
- healthy self-image
- meaningful roles
- healthy relationships
- appropriate management of pain
- handling stress in healthy ways.

Naltrexone

Naltrexone is a medication that people who have withdrawn from opioids can take for relapse prevention. It works by blocking the effects of opioids. For people who do not want medication-assisted therapy, naltrexone can support their recovery and relapse prevention (Krupitsky et al., 2010; Lobmaier et al., 2010). However, it may increase the risk of overdose if a person relapses to opioids after discontinuing naltrexone.

Options for the Person with Chronic Pain and Opioid Addiction

When prescribed appropriately and monitored carefully, opioid medications are very effective in managing pain, especially acute pain (Walwyn et al., 2010). Chronic pain is a complex condition in which the pain persists far beyond the time it takes for tissue to heal (Fishman, 2009). Chronic pain often requires a comprehensive approach to management that includes not only medications but also other interventions, such as improving conditioning through physiotherapy and supports. In addition to their pain-relieving effects, opioid medications can also cause euphoria and a sense of well-being and reduced stress, which is problematic for people at higher risk of developing opioid addiction. People with a current or past history of substance use problems are at highest risk for developing opioid addiction (National Opioid Use Guideline Group, 2010).

Opioid Addiction and Pregnancy

Women who are pregnant and addicted to opioids should be advised not to stop opioids abruptly. Abrupt cessation poses harmful risks to the woman and the fetus, as withdrawal can result in miscarriage (Kahan & Wilson, 2002). Pregnant women who are addicted to opioids and who have decided to continue with the pregnancy should be connected to their family physician for prenatal care or referred to specialized prenatal services for women with substance use problems as soon as possible. Substitution therapy with methadone is the recommended best treatment for women with opioid addiction who are pregnant. The clinician should work closely with the woman and her other care providers to support treatment (Winklbaur et al., 2008).

Considerations for Women with Opioid Addiction

Due to women's role commitments, especially those related to caregiving and child rearing, clinicians may need to modify how services and treatments are delivered for women with opioid addiction. For many women, services like inpatient medical withdrawal management or residential programs may not be feasible, unless practical issues like taking care of children while in treatment are actively addressed.

Regular, routine health care is important to address general health concerns and concerns around sexually transmitted illnesses with women with problematic opioid use. Women with opioid addiction often have irregular menstrual cycles and missed periods that become regular after withdrawal and a stretch of abstinence. Women should be informed of this change, as the risk for unplanned pregnancy is high after withdrawing from opioids (Kahan & Wilson, 2002).

The Person with High-Risk Opioid Use

Clinicians need to engage people who are not connected to any services or treatment and who have high-risk opioid use. People who take large amounts of opioids daily using unsafe intravenous practices, such as sharing injection equipment (e.g., needles, cottons, spoons), or who use in unsafe environments and who do not want formal treatment require a supportive, non-coercive engagement approach. A harm reduction approach is best, aimed at reducing the harms associated with use without necessitating quitting or abstinence. A genuine and transparent approach, demonstrating respect for the person's choices and support for his or her recovery is essential in treatment engagement and rapport. Informing the person of the real risks associated with the current pattern of use is important. Clients should be advised not to use opioids alone, and to test new batches of opioids by using very small amounts at first. They should be advised to seek medical attention in the event of overdose or withdrawal. Clinicians should also provide practical information about treatment options without being coercive. But most important in treatment engagement is developing a therapeutic relationship grounded in trust and rapport.

Revisiting the Case Study

An assessment is performed to explore Mingyu's pattern, duration and route of opioid use, as well as the nature and course of her use, looking at factors such as reasons for and consequences of use and signs of aberrant use. The counsellor explores with Mingyu the nature of her pain and the extent to which she uses opioids to manage pain. The counsellor also identifies current withdrawal symptoms and conducts a full mental status exam, paying particular attention to Mingyu's mood and level of impulsivity. Mingyu's personal history of substance use and addiction, issues of trauma and abuse and her plan to borrow medications from friends are also discussed.

Using motivational strategies, the counsellor explores with Mingyu her understanding of the risks and harms of taking another person's methadone. The counsellor helps Mingyu become aware that she has choices and would meet eligibility criteria for supervised medical withdrawal management and medication-assisted treatment. The counsellor engages Mingyu in developing a care plan by discussing with her her goals and priorities, and offers practical support for immediate concerns and priorities to build Mingyu's confidence in the value of seeking assistance. Mingyu is also encouraged to discuss her situation with her family doctor, which opens up new ways and options for assessing and managing the pain that makes her vulnerable to problematic opioid use. The counsellor offers to liaise with Mingyu's family doctor and other professionals involved in her care, and asks Mingyu to identify people who might give her social support to enhance her recovery prospects. Regardless of what Mingyu's goals and choices are around her problematic opioid use, the counsellor will continue to work with her and engage her in treatment through ongoing contact and support.

Conclusion

A person-centred or holistic approach based on a biopsychosocial model is important in guiding a comprehensive screening and assessment of people with opioid addiction. Assessment and screening should be done routinely, as opioid addiction is a chronic, relapsing condition that may be triggered by life events, as well as painful medical conditions. Assessment and treatment should address mental health diagnoses, such as depression and anxiety, and the specific risks associated with high-risk use, such as intravenous drug use and comorbid health conditions.

Practice Tips

- Seek opportunities for early treatment engagement and intervention by providing comprehensive routine screening and assessment for opioid use and other substance use problems.
- Work collaboratively using an interdisciplinary approach with existing care providers, and connect to new providers.
- Develop and employ a holistic treatment approach that considers the person's biological, psychological, social, cultural and spiritual needs, and that sees care and change as an extended and continuing process.
- Educate clients who have reduced their opioid consumption about the risks associated with loss of tolerance to opioids, particularly the risk of potentially lethal overdose if they return to their previous opioid doses.
- Take a harm reduction approach to lifestyle and behavioural issues, focusing on minimizing harmful impact, especially when clients are not committed to or able to accomplish comprehensive changes in substance use or their life situation, or where such options are not available.

- Be client-centred. Work actively with clients who have clear abstinence goals or who are committed to working on particular life issues they want to address. Be supportive and validating with clients who are ambivalent or reluctant to change, encouraging them to reduce the risk and harm related to substance use.
- Use a holistic biopsychosocial approach in your work with clients who have opioid addiction, taking into consideration the client's cultural beliefs regarding substance use.
- Build social support. Identify other people the client values as being able to play a positive role in recovery.

Resources

Publications

Center for Substance Abuse Treatment. (2008). *Medication-Assisted Treatment for Opioid Addiction in Opioid Treatment Programs Inservice Training.* Rockville, MD: Substance Abuse and Mental Health Services Administration. Retrieved from http://kap.samhsa.gov/products/trainingcurriculums/pdfs/tip43_curriculum.pdf

Handford, C., Kahan, M., Srivastava, A., Cirrone, S., Sanghera, S., Palda, V., . . . Selby, P. (2011). *Buprenorphine/Naloxone for Opioid Dependence: Clinical Practice Guidelines.* Toronto: Centre for Addiction and Mental Health. Retrieved from http://knowledgex.camh.net/primary_care/guidelines_materials/Documents/buprenorphine_naloxone_gdlns2012.pdf

National Opioid Use Guideline Group. (2010). *Canadian Guideline for Safe and Effective Use of Opioids for Chronic Non-Cancer Pain.* Hamilton, ON: Author. Retrieved from http://nationalpaincentre.mcmaster.ca/documents/opioid_guideline_part_b_v5_6.pdf

Ontario College of Physicians and Surgeons. (2011). *Methadone Maintenance Treatment Program Standards and Clinical Guidelines.* Toronto: Author. Retrieved from www.cpso.on.ca/policies/guidelines/default.aspx?id=1984

Registered Nurses' Association of Ontario. (2009). *Supporting Clients on Methadone Maintenance Treatment.* Toronto: Author. Retrieved from http://rnao.ca/bpg/guidelines/supporting-clients-methadone-maintenance-treatment

World Health Organization. (2009). *Guidelines for the Psychosocially Assisted Pharmacological Treatment of Opioid Dependence.* Geneva: Author. Retrieved from www.who.int/substance_abuse/publications/opioid_dependence_guidelines.pdf

Internet

Canadian Centre on Substance Abuse—prescription drug misuse
   www.ccsa.ca/Eng/Priorities/Prescription-Drug-Misuse/Pages/default.aspx
World Health Organization—management of substance abuse
   www.who.int/substance_abuse.en

References

Compton, W. & Volkow, N. (2006). Major increases in opioid analgesic abuse in the United States: Concerns and strategies. *Drug and Alcohol Dependence, 81*, 103–107.

Fischer, B., Patra, J., Cruz, M.F., Gittins, J. & Rehm, J. (2008). Comparing heroin users and prescription opioid users in a Canadian multi-site population of illicit opioid users. *Drug and Alcohol Review, 27*, 625–632.

Fishman, S. (2009). Opioid-based multimodal care of patients with chronic pain: Improving effectiveness and mitigating the risks. *Pain Medicine, 10* (Suppl. 12), 49–52.

Handford, C., Kahan, M., Srivastava, A., Cirrone, S., Sanghera, S., Palda, V. et al. (2011). *Buprenorphine/Naloxone for Opioid Dependence: Clinical Practice Guidelines.* Toronto: Centre for Addiction and Mental Health. Retrieved from http://knowledgex.camh.net/primary_care/guidelines_materials/Documents/buprenorphine_naloxone_gdlns2012.pdf

Hayden, E., Rehm, J., Fischer, B., Monga, N. & Adlaf, E. (2005). Prescription drug abuse in Canada and the diversion of prescription drugs into the illicit drug market. *Canadian Journal of Public Health, 96*, 459–461.

Jones, E.S. & Fiellin, D.A. (2007). Women and opioid dependence treatment: Office-based versus opioid treatment program-based care. *Substance Abuse, 28*, 3–8.

Kahan, M. & Marsh, D. (2000). Intoxication, overdose and withdrawal. In B. Brand (Ed.), *Management of Alcohol, Tobacco and Other Drug Problems: A Physician's Manual* (pp. 225–233). Toronto: Centre for Addiction and Mental Health.

Kahan, M. & Wilson, L. (2002). *Managing Alcohol, Tobacco and Other Drug Problems: A Pocket Guide for Physicians and Nurses.* Toronto: Centre for Addiction and Mental Health.

Kahan, M., Srivastava, A., Wilson, L., Gourlay, D. & Midmer, D. (2006). Misuse of and dependence on opioids: Study of chronic pain patients. *Canadian Family Physician, 52*, 1081–1087.

Krupitsky, E., Zvartau, E. & Woody, G. (2010). Use of naltrexone to treat opioid addiction in a country in which methadone and buprenorphine are available. *Current Psychiatry Reports, 12*, 448–453.

Lobmaier, P.P., Kunoe, N., Gossop, M., Katevoll, T. & Waal, H. (2010). Naltrexone implants compared to methadone: Outcomes six months after prison release. *European Addiction Research, 16*, 139–145.

Maremmani, I. & Gerra, G. (2010). Buprenorphine-based regimens and methadone for the medical management of opioid dependence: Selecting the appropriate drug for treatment. *American Journal on Addictions, 19*, 557–568.

Mattick, R.P., Breen, C., Kimber, J. & Davoli, M. (2003). Methadone maintenance therapy versus no opioid replacement therapy for opioid dependence. *Cochrane Database of Systematic Reviews.* 2003 (2): CD002209.

Miller, W. R. & Rollnick, S. (2002). *Motivational Interviewing: Preparing People for Change* (2nd ed.). New York: Guilford Press.

National Institute for Health and Clinical Excellence. (2007). *Drug Misuse: Opioid Detoxification* (Clinical guideline 52). London, United Kingdom: Author. Retrieved from http://guidance.nice.org.uk/CG52/NICEGuidance/pdf

National Opioid Use Guideline Group. (2010). *Canadian Guideline for Safe and Effective Use of Opioids for Chronic Non-Cancer Pain.* Hamilton, ON: Retrieved from http://nationalpaincentre.mcmaster.ca/documents/opioid_guideline_part_b_v5_6.pdf

Noel, L., Fischer, B., Tyndall, M.W., Bradet, D.R., Rehm, J., Brissette, S. et al. (2006). Health and social services accessed by a cohort of Canadian illicit opioid users outside of treatment. *Canadian Journal of Public Health, 97*, 166–170.

Popova, S., Patra, J., Mohapatra, S., Fischer, B. & Rehm, J. (2009). How many people in Canada use prescription opioids non-medically in general and street drug using populations? *Canadian Journal of Public Health, 100*, 104–108.

Popova, S., Rehm, J. & Fischer, B. (2006). An overview of illegal opioid use and health services utilization in Canada. *Public Health, 120*, 320–328.

Scherbaum, N. & Specka, M. (2008). Factors influencing the course of opiate addiction. *International Journal of Methods in Psychiatric Research, 17* (Suppl.), 39–44.

Walwyn, W.M., Miotto, K.A. & Evans, C.J. (2010). Opioid pharmaceuticals and addiction: The issues, and research directions seeking solutions. *Drug and Alcohol Dependence, 108*, 156–165.

Wild, T.C., el-Guebaly, N., Fischer, B., Brissette, S., Brochu, S., Bruneau J. et al. (2005). Comorbid depression among untreated illicit opiate users: Results from a multisite Canadian study. *Canadian Journal of Psychiatry, 50*, 512–518.

Winklbaur, B., Kopf, N., Ebner, N., Jung, E., Thau, K. & Fischer, G. (2008). Treating pregnant women dependent on opioids is not the same as treating pregnancy and opioid dependence: A knowledge synthesis for better treatment for women and neonates. *Addiction, 103*, 1429–1440.

World Health Organization (WHO). (2009). *Guideline for the Psychologically Assisted Pharmacological Treatment of Opioid Dependence.* Geneva: Author. Retrieved from www.who.int/substance_abuse/publications/opioid_dependence_guidelines.pdf

Zeldman, A., Ryan, R.M. & Fiscella, K. (2004). Motivation, autonomy support and entity beliefs: Their role in methadone maintenance treatment. *Journal of Social and Clinical Psychology, 23*, 675–696.

Chapter 13

Family Pathways to Care, Treatment and Recovery

Wayne Skinner, Toula Kourgiantakis and Caroline O'Grady*

OLGA AND HER CHILDREN

When Olga, a 75-year-old grandmother of four, became a client at the local addiction agency, it created a crisis in the family, particularly among her three adult children. They knew their mother had been having a hard time since their father died suddenly three years ago and that she was on an antidepressant, but they did not know she was having four drinks a day, and sometimes more. Olga's drinking problem was identified during a regular checkup with her family doctor, who acknowledged that he wished he'd asked about her drinking a few years earlier. The doctor surmised that the antidepressant hadn't been working to its full potential because of Olga's alcohol consumption. When he recommended a period of abstinence, Olga said she had tried and failed to cut back before, and would need some help. The doctor referred her to an addiction facility that offered a treatment program for older adults. Olga's children were surprised and concerned for their mother, but committed to supporting her through this difficult period. They contacted the treatment agency and asked if they could come in.

✦

DONALD AND HIS FAMILY

Wilma is a 62-year-old widow and mother of two adult children—Cathy, a highly functioning 25-year-old, and Donald, a 30-year-old who is unemployed and has severe schizoaffective disorder and an addiction to crystal methamphetamine. Donald has been attending both in- and outpatient services at various mental health institutions over the past 12 years, and for six months has been attending an outpatient program for people with schizophrenia and a psychiatric support group within a program offering treatment for

* The authors want to acknowledge with gratitude the work of Richard Boudreau in previous editions of this book. His contributions provide an inspiring foundation for the model of family care pathways we elaborate on in this chapter.

people with concurrent disorders. Wilma and Cathy have felt welcomed and accepted by the staff, but now feel they need more information and a higher level of family support from professionals and other family members experiencing similar situations. They have expressed interest in joining a family psychoeducation support group.

◆

TONY AND HIS WIFE

Tony is a 40-year-old who has had a gambling problem for more than 20 years, but his wife, Natalia, only discovered this when she received a call from the bank informing her that they were losing their home. The couple then sought services at a problem gambling program. Tony did individual and group treatment and, with the exception of one slip, had not gambled for three months. Natalia sat in on a couple of Tony's sessions with his therapist and learned about his treatment plan. She was also referred to a different therapist who helped her develop a self-care plan and more effective coping strategies. Natalia attended a family psychoeducation support group and was relieved to see that other families had been through similar experiences. Despite all of these services, the relationship between Tony and Natalia was still highly conflictual. Natalia did not trust Tony, and in turn, Tony felt that Natalia was often unjustly accusing him of things. The couple was having difficulty with household responsibilities and finances but had no problems with parenting issues (they have two children) or intimacy. Both individual therapists recommended couple therapy. The family therapist worked with Tony and Natalia for a few months and created a safe space for them to discuss difficult subjects they had been avoiding. The couple felt welcomed and involved throughout the entire treatment process, and benefited from many different types of services—problem gambling treatment, psychoeducation and support, individual counselling and couple therapy.

By the time someone with an addiction receives formal help, many other lives have already been greatly affected. The vignettes of Olga, Donald and Tony bear witness to this. For these people, the journey toward help and recovery has required travelling into the personal experience of addiction as a health issue affecting their own lives and the lives of those around them. For family and friends, seeing someone they care about seek help for an addiction problem may be another manifestation of how difficult and unmanageable things have become. At the same time, the act of getting help can also be a beginning, the start of a new journey toward health recovery and improved well-being. It also represents an admission, perhaps grudging, perhaps painful, that the person's own strengths, as well as the caring efforts of concerned others, have not been adequate to successfully deal with the problem so that professional help has become necessary.

However welcoming the helping environment may be, people seeking profes-sional help may feel they have failed to solve a problem that has become bigger than they have been able to handle. Of course, they may also see this as the opportunity to finally get help, and feel relief that experts can help them to understand and address a problem that has become progressively worse or has erupted into a crisis demanding immediate attention. All too often, families don't have positive experiences with the health care and social services world. Professional intervention can bring with it a new set of challenges and problems during this phase of the family's journey. Indeed, evi-dence indicates that clients and family members may experience stigma from the very helping professionals to whom they turn for assistance with substance use problems (Rasinski et al., 2005).

A History of Exclusion

There is a long history of excluding family members from the process of assessing and treating addiction problems. While the negative impact of addictions on the family is well documented, treatment providers tend to focus their assistance on the person with the substance use problem, giving little attention to family members (Orford, Velleman et al., 2010).

Even today, to listen to concerned family members talk about their experiences in trying to seek help for a family member is to hear all too often about how they have been ignored, avoided and excluded. They frequently report that they have been allowed no real role in the process of addiction treatment. And yet, social support—often from fam-ily members—has been shown to be a leading factor in successful treatment outcomes (O'Grady & Skinner, 2012).

All too often, addiction treatment interventions are offered in specialized settings as an episode of care—with defined beginnings and endings. Once "treated," clients return to their communities, with meagre support and weak connections to ongoing care and support, they face the formidable challenge of maintaining their treatment goals and improved, healthier functioning. Family members often have learned nothing or very little about the treatment process the person has been through, have not been engaged to determine what needs the person may have, and have not been mobilized to help support change and recovery.

As long as social support is lacking, relapse rates will continue to be higher than they should be. Yet community programs that offer continuing support usually are not inclined and do not have the resources to see addiction treatment and recovery through the inclusive lens of families and social support. Involving concerned others to build social support, particularly those who are closest to the client and most able to provide assistance, is an absent or underdeveloped element in many treatment programs—both those specialized in addictions and more broadly based community health or social services.

In this chapter, we present an approach to addiction treatment that normalizes modes of family involvement as effective, evidence-informed practices. We build on the model described by Boudreau (2004) to detail a comprehensive family-focused approach to intervention and recovery, from a family member's first contact to the ongoing challenge of preventing relapse and maintaining change by optimizing social support in the real world in which people with addiction problems live. We describe a continuum of services and supports that intentionally includes members of the social network—the client's family and circle of care and support. There are important reasons for involving families. Families are involved already. Family members may be in need of help. Families can serve as a valuable resource in the helping process. And research supports family involvement and its association with improved client treatment retention and outcome (O'Grady & Skinner, 2012).

Involving the family has the double benefit of building social support for the client and enhancing the resilience and commitment of family members to play active roles in the recovery process. Failing to involve family can compromise the best efforts of the most skilled helper to be effective therapeutically.

The Roles—and Rights—of "Family"

By "family," we mean more than blood relations or connections by marriage. We include the full social world of the client, so we extend family to mean the client's "familiars"—the people who have (already or potentially) a caring concern about that person. Family members whose presence and active involvement could interfere with the client's recovery plans and goals would not be involved. Family involvement is about including the people whose participation would constructively contribute to the client's improvement. These are the people who often already have tried to seek help on the client's behalf, who are willing and committed to playing a role in the process of change and recovery, and who—most importantly—the client wants to invite to participate in his or her recovery journey.

Anyone affected by addiction should have timely access to support and counselling. These services will sometimes need to be provided separately from or parallel to the care provided to the client. Family members may seek help at a time when the person does not want help for the issues others are concerned about. Those others can benefit from service and support: as the evidence suggests, family members can even play a role in eventually engaging the person in addiction treatment, although not in the ways that are typically dramatized on reality TV shows (Smith & Meyers, 2004; Stanton, 1997).

For more than three decades, research has been showing the important roles that families can play in addiction treatment, including improving outcomes for the person in treatment and helping to reduce the negative effects of substance use problems on other family members (Ingle et al., 2008; Velleman, 2000, 2006).

An estimated 30 to 65 per cent of adults with substance use disorders and mental illnesses live with family members (Copello et al., 2010). The ongoing shift toward community-based care for people with serious addictions and mental illnesses means that family members will be called on even more to assist with ongoing care. Although the negative impact of addiction on the family has been well documented, the predominantly individualistic approach to treatment and policy has led to a lack of understanding of the negative effects of addictions on the lives of family members. This individualistic orientation fails to tap into the constructive engagement of family members that correlates with more successful outcomes (Copello et al., 2010).

The Family Experience

The stressful experience of living with a family member who has substance use problems is associated with a number of challenging issues: unpleasant and aggressive relationships; conflict over money and possessions; preoccupation, uncertainty and worry about the person; and compromised home and family life. Other problematic issues include mental health problems, violence and abuse, neglectful parenting and social exclusion. Taken together, these issues indicate the broad range of risks to families posed by a member's substance use problems (Orford, Velleman et al., 2010).

Becoming ill is a process: it consists of events that occur in time and over time; illness can come on gradually or declare itself dramatically. By its very nature, illness is something that can impinge on our capacities and potentials. In some ways, it is harder to suffer the illness of someone else than it is to suffer our own illness. Illness can challenge us to get in touch with what is really important in life; but just as likely, illness can threaten and undermine life as we had previously known it, making us feel more afraid and more alone (O'Grady & Skinner, 2012).

Orford and Velleman (2002) identify the enormous challenges in caring for a family member with addiction and mental health problems:

- extreme isolation: in many areas there is little help available; even when help is available, some people don't know where to go for help, or are too ashamed, embarrassed or frightened to seek help
- emotional, mental and physical exhaustion
- feelings of extreme sadness, hopelessness and helplessness
- feelings of guilt, anger, bitterness and resentment
- overwhelming preoccupation with family member's health and safety
- fear of stigma by association and rejection by society.

A Family-Focused Care Pathways Model

Imagine a health and social services system that was set up to include and work with families and concerned others, whether or not the person with an addiction has presented for help. Clients would have to consent to the involvement of others in their care, and would be encouraged, as a matter of routine practice, to identify the people they would want to include. Even when the client did not want others involved, family members and concerned others could access care and support separate from the client's treatment pathways. To move beyond the compromised and comprising world of addictive behaviours, people need to achieve psychosocial integration that allows them to reach their full potential and their deeper sense of selves as members of caring communities (Alexander, 2008). To intentionally involve family members in treatment planning would shift the old care paradigm of personal recovery to a model of enhanced social connection and engagement.

O'Grady and Skinner (2012) outline the family journey from illness to recovery from addiction and co-occurring mental health problems. Figure 13-1 depicts that journey.

FIGURE 13-1: Journey as Destination

Journey into illness →	Journey through illness →	Journey into illness
Struck by lightning	Carry this albatross	Holding the hope
The ostrich thing	Double the stigma, double the pain	Coaches & kindred spirits
One roadblock after another	The conflict inside you	Thirsty for information
		Self-care virtuosos
		Families point the way

Preoccupation ————————▶ Renewal

Source: O'Grady, C. & Skinner, W.J.W. (2012). Journey as destination: A recovery model for families affected by concurrent disorders. *Qualitative Health Research, 22*, p. 1058. © SAGE Publications. Reprinted by permission.

Family members usually need to be allowed to talk about the experiences they have had on the journey into and through addiction and related problems before they can attend to the journey toward recovery. They often talk about the roadblocks they experience when they try to engage with the formal helping system. They also identify what they need from the system but often cannot get. Family members usually want to take on active roles in making their families healthier.

FIGURE 13-2: Family Care Pathways Model

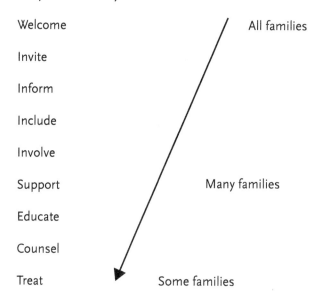

Welcoming all. The family care pathways model (see Figure 13-2) lays out a set of action terms that extends all the way from the most basic courtesies and considerations we believe *all* visitors to a health care or social service facility should receive. We organize these under the rubric "Welcome." A proactive approach to every opportunity to constructively engage family members would be informed by the four "I's": invite, inform, include and involve.

Supporting many. In the middle of this menu of family-based services is an array of supports that, if available, would be useful to *many* families affected by addiction. The supports start with routine efforts to educate and provide opportunities for peer support to family members. If "informing" provides facts and details about something, "educating" goes a step further by explaining how something is done. The distinction between telling someone to use clean needles (informing) and teaching someone how to inject safely (educating) illustrates the difference. With families, informing them that they should avoid arguing is one thing, whereas coaching them toward effective communication skills is another. Mutual aid and peer support are elements in addiction treatment that resonate as powerfully with family members as with clients themselves. Again, variations on these services and supports should be available to family members, whether or not an identified client is engaged in treatment, and even if the client does not consent to family involvement in treatment. Family members who are concerned and committed enough to want to understand and learn how they can be more effective in addressing addiction issues need to be seen as vital resources. Facilitating their access to peer support contributes to building recovery pathways that tap into family strengths and resources.

Treating some. The final cluster of services in this model of family care pathways is likely to be accessed only by *some* family members at some point along the road to recovery. These services are more formally therapeutic, where family members themselves would receive counselling and therapy for addiction-related and recovery-oriented issues. At this end of the continuum of family services and supports, the family itself may become the unit of treatment, as is common when there are intergenerational dimensions to the addiction issues. Therapy or counselling can also be used for more positive reasons, such as when the family or some of its members are so committed to a person's recovery that they want to participate actively in a program of care that will optimize the chances of a successful outcome. These other family members might recognize that the person's changing addictive behaviour creates opportunities for the family as a whole to achieve a higher level of functioning and better relationships.

WELCOMING OLGA AND HER CHILDREN

Although Olga was referred by her doctor, she was apprehensive about going to a facility that offered addiction treatment, even if it had specialized pro-gramming for older adults. When her daughters offered to go with her, she was much more receptive. Having the active interest of her adult children put Olga in an advantageous situation compared to other clients, many of whom had lost social supports. Olga attended the program, and was quite motivated to take constructive action that would ease her depression, even if it meant stopping her drinking, at least initially. Olga's doctor supported the plan and the two agreed that for the first couple of weeks, frequent but brief contact would be valuable, along with some education sessions about behavioural alternatives to substance use. Olga's daughters agreed to accompany her as needed to and from the sessions. They were invited to sit in on group-based sessions and, if Olga agreed, to join her and the therapist when they discussed their mother's progress.

Olga found that without alcohol in her system, the antidepressants were work-ing better and giving her the boost to become more physically and socially active, which meant she was spending less time alone. Olga's daughters increased their contact with her and felt rewarded to see her have better days. They felt welcome and valued in the helping process, as well as informed, and were invited to contribute suggestions as active participants. They acquired a basic understanding of alcohol and its effects, especially on older people, and an awareness of safer drinking limits. Their primary role was supportive; they credited their mother for addressing her alcohol issue, and the therapist and the treatment setting for knowing how to get organized and launch an action plan by working collaboratively with all concerned family members. The treatment process ended up being brief—about eight weeks—but Olga still receives a phone call every three months to check how things are going.

Supporting Families

Family members are important in their own right. They deserve access to group support and educational interventions that will increase their sense of empowerment and social support, and that address other factors affecting their quality of life: these interventions can reduce the sense of burden and "stigma by association," improve coping skills and enhance overall life satisfaction.

Over the past few decades, evidence-based practices have emerged to meet family members' needs for education, guidance and support (Copello et al., 2006). Various family psychoeducation programs are now offered as part of an overall clinical treatment plan, with the main focus being to improve the well-being and functioning of the client (although family members themselves experience significant benefits from such programs). While evidence-based models of family psychoeducation sometimes vary in their technical aspects, all share common features, as discussed in the next section.

Approaches to Family Support

Support-based services for families can be broadly grouped into three evidence-based types (Copello et al., 2005):

• working with family members to promote the entry and engagement of people with addictions into treatment
• involvement of family members in the care plan
• interventions responding to the needs of family members in their own right.

People who are providing emotional support, case management, financial assistance, advocacy and housing to family members with addiction problems benefit from access to support, information and resources. Family psychoeducation groups are increasingly being recognized as a valuable link in a comprehensive system of care, at all stages: assessment, pre-treatment, treatment and continuing recovery.

Combining Family Support with Psychoeducation

Emerging best practice evidence suggests that families of people with addiction and mental health problems benefit from a combination of peer support and psychoeducation tailored to their unique needs (Mueser, 2002; O'Grady & Skinner, 2012). Effective group interventions improve overall family coping and increase the sense of hope (Bloom, 1990). Client outcomes also improve when the needs of family members for information, clinical guidance and support are met (Levine & Ligenza, 2002; Mueser, 2002; Solomon et al., 1997).

Social support and psychoeducation groups can be offered to family members without the requirements of therapeutic expertise and investment of scarce resources.

These groups constitute an aspect of service and support that would allow many treatment settings a "quick win" in providing family-centred care and a sustainable resource for family members.

There are many ways clinicians can facilitate access to family psychoeducation and peer support groups: they can support and contribute to them; provide them in their own agency settings; learn where family supports resources are available in the community (e.g., 12-step groups such as Al-Anon and Gam-Anon); be aware of online supports and resources; and encourage and support families in exploring options.

Family support and psychoeducation groups share various features. They:

- combine information about substance use and related problems with training in problem solving, communication skills and developing social supports
- use the expertise of both families and professionals
- aim to reduce family stress, facilitate the development of coping skills and enhance personal empowerment for caregivers.

Successful programs have been found to offer a range of support and education benefits (Murray-Swank & Dixon, 2004). These programs:

- explore family members' expectations of the treatment and expectations for themselves and the client
- assess the strengths and limitations of the family's ability to support the client
- assist in co-ordinating elements of treatment and rehabilitation to ensure everyone works toward the same goals in a collaborative, supportive partnership
- provide information about the family member's optimum medication management and other treatment issues
- provide opportunities for professional facilitators to listen to families' concerns and involve them as equal partners in planning and delivering treatment
- help resolve family conflict by responding sensitively to emotional distress
- address participants' feelings of grief and loss
- provide an explicit crisis plan
- help improve communication among family members
- provide training for the family in structured problem-solving techniques
- encourage family members to expand their social support networks (e.g., to participate in informal family support organizations, such as the Mood Disorders Association of Canada, the Schizophrenia Society of Canada and Al-Anon).

The family plays a key part both in preventing and in intervening with substance use problems by helping to reduce risk, encourage healthy change, build resilience and support recovery.

The Evidence Base for Family Education and Support

Even brief interventions for family members, delivered in various formats, can have significant impact, generating positive changes that are maintained and that increase over time without any further formal delivery of the intervention (Velleman et al., 2011). Individualized consultation increases family members' sense of self-efficacy around supporting a loved one with serious mental illness (Velleman, 2006). Group psychoeducation also helps increase this sense of self-efficacy, particularly for family members who have never participated in a support or advocacy group.

Building Family Resilience

Including education and peer support resources for family members enhances addiction treatment, producing effects that are measurable in the family members who participate, in the family system as a whole and in the person with addiction problems (Fals-Stewart et al., 2005; Magill et al., 2010).

Family resilience can be described as family members' ability to cope with adversity, enabling them to flourish with warmth, support and cohesion. An increasingly important focus in addiction prevention and treatment will be to identify, enhance and promote family resilience. Prominent features of resilient families include positive outlook, spirituality, family member accord, flexibility, family communication, financial management, family time, shared recreation, routines and rituals, and support networks. A family resilience orientation based on the conviction that all families have inherent strengths and the potential for growth inclines the professional to focus on families' protective and recovery factors and facilitate access to community resources. The growing literature on resilience at the family level, with the identification of key factors for resilience in healthy families, offers increased support, tools and resources to health professionals working in addiction and mental health for taking a family-centred approach to treatment and recovery (Black & Lobo, 2008). This emerging evidence base is a reminder that the work of welcoming, supporting and counselling families is less about families as the source of problems and more about families as resources for change and recovery that can provide the social support that predicts better treatment outcomes.

Partnering with Families: An Illustration

At the Centre for Addiction and Mental Health in Toronto, we have been working for more than 10 years to learn how to provide, evaluate and promote peer support and psychoeducation resources for family members (O'Grady, 2005; O'Grady & Skinner, 2012). Our pilot project comparing a psychoeducation manual to a support group for family members led to the creation of the *Family Guide to Concurrent Disorders* (O'Grady & Skinner, 2007a), as well as a facilitator's guide for clinicians who want to implement peer support and education for family members (O'Grady & Skinner, 2007b). Working with colleagues around Ontario, we extended our work to 20 communities, where, in most cases, local addiction and mental health agencies collaborated in delivering education and support groups for family members. Evaluation results reinforced the key finding of the first study: when pre- and post-participation scores are compared, those participants showed measurable improvements.

Our findings (O'Grady & Skinner, 2012) confirm that participating in peer support and education groups or using the psychoeducation manual on its own are both promising tools to support family members who want to be better equipped to address addiction and co-occurring mental health problems in their families. Participants in each option:

- perceived greater social support
- felt more personal mastery and empowerment
- felt less caregiver burden
- felt more hopeful, and perceived less stigma.

Our family guide and parallel group sessions (O'Grady & Skinner, 2012) addressed the following themes:

- introduction to concurrent disorders (including pharmacotherapy and other treatment issues and approaches, stigma, other effects on the family)
- understanding substance use and mental health problems
- social support needs
- self-care for family members
- crisis management
- relapse and relapse prevention
- recovery.

More recently, we conducted a study using an Internet-based support and psychoeducational group with family members affected by addiction and mental health problems (O'Grady et al., 2010). This online group had the same positive results as our in-person groups. Not only did participants achieve significant changes for the better in terms of empowerment, social support, coping, caregiver burden, satisfaction with life, hope and stigma; participation also opened up access to family support and psychoeducation group support that otherwise is not available to most people.

Family Education and Support: Summary Points

Offering the appropriate components of family support and education appears to be an important determinant of positive outcomes for both family participants and the family member with the addiction. Important components of family support and educational interventions include providing opportunities for sharing feelings and experiences in a supportive, empowering and understanding environment with others who quickly come to be seen as "kindred spirits," and for enhancing resilience, validation and hopefulness for family participants. Effective group interventions have also been shown to improve overall family coping and increase the sense of hope.

SUPPORTING FAMILIES: DONALD'S STORY

Donald's mother, Wilma, and sister, Cathy, felt welcomed and accepted by the health professionals at their local addiction agency. When they discovered that the agency offered a 12-week family psychoeducational group, they jumped at the opportunity to get more information and a higher level of family support from professionals and others in similar situations. They used the opportunity to learn more about mental health and addiction problems and how these problems take a major toll not only on the person with the addiction and/or mental health problem, but on the family as a whole. Peer support and input led to them feeling less alone and more able to cope emotionally with the ongoing issues that arise with mental health and addiction problems. They learned how to effectively deal with the common cycle of relapse and recovery. They developed ways to do better self-care as individuals and as a family. And they applied the communication skills they learned to their interactions not just with Donald but with others, including health care providers.

Engaging People with Addictions Who Are Reluctant to Get Treatment

Most people think of TV shows such as *The Intervention* when they think about how families can intervene with a relative who has an addiction but won't seek treatment. This approach draws on the Johnson Institute Intervention model. Its dramatic staged confrontations have popular appeal in the age of reality TV, but overlook the lack of evidence to support its use.

On the other hand, there are more promising approaches that are supported by research evidence. One example is community reinforcement and family training (CRAFT), developed by Robert Meyers and colleagues in New Mexico (Smith & Meyers, 2004). Their published studies indicate that they were able to engage clients in 64 to 86 per cent of the cases they worked with. The approach works by having a "concerned significant other" try to influence the person with the substance use problem to reduce use and seek treatment. The concerned other is supported to make his or her own positive life changes, regardless of whether the person using substances enters treatment. CRAFT works with the concerned significant other to plan and implement interventions that focus on behavioural, cognitive and motivational interventions in non-confrontational ways (Smith & Meyers, 2004). Meyers and Wolfe's book, *Get Your Loved One Sober* (2004), is a practical resource for concerned others who want to use the tools themselves to help a family member.

Another promising approach is the Albany-Rochester interventional sequence for engagement (ARISE). Although it is not as well researched as CRAFT, findings suggest that its outcomes are comparable to leading approaches to engaging people with addictions in treatment while working primarily with family members other than the person with the addiction problem (Garrett et al., 1997; Lam et al., 2011; Landau et al., 2004). Although there is positive research support for CRAFT and ARISE—both methods that use less confrontation and more motivational and contingency management strategies—these clinical services are not widely available, and have not been chosen as the basis for a reality TV show.

Family Therapy

Family therapy approaches to addiction have a long lineage, going back to the 1930s, when psychodynamic approaches were used. In the 1950s, models based on family stress and coping emerged. And in the 1970s, the three major models that prevail today came on the scene: family systems models, behavioural models and the family disease model (McCrady et al., 2011). All of these represent attempts to theorize and conceptualize addiction problems and addiction treatments from family, interpersonal and social systems perspectives.

A biopsychosocial perspective on addiction applies to a family care pathways approach to addictive behaviours. Growing evidence is helping to detail how genetic factors create vulnerability to and resilience against addiction, while the family (understood in the expanded way we define it here) is the developmental environment in which a person develops from infancy through childhood and adolescence to adulthood (making it the primary site of personal development and personality formation), as well as being the social unit where values, attitudes and behaviours are modelled and learned. This means that a family-based approach can be decisive all the way along the process that starts with risk and vulnerability to addiction, to prevention and identification and, most importantly here, to treatment and recovery.

Being able to involve positive social support that is family based and understanding family challenges and issues, enhance the therapeutic opportunity to help clients move toward optimal change and recovery. Family intervention approaches not only highlight these contextual and developmental aspects of addiction problems; they also open up the question of the presence of other problems related to mental and physical health and other areas of functioning that affect well-being.

From the disease, behavioural and social systems models, Lam and colleagues (2011) identify five specific practical approaches:

- The family disease approach looks at addiction as a family disease, relying on 12-step work through Alcoholics Anonymous and other similar groups for the person with the addiction, and Al-Anon and its kindred groups for the family. Concepts such as disease, denial, co-dependence and enabling are core to this perspective, which lacks a research base.
- In family systems therapy, the therapist joins with the family to restructure alliances and interactional patterns as a way of resolving addictive behaviour. Some research supports this approach for adult drug users.

- Behavioural couple therapy is based on goal setting, behavioural alternatives and communication skills. Particularly for treating alcohol problems, there is strong evidence for improved abstinence and relationship outcomes.
- Network therapy supports the person's recovery by engaging his or her social network. Research findings support this approach for adults with alcohol problems.
- Ecological approaches, particularly multisystemic family therapy, have developed as a family-based approach for adolescents with drug problems. Multidimensional family therapy extended the systems orbit further to include school and other environments in the treatment of young people with substance use, mental health, social and legal problems.

The evidence for working with couples and significant others is actually stronger than for working with families as a whole (Miller et al., 2011), which argues for the need for further research and evaluation in developing more family-centred treatment options. Another area where family-involved treatment has proven to be particularly effective is with ethnically diverse youth who have serious substance use problems (Lam et al., 2011; Liddle et al., 2005).

Currently, less than 15 per cent of specialized addiction agencies in Canada provide any form of family counselling or other service (Beasley et al., 2012). There is now positive advice recommending a range of proven or promising therapies that build family care pathways in treatment and recovery. Whatever the approach, three areas have been identified as key to therapeutic success: helping the person with the addiction problems make healthy changes; changing the behaviour and coping patterns of family members; and modifying dysfunctional interaction patterns (McCrady et al., 2011).

Another area the counsellor needs to be skillful in assessing is violence and aggression in the family. Violence and aggression manifest in various ways, including verbal, emotional, physical and sexual abuse. Where children are the victims, counsellors are obligated to report to child welfare agencies that are charged to formally investigate these issues. By far the most common reports of family violence involve women and children as the victims. It is important in assessing toxic and abusive processes in the family to take a comprehensive approach. The processes that lead to aggressive or abusive events can be complex and involve different relationships, such as sibling to sibling, child to parent and woman to man. It is important to decide on the safety and risk issues involved in families where family violence is a factor. This is an area of work that requires extra skills and supports for the therapist, including active supervision and consultation. Rather than presuming that these factors preclude working with the family, it is worth noting that the evidence shows that family-based treatments tend to reduce family violence and increase child functioning (McCrady et al., 2011).

Addictions have a profound impact on couples and families. For family members, these difficulties can create high levels of distress (Hodgins et al., 2007), communication problems and conflict in relationships, physical and mental health problems, isolation (Dickson-Swift et al., 2005), intimacy issues, increased risks of family violence (Korman et al., 2008), parenting issues and higher rates of separation and divorce (Black et al.,

2012). Addictions often erode trust, create distance and breed conflict in relationships. Families affected by addiction often experience intense emotions, including anger, shame, guilt, fear and worry.

The relationship between family dynamics and addictive behaviour is bidirectional. While addictive behaviours can challenge and compromise family functioning and cohesion, compromised family functioning and weak cohesion may challenge healthy behaviours and encourage addiction (McCrady et al., 2011).

Family therapy can offer families a safe therapeutic space to work through difficult emotions, develop more effective communication skills, establish appropriate family roles and boundaries and rebuild relationships. Research has shown that better family functioning is linked with improved treatment outcomes (Fals-Stewart et al., 2005). Yet despite the benefits, very few treatment centres offer family or couple therapy (Beasley et al., 2012; Csiernik, 2002).

Balancing the divergent needs of family members and intense emotions and conflict can be challenging for therapists. At the same time, helping family members move from feeling overwhelmed to regaining hope and belief in the possibility of change can be incredibly rewarding. Even when reconciliation is impossible, family therapy can still succeed in helping members identify irresolvable conflicts and work toward responsible, respectful decision making and action.

The next sections provide a quick overview of some key ingredients in family therapy—assessment, alliance building and contracting. We also identify ethical issues that may arise and highlight effective therapeutic strategies.

Assessment

Couple and family therapy begin with a comprehensive initial assessment. This creates an opportunity to understand the family's current difficulties, as well as its strengths. Safety issues should be assessed as early as possible, and regularly throughout therapy. The therapist informs the family members before starting the assessment that one purpose of assessment is to ascertain whether family therapy is the best option, or whether other services or modalities may be more suitable. A well-conducted assessment enhances the family's sense of trust and safety, and helps to clarify the goals of therapy and the roles of each participant. While validating the impact addiction has had on the family, the therapist focuses more on how the addiction (rather than *person*) has affected each family member, and how the family interacts, communicates and solves problems.

The therapist starts where clients are at for the assessment, since they may each arrive with a different motivation level. It is important to find common ground, rather than trying to pull someone in the direction of the majority. The presenting problem is often a starting point and gradually the therapist broadens the focus. After the therapist has listened to each person's experience and perception of the problem, the subject can be expanded by asking about other issues that may be affecting the presenting problem or that may predate the addiction. Ideally, the therapist takes time to explore each family member's individual history, including information about family of origin, trauma history and mental health and addiction history. Although assessments tend to take more time when the family is involved, this involvement can yield useful information. Some therapists see family members separately for the assessment, although this should be done judiciously because it undermines the overall alliance with the family if members think the therapist is partial to or secretly aligned with particular members.

The therapist gathers all of the information and makes a clinical formulation highlighting the strengths and strategies the family has drawn on in the past that have been successful in coping with the problem. Focusing on what works can instil hope, which has been found to contribute to successful treatment outcomes (Sprenkle et al., 2009). Separating the problem from the person, and shifting the focus from past disappointments to present opportunities, can foster hope, increase motivation and help build a good working relationship with the family.

Building a Therapeutic Alliance

While the therapeutic alliance is important in all forms of therapy, in couple and family therapy, connecting and maintaining a working alliance with each person is especially important, since a good alliance fosters a sense of safety in therapy (Friedlander et al., 2006). Establishing a therapeutic alliance can be more challenging than in individual therapy because the family therapist must establish and maintain multiple alliances with family members who may have divergent motivations about seeking help, have different perceptions of the problem and be at different stages of change. Each family member needs to feel validated and understood. Ruptures, breaches or impasses in the therapeutic alliance can be interpreted by therapists as "resistance." Steve de Shazer (1984), the pioneer of solution-focused therapy, proposed that when the therapist experiences the client as being resistant, the therapist should reframe this as a signal that the client is feeling misunderstood. An essential task in therapeutic engagement is for the counsellor to ensure the client feels understood.

Creating a safe space in family therapy greatly enhances the quality of the therapeutic alliance. In family therapy, family members have less control over how and when information is disclosed to the therapist or to other family members. Individuals and families often feel shame, guilt, anger and frustration when facing problems related to addiction. Uncertainty and fear about what might be said in a counselling session can provoke great anxiety. For families that have experienced an addiction, the levels of emotional intensity present can interfere with alliance building. Joining with each person, including more ambivalent or reluctant members, is a fundamental task in family therapy. The therapist helps family members cope with difficult or unexpected disclosures, vulnerability and conflict. The ability to manage and effectively guide the family through these incidents builds a sense of safety, and strengthens the working alliance.

The strength of the therapeutic alliance is influenced not only by the quality of the bond between clients and therapist, but also by the therapist's understanding of the issues in the family and the goals and tasks that are contracted with the client. Creating a "shared sense of purpose" will influence the family's engagement in therapy and the alliance with the therapist (Friedlander et al., 2006). The therapist's skill at reframing contentious statements made by family members, finding common purpose and helping create unified family goals can engender hope and unity in a family that may be feeling disconnected and conflicted.

Developing Contracts and Treatment Plans

A contract or treatment plan defines the common goals identified and agreed on by the therapist and family members. Families dealing with addictions often have incongruent goals when they come to therapy. Contracting operationalizes the action steps that the therapist and family members agree on in order to reach the goals they have decided to work on. Participants negotiate what tasks need to be accomplished, by whom and by when. Doherty (2002) notes that lack of structure in family therapy is one of the most common problems among therapists, especially inexperienced ones. Contracting ideally starts during the assessment, and is reviewed and revised regularly. It outlines the treatment goals and structure (number of sessions, frequency, place, participants), role of the therapist and ethical considerations, such as confidentiality. It is common practice in couple and family therapy to contract for a specified number of sessions. For example, the therapist proposes six to eight sessions, to be renegotiated as needed. Frequency can vary, although sessions are usually weekly at the beginning of treatment.

Ethical Issues in Family Therapy

Many practice dilemmas, including ethical issues, can arise in family therapy. The most common issue is confidentiality, although there are other ambiguous quandaries, such as dual roles, documentation, role of the therapist and knowing clearly who the client is. Family therapists must adhere to the policies of the agency or hospital in which they work, and to the code of ethics and professional standards of their accreditation body. While these policies and accreditation bodies offer overarching principles and guidelines, they often do not answer specific questions that therapists have when working with families on addiction issues.

Having access to supervision and consultation is vital in any area of clinical practice, but this level of expertise is not always readily available for couple and family therapy. As the addiction field follows the evidence base, more family-based services will be available. A broader base of supervisory expertise specializing in family treatment will gradually emerge. In the meantime, therapists and agencies may need to look outside the addiction field to get the ongoing supervision and support that staff needs to develop and maintain competencies in this area. Internet-based technologies are improving access to these supports and facilitating the growth of peer communities of practice for counsellors doing couple and family therapy. In addition to clinical supervision, self-reflection, transparency, contracting and having established policies and procedures for documentation and addressing other practical issues can help therapists prevent or resolve the challenges that come with family therapy.

Therapeutic Strategies in Family Therapy

Containing intense interactions and de-escalating conflict

Many therapists worry about not being able to contain conflict and hostility that arise during family sessions. Containment is essential for family members to feel safe. Family therapists can use techniques such as softening (taking the edge off strong comments while keeping the focus on the issue) and pacing (slowing things down to allow an issue to be carefully processed, or keeping things moving by staying on task) when responding to evoked emotions, as well as interjecting and stopping hostile interactions. Not only will these techniques make sessions feel safer; they will also model ways for family members to regulate their own emotions and communicate and problem solve more effectively with other family members. Families affected by addiction are often distressed—with their distress expressing itself as emotional reactivity and volatility. While validating that the person is experiencing strong emotions, the therapist works to help the person become grounded, modelling how processes that usually race and escalate can be slowed down and take a more constructive course. Especially in families with patterns of painful and conflicted interaction, members need to feel validated, but also need to be coached on how to appropriately regulate and express emotions. The therapist skillfully acknowledges the hardships family members have endured in order to help them reassure one another that they want and are committed to rebuilding connections and making things better.

Drawing out family members who are more withdrawn

An imbalance can be created if some family members give only curt responses, while others are more involved. A member who is withdrawn can be viewed—often errone-ously by other family members—as not caring. The therapist can help the withdrawn family member identify and express his or her emotions. Some people with addiction issues may be more withdrawn and distant: they may feel that speaking is risky, makes them vulnerable and may bring to the forefront feelings of shame and guilt. They tend to respond positively when they feel more valued by their family. Therapists can reframe the behaviour of the withdrawn person positively to facilitate engagement and reduce further blame by other family members.

Slowing down the process

Going slow does not imply more therapy or longer sessions. Emotions tend to come fast: they surge and race. Many significant points can be missed in rapid and intense thera-peutic family discussions. Intense emotional discussions may not feel safe for families and may also resemble the types of interactions they have at home. If you want clients to hear, see, feel and understand what is being said or not being said during a session, slow things down by highlighting profound statements, staying focused when discussing sensitive subjects and helping each family member express and receive emotion.

Focusing on process, not content

A skilled therapist requires only a *little* bit of content to understand and focus on the process in a family. As important as it is to know *what* happened, the therapist will tend to give more attention to *how* it happened. How did the family interact? How did each family member respond? How could it have been different? How is family therapy helpful to the members of the family?

Using enactments

Enactment simply means having family members talk to one another in a therapeutic session rather than speaking only to or through the therapist. While enactments have been shown to be a core mechanism of change in family therapy, they require structure and support from the therapist; otherwise they can feel unsafe. Coach clients if they are having difficulty trying to talk to family members. Create a safe space, since clients are more emotional and vulnerable when they speak to one another. Guide couples experiencing distress during enactments.

Containing, slowing down, drawing out, focusing on process and using enactments: these illustrate some ways the couple or family therapist works in a relational context. Using these and other strategies, as well as many key skills, the therapist helps the family change unhealthy family patterns and shift from a problem-centred focus to a strengths-based one. Family members have a different interactional experience, one that is more contained, safe and purposeful. This helps a family reorganize and direct itself away from the destabilizing effects that overwhelming problems can produce. Evidence suggests that couple and family therapy can elicit significant positive changes, including more effective communication, decreased conflict and better problem solving (O'Farrell & Fals-Stewart, 2002). Family therapy can also have secondary effects on children or others who are not part of the therapy, but who are touched by the problem (Fals-Stewart et al., 2005). When terminating therapy with families that have been through a long recovery process, it is important to underline the changes and gains they have made in therapy.

TREATING TONY AND NATALIA

Tony's wife, Natalia, was the first to call the problem gambling treatment centre to inquire about services for her husband. Although the intake co-ordinator explained that Tony needed to self-refer, she spent a considerable amount of time explaining the services to Natalia and listening to her worries and frustrations. Later when Tony called, he was referred to an individual therapist who quickly understood that Tony was experiencing significant marital difficulties as a result of his gambling. The therapist encouraged him to include Natalia in part of the assessment session. The therapist also referred Natalia to an individual therapist and a four-week psychoeducational family support group, where Natalia heard more about the impact of problem gambling on the family, and learned how to establish clearer boundaries and use more effective communication strategies. The couple was having difficulty implementing these strategies consistently, so was referred to a couple and family therapist. At first, Natalia was reluctant about going, so the therapist focused extra effort on validating her feelings of betrayal, fatigue, fear and anger. She helped Tony and Natalia recall the strengths and resources they had used in the past to get through many tough times. At the end of the first session, Natalia felt more hopeful about her marriage.

Still, Natalia harboured a lot of anger because she felt Tony did not recognize the problem and its toll on their family. Tony did not feel safe about being vulnerable, since in the past when he tried to tell Natalia how sorry he was, it would come out wrong and Natalia would become infuriated. When she became angry, she would bring up a lot of the things Tony had done in the past about which he carried a lot of shame. He thought that staying quiet was a better option. The therapist helped Tony express himself and helped Natalia let her guard down and listen to her husband talk about past difficulties. Tony and Natalia learned to talk to each other and were able to work through previous unresolved issues. Their children participated in a few sessions, talking about their own fears and incidents they had witnessed. The family became more united after 14 sessions and more supportive of one another as it continued to deal with financial issues that had resulted from the gambling.

Conclusion

Family pathways to care, treatment and recovery open up the space so that addiction counsellors and their agencies can work more effectively. They allow addiction agencies to open doorways to constructive inclusion of concerned others to address the challenges of resolving addiction problems: as part of a person's treatment, as a parallel to individual treatment or as family interventions in their own right, with or without the person with the addiction being involved in care. Family pathways need to be available before, during and after addiction treatment. Although not a panacea, and not always indicated, the supportive involvement of family members and concerned others is among the most significant factors in completing treatment, adhering to goals and preventing relapse. Rather than placing responsibility for change exclusively on the shoulders of one person, family pathways to care see the client in an interpersonal context, actively mobilizing people who can play a positive role in recovery. The family's involvement does not exempt the person with the addiction from taking responsibility; rather, the family's involvement helps the person succeed with change and recovery goals. By enlisting the support of concerned others, by locating the addiction within the interpersonal context of the client's everyday life and by guiding family members through practical tasks and actions, recovery becomes a collaborative rather than solitary project, as well as a journey involving concrete and practical tasks and milestones that can be pursued together.

For many clinicians and in many treatment settings, an approach based on family care pathways represents a shift away from an interventive paradigm almost exclusively focused on the treatment of individuals toward a recovery-oriented approach that seeks to engage, support and extend the immediate social support available to people with addiction issues. Building on the family options for support and treatment that already exist, we have a continuing opportunity to develop a more robust capacity to create family care pathways that welcome and involve all families as partners in treatment and recovery, offer education and support to as many as possible, and provide formal treatment to the smaller set of families ready to take that step.

Practice Tips

- Welcome family members, informing and educating them about your agency, the problems you treat and the ways you do your work.
- Identify and affirm the family's strengths and expertise to guide treatment planning.
- Encourage families to learn more about the issues that bring a family member into treatment, drawing their attention to available resources, such as written materials, online tools, education materials and activities and peer support opportunities.
- Treat family members with dignity and respect, free of judgment or blame. Support and validate family members for the hardships they have endured as a result of the addiction. Credit them for taking the time and making the effort to participate.
- Review the rules of confidentiality when working with families. Identify real or potential problems and negotiate strategies to resolve or prevent issues of concern. While staff cannot release information about a person in their care, this does not preclude giving families general information about addiction, treatment and other services and resources available for families.

- Discuss the impact of addictions on individual family members in treatment to increase their awareness, become aware of their goals and help them rebuild significant relationships where appropriate. Helping the person with the addiction understand the family's difficulties can help repair relationships.
- Provide information sessions; individual, couple or family therapy; peer support groups; and family psychoeducation and other services families need to feel supported and learn better coping skills.
- Seek out professional education and ongoing supervision when working with families, as family work is complex and challenging, and therapists need support to address potential fatigue, frustration, countertransference and ethical dilemmas.
- Evaluate your family work by providing pre- and post-measures and other assessment and treatment tools to build evidence for the outcomes you are producing (Pinsof et al., 2012). Use these tools to give feedback and build hope with your clients.
- Educate others at your treatment centre about the importance of working with families. Form a small committee to develop workshops, discuss policies, disseminate information and identify gaps and strengths in the system.
- In a nutshell: welcome all family members, support as many as you can and offer counselling and treatment for those who are ready to take that step.

Resources

Publications

Center for Substance Abuse Treatment. (2004). *Substance Abuse Treatment and Family Therapy*. Treatment Improvement Protocol (TIP) series 39. Rockville, MD: Author. Retrieved from www.ncbi.nlm.nih.gov/books/NBK64265/pdf/TOC.pdf

O'Grady, C. P. & Skinner, W.J.W. (2007). *A Family Guide to Concurrent Disorders*. Toronto: Centre for Addiction and Mental Health. Retrieved from http://knowledgex.camh.net/amhspecialists/resources_families/Documents/Family_Guide_CD.pdf

Meyers, R.J. & Wolfe, B.L. (2004). *Get Your Loved One Sober: Alternatives to Nagging, Pleading and Threatening*. Center City, MN: Hazeldon.

Sloss. C., Buddra, S., Kelly, C., Shenfeld, J. & Tait, L. (2008). *Families CARE: Helping Families Cope and Relate Effectively. Facilitator's Manual*. Toronto: Centre for Addiction and Mental Health.

References

Alexander, B.K. (2008). *The Globalisation of Addiction: A Study in Poverty of the Spirit.* Oxford, United Kingdom: Oxford University Press.

Beasley, E., Jesseman, R., Patton, D. & National Treatment Indicators Working Group. (2012). *National Treatment Indicators Report, 2012.* Ottawa: Canadian Centre on Substance Abuse. Retrieved from www.nts-snt.ca

Black, D.W., Shaw, M.C., McCormick, B.A. & Allen, J. (2012). Marital status, childhood maltreatment, and family dysfunction: A controlled study of pathological gambling. *Journal of Clinical Psychiatry, 73,* 1293–1297.

Black, K. & Lobo, M. (2008). A conceptual review of family resilience factors. *Journal of Family Nursing, 14,* 33–55.

Bloom, J.R. (1990). The relationship of social support and health. *Social Science and Medicine, 39,* 635–637.

Boudreau, R.J. (2004). Substance use problems and the family. In S. Harrison & V. Carver (Eds.), *Alcohol & Drug Problems: A Practical Guide for Counsellors* (3rd ed., pp. 483–494). Toronto: Centre for Addiction and Mental Health.

Copello, A., Templeton, L. & Powell, J. (2010). The impact of addiction on the family: Estimates of prevalence and costs. *Drugs: Education, Prevention and Policy, 17* (Suppl. 1), 63–74.

Copello, A.G., Templeton, L. & Velleman, R. (2006). Family interventions for drug and alcohol misuse: Is there a best practice? *Current Opinion in Psychiatry, 19,* 271–276.

Copello, A.G., Velleman, R.D.B. & Templeton, L.J. (2005). Family interventions in the treatment of alcohol and drug problems. *Drug and Alcohol Review, 24,* 369–385.

Csiernik, R. (2002). Counseling for the family: The neglected aspect of addiction treatment in Canada. *Journal of Social Work Practice in the Addictions, 2,* 79–92.

De Shazer, S. (1984). The death of resistance. *Family Process, 23,* 11–17.

Dickson-Swift, V.A., James, E.L. & Kippen, S. (2005). The experience of living with a problem gambler: Spouses and partners speak out. *Journal of Gambling Issues, 13,* 1–22.

Doherty, W. (2002, November/December). Bad couples therapy: How to avoid doing it. *Psychotherapy Networker,* 26–33.

Fals-Stewart, W., O'Farrell, T.J., Birchler, G.R., Cordova, J. & Kelley, M.L. (2005). Behavioral couples therapy for alcoholism and drug abuse: Where we've been, where we are, and where we're going. *Journal of Cognitive Psychotherapy, 19,* 229–246.

Friedlander, M.L., Escudero, V. & Heatherington, L. (2006). *Therapeutic Alliances in Couple and Family Therapy: An Empirically Informed Guide to Practice.* Washington, DC: American Psychological Association.

Garrett, J., Landau-Stanton, J., Stanton, M.D., Stellato-Kabat, J. & Stellato-Kabat, D. (1997). ARISE: A method for engaging reluctant alcohol- and drug-dependent individuals in treatment. *Journal of Substance Abuse Treatment, 13* (5), 1–14.

Hodgins, D.C., Shead, N.W. & Makarchuk, K. (2007). Relationship satisfaction and psychological distress among concerned significant others of pathological gamblers. *Journal of Nervous and Mental Disease, 195*, 65–71.

Ingle, P., Marotta, J., McMillan, G. & Wisdom, J. (2008). Significant others and gambling treatment outcomes. *Journal of Gambling Studies, 24*, 381–392.

Korman, L., Collins, J., Dutton, D., Dhayananthan, B., Littman-Sharp, N. & Skinner, W. (2008). Problem gambling and intimate partner violence. *Journal of Gambling Studies, 24*, 13–23.

Lam, W.K.K., O'Farrell, T.J. & Bircher, G.R. (2011). Family therapy techniques for substance abuse treatment. In S.T. Walters & F. Rotgers (Eds.), *Treating Substance Abuse: Theory and Technique* (3rd ed., pp. 256–280). New York: Guilford Press.

Landau, J., Stanton, M.B., Brinkman-Sull, D., Ikle, D., McCormick, D., Garrett, J., et al. (2004). Outcomes with the ARISE approach to engaging reluctant drug- and alcohol-dependent individuals in treatment. *American Journal of Drug and Alcohol Treatment, 30*, 711–748.

Levine, I.S. & Ligenza, L.R. (2002). In their own voices: Families in crisis—A focus group study of families of persons with serious mental illness. *Journal of Psychiatric Practice, 8*, 344–353.

Liddle, H.A, Rodriquez, R.A., Dakof, G.A., Kanzki, E. & Marvel, F.A. (2005). Multidimensional family therapy: A science-based treatment for adolescent drug abuse. In J.L. Lebow (Ed.), *Handbook of Clinical Family Therapy* (pp. 128–163). Hoboken, NJ: Wiley.

Magill, M., Mastroleo, N.R., Apodaca, T.R., Barnett, N.P., Colby, S.M. & Monti, P.M. (2010). Motivational interviewing with significant others: Impact on treatment process and patient satisfaction and engagement. *Journal of Substance Abuse Treatment, 39*, 391–398.

McCrady, B.S., Ladd, B.O. & Hallgren, K.A. (2011). Theoretical bases of family approaches to substance abuse treatment. In S.T. Walters & F. Rotgers (Eds.), *Treating Substance Abuse: Theory and Technique* (3rd ed., pp. 224–255). New York: Guilford Press.

Meyers, R.J. & Wolfe, B.L. (2004). *Get Your Loved One Sober: Alternatives to Nagging, Pleading and Threatening*. Centre City, MN: Hazelden.

Miller, W.R., Forcehimes, A.A. & Zweben, A. (2011). *Treating Addiction: A Guide for Professionals*. New York: Guildford Press.

Mueser, K.T. (2002). A family intervention program for dual disorders. *Community Mental Health Journal, 38*, 253–270.

Murray-Swank, A.B. & Dixon, L. (2004). Family psychoeducation as an evidenced-based practice. *CNS Spectrums, 9*, 905–912.

O'Farrell, T.J. & Fals-Stewart, W. (2002). Behavioral couple and family therapy with substance abusing patients. *Current Psychiatry Reports, 4,* 371–376.

O'Grady, C.P. (2005). The impact of concurrent disorders on the family. In W.J.W. Skinner (Ed.), *Treating Concurrent Disorders: A Guide for Counsellors* (pp. 311–327). Toronto: Centre for Addiction and Mental Health.

O'Grady, C.P. & Skinner, W.J. (2007a). *A Family Guide to Concurrent Disorders.* Toronto: Centre for Addiction and Mental Health.

O'Grady, C.P. & Skinner, W.J.W. (2007b). *Partnering with Families Affected by Concurrent Disorders: Facilitator's Guide.* Toronto: Centre for Addiction and Mental Health.

O'Grady, C.P. & Skinner, W.J. (2012). Journey as destination: A recovery model for families affected by concurrent disorders. *Qualitative Health Research, 22,* 1047–1062.

O'Grady, C.P., Skinner, W.J. & Cunningham, J. (2010). A mixed method pilot study of a family concurrent disorders internet-based support / educational group. Manuscript in preparation.

Orford, J. & Velleman, R. (2002). Families and alcohol problems. In Alcohol Research Forum (Ed.), *100% Proof: Research for Action on Alcohol* (pp. 106–110). London, United Kingdom: Alcohol Concern.

Orford, J., Velleman, R., Copello, A., Templeton, L. & Ibanga, A. (2010). The experiences of affected family members: A summary of two decades of qualitative research. *Drugs: Education, Prevention, and Policy, 17* (Suppl. 1), 44–62.

Pinsof, W.M., Goldsmith, J.Z. & Latta, T.A. (2012). Information technology and feedback research can bridge the scientist-practitioner gap: A couple therapy example. *Couple and Family Psychology: Research and Practice, 4,* 253–273.

Rasinski, K.A., Woll, P. & Cooke, A. (2005). Stigma and substance use disorders. In P.W. Corrigan (Ed.), *On the Stigma of Mental Illness: Practical Strategies for Research and Social Change* (pp. 219–236). Washington, DC: American Psychological Association.

Smith, J.E. & Meyers, R.J. (2004). *Motivating Substance Abusers to Enter Treatment: Working with Family Members.* New York: Guilford Press.

Solomon, P., Draine, J., Mannion, E. & Meisel, M. (1997). Effectiveness of two models of brief family education: Retention of gains by family members of adults with serious mental illness. *American Journal of Orthopsychiatry, 67,* 177–187.

Sprenkle, D.H., Davis, S.D. & Lebow, J. (2009). *Common Factors in Couple and Family Therapy.* New York: Guilford Press.

Stanton, M.D. (1997). The role of family and significant others in the engagement and retention of drug-dependent individuals. In L.S. Oken, J.D. Blaine & J.J. Boren. (Eds.), *Beyond the Therapeutic Alliance: Keeping the Drug-Dependent Individual in Treatment* (pp. 157–180). Rockville, MD: National Institutes of Health.

Velleman, R. (2000). The importance of the family. In D. Cooper (Ed.), *Alcohol Use* (pp. 63–74). Edinburgh, United Kingdom: Radcliffe Medical Press.

Velleman, R. (2006). The importance of family members in helping problem drinkers achieve their chosen goal. *Addiction Research & Theory, 14*, 73–85.

Velleman, R., Orford, J., Templeton, L., Copello, A., Patel, A., Moore, L. et al. (2011). 12-month follow-up after brief interventions in primary care for family members affected by the substance misuse problem of a close relative. *Addiction Research & Theory, 19*, 362–374.

Chapter 14

Mutual Help Groups

John Kelly, Keith Humphreys and Julie Yeterian

Leisha is a 48-year-old single woman who entered individual outpatient treatment complaining that her alcohol use was "getting out of control." She reported a long history of heavy use since her teen years and some experimentation with sedatives and amphetamines during college. At treatment intake, she met DSM criteria for an alcohol use disorder and had an Alcohol Use Disorders Identification Test (AUDIT) score of 23 (dependent range), a Leeds Dependence Questionnaire (LDQ) score of 5 (low dependence) and a Beck Depression Inventory (BDI-II) score of 7 (few depression symptoms). She denied any prior treatment for substance use or psychiatric problems, but was taking a low dose of fluoxetine prescribed by her primary care physician for "depression and anxiety." She was involved with a number of social activities, and her social network comprised many heavy drinkers. She had a professional job with a high level of responsibility.

At the outset of treatment, Leisha was deemed to be in the "contemplation" stage of change. Motivational enhancement therapy strategies were used to help her explore her ambivalence and mobilize intrinsic resources for change. Leisha brought up the topic of Alcoholics Anonymous (AA) and asked whether the therapist thought it might help. The therapist discussed the research evidence on AA's potential benefits, including the fact that women tend to benefit as much as men and become significantly more involved. The therapist also described other potential benefits of AA, how it appears to help, and the nature and structure of meetings. Leisha expressed willingness to try two meetings during the first week of treatment. Through the online AA meeting list, two meetings were identified (including one beginners' meeting) and the therapist gave Leisha the name of a woman who was willing to serve as an AA contact and meet her at her first meeting near home.

Leisha attended the two meetings, reporting after that the personal connection helped her feel more comfortable and facilitated introductions to other members. Despite her ambivalence about quitting alcohol completely, she reported feeling "a boost" from meetings and liked many of the people she met there. Over the ensuing weeks, further attendance and involvement was encouraged and monitored in treatment. Leisha kept a diary of her reactions to her attendance. She "didn't care for" some meetings, so her therapist encouraged her to ask her AA contact to suggest meetings she might enjoy more. Leisha began to socialize a little with AA members after meetings. She continued to attend meetings, and while AA encouraged complete abstinence from alcohol and all other psychoactive substances, she continued to drink. However, her pattern of alcohol use did change, with substantial decreases in volume and intensity and a 43 per cent increase in abstinent days. Before finishing outpatient treatment, Leisha asked her AA contact to serve as her sponsor and was in daily phone contact with her.

Peer-led mutual help organizations for people with substance use disorders, such as Alcoholics Anonymous (AA), Women for Sobriety (WFS) and SMART Recovery, have grown in size and number over the past 75 years (Humphreys, 2004; Kelly & Yeterian, 2008a; White & Kurtz, 2005). Mutual help groups (sometimes referred to as self-help groups or mutual aid groups) are the most frequently sought source of help for substance-related problems in the United States (Substance Abuse and Mental Health Services Administration [SAMHSA], 2010). Clinical practice guidelines of the American Psychiatric Association and the Department of Veterans Affairs recommend referral to these groups. The widespread availability of mutual help groups in most communities, as well as flexible access to group members by phone, e-mail and texting, makes these resources well suited to addressing the chronic relapse risks associated with substance use problems (Hser & Anglin, 2011; Humphreys & Tucker, 2002).

Literature reviews identify strong evidence for the effectiveness of AA and encouraging evidence for the benefits of Al-Anon (for family members) and Narcotics Anonymous (for any drug, including alcohol). There has been very little research on 12-step alternatives, but the evidence that does exist suggests a positive relationship between participation in these groups and improved outcomes (Atkins & Hawdon, 2007). Many (though not all) of the mechanisms and types of change experienced by mutual help group members parallel those mobilized by professional treatments (Kelly et al., 2009). In addition, several recent studies testing professionally delivered interventions designed to increase client engagement with mutual help groups (i.e., 12-step facilitation [TSF]) indicate that clinicians who take an active role in facilitating client involvement can increase clients' chances for recovery (e.g., Kaskutas et al., 2009; Project MATCH Research Group, 1997; Walitzer et al., 2009). This chapter provides counsellors with background information, research evidence and clinical strategies related to helping clients make use of these empirically supported community resources.

Mutual help groups are usually formed and led by people with a common experience or problem who share their experiences and support with one another. Table 14-1 lists the six types of mutual help groups discussed in this chapter: AA and related 12-step organizations, Moderation Management (MM), Self Management and Recovery Training (SMART Recovery), Secular Organizations for Sobriety (SOS), LifeRing and WFS. We devote the most attention to AA because it is the oldest, largest and most researched mutual help organization.

TABLE 14-1

Descriptions of Mutual Help Organizations

NAME AND WEBSITE	TARGET PROBLEM	NUMBER OF GROUPS IN U.S. AND CANADA	THEORETICAL ORIENTATION	THERAPEUTIC GOAL(S)	KEY INTERVENTIONS
Alcoholics Anonymous (AA) www.aa.org	Drinking	56,000 groups in U.S. 5,800 groups in Canada Online meetings	12-step	Abstinence	Belief in higher power of individual's own choosing Sponsorship Working the steps Service to others and the group
Narcotics Anonymous (NA) www.na.org	Any drug, including alcohol	15,000 groups in U.S. 1,000 groups in Canada Online meetings			
Cocaine Anonymous (CA) www.ca.org	Cocaine/ crack	2,000 groups in U.S. 150 groups in Canada Online meetings			
Methadone Anonymous (MA) www.methadonesupport. org	Opiates	100 groups in U.S. 5 groups in Canada Online meetings			
Moderation Management (MM) www.moderation.org	Problem drinking (not dependence)	Mostly online meetings 25 groups in U.S. No groups in Canada	Cognitive-behavioural	Moderate drinking, harm reduction	30 days of abstinence Monitoring and limiting alcohol intake Awareness of triggers

NAME AND WEBSITE	TARGET PROBLEM	NUMBER OF GROUPS IN U.S. AND CANADA	THEORETICAL ORIENTATION	THERAPEUTIC GOAL(S)	KEY INTERVENTIONS
Self Management and Recovery Training (SMART Recovery) www.smartrecovery.org	All addictive behaviours	600 groups in U.S. 25 groups in Canada Online meetings	Cognitive-behavioural	Abstinence ommended, moderate use acknowledged as a possibility	Enhancing and maintaining motivation Learning to cope with urges Managing thoughts, feelings and actions Balancing short- and long-term needs
Secular Organizations for Sobriety, a.k.a. Save Ourselves (SOS) www.sossobriety.org	Alcohol and/or other drugs	115 groups in U.S. 2 groups in Canada Online meetings	Humanistic/ existential	Abstinence	Self-empowerment Specific interventions determined by individual
LifeRing http://lifering.org	Alcohol and/or other drugs	140 groups in U.S. 13 groups in Canada Online meetings	None	Abstinence	Positive reinforcement from the group Specific interventions determined by individual
Women for Sobriety (WFS) womenforsobriety.org	Alcohol	100 groups in U.S. and Canada Online meetings	Cognitive	Abstinence	13 affirmations Positive thinking Relaxation, diet, exercise Approval and encouragement from group

Alcoholics Anonymous

AA is the most widespread and well-known mutual help organization for people with substance use problems. It is estimated to have two to six million members worldwide, about half of whom live in Canada and the United States (AA, 2008; Humphreys, 2004). The 12 steps of the AA program (see Table 14-2) lead people through a series of cognitive and behavioural exercises to promote a "spiritual awakening" or "psychic change," which is AA's chief purported mechanism of recovery from alcohol addiction. These changes occur within the rich social context of the AA fellowship. In fact, research suggests that AA's ability to facilitate and mobilize social network changes is one of its main mechanisms of action (Kelly et al., 2012).

Meetings

Depending on the size of the community, the number of meetings ranges from one to many hundreds. Locations include rented rooms in church basements, hospitals and recreation centres. Phone numbers for local AA offices can be found with a quick web search or in the telephone book and can direct people to the nearest and most appropriate meeting. Like all the other mutual help organizations discussed in this chapter, AA also has a significant Internet presence that includes online meetings.

Typical format

Meetings typically last between 60 and 90 minutes and are highly varied in format and content. Some begin with a moment of silence followed by readings from AA literature, such as from the fellowship's main text, *Alcoholics Anonymous*, more commonly referred to as the "Big Book" (AA, 2001). There may also be a short prayer at the beginning of the meeting (e.g., the Serenity Prayer: "God grant me the serenity to accept the things I cannot change, the courage to change the things I can, and the wisdom to know the difference"). Meetings almost always involve some type of oral account of members' life experiences. Chips or tokens are sometimes awarded to people who have reached abstinence milestones (e.g., 30 days, one year), which some members carry with them as a recovery reminder. Because AA has a tradition of being fully self-supporting and declining outside financial contributions, a voluntary collection is taken. The main portion of the meeting focuses on a recovery topic, an AA reading or a speaker's story, which may be followed by open discussion. Meetings typically close with a prayer for those who wish to recite it.

Types of meetings

Larger communities often have AA meetings serving particular subgroups, such as women, youth and gay men or lesbians. Some offer meetings in languages other than English or French. AA meetings also vary in the level of desired anonymity ("open" vs. "closed" meetings) and format ("speaker-discussion" or "speaker only" vs. "literature-focused" meetings).

Only members or potential members may attend AA's closed meetings. Because these meetings are not accessible to the general public, participants may feel more comfortable attending and disclosing information about themselves. In contrast, anyone is welcome to attend open meetings. Family members, friends, health care professionals and students may attend to provide support or to learn more about AA.

A common type of AA meeting format is the "speaker-discussion" meeting, in which a member recounts his or her story of addiction and recovery, often including how he or she works the 12 steps in daily life. The presentation is followed by open discussion. In contrast, in a "speaker" meeting, one or several people speak at length about their recovery experiences without any discussion by other members. Recordings of speaker meetings from various 12-step organizations can be downloaded for free online.[1] Counsellors may find these recordings useful for familiarizing themselves with 12-step stories, as well as 12-step principles and practices.

Other meetings focus on AA literature such as *Living Sober* (AA, 1998), *Twelve Steps and Twelve Traditions* (AA, 1952) or the "Big Book" (AA, 2001). In these meetings, a step or chapter is read and discussed in relation to members' life experiences. These are most often closed meetings.

Guiding Principles

As an organization, AA adheres to "12 traditions," or guiding principles, which resulted from the early experiences of AA groups (AA, 1952). For example, early groups had lists of criteria for membership eligibility. This was eventually whittled down to a single requirement: "a desire to stop drinking." However, this requirement is not monitored in any way, and many people who attend may be unsure initially about stopping drinking or other drug use, or determining whether they are "alcoholic." All groups are autonomous and self-supporting financially. The collections taken at meetings pay for rent, refreshments and celebrations of abstinence, as well as maintaining the office and phones locally, regionally and internationally. Early in AA history, the organization decided not to accept contributions from people who are not AA members and to limit the yearly contributions of individual members. It was believed that too much money or property ownership (AA does not own any property) could give rise to internal disputes that would distract the organization from its primary purpose of helping others achieve sobriety (AA, 1952).

How Does AA Work?

From AA's perspective, members achieve recovery through a combination of factors, including sponsorship, working the 12 steps, belief in a "higher power" and service. Research has revealed that AA facilitates recovery through multiple mechanisms, many of which are also activated by formal treatment (Kelly et al., 2009). Most consistently

---

1 Recordings of speaker meetings from various 12-step organizations can be downloaded for free at http://xa-speakers.org.

and strongly, AA appears to work by mobilizing changes in members' social networks, for example, decreasing pro-drinking social ties and increasing pro-abstinence social ties (Bond et al., 2003; Humphreys et al., 1999; Kelly, Stout, Magill, Tonigan & Pagano, 2011). Recent empirical research also reveals that AA enhances abstinence self-efficacy, decreases negative affect, enhances psychological well-being and increases spirituality (Kelly et al., 2009; Kelly et al., 2012).

Among people with more severe alcohol problems, AA also appears to work by enhancing spiritual/religious practices, reducing depression and increasing people's confidence in their ability to cope with negative affect (Kelly et al., 2012; Kelly, Stout, Magill & Tonigan, 2011; Kelly, Stout, Magill, Tonigan & Pagano, 2011; Morgenstern et al., 1997; Robinson et al., 2011; Zemore, 2007). It is likely that AA works differently for different people, as their needs vary greatly depending on life circumstances, substance use history and social supports.

Sponsorship

Sponsors are mentors who, by virtue of well-established abstinence and adjustment to sobriety, serve as models and provide help to those they sponsor. They share how they use the tools of the program to help them cope effectively without drinking. The relationship is one of trust and acceptance, which develops over time.

Newcomers are encouraged to seek out an established member with whom they believe they could feel comfortable and whose sober lifestyle they admire. Newcomers then ask the person to serve as a sponsor. AA recommends that the sponsor and the sponsored person be of the same sex to avoid potential romantic complications (AA, 1994). For people who are gay or lesbian, this may mean someone of the opposite sex.

Sponsored people who have abstained from alcohol for at least several months and have worked the 12 steps are often encouraged to become sponsors themselves. Research has shown that both having a sponsor during early recovery (Subbaraman et al., 2011; Tonigan & Rice, 2010) and serving as a sponsor (Crape et al., 2002; Cross et al., 1990) are strongly associated with abstinence.

Working the 12 steps

AA's 12 steps are suggested as a means to achieve both abstinence and sobriety, characterized by subjective well-being, spiritual growth, better interpersonal relationships and improved quality of life (AA, 2001). Only the first step mentions alcohol, indicating that attaining abstinence is only the initial goal of AA membership. The steps are actually 12 statements describing the sequential process of how AA's first 100 members achieved sobriety. Table 14-2 lists the 12 steps, as they are stated in the 12-step literature, followed by our interpretations of the broader themes on which each step is based, as well as the therapeutic outcomes that should result from successfully completing each step. Completion of all the steps is the suggested (though not mandated) path to sobriety.

TABLE 14-2

Interpretation and Potential Therapeutic Outcome of AA's 12-step Process

STEP	THEME	MEANING	THERAPEUTIC OUTCOME
1. We admitted we were powerless over alcohol—that our lives had become unmanageable.	Surrender	Acknowledgment of repeated failed attempts to stop alcohol use and of the causal connection between alcohol use and presenting problems.	Psychological relief; liberation
2. Came to believe that a power greater than ourselves could restore us to sanity.	Open-mindedness	Recovery is possible and attending AA meetings can lead to changes that will facilitate recovery.	Instillation of hope
3. Made a decision to turn our will and our lives over to the care of God, *as we understood him.*	Willingness	Make a decision to trust the AA process and begin working through the rest of the steps.	Self-efficacy
4. Made a searching and fearless moral inventory of ourselves.	Self-assessment and appraisal	Uncovering festering sources of guilt, shame and anger facilitates insight into areas of dissatisfaction and of potential relapse risk.	Insight
5. Admitted to God, to ourselves and to another human being the exact nature of our wrongs.	Self-forgiveness	Discussing step 4, self-assessment, with another human being lessens guilt and shame and promotes a more balanced and objective view of oneself.	Reduced shame and guilt

STEP	THEME	MEANING	THERAPEUTIC OUTCOME
6. Were entirely ready to have God remove all these defects of character.	Readiness to change	Recognizing that the problems uncovered during the self-assessment phase (steps 4 and 5) are clearly related to relapse risk and must be dealt with.	Cognitive consonance
7. Humbly asked God to remove our shortcomings.	Humility	Genuine willingness to be rid of the problematic attitudes and behaviours that have led, and may again lead, to drinking.	Cognitive consonance
8. Made a list of all people we had harmed and became willing to make amends to them all.	Taking responsibility and forgiving others	Genuine willingness to forgive personal harms caused by others and to take responsibility for the harms one has inflicted on others.	Peace of mind
9. Made direct amends to such people whenever possible except when to do so would injure them or others.	Restitution to others	Making direct amends to others, except when such contact would exacerbate the problem or create new difficulties.	Peace of mind, self-esteem
10. Continued to take personal inventory, and when we were wrong, promptly admitted it.	Emotional balance	Practising self-monitoring and self-appraisal on a daily basis and correcting any new problems quickly.	Affect self-regulation

STEP	THEME	MEANING	THERAPEUTIC OUTCOME
11. Sought through prayer and meditation to improve our conscious contact with God, as we understood him, praying only for knowledge of his will for us and the power to carry that out.	Connected-ness and emotional balance	Strengthening faith and spirituality by regular prayer and meditation, loosely defined.	Awareness, psychological well-being
12. Having had a spiritual awakening as the result of these steps, we tried to carry this message to alcoholics and to practise these principles in all our affairs.	Positive emotion, joyful living, helping others achieve recovery	Having experienced the cognitive, affective and behavioural changes as a function of completing the prior steps, it is now time to strengthen and maintain one's own recovery by helping other alcoholics.	Self-esteem and mastery

Source: Kelly, J.F. & McCrady, B.S. (2008). Twelve-step facilitation in non-specialty settings. *Recent Developments in Alcoholism*, *18*, 321–346. Adapted with permission.

Belief in a higher power

AA encourages members to develop a concept of a "higher power." What that higher power means to AA members varies widely. For some, their higher power represents a God of their religious background. For others, their AA group becomes their higher power, referred to by some as "Group of Drunks" ("GOD"). Others rely simply on "Good Orderly Direction" as their higher power. AA includes many members in recovery who are atheists or agnostics (Tonigan et al., 2002) and indeed in some locations, such as Sweden, such members are a majority (see Mäkelä et al., 1996). Half of AA's original membership was in this category (AA, 2001). Although less religiously involved people may be more likely to drop out of 12-step groups (Kelly & Moos, 2003), those who continue appear to benefit as much as those who are more religious (Winzelberg & Humphreys, 1999).

While the concept of a higher power may be off-putting to some potential AA members, others may find that ceasing efforts to control all aspects of their lives paradoxically increases their sense of control over alcohol and their lives, and provides a greater sense of freedom.

Service

Service work can take many forms—from helping to set up meetings, to making coffee, being responsible for literature or looking after the group's finances. It can also involve serving as the secretary of a meeting or being the group representative at regional events. These activities may increase self-esteem and confidence among members, and enhance social integration, as well as decreasing self-centredness, which AA considers a barrier to attaining sobriety. Service is seen as an essential part of recovery, in that it helps members become more responsible for their personal success, as well as that of the fellowship. Recent research has linked AA-related helping to improved substance use outcomes (see Pagano et al., 2011, for a review).

Resistance to AA

Counsellors or clients may object to some aspects of the AA program. They may find the spiritual approach unfamiliar, too religious or not religious enough. Some people may find it objectionable to attend meetings with "alcoholics." They may not want to be in church basements or in groups. They may find meetings monotonous, boring or ritualistic. They may express fears of becoming dependent on AA and their higher power. They may still want to drink alcohol or use other drugs. They may fear being told they must stop taking prescribed medication (e.g., antidepressants). Some people are unwilling to believe they are "powerless over alcohol." Some of these objections are specific to AA, while others represent a client's general reluctance to engage in any form of mutual help or continuing care. Importantly, there are now evidence-based strategies that clinicians can use to help clients consider and overcome many of these barriers. (For a review of these strategies, see Kelly & Yeterian, 2011.)

Other 12-Step Organizations

Other 12-step organizations have been formed based on the AA model, including Narcotics Anonymous (NA), Cocaine Anonymous (CA) and Methadone Anonymous (MA) (see Table 14-1). These organizations are less widespread than AA. They are designed to serve the different needs of their members. For example, NA focuses on recovery from any drug addiction, including alcohol. Methadone Anonymous provides support to people who are using methadone to aid their recovery and who may feel unwelcome in traditional 12-step meetings that focus on total abstinence from all substances (Gilman et al., 2001).

Many members of these groups also attend AA, where they may find people who have been abstinent longer, giving them the hope and example that newcomers seek, while also receiving help for concurrent alcohol use. More often than not, CA and NA members also have alcohol use problems. Although a person's primary drug of choice may not exactly match that of a specific 12-step fellowship, the person can still benefit from attending (Weiss et al., 2000).

Moderation Management

Moderation Management (MM) is the only mutual help organization that targets people whose drinking problems have never reached the point of dependence (Kishline, 1994). MM is also the only mutual help group that does not advocate complete abstinence from alcohol (Kelly & Yeterian, 2008a). Instead, its main aim is to help people who have drinking problems but are not addicted to return to moderate levels of consumption. MM's current North American membership is not precisely known, but is estimated to be between 3,000 and 4,000 people (J. Mergens, personal communication, April 19, 2012), with most of the mutual support being provided through online meetings (Kelly & Yeterian, 2008a; Lembke & Humphreys, 2012). Survey research indicates that the typical MM member is Caucasian, well educated and employed; most members show no signs of physical dependence on alcohol and do not use illicit drugs (Humphreys & Klaw, 2001).

MM encourages people who are concerned about their drinking to take action to change as soon as possible, before drinking problems become severe (MM, 1996). It advocates a 30-day period of complete abstinence, followed by a carefully self-monitored return to drinking. MM also encourages abstinence as a "fall-back if moderation doesn't work" (MM, n.d., p. 4). For guidance through the change process, MM provides a nine-step program, which provides information about alcohol, moderate drinking guidelines and limits, drink-monitoring exercises, goal-setting techniques and self-management strategies.

SMART Recovery

Self Management and Recovery Training (SMART Recovery) is an outgrowth of another mutual help organization, Rational Recovery. SMART Recovery has more than 600 groups throughout the world, most of them in the United States (Allwood & White, 2011). Lately, it has expanded particularly dramatically in the United Kingdom, where dozens of groups have formed in recent years. SMART Recovery is based on a cognitive-behavioural model and is centred on four main themes:
1.   enhancing and maintaining motivation to abstain
2.   coping with urges

3. managing thoughts, feelings and behaviour
4. balancing momentary and enduring satisfactions.

When success is achieved, graduates may choose to leave or stay with their group to help others (SMART Recovery, 1996).

Meetings

Ten to 12 people usually attend meetings, which are led by trained facilitators who are not required to be in recovery themselves and who may be professionals (Horvath & Yeterian, 2012). Each group has a professional therapist advisor who may or may not attend every meeting. This person is available to the facilitator for guidance in group functioning, to teach a new strategy or to be available if a member is in trouble. With greater professional involvement than most other mutual help groups, SMART Recovery might be considered a somewhat different form of help than other purely non-professional groups.

Groups meet once or twice weekly with the aim of helping members gain more control over their thinking, emotions and behaviour, and develop effective relapse-prevention skills. Meetings last 90 minutes and begin with a brief introduction, a 10- to 20-minute check-in and a brief agenda-setting period. The next 40 to 50 minutes are designated as "working time," when members may talk about their experiences with recovery and relapse, discuss strategies for avoiding relapse and analyze their thinking (Bishop, 1995). Social skills training and role-playing may be part of the program. Cross-talk is encouraged, with members confronting others when they want them to recognize the irrationality of their thinking and behaviour. At the end of the meeting, a collection is taken to defray costs, followed by a 15-minute check-out period. Members may exchange phone numbers to keep in touch between meetings.

Resistance to SMART Recovery

Bishop (1995) reports that, because of the emphasis on rationality and the absence of a spiritual focus, many people find SMART Recovery helpful, whereas others find the confrontation upsetting. Some people attend both AA and SMART Recovery. Others who have tried SMART Recovery find it "as unsatisfactory as AA," which may reflect a generalized aversion to groups or to stopping alcohol consumption (Bishop, 1995).

Secular Organizations for Sobriety

Secular Organizations for Sobriety (SOS), also known as "Save Our Selves," "a self-empowerment approach to sobriety," is a network of groups with the sole aim of helping people maintain their recovery from alcohol problems. Precise estimates of SOS's current membership and group prevalence are difficult to find, but the network's website lists approximately 120 meetings in the United States and Canada, along with several online support forums and chat rooms. SOS is an alternative for people who are uncomfortable with the spiritual content of 12-step programs. It credits the individual with achieving and maintaining abstinence and encourages using the scientific method to understand alcohol problems. Like AA, SOS expresses no opinion on external social or political matters.

Meetings

SOS groups have a maximum of 20 people and leadership is shared. The meeting structure and format are established by the group. Members are expected to choose non-destructive, rational and sober approaches to living the "good life" (SOS, 1996). Abstinence anniversaries are acknowledged. New members are encouraged to attend meetings at least once a week for the first six months, followed by "booster" meetings as needed. Pamphlets and books are available at meetings, and the SOS National Clearinghouse publishes a quarterly newsletter.

LifeRing

Formed in 1999, LifeRing is one of the newest mutual help groups, with about 140 groups in four countries and 16 online forums and e-mail lists. More than half of the North American LifeRing groups are in northern California. Like SOS, LifeRing takes a secular approach to addiction recovery and encourages participants to figure out their own path to recovery from alcohol and other drugs. LifeRing emphasizes positive reinforcement from the group and personal responsibility for sobriety as key mechanisms of change. Its "3-S" philosophy is:
1. sobriety (i.e., "We do not drink or use, no matter what")
2. secularity (i.e., members' religious beliefs, or lack thereof, remain private and are not related to program or meeting content)
3. self-help (i.e., recovery depends on the motivation and effort of the individual, rather than a particular theoretical model or set of steps). (White & Nicolaus, 2005)

Meetings

LifeRing groups typically meet for one hour per week. Meetings are led by "convenors," or lay people in recovery. Format varies, but usually includes a discussion of each participant's past week and that person's planning for sobriety in the coming week. Discussing distant substance use histories is discouraged. In contrast to AA and other 12-step fellowships, non-confrontational "cross-talk" (talking directly to and receiving feedback from other members during the meeting) is encouraged and members are encouraged to be in touch with one another between meetings. Group members provide positive reinforcement to one another during meetings.

Women for Sobriety

Women for Sobriety (WFS) was established in 1975 by Jean Kirkpatrick, a woman in recovery, who found that AA did not meet all her needs. She believed that women need their own groups, free from men and role expectations, in which to share their experiences. Today, WFS has about 100 active face-to-face groups in the United States and Canada, with additional groups in Australia, Finland, Iceland and other countries (Fenner & Gifford, 2012). This represents a slight decline in size since WFS was last surveyed in the early 1990s (Kaskutas, 1992).

The WFS program "is an affirmation of the value and worth of each woman," as reflected in its 13 statements of acceptance (see Table 14-3). WFS members believe that a person's dependence on alcohol, acquired to overcome stress, loneliness and emotional deprivation, must be resolved through abstinence and personal change. Through the program, women learn to see themselves as able to overcome their drinking and other problems. Changes are reinforced by the group.

TABLE 14-3
Women for Sobriety 13 Statements of Acceptance

1. I have a life-threatening problem that once had me.
2. Negative thoughts destroy only myself.
3. Happiness is a habit I will develop.
4. Problems bother me only to the degree I permit them to.
5. I am what I think.
6. Life can be ordinary or it can be great.
7. Love can change the course of my world.
8. The fundamental object of life is emotional and spiritual growth.
9. The past is gone forever.
10. All love given returns.
11. Enthusiasm is my daily exercise.
12. I am a competent woman and have much to give life.
13. I am responsible for myself and for my actions.

Source: Women for Sobriety. (n.d.). Reprinted with permission from www.womenforsobriety.org/wfs_program.html.

Meetings

Eight to 12 women usually attend meetings. The discussion or "conversation" is led by one of the members (Kirkpatrick, 1978). Most groups meet once a week. Membership is open to any woman who has a problem with alcohol and wants to stop drinking. Unlike in AA, a recital of a woman's drinking history is not required, since there are no open speaker meetings.

As with other mutual help organizations, in the absence of a local WFS group, women can seek support through the online WFS recovery community. Literature, workbooks, DVDs and audio recordings are also available from the WFS website.

Research on Mutual Help Groups

As mentioned, most research on mutual help groups has been conducted on AA and similar 12-step programs because of their sheer size and influence. Although there is a lack of empirical research on non–12-step mutual help organizations, anecdotal reports and the theory of group dynamics suggest they may hold similar promise (Yalom & Leszcz, 2005). The following section examines the effectiveness of mutual help groups in "real world situations"; their cost-effectiveness; and their efficacy, as determined in randomized controlled trials of TSF interventions.

Effectiveness

Hundreds of empirical studies on AA have been summarized in several meta-analyses (Emrick et al, 1993; Kownacki & Shadish, 1999; Tonigan et al., 1996), as well as in one Cochrane review (Ferri et al., 2006). These reviews have found that AA is associated with a moderate effect on substance use that is on par with professional treatment, unless the outcome of interest is abstinence, in which case AA tends to outperform professional ambulatory treatments alone. The effect holds even when accounting for other factors related to improved outcomes, such as motivation (McKellar et al., 2003). Most of the existing research is based on treated samples (i.e., individuals who had received or were receiving professional treatment). Importantly, it appears that the combination of AA plus professional treatment is more potent than either one alone (Fiorentine & Hillhouse, 2000), and that people who try to change their substance use without any type of help tend to have the worst outcomes (Timko et al., 2000). For some people, however, participating in a mutual help group alone is effective (McKellar et al., 2003; Moos & Moos, 2006; Timko et al., 2000).

Cost-Effectiveness

Involvement in 12-step organizations can reduce the need for more costly professional treatments while simultaneously improving outcomes. Humphreys and Moos
(1996) found that people who attended only AA had overall treatment costs that were
substantially lower than those of people who attended outpatient treatment, at no detriment to their substance use outcomes and despite experiencing more drinking-related
consequences at the beginning of the study. Similarly, a study of more than 1,700
substance-dependent males found that those who were treated in 12-step programs
participated in community-based 12-step meetings much more than those treated
under a cognitive-behavioural therapy (CBT) model, which translated into a two-year
savings of more than US\$7,000 per person, again without compromising abstinence
rates (Humphreys & Moos, 2001; 2007). In fact, those from 12-step treatments had one
third higher rates of abstinence than those who had received CBT, despite the similarity of groups at baseline. Empirical research supports the common sense notion that
participating in low-cost community resources can reduce the need for more expensive
professional treatments, thereby reducing treatment costs overall.

Efficacy

It would not be appropriate to study the efficacy of mutual help groups using randomized controlled trials (where participants would be randomly assigned to attend mutual
help groups or not), since real-world mutual help groups are attended voluntarily and do
not follow standardized procedures. However, efficacy trials have been conducted on professional interventions, namely TSF, that are designed to increase clients' involvement in
mutual help groups. Project MATCH (1993) has been the largest of these studies, with
1,726 male and female participants. In Project MATCH, TSF treatment was compared to
motivational enhancement therapy (MET) and CBT. Results revealed that TSF increased
12-step group attendance and was as effective as CBT and MET at reducing the quantity and frequency of alcohol use post-treatment, and at one- and three-year follow-ups.
Moreover, TSF was superior to CBT and MET at increasing rates of continuous abstinence (Tonigan et al., 2003).

Similar findings have been demonstrated in other randomized controlled trials
that use various forms of TSF. These studies consistently show that TSF interventions
produce substance use outcomes that are superior to control conditions (Kaskutas et
al., 2009; Litt et al., 2009; Timko et al., 2006; Walitzer et al., 2009). As a result of this
growing empirical support, TSF was recently recognized as a "well supported treatment"
by Division 12 of the American Psychological Association and was added to SAMHSA's
National Registry of Evidence-Based Practices and Programs in 2008.

Concerns with Specific Populations

Clients with Comorbid Psychiatric Disorders

Some counsellors express concern about whether substance-focused mutual aid groups are appropriate for people with comorbid substance use and mental health problems. The principal fear is that group members may persuade these clients to stop taking their psychotropic medication. Research in this area is scarce, but suggests that a small minority of substance-focused mutual help group members oppose medication use (Rychtarik et al., 2000; Tonigan & Kelly, 2004). Even so, many people with comorbid disorders may benefit from attending mutual help groups, so counsellors may wish to prepare them to cope with potential opposition to psychotropic or anti-dipsotropic medication (i.e., medication intended to help a person reduce or eliminate alcohol consumption), such as naltrexone. Furthermore, there is no evidence that 12-step members are any more skeptical of psychotropic medication than anyone else; they may even be less so.

How much people with comorbid problems attend and benefit from mutual help groups may depend on the particular combination of problems. For example, people with substance use problems and posttraumatic stress disorder appear to participate in and benefit from 12-step groups as much as people with substance use problems alone (Ouimette et al., 2001). In contrast, people with substance dependence and psychotic disorders such as schizophrenia may have difficulty fitting in at meetings and may not benefit as much as others (Bogenschutz & Akin, 2000). The same may be true with severe major depressive disorder (Kelly et al., 2003). Thus, different subgroups will vary in how well they fit into groups and how much benefit they receive. Newer mutual help organizations such as Double Trouble in Recovery and Dual Recovery Anonymous may be a better fit for clients with concurrent disorders (for a review, see Kelly & Yeterian, 2008b).[2] These groups focus on both substance use and mental health problems, and so may be a better fit for clients with concurrent disorders; for example, they explicitly encourage members to take their medication.

Youth

Some counsellors who work with adolescents and young adults are concerned that most mutual help groups are geared toward an older demographic (i.e., people in their 40s). Compared to adults, young people tend to have less severe addictions, which may make abstinence-focused groups less appealing to them. Young people also face different life-stage challenges and are less likely to have marital or employment concerns. Nevertheless, adolescents and young adults have been shown to attend and benefit from mutual help groups (Alford et al., 1991; Chi et al., 2009; Kelly et al., 2002; Kelly et al.,

---

2   For more information about Double Trouble in Recovery, visit www.doubletroubleinrecovery.org. For more information about Dual Recovery Anonymous, visit http://draonline.org.

2008; Kelly, Dow et al., 2010; Kennedy & Minami, 1993). Youth may benefit more if they attend meetings at which others of their age are present (Kelly et al., 2005). Given the potential benefit of mutual aid groups, counsellors should direct youth to 12-step young people's meetings whenever possible.

Conclusion

Various substance-focused mutual help organizations exist and are growing in both size and variety (Kelly & White, 2012). Current evidence suggests that people who attend 12-step groups such as AA or NA have significantly better outcomes than people who do not attend these groups. Other non-12-step mutual help groups may confer similar benefits, but await more formal investigation. Discussing alternatives with clients and facilitating their exposure to other options may increase the likelihood that clients will engage in and benefit from mutual help groups (Kelly & White, 2012). This involvement, in turn, significantly increases the chances that clients will initiate and sustain recovery, especially after counselling ends.

Practice Tips

Despite encouragement from their counsellors, many clients decide not to attend mutual help groups, or they drop out too quickly to realize benefits (Kelly & Moos, 2003; Tonigan et al., 2003). However, clinicians can affect the likelihood that their clients will become and stay involved in these groups, thus increasing their chances for sustained recovery. The following tips suggest how clinicians can facilitate mutual help group attendance.

- Recognize the validity and importance of mutual aid groups. Preconceived notions or occasional negative anecdotes can cloud the counsellor's views on mutual help groups. However, a large body of empirical research suggests that these groups can be as helpful as professional treatment. It is important to recognize the value of these free, long-term and easily accessible resources and to communicate their value to clients.
- Visit and become familiar with local mutual help groups. The descriptions in this chapter may be informative, but counsellors often feel more confident discussing mutual help groups with clients if they themselves have attended. Counsellors who are not themselves in recovery or seeking help for a substance use problem should attend meetings that are open to the public (designated as "O" in 12-step meeting lists). Becoming familiar with the formats, types and sizes of meetings can help counsellors assist their clients in making informed choices about which groups to attend.

- Make contacts and actively facilitate attendance. Keep in touch with former clients who attend mutual help groups and develop a list of people who volunteer to take a client to his or her first meeting. Be willing to put clients in contact with mutual aid group members through counselling sessions, as this can be very influential in a client's decision to attend (Sisson & Mallams, 1981; Timko et al., 2006).
- Ask clients to become involved in mutual help groups early in their therapy and follow up with them. This strategy allows the client to get used to the groups and discuss concerns before counselling ends. Some counsellors ask clients to keep a journal of their experiences at meetings for discussion in sessions. Counsellors should encourage clients to attend at least two or three meetings per week, as this has been associated with a decreased likelihood of relapse (Etheridge et al., 1999; Kelly et al., 2006; Kelly et al., 2008).
- Direct clients to suitable meetings and prepare them for what to expect. When recommending meetings to clients, it is best to have a sense of which groups may be a good fit. For example, if you are working with adolescents or young adults, suggest meetings where other young people may be present (e.g., young people's AA meetings). If you are working with clients with concurrent substance use and mental health problems, direct them to "dual recovery" meetings, meetings that are more "medication friendly" or meetings where other people with concurrent issues will be present to provide support. It is wise to discuss the potential barrier of "poor fit" at the outset of counselling, while emphasizing that clients should be persistent in seeking a group that is a good fit for them.
- Emphasize the diversity of meetings. The character, philosophy and membership of different organizations can vary, as can different group meetings within the same organization. Thus, it is important to tell clients that if they don't like the first meeting they attend, they should still try other meetings and not use this single experience to justify rejecting mutual group involvement altogether.

Resources

Publications

Humphreys, K. (2004). *Circles of Recovery: Self-Help Organizations for Addictions.* Cambridge, United Kingdom: Cambridge University Press.

Humphreys, K. & Moos, R.H. (2007). Encouraging post-treatment self-help group involvement to reduce demand for continuing care services: Two-year clinical and utilization outcomes. *Alcoholism: Clinical and Experimental Research, 31,* 64–68.

Kelly, J.F., Magill, M. & Stout, R.L. (2009). How do people recover from alcohol dependence? A systematic review of the research on mechanisms of behavior change in Alcoholics Anonymous. *Addiction Research and Theory, 17,* 236–259.

Kelly, J.F. & White, W. (2012). Broadening the base of addiction mutual-help organizations, *Journal of Groups in Addiction and Recovery, 7,* 82–101.

White, W. (2009). *Peer-Based Addiction Recovery Support: History, Theory, Practice, and Scientific Evaluation.* Chicago: Great Lakes Addiction Technology Transfer Center, and Philadelphia Department of Behavioral Health and Mental Retardation Services.

Internet

Faces & Voices Guide to Mutual Aid Resources
www.facesandvoicesofrecovery.org/resources/support/index.html

References

Alcoholics Anonymous (AA). (1952). *Twelve Steps and Twelve Traditions.* New York: Author.

Alcoholics Anonymous (AA). (1994). *Questions and Answers on Sponsorship.* New York: Author.

Alcoholics Anonymous (AA). (1998). *Living Sober: Some Methods AA Members Have Used for Not Drinking.* New York: Author.

Alcoholics Anonymous (AA). (2001). *Alcoholics Anonymous: The Story of How Thousands of Men and Women Have Recovered from Alcoholism* (4th ed.). New York: Author.

Alcoholics Anonymous (AA). (2008). *Alcoholics Anonymous 2007 Membership Survey.* New York: Author.

Alford, G.S., Koehler, R.A. & Leonard, J. (1991). Alcoholics Anonymous–Narcotics Anonymous model inpatient treatment of chemically dependent adolescents: A 2-year outcome study. *Journal of Studies on Alcohol, 52,* 118–126.

Allwood, S. & White, W. (2011). *A Chronology of SMART Recovery®.* Retrieved from www.williamwhitepapers.com/chronologies

Atkins, R.G. & Hawdon, J.E. (2007). Religiosity and participation in mutual-aid support groups for addiction. *Journal of Substance Abuse Treatment, 33,* 321–331.

Bishop, F.M. (1995). Rational-emotive behavior therapy and two self-help alternatives to the 12-step model. In A. Washton (Ed.), *Psychotherapy and Substance Abuse: A Practitioner's Handbook* (pp. 141–160). New York: Guilford Press.

Bogenschutz, M.P. & Akin, S.J. (2000). 12-step participation and attitudes toward 12-step meetings in dual diagnosis patients. *Alcoholism Treatment Quarterly, 18* (4), 31–45.

Bond J., Kaskutas, L.A. & Weisner, C. (2003). The persistent influence of social networks and Alcoholics Anonymous on abstinence. *Journal of Studies on Alcohol, 64,* 579–588.

Chi, F.W., Kaskutas, L.A., Sterling, S., Campbell, C.I. & Weisner, C. (2009). Twelve-step affiliation and 3-year substance use outcomes among adolescents: Social support and religious service attendance as potential mediators. *Addiction, 104,* 927–939.

Crape, B.L., Latkin, C.A., Laris, A.S. & Knowlton, A.R. (2002). The effects of sponsorship in 12-step treatment of injection drug users. *Drug and Alcohol Dependence, 65,* 291–301.

Cross, G.M., Morgan, C.W., Mooney, A.J., Martin, C.A. & Rafter, J.A. (1990). Alcoholism treatment: A ten-year follow-up study. *Alcoholism: Clinical and Experimental Research, 14,* 169–173.

Emrick, C.D., Tonigan, J.S., Montgomery, H. & Little, L. (1993). Alcoholics Anonymous: What is currently known? In B.S. McCrady & W.R. Miller (Eds.), *Research on Alcoholics Anonymous: Opportunities and Alternatives* (pp. 41–76). Piscataway, NJ: Rutgers Center of Alcohol Studies.

Etheridge, R.M., Craddock, S.G., Hubbard, R.L. & Rounds-Bryant, J.L. (1999). The relationship of counseling and self-help participation to patient outcomes in DATOS. *Drug and Alcohol Dependence, 57,* 99–112.

Fenner, R.M. & Gifford, M.H. (2012). Women for Sobriety: Adaptations over time—over 35 years of challenges, changes, and continuity. *Journal of Groups in Addiction and Recovery, 7,* 142–170.

Ferri, M., Amato, L. & Davoli, M. (2006). Alcoholics Anonymous and other 12-step programmes for alcohol dependence. *Cochrane Database of Systematic Reviews, 2006* (3). doi: 10.1002/14651858.CD005032.pub2

Fiorentine, R. & Hillhouse, M.P. (2000). Drug treatment and 12-step program participation: The additive effects of integrated recovery activities. *Journal of Substance Abuse Treatment, 18* (1), 65–74.

Gilman, S.M., Galanter, M. & Dermatis, H. (2001). Methadone Anonymous: A 12-step program for methadone maintained heroin addicts. *Substance Abuse, 22,* 247–257.

Horvath, A.T. & Yeterian, J.D. (2012). SMART Recovery: Self-empowering, science-based recovery support. *Journal of Groups in Addiction and Recovery, 7,* 102–117.

Hser, Y. & Anglin, M.D. (2011). Addiction treatment and recovery careers. In J.F. Kelly & W.L. White (Eds.), *Addiction Recovery Management: Theory, Research, and Practice* (pp. 9–29). New York: Humana Press.

Humphreys, K. (2004). *Circles of Recovery: Self-Help Organizations for Addictions.* Cambridge, United Kingdom: Cambridge University Press.

Humphreys, K. & Klaw, E. (2001). Can targeting non-dependent problem drinkers and providing internet-based services expand access to assistance for alcohol problems? A study of the Moderation Management mutual help/mutual help organization. *Journal of Studies on Alcohol, 62,* 528–532.

Humphreys, K., Mankowski, E., Moos, R.H. & Finney, J.W. (1999). Do enhanced friendship networks and active coping mediate the effect of self-help groups on substance use? *Annals of Behavioral Medicine, 21,* 54–60.

Humphreys, K. & Moos, R.H. (1996). Reduced substance-abuse–related health care costs among voluntary participants in Alcoholics Anonymous. *Psychiatric Services, 47,* 709–713.

Humphreys, K. & Moos, R.H. (2001). Can encouraging substance abuse patients to participate in self-help groups reduce demand for health care? A quasi-experimental study. *Alcoholism: Clinical and Experimental Research, 25,* 711–716.

Humphreys, K. & Moos, R.H. (2007). Encouraging post-treatment self-help group involvement to reduce demand for continuing care services: Two-year clinical and utilization outcomes. *Alcoholism: Clinical and Experimental Research, 31,* 64–68.

Humphreys, K. & Tucker, J. (2002). Towards more responsive and effective intervention systems for alcohol-related problems. *Addiction, 97,* 126–132.

Kaskutas, L.A. (1992). *An analysis of Women for Sobriety. Dissertation Abstracts International, 54* (06). (UMI No. 9330441).

Kaskutas, L.A., Subbaraman, M.S., Witbrodt, J. & Zemore, S.E. (2009). Effectiveness of making Alcoholics Anonymous easier: A group format 12-step facilitation approach. *Journal of Substance Abuse Treatment, 37,* 228–239.

Kelly, J.F., Brown, S.A., Abrantes, A., Kahler, C.W. & Myers, M.G. (2008). Social recovery model: An 8-year investigation of adolescent 12-step group involvement following inpatient treatment. *Alcoholism: Clinical and Experimental Research, 32,* 1468–1478.

Kelly, J.F., Dow, S.J., Yeterian, J.D. & Kahler, C. (2010). Can 12-step group participation strengthen and extend the benefits of adolescent addiction treatment? A prospective analysis. *Drug and Alcohol Dependence, 110* (1–2), 117–125.

Kelly, J.F., Hoeppner, B., Stout, R.L. & Pagano, M. (2012). Determining the relative importance of the mechanisms of behavior change within Alcoholics Anonymous: A multiple mediator model. *Addiction, 107,* 289–299. doi: 10.1111/j.1360-0443.2011.03593.x

Kelly, J.F., Magill, M. & Stout, R.L. (2009). How do people recover from alcohol dependence? A systematic review of the research on mechanisms of behavior change in Alcoholics Anonymous. *Addiction Research and Theory, 17,* 236–259.

Kelly, J.F., McKellar, J.D. & Moos, R.H. (2003). Major depression in patients with substance use disorders: Relationship to 12-step self-help involvement and substance use outcomes. *Addiction, 98,* 499–508.

Kelly, J.F. & Moos, R.H. (2003). Dropout from 12-step self-help groups: Prevalence, predictors and counteracting treatment influences. *Journal of Substance Abuse Treatment, 24*, 241–250.

Kelly, J.F., Myers, M.G. & Brown, S.A. (2002). Do adolescents affiliate with 12-step groups? A multivariate process model of effects. *Journal of Studies on Alcohol, 63*, 293–304.

Kelly, J.F., Myers, M.G. & Brown, S.A. (2005). The effects of age composition of 12-step groups on adolescent 12-step participation and substance use outcome. *Journal of Child & Adolescent Substance Abuse, 15* (1), 67–76.

Kelly, J.F., Stout, R.L., Magill, M. & Tonigan, J.S. (2011). The role of Alcoholics Anonymous in mobilizing adaptive social network changes: A prospective lagged mediational analysis. *Drug and Alcohol Dependence, 114* (2–3), 119–126.

Kelly, J.F., Stout, R.L., Magill, M., Tonigan, J.S. & Pagano, M.E. (2011). Spirituality in recovery: A lagged mediational analysis of Alcoholics Anonymous' principal theoretical mechanism of behavior change. *Alcoholism: Clinical and Experimental Research, 35*, 454–463.

Kelly, J.F., Stout, R., Zywiak, W. & Schneider, R. (2006). A 3-year study of addiction mutual-help group participation following intensive outpatient treatment. *Alcoholism: Clinical and Experimental Research, 30*, 1381–1392.

Kelly, J.F. & White, W. (2012). Broadening the base of addiction mutual-help organizations, *Journal of Groups in Addiction and Recovery, 7*, 82–101.

Kelly, J.F. & Yeterian, J.D. (2008a). Mutual-help groups. In W. O'Donohue & J.A. Cunningham (Eds.), *Evidence-Based Adjunctive Treatments* (pp. 61–105). New York: Elsevier.

Kelly, J.F. & Yeterian, J.D. (2008b). Mutual-help groups for dually diagnosed individuals: Rationale, description, and review of the evidence. *Journal of Groups in Addiction and Recovery, 3*, 217–242.

Kelly, J.F. & Yeterian, J.D. (2011). The role of mutual-help groups in extending the framework of treatment. *Alcohol Research & Health, 33*, 350–355.

Kennedy, B.P. & Minami, M. (1993). The Beech Hill Hospital/Outward Bound Adolescent Chemical Dependency Treatment Program. *Journal of Substance Abuse Treatment, 10*, 395–406.

Kirkpatrick, J. (1978). *Turnabout: Help for a New Life*. New York: Doubleday.

Kishline, A. (1994). *Moderate Drinking: The Moderation Management Guide for People Who Want to Reduce Their Drinking*. New York: Crown.

Kownacki, R.J. & Shadish, W.R. (1999). Does Alcoholics Anonymous work? The results from a meta-analysis of controlled experiments. *Substance Use & Misuse, 34*, 1897–1916.

Lembke, A. & Humphreys, K. (2012). Moderation Management: A mutual help organization for problem drinkers who are not alcohol dependent. *Journal of Groups in Addiction and Recovery, 7*, 130–141.

Litt, M.D., Kadden, R.M., Kabela-Cormier, E. & Petry, N.M. (2009). Changing network support for drinking: Network support project 2-year follow-up. *Journal of Consulting and Clinical Psychology, 77,* 229–242.

Mäkelä, K., Arminen, I., Bloomfield, K., Eisenbach-Stangl, I., Helmersson Bergmark, K., Mariolini, N. et al. (1996). *Alcoholics Anonymous as a Mutual Help Movement: A Study in Eight Societies.* Madison, WI: University of Wisconsin Press.

McKellar, J.D., Stewart, E. & Humphreys, K.N. (2003). Alcoholics Anonymous involvement and positive alcohol-related outcomes: Cause, consequence, or just a correlation? A prospective 2-year study of 2,319 alcohol-dependent men. *Journal of Consulting and Clinical Psychology, 71,* 302–308.

Moderation Management (MM). (1996). *Moderate Drinking.* Ann Arbor, MI: Author.

Moderation Management (MM). (n.d.). *Guide to Moderation Management Steps of Change.* Retrieved from www.moderation.org/about_mm/steps_of_change.shtml

Moos, R.H. & Moos, B.S. (2006). Participation in treatment and Alcoholics Anonymous: A 16-year follow-up of initially untreated individuals. *Journal of Clinical Psychology, 62,* 735–750.

Morgenstern, J., Labouvie, E., McCrady, B.S., Kahler, C.W. & Frey, R.M. (1997). Affiliation with Alcoholics Anonymous after treatment: A study of its therapeutic effects and mechanisms of action. *Journal of Consulting and Clinical Psychology, 65,* 768–777.

Ouimette, P., Humphreys, K., Moos, R.H., Finney, J.W., Cronkite, R. & Federman, B. (2001). Self-help group participation among substance use disorder patients with posttraumatic stress disorder. *Journal of Substance Abuse Treatment, 20,* 25–32.

Pagano, M.E., Post, S.G. & Johnson, S.M. (2011). Alcoholics Anonymous–related helping and the helper therapy principle. *Alcoholism Treatment Quarterly, 29* (1), 23–34.

Project MATCH Research Group. (1993). Project MATCH (Matching Alcoholism Treatment to Client Heterogeneity): Rationale and methods for a multisite clinical trial matching patients to alcoholism treatment. *Alcoholism: Clinical Experimental Research, 17,* 1130–1145.

Project MATCH Research Group. (1997). Matching alcoholism treatments to client heterogeneity: Project MATCH posttreatment drinking outcomes. *Journal of Studies on Alcohol, 58,* 7–29.

Robinson, E.A.R., Krentzman, A.R., Webb, J.R. & Brower, K.J. (2011). Six-month changes in spirituality and religiousness in alcoholics predict drinking outcomes at nine months. *Journal of Studies on Alcohol and Drugs, 72,* 660–668.

Rychtarik, R.G., Connors, G.J., Dermen, K.H. & Stasiewicz, P.R. (2000). Alcoholics Anonymous and the use of medications to prevent relapse: An anonymous survey of member attitudes. *Journal of Studies on Alcohol, 61,* 134–138.

Secular Organizations for Sobriety (SOS). (1996). *The Sobriety Priority.* Buffalo, NY: Author.

Sisson, R.W. & Mallams, J.H. (1981). The use of systematic encouragement and community access procedures to increase attendance at Alcoholic Anonymous and Al-Anon meetings. *American Journal of Drug and Alcohol Abuse, 8,* 371–376.

SMART Recovery. (1996). *Alcohol or Drug Problem? Now There Is a Scientific Alternative.* Beachwood, OH: Alcohol and Drug Abuse Mutual Help Network.

Subbaraman, M.S., Kaskutasa, L.A. & Zemore, S. (2011). Sponsorship and service as mediators of the effects of Making Alcoholics Anonymous Easier (MAAEZ), a 12-step facilitation intervention. *Drug and Alcohol Dependence, 116,* 117–124.

Substance Abuse and Mental Health Services Administration (SAMHSA). (2010). *Results from the 2009 National Survey on Drug Use and Health: Volume I. Summary of National Findings.* Rockville, MD: Author. Retrieved from www.samhsa.gov/data/NSDUH/2k9NSDUH/2k9Results.htm

Timko, C., DeBenedetti, A. & Billow, R. (2006). Intensive referral to 12-step self-help groups and 6-month substance use disorder outcomes. *Addiction, 101,* 678–688.

Timko, C., Moos, R.H., Finney, J.W. & Lesar, M.D. (2000). Long-term outcomes of alcohol use disorders: Comparing untreated individuals with those in Alcoholics Anonymous and formal treatment. *Journal of Studies on Alcohol, 6,* 529–540.

Tonigan, J.S., Connors, G.J. & Miller, W.R. (2003). Participation and involvement in Alcoholics Anonymous. In T. Babor & F. DelBoca (Eds.), *Treatment Matching in Alcoholism* (pp. 184–204). New York: Cambridge University Press.

Tonigan, J.S. & Kelly, J.F. (2004). Beliefs about AA and the use of medications: A comparison of three groups of AA-exposed alcohol dependent persons. *Alcoholism Treatment Quarterly, 22* (2), 67–78.

Tonigan, J.S., Miller, W.R., & Schermer, C. (2002). Atheists, agnostics and Alcoholics Anonymous. *Journal of Studies on Alcohol, 63,* 534–541.

Tonigan, J.S. & Rice, S.L. (2010). Is it beneficial to have an Alcoholics Anonymous sponsor? *Psychology of Addictive Behaviors, 24,* 397–403.

Tonigan, J.S., Toscova, R. & Miller, W.R. (1996). Meta-analysis of the literature on Alcoholics Anonymous: Sample and study characteristics moderate findings. *Journal of Studies on Alcohol, 57,* 65–72.

Walitzer, K.S., Dermen, K.H. & Barrick, C. (2009). Facilitating involvement in Alcoholics Anonymous during out-patient treatment: A randomized clinical trial. *Addiction, 104,* 391–401.

Weiss, R.D., Griffin, M.L., Gallop, R., Luborsky, L., Siqueland, L., Frank, A. et al. (2000). Predictors of self-help group participation in cocaine dependent patients. *Journal of Studies on Alcohol, 61,* 714–719.

White, W. & Kurtz, E. (2005). *The Varieties of Recovery Experience.* Chicago, IL: Great Lakes Addiction Technology Transfer Center.

White, W. & Nicolaus, M. (2005). Styles of secular recovery. *Counselor, 6* (4), 58–61.

Winzelberg, A. & Humphreys, K. (1999). Should patients' religiosity influence clinicians' referral to 12-step self-help groups? Evidence from a study of 3,018 male substance abuse patients. *Journal of Consulting and Clinical Psychology, 67,* 790–794.

Yalom, I.D. & Leszcz, M. (2005). *The Theory and Practice of Group Psychotherapy* (5th ed.). New York: Basic Books.

Zemore, S. (2007). A role for spiritual change in the benefits of 12-step involvement. *Alcoholism: Clinical and Experimental Research, 31* (Suppl. 3), 76–79.

Chapter 15

A Digital Future: How Technology Is Changing Addiction Recovery

Sylvia Hagopian, Anne Ptasznik, Paul Radkowski and Monique Peats

Technology is providing a fascinating means to expand treatment, education and support for people with addictions, as well as their families. As users become increasingly "techno-savvy," so too are health care options rapidly expanding to meet users' needs.

People can now use smartphones to monitor patterns and triggers to their substance use. They can Skype their therapist while on holiday. They can download homework to help them practise coping strategies or listen to prerecorded psychoeducational videos. They can also interact with bloggers with similar addictions, and with families seeking support and information through the same online forums, discussion boards and networks.

This range of online options reflects people's increased comfort and use of the Internet. According to Newbold and Campus (2011), "More and more users are turning to social media for health information, advice and support" (p. 18). Conversations about health and wellness, treatment and care are happening online. Research by ComScore (2012) has found that, at 45 hours a month, Canadians spend more time online than any other Internet users.

This chapter includes four sections: Sylvia Hagopian introduces us to the range of Internet and mobile apps now available, and looks at existing research on the effectiveness of various options, and the barriers and benefits to their use. Anne Ptasznik examines how bloggers are using their online writing as a way to gain support from others with similar issues, reflect on their own struggles and recovery, and educate the public with anti-stigma messages about addiction. Paul Radkowski and Monique Peats describe how the Life Recovery Program they founded offers a range of online modalities to support people with addiction and mental health issues. And finally, Hagopian reflects on future directions in the field.

We are finally catching up to what clients and families have built online in their search for information and support. Many options for supporting and treating people with addiction and mental health problems are being offered as an adjunct to "face-to-face" time; in other cases, online chatting, blogging and other interventions are the only options for people with certain disabilities, people living in remote areas or people isolated by stigma.

Consider this chapter as an introduction to mobile and web-based technology. No doubt, by the next edition of this book, the application of these interventions, and the range of what is possible, will make current applications and other technological tools obsolete. In the years to come, we will develop much more sophisticated approaches to addressing many existing barriers, such as confidentiality and privacy issues, and restrictions imposed by literacy and language differences. But regardless of the sophistication of technology, people will always need "face time": to sit in a room with others, make eye contact, express themselves through their body language—and get immediate help in a crisis.

The Evolution of Web and Mobile Health Care Devices

Sylvia Hagopian

People are increasingly turning to the Internet as a medium through which to obtain information and guidance in dealing with their health concerns. In response, health care institutions are offering more applications and psychoeducational material through the Internet and mobile devices. The terms *e-disease management, e-health, telehealth* and *e-therapy* are commonly used to define this category of web and mobile health care intervention. These interventions vary in technological sophistication, client anonymity and degree of interaction. Some communication strategies are synchronous or in real time (e.g., Internet, online chat, instant and text messaging, video or web-conferencing, telephone), while others are asynchronous or posted and read at different times (e.g., e-mail, discussion boards, online forums, text messaging, comments on blogs). These tools include everything from assessment and diagnostic modules, to sophisticated monitoring tools and alert systems that integrate directly with a patient's electronic health record. These resources are often "bundled" with web content, interactive web tools (e.g., peer-support discussion boards, online forums), cognitive-behavioural learning modules and mobile applications.

Applications (commonly known as "apps") are computer software that helps end users accomplish a certain task. In 2007, Apple Inc. launched the iPhone and allowed external companies to develop apps that could be used with the iPhone interface. As a result, the popularity of this smartphone exploded. Besides Apple, other operating systems provided by BlackBerry and Android are flooding the market with their own versions of mobile phones and tablet computers. Today there are more than 300,000 iPhone apps—and more than 13,000 health apps in Apple's App Store, according to a MobiHealthNews report (Dolan, 2011). Within e-health, mobile apps have been developed to help people keep addiction journals, schedule peer-support meetings, track their substance use and identify substance use patterns and triggers.

E-health tools have proliferated for many reasons, including:

- administrative need for more time- and cost-effective interventions
- increasing affordability and availability of Internet and technology solutions
- patients' demand for increased autonomy and control over their own care
- industry-driven marketing.

Another catalyst for developing e-health interventions is to offer options in the continuum of supports and services for people who aren't able or willing to access face-to-face treatment for addiction. Research has shown that only about one in 10 gamblers with a lifetime diagnosis of gambling dependence will ever seek treatment (Cunningham, 2005). A key motivation for developing Internet and mobile-based tools is the desire to reach out to people with addictions who are not accessing traditional forms of treatment, whether due to stigma, mobility issues, geographic barriers or other reasons.

Evidence for Technology-Based Interventions

Research into the effectiveness of computer and mobile technology in the treatment of addiction and mental health issues has been limited. However, research across the technological spectrum is expanding quickly as software costs become more competitive and hardware costs become more affordable. Technological advancements are giving clinical researchers the opportunity to develop, implement and test an array of web and mobile applications.

According to Monaghan and Blaszczynski (2009):

> Preliminary evidence shows that Internet therapy and other online interventions are more effective than no treatment, and may be as effective as face-to-face therapy for a large range of mental health disorders, including treatment of substance use addictions and problem gambling. (p. 5)

The best evidence for the efficacy of such online interventions tends to come from randomized controlled trials, although there are relatively few. However, promising research is emerging in the following areas:

- text messaging to discourage alcohol consumption (Suffoletto et al., 2012)
- web-based personalized feedback interventions for problem gambling (Cunningham et al., 2011)
- psychoeducational web tools to educate people about mood disorders (Smith et al., 2011)
- online peer support programs for smoking cessation (Graham et al., 2011)
- smartphones and image applications to treat social anxiety (Enock et al., n.d.)
- e-therapy and problem gambling (Monaghan & Blaszczynski, 2009).

Each form of communication has advantages and disadvantages, which should be considered when determining the best way to serve people with addictions (Center for Substance Abuse Treatment, 2009). Research into the effectiveness and clinical appropriateness of e-health tools will be crucial as governments and other sectors continue to finance the development of innovative health care applications.

The focus of research may well turn from debating the effectiveness of online interventions to exploring how to retain participants in treatment; in other words, how to reduce attrition rates and improve the efficacy of these web-based treatment programs (Postel et al., 2011). Future research may also explore self-directedness in online interventions.

Barriers and Considerations

Self-directed web and mobile interventions for addictions are not suitable for everyone. People who are in crisis or at immediate risk of harming themselves or others shouldn't rely on this method of communication for seeking help. Since inputs or "posts" are often made anonymously, using asynchronous tools, this delays and prevents therapists from responding quickly and efficiently in an emergency. Access to online or mobile tools and applications may also be a barrier, particularly for people who are under-housed or homeless, people from remote communities with limited access to the Internet, people with literacy or language barriers and people with certain disabilities. These tools are meant to enhance a well-established program, not be a substitute for it, but the field is still developing and more research is needed (LeGrow & Metzger, 2001).

Psychoeducational tools may assist therapists in their practice by allowing clients to access web and mobile activities between clinical sessions. If a therapist decides that a particular web- or mobile-based tool can be used with clients as an adjunct to treatment, the therapist should first know the reputation of the organization responsible for developing the tool, and consider the following issues before recommending it:

- Is there a fee for use or service?
- Are the online resources credible and informed by research?
- Is the organization for profit or not for profit?
- Where will personal health information be stored?
- How is privacy protected?
- Who funds the development and ongoing hosting of these tools?
- Will there be regular reviews of content and improvements?
- What was the rationale for developing the tool?

With thousands of health care consumer applications available on the web and via mobile devices, health professionals and clients should also consider the reliability of the medical and health information within these applications.

The health care community is seeing immense potential and opportunities for using technology to interact with and support clients. As opposed to purchasing or licensing pre-built tools to integrate into their programs, institutions might consider developing a suite of their own e-health tools. Benefits of developing these tools in house include more control over data transmission, storage and privacy; better integration with existing technological platforms; and the ability to self-support upgrades and improvements. Also, all intellectual property rights would belong to the organization, allowing it to more easily customize the tool based on treatment needs. Organizations that are considering this venture should first think about various issues. Although not exhaustive, this list highlights some important considerations:

Resources: Does the organization have the capacity to develop or host a program, including all the safeguards required to provide a database and storage environment that are safe from external threats, such as security breaches? Can the organization supply a front-line helpdesk function that can assist with tasks as simple as password resets, to more complicated therapeutic functional support roles?

Identification and verification of users: With face-to-face treatment, a client's identity can be easily verified. However, with remote systems using the Internet and chat or e-mail, for example, how can the clinician verify that the person he or she is communicating with is indeed the client? Because user names and passwords can easily be shared or accidently exposed, this is an important privacy consideration for both the organization and the clinician.

Privacy: Programs often allow end-users to save their session information locally onto their computer hard drives, or convert their self-help work into printable formats for saving and sharing. This may pose a challenge in adhering to rigorous standards for protecting and sharing personal health information. It is very easy to forward an e-mail to a third party or inadvertently forget to log out of a computer. Where do the responsibilities of the organization for protecting privacy end and the due diligence of end-users begin? The organization needs to conduct a thorough legal, privacy impact and threat risk assessment for each technological service developed.

Non-verbal communication: Many e-health programs include contact with a therapist through web chat or e-mail correspondence. But can clinicians adequately provide treatment if they are unable to interpret the body language or non-verbal cues that are prevalent in face-to-face sessions? Does the long silence in a chat session mean the client is upset and unsure of how to respond, or has the client wandered away from the computer? Can the lack of e-mail response be due to a technology glitch, or is the client not interested in continuing treatment? These are just a few examples of possible limitations to e-therapy, although barriers have been addressed in the literature.

Language barriers: How will the organization provide services that accommodate non-English–speaking clients? Have the resources been culturally adapted, and have they been adequately tested with other cultural groups? Organizations are investing more and more time and resources in providing culturally competent care. How will e-health solutions adapt to deliver this care? Even English-speaking end-users will vary in language ability and writing skills. People unaccustomed to communicating in English, or to typing or the web may need a completely different set of communication standards.

Jurisdictional and licensing boards: Most helping professionals, such as doctors, social workers and psychologists, operate under licensing bodies. Licensing boards provide practitioners with a code of ethics, practice standards and regulation requirements. These standards are often bound to a province or jurisdiction. Addiction professionals should confirm with their licensing bodies that they are still protected if they choose to use an e-health intervention with their clients. To address jurisdictional practice limits, helping professionals will also need to know where their clients live. This can be a challenge, since client verification and identification may not be completely reliable and clinicians may not be covered for liability, for example, if clients live outside their professional jurisdiction.

Significant upfront costs and resource allocation are needed to develop e-health tools. The demand for these services will continue to put pressure on the system to provide increasingly innovative options in the continuum of supports and services for people with addiction and mental health problems. Growing research demonstrates that the benefits of e-health tools for clients, families and helping professionals is definitely worth this initial investment.

Bloggers Create Communities of Support—but with Some Risks

Anne Ptasznik

Ron Grover believes that blogging saved both his life and his marriage. He and his wife had been struggling to deal with their son's addiction for years, without getting the support they needed. "This is hard on a marriage, and hard on parents," he says. "It got to the point where there were no other options. I'd gone to AA [Alcoholics Anonymous], Al-Anon [for friends and family of problem drinkers], Nar-Anon [for friends and family of people with an addiction], and it wasn't helping. I'd read books and I'm not a therapist, counsellor-type guy." Grover, who has a high-school education, hated English and writing in school, but still turned to blogging as an outlet: "The blog was a way for me to communicate what was going on inside of me, what I felt, what I thought."

Journalling and writing have long been used in psychotherapy, based on the principle that emotions and experiences can be better "understood, mastered and assimilated when explored through language," says Dr. John Suler. Suler, a psychology professor at Rider University in Lawrenceville, New Jersey, is the author of the online book *The Psychology of Cyberspace*, originally published in 1996, and expanded and revised since then. But while many psychotherapies encourage people to talk about their issues, Suler says that for some people, putting words to their experience is easier in writing. Journals can be used as a coping tool, as well as a mechanism to reflect on life, gain insight and reduce psychological stress by venting and processing emotional situations (Baker & Moore, 2008a).

Journal writing is fundamentally different from blogging in that it can be kept private. Most people blog to share their expertise and experience with others, according to the *State of the Blogosphere 2011* report (Technorati Media, 2011). But bloggers like Grover, who expose their personal concerns to family, friends, neighbours and even employers, may, as a result, face discrimination and even abuse. Still, research has shown that many people use their blog as a personal diary and emotional outlet, as was found in a content analysis of MySpace blogs published in the journal *CyberPsychology & Behavior* (Fullwood et al., 2009). Almost 50 per cent of people posting entries on Internet blogs or weblogs did so as a form of self-therapy, according to the 2005 AOL Blog Trends Survey (Tan, 2008). While people who blog about their addiction, or that of a family member, may be particularly exposed to stigma, this does not deter the many people who are blogging about addiction recovery on Blogger, WordPress and other blogging sites.

So, considering the risks, what motivates people to write publicly about their struggles?

Anticipating an audience and writing for that audience stimulates a valuable process of "trying to see oneself more objectively [through other people's eyes]," says Suler. "There's also the added benefit of people supporting the blogger via e-mail or other messaging, and of others with similar issues offering advice and empathy. Essentially, the blogging community can become like a self-help/support group." Some bloggers also use the medium to educate the public and fight stigma. Some even take their sharing offline and speak to community groups and schools about their experiences with recovery.

Ashley McGowan is a community support manager with Evolution Health, a Toronto-based company that develops evidence-based software to support behavioural change. The software, including both free beta programs and licensed commercial versions, incorporates blogs and discussion forums, which are moderated by a team of health educators managed by McGowan. McGowan says that members of the company's online communities generally use the blogs to "let loose" in a way they may feel self-conscious doing in the discussion forums. Members also use their blogs as a daily tracking tool, for example, to document their quitting efforts on the smoking cessation site. The blogs can then be used as an encouraging self-reminder: if tempted to smoke, bloggers can look back at their postings and see that they can get through the cravings and withdrawal symptoms. Members also receive supportive comments and benefit altruistically when they see how their blogs are giving support to other members who read and see what they went through while quitting.

Grover says that he would review his own postings to reinforce the actions he needed to take around his son's addiction. "I had it written down and I would have to hold myself to what I was saying," he says. "There were people out there who commented who had been where I was at. It's kind of like an online Nar-Anon meeting. They would talk with me and make a comment, and I would write back and interact with them."

Support became particularly important for Grover and his wife when they began repeatedly bailing their son out of jail, only to have him end up back in jail shortly after being released. Grover's blog readers advised that his son was better off in jail. "When you are talking about your own son, your own blood, it's hard to make that real life, but when I wrote it down, I'd say, 'Remember you already thought this through and it's safer for him to be in jail than it is searching out a drug dealer with a gun in his belt and heroin.'" When Grover and his wife wouldn't pay a $50 bail bond, their son ended up in jail for 11 days. People commented that Grover was right on target. "It's always good to have reassurance that you're moving in the direction that you need to move to," Grover says.

Emily Jones* blogs about her recovery in AA. She says that blogging has helped her sobriety because it has forced her to reread the AA literature. "It has allowed me the privilege of meeting other bloggers around the country," she says. "We have formed friendships that I would have never thought possible." One person even picked up Jones from the airport in a foreign city and drove her to her hotel. She felt she could judge the person trustworthy by the fact that he "posted on his blog without fail, before 5 a.m., 365 days a year, for many years."

Recent research has corroborated the benefits of blogging as a means of social support. An online survey of about 300 bloggers published in *Cyberpsychology, Behavior, and Social Networking* (Hollenbaugh, 2011) identified seven motives for maintaining a blog, with the highest scores relating to helping others or forming social connection. A study of 58 MySpace users found that bloggers' social integration, trust in others and friendship satisfaction increased significantly compared to that of non-bloggers (Baker & Moore, 2008b). The researchers concluded that bloggers benefit from perceived social support.

Researchers at the University of Haifa in Israel conducted one of the first studies to proactively implement blogging as an intervention. Published in *Psychological Services* (Boniel-Nissim & Barak, 2011), the study examined the therapeutic value of blogging for adolescents with social and emotional difficulties. The researchers randomly assigned students to six groups. Two groups blogged about thoughts and feelings about their social circumstances and interpersonal relationships. Participants in one group left their blogs open to online responses; the blogs of the other group were closed. Two groups were free to blog on any subject they wanted; the fifth group kept a computer diary, and the sixth, which served as a non-treatment control group, did not write at all.

The study results showed that the young people who experienced the greatest positive change were those who blogged about their social and emotional difficulties. Bloggers who accepted comments benefited the most. The authors say these findings highlight the important roles of social visibility and feedback that characterize blogging. (The researchers did supervise all blog posts and comments and deleted or asked bloggers to delete any potentially harmful text, but very few deletions were required.)

Being more open on a blog and in a community forum can help some people gain confidence to be more open in their real lives, according to McGowan. One potential pitfall, however, is if bloggers, who may be emotionally vulnerable, post in the belief that

---

* not her real name

they will acquire new friends and "likes," and then become defeated if that does not happen. They may internalize any negative comments they receive, making the experience counterproductive, she says. She adds that discussion forums may be a better option for these people to get support.

Blogs can also be used to express thoughts that come up in therapy. Suler says that although blogs are public, he first asks clients for permission to read their postings and encourages them to discuss their blogs with him if the content is relevant to the therapy.

An additional motivation beyond self-observation and social support for some bloggers can be the opportunity to educate the public. In her blog, Jones tries to counter the negative misinformation about AA and the belief that people need to spend thousands of dollars in treatment to get sober. She hopes her blog can "encourage people to go to AA, ask God for help, jump in with both feet and get sober!"

She knows that her blog was a catalyst for one woman to go to AA. The woman has now been sober for six years. "This is definitely the highlight of blogging for me!" says Jones.

Addressing stigma is the main reason why Grover, who originally blogged anonymously, began to use his real name and e-mail on his blog and post personal photographs. While he is not a "super private person," and had supportive colleagues who knew about his son's addiction and difficulties with the law, his wife works in a large company and did not want to go public.

But after being told that addiction is a disease like diabetes, Grover reconsidered using his real name. He began to ask himself, "If this is a disease, why am I hiding?" He saw that remaining secretive would not help improve the situation for people with addiction, including his son: "I don't like what he's doing, but I've never been ashamed of any of my kids. If this is a disease, let's go public with it," Grover declared. So he talked it over with his wife. She agreed, and they posted their picture and e-mail address on the blog.

Grover, whose son has now stopped all substance use, appreciates that his experiences can benefit others. He considers his blogging to be a form of community service and responds to everyone who e-mails him. "I know how dark of a place it is when you think you're going to lose your child or something is taking them over that you can't do anything about," he says. "If somebody is so desperate that they would write a stranger and tell them all these intimate things about what's going on in their lives, they deserve an answer [to their e-mail]."

But blogging still has its risks. Grover has often been criticized and called a "bad parent." If people are "writing from the heart," he says, he does not mind negative comments. But as Suler warns, not everyone online is supportive or benign. "People do all sorts of acting out in cyberspace, and they are looking for targets," he says. Transference reactions, where people misperceive others based on their own needs and fears, are common, and Suler says bloggers can easily become the target of these hostilities.

Jones, who began blogging when she was 21 years sober, says, "Blogging is a tough business. I would not recommend it to one who is newly sober unless they have a very tough skin." She stopped allowing anonymous comments after someone left some particularly mean-spirited ones.

To help safeguard privacy, members of Evolution Health communities are advised upon registration not to use an e-mail containing a company name or a name that is otherwise recognizable, and not to post any identifying information. Trevor van Mierlo, CEO of Evolution Health, warns that once people post on the Internet, they have no control over what happens to that information. He says that on some commercial blogging sites, the way this lack of control manifests is through advertising relating to the person's content; for example, an electronic cigarette ad may pop up automatically if the person blogs about his efforts to quit smoking. This makes it appear as though the blogger is endorsing the product.

Grover says people need to consider how private they want to be. He knows that some bloggers do not even tell their family members. He advises that if people want to remain anonymous, they need to be very careful about not disclosing where they live and any other personal details.

One thing Grover never even considered when he started blogging was all the time it would take, which has included responding to invitations to speak at high schools and parenting groups. Still, Grover recommends blogging. "To me this is just a journal on steroids. I'm writing my thoughts, my beliefs, whether right or wrong, what I've done, my experiences, just like a journal or a diary, except I have the benefit of thousands of people reading this and writing their comments. I have the benefit of all that wisdom, of people farther along in the process, and from people just beginning."

The Life Recovery Program

Paul Radkowski and Monique Peats

Online programs are increasingly being accepted as viable options to support, provide psychoeducation and offer treatment to people with mental health and addiction issues, a finding that is being supported by much of the current research. Online treatment programs have the advantage over face-to-face programs of being easy to access; eliminating issues of stigma; and providing clients with autonomy, empowerment and the ability to participate in recovery at their own pace.

Cunningham and colleagues (2010) affirm that trials of computer-based interventions for different health behaviours and interventions provide "significant evidence for their efficacy" (p. 1). A meta-analysis also suggests that minimal contact computer-delivered treatments that can be accessed via the Internet may represent a cost-effective means of treating uncomplicated substance use problems and related issues (Rooke et al., 2010).

The Life Recovery Program[1] (LRP) is an award-winning program that uses online modalities to support people who have addiction and mental health issues. The program

---

1 For more information about the Life Recovery Program, visit www.liferecoveryprogram.com.

is unique in that it also provides psychoeducation and support to friends and family, and is based in a trauma-informed approach. (For more on trauma-informed care, see Chapter 17.)

As a video-based addiction and mental health recovery program, the LRP integrates materials and resources used by many inpatient addiction treatment centres. It offers an evidence-informed holistic approach that recognizes the biological, spiritual and psychosocial influences of addiction. It includes supportive homework downloads that enable clients to practise and review new coping strategies; weekly e-mails that encourage such things as seeking an accountability partner (e.g., AA, a friend, counsellor, pastor); summaries and reiteration of key messages from the most recent lesson in the program; and pre-recorded psychoeducational videos. The program also provides clients with various grounding techniques to help them develop healthy and consistent coping strategies. Several LRP e-books explain the role of trauma and stress in mental health and addictive patterns of behaviour.

The interactive part of the program is a clinician-moderated peer-support forum enabling participants to experience immediate support and resources through anonymous interaction with other people dealing with mental health and addiction issues—from substance use and behavioural or process addictions to self-cutting, disordered eating, gambling, toxic relationships, anger, chronic stress, trauma and impulse control issues. Resources are provided throughout the recovery program and are used to reinforce the message of recovery and healing by addressing such issues as the role of addictions and concurrent mental health issues among people with addictive patterns of behaviour.

The need for programs like LRP was highlighted by findings from the U.S. 2005 National Comorbidity Survey Replication Study in the United States, which revealed a six- to 23-year delay between the onset of a mental health issue and receiving treatment (Wang et al., 2005). Many people do not seek treatment due to lack of resources, difficulty in accessing services and stigma. Despite greater awareness of mental health issues, people are more comfortable sharing about a health issue such as diabetes or cancer than a diagnosis of depression or anxiety. Consequently, self-medication through various addictive substances or behaviours can become the treatment modality, with potentially destructive results. The study found that because 75 per cent of all lifelong mental illnesses occur before age 24, many people adopt unhealthy coping strategies, including using substances, to cope with mental health issues, which often result in other problems.

The Internet eliminates accessibility issues by providing a 24/7 option that enables people to get help when they need it, wherever they are. The LRP and other computer-based options make sense in this current technological age, among a generation that searches the Internet for information about every aspect of life, including health and wellness.

A major challenge faced by the LRP in providing a comprehensive computer-based option of support has been to address people's confusion or misconceptions about the role and purpose of the program. Some people mistakenly assume that we provide e-counselling and live interactive video exchange; others fear that this online program is trying to replace traditional treatment options. Because the LRP does not include e-counselling, it is not bound by the same legalities and liabilities, and has the advantage of being accessible anywhere in the world, at any time. The ongoing journey of the LRP has been to dispel these myths, and to educate, share and communicate the effectiveness of this unique yet comprehensive online program.

Because LRP is an online modality, it can be used by a variety of people for many different purposes, such as support for someone waiting for treatment (which can range from months to years) or a stand-alone option for someone who wants anonymity and who is unable or not ready to engage in face-to-face treatment. The program can also be used as a relapse prevention resource and support for someone recently coming out of treatment. It is designed to fill current service gaps—not to replace existing modalities of support for mental health and addiction treatment.

A content analysis of the LRP revealed that more than 80 per cent of participants were able to view their lives differently, manage their moods through self-regulation and decrease or stop their addictive behaviours as they developed new ways of coping. Twenty-seven per cent of active members chose to sign up and pay to go through the entire six-month program (which remains available for one year) for a second time, thus decreasing their likelihood of relapse. A positive shift in self-talk revealed an increase in self-awareness and meta-cognitive abilities. Also noted were clients' increased use of alternative resources, such as support groups and therapists, where some had been fearful of using them in the past.

The recent research findings for this emerging modality are promising. It will be interesting to see if and how the Internet becomes a modality to keep some of the most common mental health and addiction concerns in a preclinical, preventative phase before more serious symptoms emerge. It will also be interesting to see to what degree such a modality could be used to reduce some of the most severe symptoms experienced by people with mental health and addiction issues.

The LRP has been peer-reviewed and was recognized in 2008 for its comprehensiveness and innovation through the International Association of Addictions and Offender Counselors' Outstanding Addictions Professional Award. The program was also awarded the Outstanding Mental Health Award from the Ontario Association of Counsellors, Consultants, Psychometrists and Psychologists in 2011.

Conclusion

There is no question that e-health tools will continue to gain popularity and be widely adopted. The general public will look for more sophisticated apps that will help them manage their health concerns from the convenience of their home computer and mobile devices, and institutions will look for solutions that also integrate data seamlessly into their electronic health records.

The trend will be to develop more tablet computer applications, such as highly portable computers that can be used by a patient's bedside, making them popular with helping professionals. Addiction therapists can use these portable devices with clients to complete assessments and access treatment planning tools. Busy helping professionals find the convenience of tablets very appealing because they can use them to quickly and easily access patient records, screening instruments, drug information, anatomy programs, medical encyclopedias and more.

More technology companies and system integrators are investing in the future of e-health with dedicated teams and divisions focused on helping institutions fulfil their objectives of providing better access to care. The demand for more e-health applications will certainly increase as a new generation of digital citizens comes of age, which is accustomed to—and expects—the conveniences of online and mobile delivery mechanisms for retail and commerce, communication and health care. With telemedicine and telepsychiatry's fairly long tradition of delivering health (including mental health) services to remote populations, e-health could be regarded as building on this tradition. As health care system costs continue to rise and one-on-one clinician-patient relationships become scarcer, innovative new tools will be a welcome addition to the continuum of care.

Resources

Publications

Barak, A., Klein, B. & Proudfoot, J.G. (2009). Defining Internet-supported therapeutic interventions. *Annals of Behavioral Medicine, 38*, 4–17.

Center for Substance Abuse Treatment. (2009). *Considerations for the Provision of E-Therapy*. Rockville, MD: Author. Retrieved from http://store.samhsa.gov/shin/content//SMA09-4450/SMA09-4450.pdf

LeGrow, G. & Metzger, J. (2001). *E-Disease Management*. [Report prepared for the California Healthcare Foundation]. Oakland, CA: First Consulting Group. Retrieved from www.chcf.org/~/media/MEDIA%20LIBRARY%20Files/PDF/E/PDF%20EDiseaseManagement.pdf

Internet

Human Services Information Technology Applications
www.husita.org

International Society for Mental Health Online
www.ismho.org

International Society for Research on Internet Interventions
www.isrii.org

References

Baker, J.R. & Moore, S.M. (2008a). Distress, coping and blogging: Comparing new Myspace users by their intention to blog. *CyberPsychology & Behavior, 11*, 81–85. doi: 10.1089/cpb.2007.9930

Baker, J.R. & Moore, S.M. (2008b). Blogging as a social tool: A psychosocial examination of the effects of blogging. *CyberPsychology & Behavior, 11*, 747–749. doi: 10.1089/cpb.2008.0053

Boniel-Nissim, M. & Barak, A. (2011). The therapeutic value of adolescents' blogging about social-emotional difficulties. *Psychological Services*. doi: 10.1037/a0026664

Center for Substance Abuse Treatment. (2009). *Considerations for the Provision of E-Therapy*. Rockville, MD: Author. Retrieved from http://store.samhsa.gov/shin/content//SMA09-4450/SMA09-4450.pdf

ComScore. (2012). *2012 Canada Digital Future in Focus*. Retrieved from www.comscore.com/Insights/Presentations_and_Whitepapers/2012/2012_Canada_Digital_Future_in_Focus

Cunningham, J.A. (2005). Little use of treatment among problem gamblers. *Psychiatric Services, 56*, 1024–1025.

Cunningham, J.A., Hodgins, D. & Toneatto, T. (2011). Pilot study of an Internet-based personalized feedback intervention for problem gamblers. *Journal of Gambling Issues, 26*, 3–10.

Cunningham, J.A., Wild, C.T., Cordingley, J., Van Mierlo, T. & Humphreys, K. (2010). Twelve-month follow-up results from a randomized controlled trial of a brief personalized feedback intervention for problem drinkers. *Alcohol and Alcoholism*. doi: 10.1093/alcalc/agq009

Dolan, B. (2011, September 22). Report: 13K iPhone consumer health apps in 2012. Retrieved from http://mobihealthnews.com/13368/report-13k-iphone-consumer-health-apps-in-2012/

Enock, P. & McNally, R. (n.d.). Handheld Training Study (Smart-phone anxiety study). Harvard University, Department of Psychology. Retrieved from http://handheldtrainingstudy.com/

Fullwood, C., Sheehan, N. & Nicholls, W. (2009). Blog function revisited: A content analysis of MySpace blogs. *CyberPsychology & Behavior, 12.* doi: 10.1089/cpb.2009.0138

Graham, A.L., Papandonatos, G.D., Kang, H., Moreno, J.L. & Abrams, D.B. (2011). Development and validation of the online social support for smokers scale. *Journal of Medical Internet Research, 13* (3), e69. doi: 10.2196/jmir.1801

Hollenbaugh, E.E. (2011). Motives for maintaining personal journal blogs. *Cyberpsychology, Behavior, and Social Networking, 14,* 13–20. doi: 10.1089/cyber.2009.0403

LeGrow, G. & Metzger, J. (2001). *E-Disease Management* [Report prepared for the California Healthcare Foundation]. Oakland, CA: First Consulting Group. Retrieved from www.chcf.org/~/media/MEDIA%20LIBRARY%20Files/PDF/E/PDF%20EDiseaseManagement.pdf

Monaghan, S. & Blaszczynski, A. (2009). *Internet-Based Interventions for the Treatment of Problem Gambling.* Toronto: Centre for Addiction and Mental Health.

Newbold, B.K. & Campos, S. (2011). *Media and Social Media in Public Health Messages: A Systematic Review.* Retrieved from www.mcmaster.ca/mieh/documents/publications/Social%20Media%20Report.pdf

Postel, M.G., de Haan, H.A., ter Huurne, E.D., van der Palen, J., Becker, E.S. & de Jong, C.A. (2011). Attrition in web-based treatment for problem drinkers. *Journal of Medical Internet Research, 13* (4), e117. doi: 10.2196/jmir.1811

Rooke, S., Thorsteinsson, E., Karpin, A., Copeland, J. & Allsop, D. (2010). Computer-delivered interventions for alcohol and tobacco use: A meta-analysis. *Addiction, 105,* 1381–1390. doi: 10.1111/j.1360-0443.2010.02975.x

Smith, D.J., Griffiths, E., Poole, R., Di Florio, A., Barnes, E., Kelly, M.J. et al. (2011). Beating bipolar: Exploratory trial of a novel Internet-based psychoeducational treatment for bipolar disorder. *Bipolar Disorders, 13,* 571–577. doi: 10.1111/j.1399-5618.2011.00949.x

Suffoletto, B., Callaway, C., Kristan, J., Kraemer, K. & Clark, D. (2012). Text-message–based drinking assessments and brief interventions for young adults discharged from the emergency department. *Alcoholism: Clinical and Experimental Research, 36,* 552–560. doi: 10.1111/j.1530-0277.2011.01646.x

Suler, J. (1996). *The Psychology of Cyberspace.* Retrieved from http://users.rider.edu/~suler/psycyber/psycyber.html

Tan, L. (2008). Psychotherapy 2.0: MySpace® blogging as self-therapy. *American Journal of Psychotherapy, 62* (2), 143–163.

Technorati Media. (2011). *State of the Blogosphere 2011.* Retrieved from http://technorati.com/social-media/feature/state-of-the-blogosphere-2011/

Wang, P.S., Berglund, P., Olfson, M., Pincus, H.A., Wells, K.B. & Kessler, R.C. (2005). Failure and delay in initial treatment contact after first onset of mental disorders in the National Comorbidity Survey Replication. *Archives of General Psychiatry, 62,* 603–613.

SECTION 3

SPECIAL ISSUES AND CONSIDERATIONS

Chapter 16

Concurrent Disorders

Andrea Tsanos

> Marcello is a 35-year-old man who has been struggling with alcohol problems and concurrent social anxiety and depression. He has a history of political affiliations in his native Guatemala that resulted in his being tortured, and then having to flee to Canada as a political refugee. Marcello is not able to return to, call or write to his family back home for fear that he will be discovered, so his move has represented considerable loss.
>
> Marcello has found assimilation into Canadian culture to be a challenge. This, combined with posttraumatic stress disorder (PTSD) symptoms related to his torture, has led to drinking 40 ounces of tequila daily. Drinking helps numb Marcello's symptoms and helps him to cope with social isolation and missing his country and family. Marcello also drinks to help him function in social settings, since he finds group settings and relating with women extremely anxiety-evoking. His greatest fear is that women will think he is "weak as a man." While drinking helps him cope with depression and anxiety, it has resulted in hangovers, work-related problems such as absenteeism and decreased performance, and financial strain from spending considerable money on alcohol.
>
> Marcello explained that in his culture, there is an expectation that he "should have been married with children by now." He describes feeling profound shame and stigma when he meets anyone from the Spanish-speaking community because he has not achieved these goals, so he often avoids people. In Marcello's culture, men must never appear to be weak, so it is a significant challenge for him to seek therapy and disclose his problems. Discussing personal vulnerabilities reflects a lack of machismo and carries a very negative judgment.

Co-occurring substance use and mental health issues frequently present themselves in clinical practice. If you are working with clients with substance use or mental health issues, then you are likely already working with clients who have both issues, called *concurrent disorders*. Experiencing a single problem, such as addiction, is challenging in and of itself, but when a person has more than one problem (and in some cases multiple problems, as with Marcello), naturally, the challenge is exacerbated.

Given our still fragmented systems of care, as well as the frequent crises and relapses that often characterize addiction and mental health issues, people with concurrent disorders remain a complex client population to serve. But it is important to recognize that *there is help*, and equally important, *there is hope*; and working within an evidenced-based or best practices "integrated treatment" approach offers the best chance for recovery.

Defining Concurrent Disorders

A number of terms exist to describe concurrent disorders, depending on the jurisdiction and context. In Ontario, the Ministry of Health and Long-Term Care uses the term *concurrent disorders* to refer to co-occurring addiction and mental health problems. The Canadian Centre on Substance Abuse ([CCSA], 2010) offers the following definition: "The term *concurrent disorders* is used to describe the situation where a person has both a mental health and a substance use problem" (p. 1).

A broader definition of addiction encompasses not only addiction to substances, but addiction to certain behaviours, such as excessive gambling, shopping, eating, sex, and computer and video game playing. (For more about behavioural or process addictions, see Chapter 20.) While these behavioural or process addictions also frequently co-occur with mental health problems, current definitions of concurrent disorders are limited to substance use disorders. However, these other addictions are increasingly being recognized as important subgroups to be mindful of, and may factor into a new and broadened iteration of the definition of concurrent disorders in the coming years.

In fact, Smith (2012) has indicated that recent developments in brain science influenced the DSM-5 Task Force to suggest a new category called "addictions and related disorders," which would encompass both substance-related and behavioural/process addictions. This change would have represented an expansion of the current definition of addiction based on the understanding that both psychoactive drugs and certain behaviours produce a surge of dopamine in the midbrain, illustrating a biological substrate for addictive behaviour. However, the recently released DSM-5 (APA, 2013a) has ultimately landed on new terminology that collapses the former DSM diagnostic categories of substance abuse and substance dependence into one category called "substance use disorder," along with another non-substance category related to behavioural disorder called "gambling disorder," which in previous editions was called "pathological gambling." In the DSM-5, substance use disorder and gambling disorder are contained in a chapter called "Substance Use Disorders and Addictive Disorders," even though gambling disorder remains the only non-substance addictive disorder included at present. While there was pressure from clinicians to add Internet use disorder and other behavioural addictions, "Internet use disorder" was deemed an area within DSM-5 for conditions requiring further study before they would be considered disorders per se, which is hoped will encourage further research on the condition (APA, 2013b).

Other terms for concurrent disorders

Other terms for concurrent disorders have been, and still are, used in other settings and by different groups. Some professional groups still use pejorative terms. The following list clarifies some of the confusion around terminology:

Comorbid disorders: a medical term used to describe the presence of more than one significant health problem

CAMI (Chemically abusing mentally ill): people whose primary problem is substance use who also have mental illness

MICA (Mentally ill chemical abuser): people whose primary problem is mental illness who have co-occurring substance use problems

SAMI (Substance abusing mentally ill): people with a substance use problem concurrent with a serious and persistent mental illness

Dual diagnosis / dual disorders: used outside of Ontario, including the United States, to describe concurrent disorders. In Ontario, dual diagnosis refers to co-occurring developmental and psychiatric disorders.

Double trouble: sometimes used by people with co-occurring substance use and mental health problems to refer to their own experiences.

Subgroups

A wide variety of psychiatric disorders exists, each of which can play a role in the experience of concurrent disorders. Similarly, a wide range of psychoactive substances is available, each of which can be used alone, or in combination. These substances include:
- stimulants (e.g., amphetamines, cocaine, caffeine, nicotine)
- sedatives (e.g., alcohol, barbiturates, benzodiazepines, inhalants)
- opioids (e.g., heroin, morphine)
- hallucinogens (e.g., cannabis, LSD, PCP).

Accordingly, the term concurrent disorders can be applied to various combinations or subgroups of substance use and mental health problems, such as:
- anxiety disorder (e.g., panic disorder) and concurrent benzodiazepine misuse
- mood disorder (e.g., major depressive disorder) and concurrent alcohol use disorder
- psychotic disorder (e.g., schizophrenia) and concurrent cannabis use disorder
- eating disorder (e.g., bulimia nervosa) and concurrent cocaine use disorder
- personality disorder (e.g., borderline personality disorder) and concurrent opioid (e.g., OxyContin) addiction.

The diversity of combinations underscores the fact that people with concurrent disorders are far from being a homogeneous group.

A CCSA (2009) report on concurrent disorders designated five general concurrent disorder subgroups to help clarify and categorize the most common combinations of concurrent disorders:

1. Mood disorders and substance use disorders. People with mood disorders are more likely to use substances; conversely, people who use substances are more likely to experience mood disorders (e.g., bipolar disorder, major depressive disorder, dysthymia, cyclothymia).

2. Anxiety and substance use disorders. People with anxiety disorders have two to five times the risk of having a problem with alcohol or other drugs.

3. Stress, trauma and substance use disorders. The experience of a traumatic event significantly increases the risk of alcohol and other drug use. Substance use can lead to new traumatic experiences, which can subsequently lead to further substance use, thus perpetuating the "stress–substance use" cycle.

4. Psychosis and substance use disorders. The rate of substance use disorders among people with psychotic disorders is roughly 50 per cent, which is much higher than in the general Canadian population.

5. Impulsivity and substance use disorders. Difficulties with impulse control, such as the tendency to act without planning, forethought or restraint, represent the single foremost predictor of developing a substance use problem.

An earlier Health Canada (2002) report also described five general subgroups, with some of the same classifications as the 2009 CCSA report, but added some slightly different classifications. These included:

- eating disorders and substance use disorders
- personality disorders and substance use disorders.

CCSA (2009) organized its five classifications based on more recent conceptualizations of concurrent disorders. Examples of such advances in understanding are:

- recognition of the episodic nature of psychosis (versus the earlier Health Canada [2002] category "Serious and persistent mental illness")
- division of the "mood and anxiety disorders" category into two distinct categories (rather than treating them as an amalgamated subgroup as did the Health Canada [2002] report).

While such subgroup distinctions enhance our general understanding of concurrent disorders, each main category can be further subdivided into the specific sub-level of disorders (e.g., within the broad subgroup of anxiety disorders and substance use disorders: panic disorder and alcohol dependence).

This truly is a heterogeneous population characterized by clinical complexity. Understanding the various diagnostic subgroups is important, since each one points to a subgroup-specific etiology and corresponding treatment recommendation. For example, with concurrent PTSD and substance use disorder, a careful integrated approach is the recommended treatment plan (Brown et al., 1998; Evans & Sullivan, 1995; Najavits, 2002, 2003). Targeting the substance problem without attending to the PTSD symptoms may cause the client's psychological functioning to worsen; conversely, if the PTSD symptoms are targeted without addressing the substance use, the client may feel at risk of using substances to cope.

Beyond this understanding of concurrent disorders subgroups, however, it is equally important that health care providers recognize each client's unique characteristics and experiences. For example, one person's alcohol use disorder and concurrent major depressive disorder might be characterized by:

- depressed mood
- thoughts of suicide
- loss of appetite
- insomnia.

Another person with these identical concurrent diagnoses might experience a depressive episode that is characterized by a different set of depressive symptoms that includes:

- loss of interest or pleasure in usual activities
- a sense of worthlessness and/or inappropriate guilt
- overeating
- excessive sleeping.

While both scenarios involve depression, the lived experiences of these two people will be qualitatively different. In addition, the particular depressive symptoms that may trigger drinking might also be entirely different; for example, thoughts of suicide with a plan and intent versus a sense of worthlessness without suicidal ideation. These symptoms naturally pose different levels of risk and thus warrant different interventions.

Complexity

To further add to the diversity and complexity of this client population, it is important to recognize that people with concurrent disorders may have more than one mental health concern and more than one substance use problem at a given time.

A common example of concurrent disorders is PTSD arising from the experience of childhood sexual abuse, and co-occurring with alcohol and/or opiate addiction to cope with distressing PTSD symptoms, such as flashbacks and persistent, frightening intrusive thoughts related to the event. People who have experienced trauma often self-medicate with substances to numb or escape from the emotional pain (Najavits, 2004).

Severity

People with concurrent disorders may experience differing levels of severity of their substance use and mental health problems. The possible combinations are depicted in Figure 16-1.

FIGURE 16-1: Four-Quadrant Model: Co-occurring Disorders by Severity

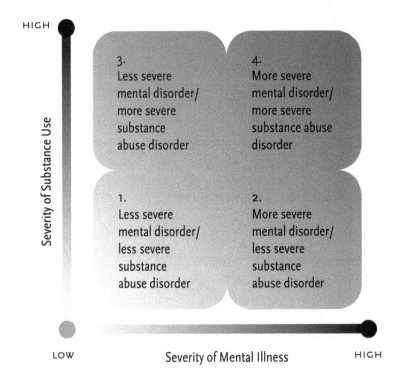

FIGURE 16-1: Four-Quadrant Model: Co-occurring Disorders by Severity

Source: Concurrent Disorders Ontario Network. (2005). *Concurrent Disorders Policy Framework*, p. 19. www.ofcmhap.on.ca/sites/ofcmhap.on.ca/files/-CDpolicy%20final.pdf.

Figure 16-2 illustrates the locus of care that each quadrant of severity points to (i.e., in which setting the client would best be managed). For example, an individual with concurrent disorders characterized by high substance use severity but low mental illness severity might best be treated in an addiction setting, whereas an individual with high mental illness severity but low addiction severity might best be treated within a mental health setting. An individual with concurrent disorders characterized by high substance use severity as well as high mental illness severity might best be treated within a truly integrated concurrent disorders treatment setting.

FIGURE 16-2: Four-Quadrant Model for Assessment of Concurrent Disorders Subtypes and Treatment Planning

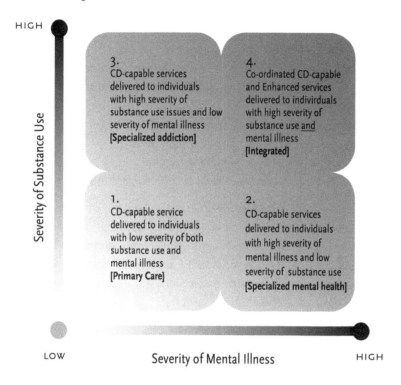

HIGH

Severity of Substance Use

3.
CD-capable services delivered to individuals with high severity of substance use issues and low severity of mental illness
[Specialized addiction]

4.
Co-ordinated CD-capable and Enhanced services delivered to indivirduals with high severity of substance use and mental illness
[Integrated]

1.
CD-capable service delivered to individuals with low severity of both substance use and mental illness
[Primary Care]

2.
CD-capable services delivered to individuals with high severity of mental illness and low severity of substance use
[Specialized mental health]

LOW   Severity of Mental Illness   HIGH

Source: Adapted from Substance Abuse and Mental Health Services Administration (2002).

The model presented in Figure 16-2 suggests that the notion of severity (of the client's substance use and mental health problems) determines where clinical service would ideally be provided. The model is fluid, meaning that clients can move back and forth within quadrants depending on the severity of their illness and the overall status of their recovery.

Prevalence

Providing treatment for clients with concurrent disorders can be challenging: they have higher rates of relapse for both substance use and psychiatric problems than people with a single disorder. When someone has a substance use problem, the risk of developing a concurrent mental health problem is increased; conversely, a person with a mental health problem is at increased risk of developing a concurrent substance use problem.

Earlier epidemiological data indicated that about half of people with either a mental health or substance use disorder have had problems in the other domain at some point in their lives (Health Canada, 2002; Kessler et al., 2005; Regier et al., 1990). Interestingly, more recent Ontario-specific data has cited different rates, depending on the treatment setting, gender and type of mental health population. Rush and Koegl (2008) found that:

- **about 20 per cent** of Ontarians treated for mental health issues in Ontario hospitals and mental health clinics were found to have had a co-occurring substance use problem
- within Ontario substance use service settings, prevalence rates were as high as **70 to 80 per cent**
- within mental health settings, the prevalence of concurrent disorders was **15 to 20 per cent** (which appears low compared to earlier data and to rates within substance use settings). These rates increase when looking at specific subsets of the mental health treatment population:
  - 55 per cent among young males in treatment
  - 28 per cent in those receiving specific inpatient care
  - 34 per cent for people with personality disorders
  - as high as 75 per cent in forensic and correctional settings (Ogloff, et al., 2006).

While statistics on concurrent disorders vary because of different sampling and statistical methodologies, prevalence rates within mental health and addiction clinical settings are generally higher than in non-clinical community samples. The 2002 Canadian Community Health Survey (Rush et al., 2008) found that almost two per cent of the general population experienced co-occurring disorders within the 12-month period prior to participating in the survey. However, since several disorders known to highly co-occur with substance use disorders (e.g., PTSD) were excluded from this survey methodology, these Canadian rates are thought to be at the lower end of the range of that which is reported internationally. The researchers note that the figure of two per cent more specifically represents the rate at which mood or anxiety disorders co-occur with substance use problems.

This recent data challenges us to reflect on the 50 per cent prevalence rate that is often assumed for concurrent disorders, and to consider how specific types of disorders influence this statistic. For instance, as already noted, there is a high overlap between PTSD and substance use disorders, particularly for women, with rates estimated between 30 and 75 per cent (Brady et al., 1994; Jacobsen et al., 2001; Najavits et al., 1997). However, among women in treatment for substance use disorders, the rate jumps to 86 to 90 per cent (Najavits, 2002).

Index of Suspicion

Given the prevalence rates of concurrent disorders within clinical treatment settings, and within addiction treatment settings especially, concurrent disorders "should be expected, rather than considered the exception" (Minkoff, 2001a). This means that when a client seeks service for either a mental health or addiction problem, service providers should have a high index of suspicion for the possibility that concurrent disorders exist (rather than a single problem alone for which the client has sought treatment). The Toronto Drug Strategy Advisory Committee (2005) identified more vulnerable populations with higher-than-average levels of substance use and concurrent disorders for which a high index of suspicion is recommended. These include:

- homeless youth and adults
- lesbian, gay, bisexual, transsexual, transgendered or queer (LGBTTQ) youth and adults
- Aboriginal people
- people involved in the sex trade industry
- people in detention centres and prisons
- people with mental health problems.

Making it common practice to screen for concurrent disorders could help practitioners better identify and engage clients with concurrent disorders, and develop plans for further assessment and treatment.

Issues and Impacts for People with Concurrent Disorders

How people are affected by concurrent disorders depends on various factors, including the combination of the problems and their severity (O'Grady & Skinner, 2007). According to Minkoff (2000), people with concurrent disorders tend to do worse and have poorer outcomes overall compared with people who have only one disorder. They also tend to be heavy users of services, are highly crisis prone and tend not to seek the help they need (Minkoff, 2000). People with concurrent disorders, whether in treatment or not, are at higher risk of:
- being stigmatized at many levels
- homelessness
- victimization
- relapse
- re-hospitalization
- physical health problems
- HIV infection
- financial problems
- legal problems and incarceration
- family violence
- suicide.

Barriers for Diverse Client Populations

Clients who come from ethnocultural, racialized and other diverse backgrounds may experience even greater barriers to treatment because of cultural taboos and higher degrees of distrust or even hostility toward mainstream institutions. Many specialty treatment settings have restrictive treatment-entry requirements that are difficult to navigate. Different cultural beliefs about mental health and substance use problems can also inform how individuals and their families understand these issues. Not having services that offer specific ethnocultural approaches to care, or not having services offered in various languages, can be barriers to care. (For more about diversity and equity competencies in addiction treatment, see Chapter 3.)

Stigma and Misconceptions Surrounding Concurrent Disorders

Society has a long history of people—including health care providers—holding negative views of people who have mental health or addiction problems. People with mental health and addiction issues are often judged and labelled as scary or dangerous, deficient in some way, of lower moral stature than the general public, strange, weak, less deserving than others, unable to be helped, lazy, out of control, worthless and incompetent. This stigma is difficult enough for someone with just one disorder to face; for people with concurrent disorders, the stigma of having both a mental health and a substance use disorder is like having a "double stigma," or multiple layers of stigma.

The impact of this kind of stigma can be devastating. Stigma can lead to feelings of shame, isolation, poor self-esteem, low self-confidence, a reduced likelihood of seeking help, secrecy regarding symptoms and loss of hope for recovery. According to Torrey (1994), "some individuals with a serious mental illness say that the stigma is worse than the disease itself" (p. 653).

Even health care providers can be guilty of stigma. Most receive their education and training in either addiction or mental health, not both. This has led to a fragmentation in clinicians' minds as to what kinds of issues they feel comfortable dealing with. This perception is reflected in statements such as:

> *"It's not my role to work with concurrent disorders."*

> *"I'm not an expert in the area of concurrent disorders, so there's nothing I can do."*

> *"It's too time-consuming to work with clients with concurrent disorders."*

> *"We can't work with someone who is actively using substances."*

> *"I can't work with someone who does not have abstinence as a goal."*

> *"The patient has to want to make a change but he doesn't, so there's nothing I can do."*

> *"These people are hopeless."* (i.e., feeling pessimistic about the likelihood that the client can get better)

> *"Substance use is a moral defect, character flaw or individual failing."* (i.e., being judgmental about substance use)

How we feel about people with mental health and/or addiction issues influences how we interact and work with them. Skinner (2005) describes how mental health professionals and addiction professionals may have different attitudes toward the issues each works with:

> Although [mental health and addiction issues] both can be chronic and relapsing health problems, people tend to make a distinction between the two. Some mental health workers, for example, may see people's psychiatric problems as real illnesses, and their substance use problems as intentional behaviour. Addiction workers, on the other hand, may firmly believe that most people can recover from substance use problems, but think people with serious mental health problems are not capable of significant change. As more mental health and addiction workers learn to work with clients with co-occurring problems, and their understanding of the relationship between substance use and mental health problems increases, client care will become more responsive and effective. (p. xviii)

System Issues and Navigating Access to Specialized Services

Historically, mental health and addiction services have been organized separately, with each system designed to provide care for either the addiction or the mental health issue, but not both. This has led to fragmented care, creating inefficiencies in the system and contributing to poor treatment outcomes:

> Often [clients with concurrent disorders] are shuttled back and forth, or they fall through the cracks of the system and are lost to treatment, or they are treated in both [psychiatric and substance use] clinics with conflicting methods and confusing effects. (Gottheil et al., 1980, p. xii)

These clients, many of whom have multiple, complex problems, are often lost in a system that is not well integrated, and fall through the cracks. One consumer describes the experience:

> I've gotten help for each individual thing but to get help for, like [both] at the same time, you fall between the cracks and if one of your disorders is worse than another, and then one doctor thinks you're seeing somebody else, basically nobody's helping you, nobody follows up, you kind of disappear in there. (Health Canada, 2002, p. 74)

Fortunately, things are starting to change. At the international, national and provincial levels, efforts are underway to co-ordinate systems and better integrate mental health and addiction treatment. In Ontario, the government's aim is "to integrate mental health and addiction services with the rest of the health system—to make every door the right door" (Ministry of Health and Long-Term Care, 2009, p. 9).

The mental health and addiction services systems are still working toward improved access and integration across and within their settings. There are not enough treatment programs, psychiatrists and other specialists who provide services for people with concurrent disorders, and long wait-lists to access these services are common.

When mental health and addiction agencies do exist in particular communities, people with concurrent disorders are often ineligible for one service or the other, because admission criteria exclude people with co-occurring disorders. It can feel overwhelming trying to find the right point of entry. While the Ontario government is calling for reducing the barriers to accessing mental health and addiction services, the reality of change is that it is slow and takes time.

Rush and Nadeau (2011) describe the need for the system to have a much broader integrated response to better serve people with concurrent disorders. They argue that we can no longer look at only specialized mental health and addiction treatment services to provide support for people with concurrent disorders; rather, we must look toward a more comprehensive network of supports with multiple systems, including primary care, hospitals and emergency services, as well as the justice, housing, school, social assistance and street services systems.

Approaches to Care

Skinner (2005) explains why it is important for service providers across a diverse range of settings to understand concurrent disorders:

> If you work with clients who have substance use or mental health problems, you are undoubtedly already working with people who have concurrent disorders. If you are committed to understanding and working with clients as whole persons, then you need to understand what these problems are, how they co-occur and how you can help.

> Leaving this work to specialists in concurrent disorders is not enough. People in all kinds of helping roles can provide support—people who work in the addiction and mental health systems, obviously, but also people working in other domains, such as criminal justice and corrections, health care, child welfare and family service, employee assistance programs and education. (p. xiv)

Screening

Clients enter "the system" through different entry points—addiction and mental health agencies, emergency and crisis services, corrections, homeless shelters and primary care settings. The concept of "no wrong door" (Center for Substance Abuse Treatment [CSAT], 2005) emphasizes the principle that the health-care delivery system and all treatment providers

> have a responsibility to address the range of client needs wherever and whenever a person presents for care. When clients appear at a facility that is not qualified to provide some type of needed service, those clients should carefully be guided to appropriate, cooperating facilities with followup by staff to ensure that clients receive proper care. (p. 11–12)

For the client, every "door" in the health-care delivery system should be the "right door."

The concept of "no wrong door" represents the ultimate goal shared by both the addiction and mental health systems—to provide a welcoming environment wherever clients enter the system, providing services in a more seamless and timely fashion.

The available resource capacity (e.g., staff time, appropriate training, availability and mandate of screening tools) for identifying concurrent disorders varies from agency to agency, as does the professional competence of staff. However, regardless of resources and expertise, all clinicians can serve clients better if they can recognize concurrent disorders. (For more information on screening, see Chapter 8.)

Screening best practices

The function of screening is to raise red flags that alert the service provider to the possible need for more detailed assessment and treatment planning around possible mental health and/or substance use issues.

With screening, a small investment of time can make a major difference. Screening does not have to be a complicated or formal process; for busy health care practitioners, screening methodologies need to be user friendly and suitable to the environment and context.

Screening for concurrent disorders is important given the prevalence of co-occurring mental health problems in people with substance use concerns, and of substance use problems in people with mental health issues. Clients often do not disclose to the health care provider that they have mental health and substance use issues and that they are interested in getting help. In fact, because of stigma and other fears about negative consequences, people with concurrent disorders often intentionally hide these problems. Health care providers can best help clients when they have comprehensive information. Screening is the first step in this process.

Health Canada (2002) recommends that *all* people seeking help from mental health or substance use services be systematically screened for concurrent disorders.

This involves two levels. At Level I, clinicians proceed with the index of suspicion (described earlier) and ask non-threatening, straightforward questions. At Level II, clinicians use validated instruments that are quick and easy to administer.

In an ideal world, the most reliable screening and assessment occur if the client has detoxified from all psychoactive substances that are not medically necessary. The service provider should explain to the client that substance use can confound or even exacerbate the mental health condition and thus should be avoided (or at least minimized).

Navigating Screening Options for Concurrent Disorders (Centre for Addiction and Mental Health, 2006) states that screening methods should be brief, valid and reliable, and have sensitivity and specificity. The guide identifies numerous ways to screen for mental health or substance use problems, including:

- rating the probability of a client having a co-occurring disorder
- asking the client a few direct questions
- using brief screening tools.

Toxicology screening is another mechanism for screening for substance use; however, it alone cannot be used to make diagnoses.

Probability ratings

Clinicians should be aware of the many health and social factors often related to substance use and mental health problems that can indicate the need for further assessment (Skinner, 2005). Health Canada (2002) lists the following indicators of substance use problems:

- housing instability
- difficulty budgeting funds
- symptom relapses apparently unrelated to life stressors
- treatment non-compliance
- prostitution
- social isolation
- violent behaviour or threats of violence
- pervasive, repeated social difficulties
- sudden unexplained mood shifts
- legal problems
- cognitive impairments
- suicidal ideation or attempts
- employment difficulties
- repeated self-harm in the absence of clear, situationally relevant stressors.

Because clients do not always identify either the substance use or mental health difficulty as a presenting problem, practitioners should consider the reason the person is making contact and presenting for treatment, and be alert to possible indications of an underlying mental health or substance use issue. Skinner (2005) identified various presentations that may be the client's primary concern and that could warrant further investigation into possible mental health or substance use issues. These include:

- physical traumas, such as falls, fractures or burns
- suicide attempts
- incidents of domestic violence
- physical aggression or public disturbance
- truancy, vagrancy, homelessness, social isolation or family abandonment.

Asking a few direct questions

A very direct approach is to ask the client three key questions that can help elicit more information, without judgment and without relying on formal psychometric screening tools. This approach is often used in screening for other health care issues.

Health Canada–recommended screening questions

Health Canada (2002) recommends the following three screening questions related to substance use and recommends further investigation if the client responds "yes" to one or more questions:

1. "Have you ever had any problems related to your use of alcohol or other drugs?"
2. "Has a relative or friend, or a doctor or other health worker, been concerned about your drinking or other drug use, or suggested you cut down?"
3. "Have you ever said to another person, 'I don't have a problem' (with alcohol or other drugs) when, around the same time, you wondered whether you did have a problem?" (pp. 31–32)

Health Canada recommends asking the following three questions to screen for mental health problems, and suggests further investigation if a client responds "yes" to one or more questions:

1. "Have you ever been given a mental health diagnosis by a qualified mental health professional?"
2. "Have you ever been hospitalized for a mental health–related illness?"
3. "Have you ever harmed yourself or thought about harming yourself, but not as a direct result of alcohol or other drug use?" (p. 37)

As part of a comprehensive screening process, consider who might serve as collateral sources of information. Family members, friends and other health care and service providers in the client's circle of care can provide information.

Basic screening questions elicit a "yes" or "no" answer: Does the person presenting for help with a substance use or mental health problem show signs of a possible concurrent mental health or substance use problem? The screening process does not necessarily identify what kind of problem the person might have, or how severe or serious it might be; rather, it determines whether further assessment is warranted. Compared to more structured approaches, such as using screening tools, standard assessment practices based solely on interviews do a relatively poor job of identifying co-occurring problem areas outside the realm of the presenting concerns and symptoms.

Screening tools

Screening tools provide more objective measures of the possibility of mental health and substance use issues than the methods discussed earlier. Validated screening tools can be used in a standardized way within and across practice settings. However, since there is not one particular tool that is the recommended "magic bullet" for all settings or service environments, it is still valuable to:

- approach people with substance user and/or mental health issues with a high index of suspicion about the presence of a concurrent disorder
- find ways to incorporate some simple questions
- use your best clinical judgment to complement any screening tools already in use within your own setting.

The Global Appraisal of Individual Needs—Short Screener (GAIN-SS) (Dennis et al., 2006) is a self-administered 19-item screening tool. It identifies people who are likely to have a substance use or mental health disorder and who thus should undergo a fuller, more comprehensive assessment. The GAIN-SS is used by several local health integration networks (LHINs) across Ontario in various community and hospital settings. (See Chapter 8 for examples of other screening tools.)

One barrier to regularly screening for substance use and mental health issues is care providers' own limitations in being able to assess and further manage people who screen positive. Although specialty services are limited and have wait-lists, care providers can refer clients with more complex or specialized needs to these services. In an ideal system, collaborations and partnerships would be developed between clinicians within their own settings, and with the specialized addiction and mental health services that exist, as well as with other key sectors, such as emergency departments, housing agencies and other social services.

Minkoff (2001b) describes the agency capability framework, which calls on all services and sectors to be "CD capable" to at least some degree:

- Mental health services: provide universal screening for substance use problems/ disorders
- Addiction services: provide universal screening for mental health problems/disorders
- Tailor approach/tools to different settings and the time and resources available.

Accordingly, basic-level capacity includes systematic screening, with referral links in place for follow-up assessment and treatment planning.

Assessment

When screening indicates that a person may have a concurrent disorder, further assessment is needed. Both screening and assessment should be viewed as an ongoing process, rather than as discrete, single events that happen at intake or at the beginning of a new treatment relationship. Concurrent disorders can be complex, and it often takes time for a clear picture to emerge. Clients with concurrent disorders are a heterogeneous group, with defining features or presenting diagnostic profiles that can change over time. Every client has a unique situation that requires different levels of intervention.

Although care providers screen for mental health and addiction issues, conducting comprehensive concurrent disorders assessments may be beyond the scope of a primary health care provider or a community-based care environment.

A comprehensive assessment includes assessing substance use and mental health problems and their relationship, as well as motivation to change and psychosocial functioning. Skinner (2005) identified the following domains to include when conducting a comprehensive assessment of concurrent disorders:

- estimation of the severity of substance use, including types of substances used, quantity and frequency, as well as the severity of the mental health problem
- assessment for additional problem areas that can affect treatment planning and effectiveness (e.g., physical health; occupation; access to housing, food, income, employment or schooling; social support, legal issues; family relationships; risks of victimization and overall safety)
- the client's understanding of the effects of substance use
- any vulnerabilities or barriers the client identifies (i.e., factors that would interfere with treatment)
- the client's readiness to make changes to substance use and engage in treatment.

In addition to helping form a diagnosis and inform treatment planning, an assessment can also be used to:

- build a therapeutic alliance with the client
- allow the collection of a thorough history of the client
- allow the practitioner and client to discuss the consequences of substance use and mental health problems, as well as concerns in other areas, such as work, housing and relationships
- allow for crisis management and stabilization
- serve as baseline information to compare with results at end of treatment to determine if or how the client has changed over time and over the course of treatment
- provide opportunities for the client to better understand his or her problems
- investigate the causes of and interrelationship between a client's mental health and substance use disorders.

See Chapter 8 on screening and assessment for more detail on individual considerations in addiction assessment.

Assessing the relationship between concurrent problems

Assessing concurrent disorders can feel like trying to put together a difficult puzzle. Clinicians need to address the nature and extent of both the presenting mental illness and the substance use issue, as well as the ways in which they affect and interact with each other. For instance, which came first? Did psychiatric symptoms develop during a period of substance intoxication or withdrawal? Do the symptoms resolve with abstinence? Did the substance use precede the mental health symptoms?

It is important to attend to all the possible ways the substance use symptoms can interrelate with mental health symptoms, and to determine the type of functional relationship that exists between the two. The assessment process can be particularly challenging because the symptoms of substance use and withdrawal issues, and the symptoms of mental health disorders, can mimic, mask, trigger or exacerbate one another.

Some questions to consider:

1. What is the temporal relationship between symptoms?
   - Which predated the other?
   - Are psychiatric symptoms present at the same time as substance use / withdrawal symptoms?
2. How does the substance use affect the psychiatric symptoms?
   - Worsen?
   - Relieve?
   - No effect?
3. What happens to the psychiatric symptoms during periods of abstinence?
   - Improve?
   - Worsen?

TABLE 16-1

Etiological Models of Concurrent Disorders

MODEL	DEFINITION	CLINICAL EXAMPLE
Self-medication hypothesis (Khantzian et al., 1974, 2003)	Substance use is a coping response for mental health symptoms.	Self-medication of panic symptoms with alcohol Crack-cocaine used to escape feelings of boredom
Substance-induced	Mental health symptoms are the result of chronic or excessive substance use or withdrawal.	Cocaine-induced depression Marijuana-induced psychosis

The two models presented in Table 16-1 represent the predominant theories for understanding concurrent disorders comorbidity and relate to all combinations of concurrent disorders. The etiological model can be refined as new information emerges over the ongoing assessment process. For the concurrent disorders subpopulation of people with severe mental illness/psychosis, the model presented in Table 16-2 is more compelling.

TABLE 16-2

Etiological Model for Concurrent Major and Severe Mental Illness and Substance Use Disorder

MODEL	DEFINITION	CLINICAL EXAMPLE
Shared/common vulnerability hypothesis (Valkow, 2009)	A shared or common vulnerability referred to as the "vulnerable brain" exists where the person has a "supersensitivity" arising from shared bio-genetic traits (e.g., dopamine, GABA) seen in both the psychotic disorder and the substance use disorder.	A person who has a psychotic disorder (e.g., schizophrenia) who is also dependent on cannabis and crack-cocaine. The person has a biological vulnerability to dopamine receptors for the development of: (a) a major mental health disorder (in this case schizophrenia) and (b) having a supersensitivity to the effects of substances on the brain—with greater liability to developing addiction/dependence and experiencing negative consequences from use (e.g., psychosis).

Other important factors for assessment:

- Know about different drugs the client is taking and recognize symptoms of psychiatric disorders that may be drug induced. (Drugs that can cause psychiatric disorders and their main symptoms may be induced by various psychotropic substances: differentiate between primary psychiatric disorders and those that are substance induced.)
- Recognize the signs and symptoms of intoxication and withdrawal from various substances.
- Determine whether there is a family history of mental health or substance use disorders.

Diversity considerations

Given our diverse communities, both locally and nationally, clinicians must be sensitive to and respect clients' unique cultural issues and needs. Cultural competence is associated with improved quality of care, as well as improved health outcomes for racialized and underserved populations (Anderson et al., 2003; Shaw-Taylor & Benesch, 1998).

A culturally competent clinician recognizes and respects that clients have diverse values, beliefs and understanding of mental health and substance use issues that are culturally based and culturally defined, and considers these factors in the assessment process. For example, how people understand and interpret their mental health symptoms or how they understand the concept of a "drug" can vary across cultures, as can social and cultural norms about the use of alcohol or other drugs. (See Chapter 3 for more on diversity issues in addiction treatment.)

Treatment Philosophy and Key Principles

When people with concurrent disorders seek help, treatment all too often targets only one of their problems as their primary concern. While helping clients to address one key problem (e.g., alcohol) can mobilize a process of change that ultimately benefits the co-occurring problem (e.g., depression), taking this fragmented and compartmentalized approach may in fact not be helpful to the concurrent problem, and may even exacerbate both problems. To best help clients, clinicians need to look at the person as a whole, and seek to understand how that person's problems overlap with or influence, mask or exaggerate one another.

Treatment for concurrent disorders should take a client-centred approach that is tailored to the specific needs of each client. It can involve psychosocial approaches and counselling, pharmacological management or both. While there are particular recommended interventions based on evidence and best practices for particular types of concurrent disorders, the overall philosophy cuts across all types of concurrent disorders. Minkoff (2000) identifies the following overarching elements of concurrent disorders treatment that form a framework and values base from which clinicians can approach their work:
- creation of an empathic, hopeful, continuous treatment relationship
- recognition that treatment may involve multiple treatment episodes over time
- development of an integrated treatment plan in which there is co-ordination of care
- recognition of the importance of maintaining alliance and engagement with the client.

Integrated treatment

Health Canada's (2002) best practice recommendations for concurrent disorders suggest that treatment should be integrated and individualized to the specific needs and context of the client, and should include support for immediate problem resolution, longer-term monitoring, support and rehabilitation. More recently, CCSA (2009) identified emerging research and clinical advances in treating concurrent disorders in Canada.

Although the interconnectedness of substance use and mental health problems has become better understood over the years, the notion of actually integrating treatment has only more recently received attention.

Treatment models have historically taken a sequential approach (i.e., "Go and take care of your addiction first, and once that's dealt with, come back for counselling for your depression"). People seeking mental health treatment have often been rejected once their substance use has been disclosed; conversely, people seeking addiction treatment have often been excluded when they have revealed having a psychiatric diagnosis or using prescribed psychotropic medication.

At best, some clients have received parallel treatment—obtaining mental health treatment from one place and substance use treatment from another. Within this model, there is typically no connection or communication between the two services.

It is only in the past 20 years that research has focused on clinical outcomes for clients with concurrent disorders and that clinicians have begun to develop and implement more co-ordinated, comprehensive and integrated treatments. Integrated treatment combines interventions for mental health and substance use problems concurrently, in two ways (Health Canada, 2002):

1. **Program integration**. One clinician or one team provides mental health and substance use treatment within the same setting or "under one roof." Ideally, the team comprises professionally trained addiction and mental health clinicians (including physicians, where pharmacotherapy is involved), whose work is augmented by client participation in mutual aid groups, if required or desired.

2. **System integration**. Enduring linkages between service providers / treatment units are established. This is similar to the parallel treatment model, but is enhanced by a commitment to communication and co-ordination between providers from addiction and mental health services within the overall system, ideally co-ordinated by one case manager (who has major responsibility for the case).

Regardless of which model is used, the overall goal within integrated treatment is to ensure that clients receive a consistent explanation of their issues and a coherent prescription for treatment, rather than a contradictory set of messages from different care providers.

Equally important is that all diagnoses are considered primary, thus eradicating the historical primary/secondary distinction, and eliminating the bias toward addressing just one of the problems within the complex interplay of concurrent disorders. Within an integrated approach, clients report finally feeling understood and feeling they are in the right place.

Minkoff (2000) outlines the seven principles of integrated treatment for a more successful therapeutic outcome:

1. comprehensive programs and services
2. continuity of treatment over time
3. accessibility in the location of services, and flexible hours and service delivery
4. acceptance by practitioners of both the mental health and addiction issues
5. a sense of optimism about the possibility of recovery, even for clients with very severe or complex problems
6. individualized treatment (tailored to individual needs)
7. culturally competent treatment.

Practice implications

Various mental health and addiction agencies in North America have endorsed the development of concurrent disorder capability. For example, the U.S. Substance Abuse and Mental Health Services Administration (SAMHSA, 2002) has identified co-occurring disorders as a top priority with which all clinicians should become "CD informed" and "CD capable" in their practice. At a macro level, agencies and programs as a whole can work to meet criteria to be CD capable at the program level; at the micro service level, individual clinicians can strive to attain concurrent disorder competence at a basic level (Level I) or a more advanced level (Level II).

CD competencies (levels I & II)

While the level of complexity of concurrent disorders seen in a given health care setting may be different from that seen in a tertiary care or specialized care setting, most people with mental health and substance use issues have mild to moderate substance use and mental health problems (Skinner, 2005), and likely have been seen by a community health care provider before they seek service from a tertiary care setting. Given that we are striving toward a more integrated health care system for clients, health care providers should develop at least a basic level of skill at identifying, assessing and working with clients with concurrent disorders.

Minkoff (2001b) uses the following terminology to describe different levels of concurrent disorder (CD) capability at the agency or program level, based on the American Society of Addiction Medicine's patient placement criteria (Mee-Lee, 2001):

- **CD capable:** ability to meet the needs of clients with substance abuse and relatively stable mental health disorders
- **CD enhanced:** ability to meet the needs of clients with substance abuse and unstable or disabling mental health disorders.

In specialized mental health and/or addiction settings, Level I competencies and capabilities include those outlined in Table 16-3.

TABLE 16-3

Level I: CD-Capable Capacities and Competencies

Capacities	Ability to provide a minimal level of integrated mental health and addiction services for clients who also present with concurrent mental health problems.
	CD-capable addiction clinicians can help clients with concurrent mental health issues of low severity.
	CD-capable mental health clinicians can help clients with concurrent substance use problems of low to moderate severity.

Competencies	Clinicians have knowledge and skill at the individual practitioner level in the following areas: • attitudes and values about addiction and mental illness (including understanding the impact of stigma) • identification/screening for concurrent disorders • assessment • treatment planning • provision of Level I individual and group treatment interventions (e.g. motivational interviewing, harm reduction, relapse prevention) for clients with concurrent disorders of a low to moderate severity • case management and supportive care • referral mechanisms (for clients who require more specialized Level II care).

Source: Concurrent Disorders Training Strategy Work Group. (2004). *Enhancing Concurrent Disorders Knowledge in Ontario: A Report of the Concurrent Disorders Training Strategy Work Group.* Adapted with permission from the Centre for Addiction and Mental Health.

Level II competencies and capabilities for specialized mental health and/or addiction settings are presented in Table 16-4.

TABLE 16-4

Level II: CD-Enhanced Capacities and Competencies

Capacities	Ability to provide fully integrated mental health and addiction treatment to individuals with a high severity of both issues. CD-specialized clinicians have expertise in comprehensive assessment, treatment and support for concurrent disorders populations, such as people with eating disorders and addiction, borderline personality disorder and addiction, trauma and addiction, schizophrenia and addiction, and others.
Competencies	All Level I competencies, plus the ability to: • administer specialized assessment methods (e.g., Structured Clinical Interview for DSM and procedures • deliver specialized evidence-based therapies (e.g., Seeking Safety, dialectical behaviour therapy; cognitive-behavioural therapy) as developed for targeted concurrent disorders problems • provide specialized consultation to Level I staff • provide clinical training and education in topics relating to the assessment and treatment of concurrent disorders • collaborate on or conduct clinical research in concurrent disorders.

Source: Concurrent Disorders Training Strategy Work Group. (2004). *Enhancing Concurrent Disorders Knowledge in Ontario: A Report of the Concurrent Disorders Training Strategy Work Group.* Adapted with permission from the Centre for Addiction and Mental Health.

CSAT (2005) has also delineated a set of core competencies in mental health for addiction clinicians to help them work with clients with concurrent disorders. The competencies lie on a continuum ranging from basic to intermediate to advanced.

Because of the complexity of concurrent disorders, working collaboratively and having access to peer, team and specialist clinical consultation can be a vital asset to clinicians on the front lines working to enhance their concurrent disorders competence. Having a culture that supports clinical consultation and supervision and that encourages concurrent disorders staff development and capacity building can serve as a stabilizing and supportive platform for clinicians to be more effective with clients.

Psychosocial treatment

The following is a list of commonly used psychosocial treatments.

Psychoeducation
- teaching clients and their families about mental health and substance use issues.

Psychotherapy (individual and group therapy)
- CD-adapted motivational interviewing (Miller & Rollnick, 2009)
- CD-adapted structured relapse prevention (Herie & Watkin-Merek, 2006)
- cognitive-behavioural therapy
    - integrated group therapy (Weiss et al., 2007) for concurrent bipolar and substance use disorder
    - Seeking Safety (Najavits, 2003). This CBT approach has a strong evidence base for people with PTSD and substance use issues[1]
- dialectical behaviour therapy (for concurrent borderline personality disorder and substance use disorder, and for concurrent borderline eating disorder and substance use disorder)[2]
- interpersonal group therapy (Malat & Leszcz, 2005; Sciacca, 2011).

Family support and inclusion
- working with families who are providing care to someone with a concurrent disorder to develop strategies and treatment planning that supports the individual's recovery
- offering support to families while working with them around treatment planning (O'Grady & Skinner, 2007).

Peer support

Consumer-led peer support and mutual aid / self-help groups provide opportunities for people with concurrent disorders to share, connect and learn from one another (Hamilton & Samples, 1995). Examples of mutual aid groups include Double Trouble in

---

1 For more information about Seeking Safety, visit www.seekingsafety.org.
2 For more information about dialectical behaviour therapy, visit www.behavioraltech.org.

Recovery (Vogel, 2010) and the web-based mutual aid group Dual Recovery Anonymous[3] for those who have computer skills and Internet access. Concurrent disorders–focused mutual aid groups can be a useful supplement to treatment for the following reasons:

- There is no charge for affiliation, so money is not a barrier.
- Members can attend as often as needed, for as long as desired.
- There is a social network of welcoming people who share common goals.
- A sponsor system is available for 24-hour support.
- Meetings can help to reduce boredom, provide more structure and minimize the risk of relapse.

Case management

According to SAMHSA (2000), case management involves:

- planning or co-ordinating a package of health and social services to meet a particular client's needs
- ensuring that clients get whatever services they need in a co-ordinated, effective and efficient manner
- helping clients who need assistance from several helpers at once
- monitoring, tracking and providing support throughout treatment and after
- helping the client re-establish an awareness of internal resources such as intelligence, competence and problem-solving abilities
- establishing and negotiating lines of operation and communication between the client and external resources
- advocating with external resources to enhance the continuity, accessibility, accountability and efficiency of those resources (p. 2).

Pharmacological interventions

Pharmacological interventions are an evidence-based treatment or adjunct in the treatment of some concurrent disorders; however, a full review of such medications is well beyond the scope of this book and can be found elsewhere.[4]

Abstinence

Treating substance use problems in the context of concurrent disorders can feel overwhelming. Clinicians naturally have the best interests of clients at heart and want clients to make the healthiest choices possible. For most clients, abstinence from substances, and taking psychiatric medication regularly and as prescribed would be the most reasonable goals for a successful outcome. However, if the clinician frames abstinence as the only acceptable goal for coping with a substance use problem, some clients may feel

---

3 For more information about Dual Recovery Anonymous, visit www.draonline.org.
4 *Concurrent Substance Use and Mental Health Disorders: An Information Guide* (2010) provides an overview of pharmacotherapies for concurrent disorders. The guide can be found at http://knowledgex.camh.net/amhspecialists/resources_families/Documents/concurrent_guide_en.pdf.

discouraged and ill-prepared to give up substances altogether. Because of the chronic, relapsing and remitting nature of substance use and mental health problems, it is unrealistic to expect clients to accept such an extreme goal immediately, although some clients do enter treatment with this readiness and willingness to try.

Strategies for achieving abstinence include:

- stopping cold turkey (this may involve setting a pre-planned quit date)
- tapering quantity and frequency according to a schedule
- following a medically assisted withdrawal management protocol (if warranted), either undertaken as an outpatient or an inpatient depending on level of need and preference
- using an evidenced-based pharmacotherapy as an adjunct to counselling. In Ontario, evidence-based medications are available for the treatment of alcohol dependence (e.g., naltrexone [Revia], disulfiram [Antabuse] or acamprosate [Campral]); opioid dependence (e.g., methadone); and tobacco dependence (e.g., bupropion [Zyban, Wellbutrin] and varenicline [Champix])[5]
- taking a "drug holiday" (a short-term abstinence from one or more drugs). This is often less overwhelming and intimidating than setting a goal of long-term abstinence from *all* drugs, which can feel like a "forever" goal.

In Prochaska and DiClemente's (1984) Stages of Change model, relapse is identified as its own stage. Framed as a "normal" and common part of the change process, the relapse can be used as an opportunity to discuss what led up to and triggered a return to substance use, so the client can learn from the experience and identify what he or she can do differently if a similar situation arises in the future.

Thus, despite the recognized value of abstinence as an "ideal" goal, most clinicians in the field acknowledge the realities of the challenges many clients with concurrent disorders have in attaining abstinence, or in feeling sufficiently motivated to even try to attain it. Despite the challenges, clinicians need to continue to work with these clients, even if—or especially when—they are not able to refrain from substance use. Viewing concurrent disorders with this understanding helps clinicians, clients and their families realize that these are chronic, recurring problems, with no magic bullet solution.

Harm Reduction

The harm reduction model offers the opportunity for flexible goal choice (that may or may not involve abstinence). In practical terms, this means that if a client is not ready or interested in pursuing abstinence as a goal, other goals can be considered. A far more effective strategy involves "working where the client is at," recognizing the importance of engagement and knowing that goals are not static and can change over time. The following are examples of different substance use goals a client may consider within a harm reduction approach:

- abstinence from one drug (e.g., cocaine), but not all drugs (e.g., tobacco).

---

5 For more information about pharmacotherapies that support abstinence, see the *Primary Care Addiction Toolkit* at http://knowledgex.camh.net/primary_care/toolkits/addiction_toolkit/Pages/default.aspx.

- setting a goal for reducing the quantity and frequency of substance use to try to minimize or circumvent negative consequences (e.g., to drink no more than one drink, once a week). People with concurrent disorders, especially those who have more severe forms of dependence, are not as successful at being able to limit their use, but for many clients, having the opportunity to try moderation and reduction can be a useful avenue for then exploring motivation to rethink the value of an abstinence goal. (For more about harm reduction, see Chapter 4.)

A Blended Approach

A blended approach involves having abstinence as the overarching goal, but then using harm reduction strategies in the event of relapse (e.g., no re-use of needles if using).

The "No-Change" Goal

This is a bare-minimum goal designed especially for clients who are mandated into treatment or who do not see their substance use as a problem: the client agrees to at least *monitor* and *discuss* substance use. With this low-threshold goal, there is no requirement to make a change to substance use, but the client must be willing to attend counselling and to monitor and discuss substance use. This enhances the client's awareness and insight during the initial engagement phase, leading to a positive shift in motivation or readiness to change.

Revisiting the Case Study

Returning to the case of Marcello that opened this chapter, imagine you are the worker who is seeing Marcello for the first time for an assessment. As you consider his case, try to apply the concepts you have learned to answer the following questions:

1. What are the various concurrent disorder issues Marcello is experiencing?
2. What etiological model(s) appear(s) to be at play (i.e., how do Marcello's substance use and mental health issues interact and influence one another)?
3. What should you do (or consider) to ensure that Marcello receives care from a culturally sensitive perspective?
4. What assessment questions or tools would you want to use?
5. What should the treatment plan consist of to ensure Marcello receives integrated evidenced-based care for concurrent disorders?

Conclusion

Addiction and mental health care providers have long worked with clients with concurrent disorders, despite often not having the knowledge, skills or resources to work effectively with such complex problems. While integrated services for concurrent disorders are still uncommon in many communities, what is encouraging is that they are indeed growing. Treatment providers are becoming increasingly aware of the importance of screening clients for concurrent disorders and, where identified, providing or linking clients to integrated treatment, where available. With a more collaborative, integrative approach to treating concurrent disorders, the hope is that clinicians will be better prepared to welcome the challenges—and the opportunities—of working with these clients.

Practice Tips

- Embrace the "no wrong door" philosophy.
- Adopt a high index of suspicion for concurrent disorders.
- Engage in systematic screening of concurrent disorders.
- Practise integrated treatment.
- View relapse as a learning opportunity when it occurs.
- Create opportunities for repeated engagement.

Resources

Publications

Canadian Centre on Substance Abuse (CCSA). (2009). *Substance Abuse in Canada: Concurrent Disorders*. Ottawa: Author. Retrieved from www.ccsa.ca/2010%20 CCSA%20Documents/ccsa-011811-2010.pdf

Centre for Addiction and Mental Health. (2006). *Navigating Screening Options for Concurrent Disorders*. Toronto: Author. Retrieved from http://knowledgex.camh.net/ amhspecialists/Screening_Assessment/screening/navigating_screeningcd/Pages/ default.aspx

Mueser, K.T., Noordsy, D.L., Drake, R.E., Fox, L. & Barlow, D. (Eds.). (2003). *Integrated Treatment for Dual Disorders: A Guide to Effective Practice*. New York: Guilford Press.

Skinner, W.J.W. (2005). *Treating Concurrent Disorders: A Guide for Counsellors*. Toronto: Centre for Addiction and Mental Health.

Substance Abuse and Mental Health Services Administration. (2002). *Report to Congress on the Prevention and Treatment of Co-occurring Substance Abuse Disorders and Mental Disorders*. Rockville, MD: Author. Retrieved from www.samhsa.gov/reports/ congress2002/CoOccurringRpt.pdf

References

American Psychiatric Association (APA). (2013a). *Diagnostic and Statistical Manual of Mental Disorders* (5th ed.). Washington, DC: Author.

American Psychiatric Association (APA). (2013b). DSM-5 Facts. Washington, DC: Author. Retrieved from http://dsmfacts.org

Anderson, L.M., Scrimshaw, S.C. & Fullilove, M.T. (2003). Culturally competent healthcare systems: A systematic review. *American Journal of Preventive Medicine, 24,* 68–79.

Brady, K., Killeen, T., Saladin, M., Dansky, B. & Becker, S. (1994). Comorbid substance abuse and posttraumatic stress disorder: Characteristics of women in treatment. *American Journal on Addictions, 3,* 160–164.

Brown, P.J., Stout, R.L. & Gannon-Rowley J. (1998). Substance use disorder–PTSD comorbidity. Patients' perceptions of symptom interplay and treatment issues. *Journal of Substance Abuse Treatment, 15,* 445-448.

Canadian Centre on Substance Abuse (CCSA). (2009). *Substance Abuse in Canada: Concurrent Disorders.* Ottawa: Author. Retrieved from www.ccsa.ca/2010%20 CCSA%20Documents/ccsa-011811-2010.pdf

Canadian Centre on Substance Abuse (CCSA). (2010). *Substance Abuse in Canada: Concurrent Disorders. Highlights.* Ottawa: Author. Retrieved from www.ccsa. ca/2010%20CCSA%20Documents/ ccsa-011813-2010.pdf

Center for Substance Abuse Treatment (CSAT). (2000). *Changing the Conversation— Improving Substance Abuse Treatment: The National Treatment Plan Initiative.* Rockville, MD: Author. Retrieved from http://atforum.com/SiteRoot/pages/ addiction_resources/Natxplan%201.pdf

Center for Substance Abuse Treatment (CSAT). (2005). *Substance Abuse Treatment for Persons with Co-occurring Disorders.* Treatment Improvement Protocol (TIP) series 42. Rockville, MD: Author. Retrieved from www.ncbi.nlm.nih.gov/books/ NBK64197/pdf/TOC.pdf

Centre for Addiction and Mental Health. (2006). *Navigating Screening Options for Concurrent Disorders.* Toronto: Author. Retrieved from http://knowledgex.camh.net/ amhspecialists/Screening_Assessment/screening/navigating_screeningcd/Pages/ default.aspx.

Concurrent Disorders Ontario Network. (2005). *Concurrent Disorders Policy Framework.* Retrieved from www.ofcmhap.on.ca/sites/ofcmhap.on.ca/files/-CDpolicy%20final.pdf

Dennis, M.L., Chan, Y-.F. & Funk, R.R. (2006). Development and validation of the GAIN Short Screener (GAIN-SS) for psychopathology and crime/violence among adolescents and adults. *American Journal on Addictions, 15* (Suppl. 1), 80–91.

Evans, K. & Sullivan, J.M. (1995). *Treating Addicted Survivors of Trauma.* New York: Guilford Press.

Gottheil, E., McLellan, A.T. & Druley, K.A. (1980). *Substance Abuse and Psychiatric Illness.* New York: Pergamon Press.

Hamilton, T. & Samples, P. (1995). *The 12 Steps and Dual Disorders*. Center City, MN: Hazelden.

Health Canada. (2002). *Best Practices: Concurrent Mental Health and Substance Use Disorders*. Ottawa: Author. Retrieved from www.hc-sc.gc.ca/hc-ps/pubs/adp-apd/bp_disorder-mp_concomitants/index-eng.php

Herie, M. & Watkin-Merek, L. (2006). *Relapse Prevention: An Outpatient Counselling Approach* (2nd ed.). Toronto: Centre for Addiction and Mental Health.

Jacobsen, L., Southwick, S. & Kosten, T. (2001). Substance use disorders in patients with posttraumatic stress disorder: A review of the literature. *American Journal of Psychiatry, 158*, 1184–1190.

Kessler, R.C., Berglund, P., Demler, O., Jin, R., Merikangas, K.R. & Walters, E.E. (2005). Lifetime prevalence and age-of-onset distributions of DSM-IV disorders in the National Comorbidity Survey replication. *Archives of General Psychiatry, 62*, 593–602.

Khantzian, E.J. (2003). The self-medication hypothesis revisited: The dually diagnosed patient. *Primary Psychiatry, 10*, 47–48, 53–54.

Khantzian, E.J., Mack, J.E. & Schatzberg, A.F. (1974). Heroin use as an attempt to cope: Clinical observations. *American Journal of Psychiatry, 131*, 160–164.

Malat, J. & Leszcz, M. (2005). Interpersonal group therapy for alcohol dependence. In W. Skinner (Ed.), *Treating Concurrent Disorders: A Guide for Counsellors*. Toronto: Centre for Addiction and Mental Health.

Mee-Lee, D. (2001) *ASAM PPC-2R: ASAM Patient Placement Criteria for the Treatment of Substance-Related Disorders* (2nd ed. rev.). Chevy Chase, MD: American Society of Addiction Medicine.

Miller, W.R. & Rollnick, S. (2009). Ten things that motivational interviewing is not. *Behavioural and Cognitive Psychotherapy, 37*, 129–140.

Ministry of Health and Long-Term Care, Ontario. (2009). *Every Door Is the Right Door: Towards a 10-Year Mental Health and Addictions Strategy*. Toronto: Author. Retrieved from http://health.gov.on.ca

Minkoff, K. (2000). An integrated model for the management of co-occurring psychiatric and substance disorders in managed care systems. *Disease Management & Health Outcomes, 8*, 251–257.

Minkoff, K. (2001a). Developing standards of care for individuals with co-occurring psychiatric and substance use disorders. *Psychiatric Services, 52*, 597–599.

Minkoff, K. (2001b). *Behavioral Health Recovery Management Service Planning Guidelines for Co-occurring Psychiatric and Substance Use Disorders*. Chicago: Illinois Department of Human Services.

Najavits, L.M. (2002). *Seeking Safety: A Treatment Manual for PTSD and Substance Abuse*. New York: Guilford Press.

Najavits L.M. (2003). Seeking Safety: A new psychotherapy for posttraumatic stress disorder and substance use disorder. In P. Ouimette & P. Brown (Eds.), *Trauma and Substance Abuse: Causes, Consequences, and Treatment of Comorbid Disorders* (pp. 147–170). Washington, DC: American Psychological Association Press.

Najavits, L.M. (2004). Assessment of trauma, PTSD, and substance use disorder: A practical guide. In J.P. Wilson & T.M. Keane (Eds.), *Assessment of Psychological Trauma and PTSD* (pp. 466–491). New York: Guilford Press.

Najavits, L.M., Weiss, R.D. & Shaw, S.R. (1997). The link between substance abuse and posttraumatic stress disorder in women: A research review. *American Journal on Addictions 6*, 273–283.

Ogloff, J.R., Lemphers, A. & Dwyer, C. (2006). Dual diagnosis in an Australian forensic psychiatric hospital: Prevalence and implications for services. *Behavioral Sciences and the Law*, 22, 543–562.

O'Grady, C. & Skinner. W.J. (2007). *A Family Guide to Concurrent Disorders*. Toronto: Centre for Addiction and Mental Health.

Prochaska, J. & DiClemente, C. (1984). *The Transtheoretical Approach: Crossing Traditional Boundaries of Therapy*. Homewood, IL: Dow Jones-Irwin.

Regier, D.A., Farmer, M.E. & Rae, D.S. (1990). Comorbidity of mental disorders with alcohol and other drug abuse: Results from the epidemiologic catchment area study. *JAMA, 264*, 2511–2518.

Rush, B.R. & Koegl, C. (2008). Prevalence and profile of people with co-occurring mental and substance use disorders within a comprehensive mental health system. *Canadian Journal of Psychiatry, 53*, 810–821.

Rush, B.R. & Nadeau, L. (2011). Integrated service and system planning debate. In D. Cooper (Ed.), *Responding in Mental Health–Substance Use* (pp. 148–175). London, United Kingdom: Radcliffe Publishing.

Rush, B.R., Urbanowski, K. Bassani, D. Castel, S. Wild, T.C., Strike, C. et al. (2008). Prevalence of co-occurring substance use and other mental disorders in the Canadian population. *Canadian Journal of Psychiatry, 53*, 800–809.

Sciacca, K. (2011). Integrated group treatment for people experiencing mental health–substance use problems. In D. Cooper (Ed.), *Intervention in Mental Health–Substance Use* (pp. 114–127). London, United Kingdom: Radcliffe Publishing.

Shaw-Taylor, Y. & Benesch, B. (1998). Workforce diversity and cultural competence in healthcare. *Journal of Cultural Diversity, 5*, 138–146.

Skinner, W.J.W. (Ed). (2005). *Treating Concurrent Disorders: A Guide for Counsellors*. Toronto: Centre for Addiction and Mental Health.

Smith, D.E. (2012). The process addictions and the new ASAM definition of addiction. *Journal of Psychoactive Drugs, 44* (1), 1–4.

Substance Abuse and Mental Health Services Administration (SAMHSA). (2000). *Case Management for Substance Abuse Treatment: A Guide for Treatment Providers*. Rockville, MD: Author. Retrieved from http://kap.samhsa.gov/products/brochures/pdfs/TIP_27_Desk_Reference.pdf

Substance Abuse and Mental Health Services Administration (SAMHSA). (2002). *Report to Congress on the Prevention and Treatment of Co-occurring Substance Abuse Disorders and Mental Disorders*. Rockville, MD: Author. Retrieved from www.samhsa.gov/reports/congress2002/CoOccurringRpt.pdf

Toronto Drug Strategy Advisory Committee. (2005). *Appendix E—Substance Use in Toronto: Issues, Impacts and Interventions. An Environmental Scan Prepared for the Toronto Drug Strategy Initiative.* Retrieved from www.toronto.ca/health/drugstrategy/pdf/tds_appendix_e.pdf

Torrey, E.F. (1994). Violent behaviour by individuals with serious mental illness. *Hospital and Community Psychiatry, 45,* 653–662.

Valkow, N. (2009). Substance use disorder in schizophrenia: Clinical implications of co-morbidity. *Schizophrenia Bulletin, 35,* 469–472.

Vogel, H. (2010). *Double Trouble in Recovery: Basic Guide.* Center City, MN: Hazelden.

Weiss, R.D., Griffin, M.L., Kolodziej, M.E., Greenfield, S.F., Najavits, L.M., Daley, D.C. et al. (2007). A randomized trial of integrated group therapy versus group drug counseling for patients with bipolar disorder and substance dependence. *American Journal of Psychiatry, 164,* 100–107.

Chapter 17

Working with Clients Who Have Histories of Trauma

Tammy MacKenzie, Robin Cuff and Nancy Poole

Magda is 38 years old, and has two children who are not in her care. She has a 15-year history of substance use problems, which started with alcohol and now include alcohol, benzodiazepines and, most recently, Percocet. Her children's child welfare worker referred her to an addiction treatment agency where she was given information over the phone about how she could "get started." After Magda missed her assessment appointment (she used the night before and was unable to "pull herself together"), the receptionist informed her that she would be placed at the bottom of the waiting list if she missed another appointment. A few days later—after missing her second assessment appointment—Magda called the agency again and was told that, since she had missed two appointments, she would now move to the bottom of the waiting list. Magda, disappointed with herself, went on a two-week binge.

Six weeks later, Magda received a call from the agency and was told that there was a cancellation and she could attend an assessment appointment the next day. Magda attended the appointment. She was accepted into the residential program, but she left the appointment feeling quite overwhelmed by the experience. She was given an admission date and told that she would receive an information package before she entered the program in six weeks. A week before her start date, she received the package in the mail that included the "rules" for her stay in treatment. Magda was concerned that she would have to share a washroom and bedroom. She worried that her roommates would be upset by her insomnia and night terrors, and she was concerned about having to share a washroom.

Staff were warm and welcoming when Magda arrived, but her anxiety increased when they took her belongings into another room to be searched and left her in the reception waiting area. In the program, Magda really enjoyed the psychoeducational modules and felt a connection with her primary therapist. However, she had some difficulty with the process groups, especially when called on to share. Staff felt that Magda was not "working the program" and that they were "working harder than she was," as she was not participating by sharing with the group. They also felt she was disrespectful to staff and fellow clients by consistently being late, despite constant reminders.

In the second week, Magda was asked to leave because staff felt she was not "group ready": they said she wasn't following the rules, was disrespecting other group members and had not disclosed two relapses with Gravol. Staff were aware that she had disclosed trauma in her assessment; however, they did not address it, as Magda had said it did not affect her anymore, and the agency philosophy was to deal with the addiction first and then deal with other issues.

This chapter focuses on the prevalence of trauma among people in treatment for substance use problems. We describe the effects of trauma, and the implications of our work with people who have co-existing substance use problems and experiences of trauma and violence. Throughout the chapter, we use a case study to illustrate the considerations and strategies in working with trauma survivors in substance use treatment settings.

We have become increasingly aware of the powerful impact of traumatic experiences on health and adaptive functioning. Much of the early knowledge about the effects of traumatic events came from people treating war veterans and concentration camp survivors, most of whom were men. The focus expanded in the early 1970s, when the women's movement began to address violence against women and children. Feminist Judith Herman's groundbreaking book *Trauma and Recovery* (1992) greatly advanced our understanding of the multi-layered nature of trauma and recovery, and galvanized action on support and treatment.

This greater awareness of trauma's pervasiveness in the lives of people with substance use and mental health concerns has been accompanied by a better understanding of trauma's potential negative impact on present functioning. We are making advances in designing a continuum of care within mental health and addiction services to prevent further traumatization, and to support and treat survivors of trauma. With contributions from neurobiology, psychology, health equity research and organizational development and health systems planning, we are identifying comprehensive approaches to trauma-informed and trauma-specific interventions.

Connecting the Experience of Trauma with Substance Use Problems

Defining Trauma

Common to definitions of trauma is the understanding that trauma is the result of overwhelming experiences—war, natural disaster, accident or crime; physical, sexual or emotional abuse; or neglect. Herman (1992) describes psychological trauma as an "affliction of the powerless. At the moment of trauma, the victim is rendered helpless by overwhelming force. Traumatic events overwhelm the ordinary systems of care that give people a sense of control, connection and meaning" (p. 33).

Most people who experience a traumatic event are able to integrate the experience and move ahead with their lives. However, some people are unable to achieve this integration and begin to develop the specific patterns of avoidance and hyperarousal that are associated with posttraumatic stress disorder (PTSD). In the *Diagnostic and Statistical Manual of Mental Disorders* ([DSM-IV-TR], American Psychiatric Association [APA], 2000), the criteria used to assign a diagnosis of PTSD were grouped around three clusters of symptoms: intrusive re-experiencing, avoidance and numbing, and increased arousal. In the newly released DSM-5 (APA, 2013), these three areas have been divided into four clusters: intrusion, avoidance, negative alterations in cognitions and mood, and alterations in arousal and reactivity.

Despite their differences, the terms "violence," "trauma," "abuse" and "posttraumatic stress disorder" often are used interchangeably. Trauma expert Stephanie Covington argues that one way to clarify these terms is to think of trauma as a response to violence or some other overwhelmingly negative experience that can but does not necessarily result in PTSD (Covington, 2003, p. 5). Trauma is both an event and a particular response to an event.[1]

Trauma can vary in magnitude, complexity, frequency, duration and interpersonal or external source. Simple- or single-incident trauma relates to an unexpected and overwhelming event such as an accident, natural disaster, single episode of abuse or assault, sudden loss or witnessing violence. Complex or repetitive trauma is a response to ongoing abuse, domestic violence, war, ongoing betrayal or disconnection from one's culture, and often involves being trapped emotionally and/or physically. Developmental trauma results from exposure to early trauma (as infants, children and youth) that involves neglect, abandonment, physical abuse or assault, sexual abuse or assault, emotional abuse, witnessing violence or death and/or coercion or betrayal.

---

1 Psychologist Lori Haskell has contributed greatly to our understanding of trauma and its relevance for the substance use field. She has worked with the Centre for Addiction and Mental Health to produce pamphlets that describe in simple language the effects of trauma (*Common Questions about Trauma*, 2000; *Women: What Do These Signs Have in Common? Recognizing the Effects of Abuse-Related Trauma*, 2004); booklets that describe the importance of integrated support for women (*Bridging Responses: A Front-Line Worker's Guide to Supporting Women Who Have Post-Traumatic Stress*, 2001; *Women, Abuse and Trauma Therapy*, 2004); and a book that provides more in-depth strategies for trauma-related practice (*First Stage Trauma Treatment: A Guide for Mental Health Professionals Working with Women*, 2003). These resources are available through www.camh.ca or http://knowledgex.camh.net.

Prevalence of Trauma and Substance Use Problems

Clinical literature has established clear links between substance use problems and a history of trauma (see Bonin et al., 2000; Mills et al., 2005; Najavits et al., 2003; Ouimette et al., 2000; Wu et al., 2010). These and other studies place the prevalence of trauma histories among people receiving substance abuse treatment between 25 and 90 per cent, depending on the treatment setting, the manner and timing of screening and specific client characteristics.

Women

Among those seeking help for substance use problems, women report past abuse much more frequently than men. In fact, most women in substance use treatment programs report physical and/or sexual abuse over their lifetime, and about one quarter have received a diagnosis of PTSD (Poole, 2007; Savage et al., 2007).

Men and gender differences

Men experience physical abuse more often than sexual abuse, while women report a higher level of sexual victimization and more abuse, both physical and sexual (Ouimette & Brown, 2002). In a U.S. National Comorbidity Study that surveyed a sample of adults in the general population, the estimated lifetime exposure to severe traumatic events was 61 per cent in men and 51 per cent in women (Kessler et al., 1995). Men's experiences of trauma that were most likely to result in PTSD included rape, combat exposure, childhood neglect and childhood physical abuse. Women were more likely than men to develop stress symptoms following rape, sexual molestation and physical attack, being threatened with a weapon or childhood physical abuse. Although men were more likely than women to be exposed to traumatic conditions, women were twice as likely to develop symptoms of PTSD (10 per cent versus five per cent), related to their much higher likelihood of being sexually assaulted. Women are also more prone to long-term alterations in their stress systems, conferring increased vulnerability to adverse trauma-related health outcomes (MacMillan et al., 2001).

Youth

Ballon and colleagues (2001) evaluated the prevalence of reported physical and sexual abuse among youth with substance use problems and found that 50 per cent of females reported having been sexually abused, compared with 10.4 per cent of their male counterparts. Similarly, 50.5 per cent of females had a history of physical abuse, compared with 26 per cent of males. Of those who cited a history of abuse, more females (64.7%) than males (37.9%) reported using substances to cope with this trauma.

Aboriginal people

Haskell and Randall (2009) describe how historical trauma experienced by Aboriginal people in Canada flows from "an unfortunately long list of events" (p. 68), including colonialism, residential schools, loss of custody of children, loss of land and racism. Given the very high prevalence of historical and contemporary trauma experienced by Aboriginal people, Haskell and Randall (2009) argue for a much broader framework that includes an understanding of the social context of trauma and trauma-informed programs to treat alcohol and other substance use issues.

Many people with substance use problems, such as refugees; veterans; people with disabilities; and gay, lesbian, bisexual and trans people, have unique overlapping experiences of trauma. (For the latter group, see Chapter 25 on sexual orientation and gender identity.)

Effects of Trauma

Clients with a trauma history often have a complex array of symptoms. Some clients report intrusive experiences, such as memories of the traumatic episode, distressing dreams or reliving the experience as though it were happening in the present (flashbacks). Others avoid feelings and appear to lack access to their emotions. They may appear emotionally numb or detached from their feelings and actively use distractions to avoid experiencing feelings, especially as they relate to the traumatic experience. Other symptoms include hypervigilance (e.g., having a sense of a dangerous presence), hyperarousal, irritability and exaggerated startle response. Many clients report great difficulty concentrating. They often shift rapidly from a state of emotional constriction to one of hyperarousal and have difficulty moderating their emotional states.

For trauma survivors, substances can, in the short term, be very effective in modulating mood. For example, people who present with a flat affect may use cocaine and other stimulants to increase their energy level and concentration and decrease their sense of emotional numbness. Others may use depressants such as alcohol, heroin and benzodiazepines to decrease their physical, emotional and cognitive states of hyperarousal. These substances may temporarily help to decrease their anxiety and pervasive perception of danger.

Integrated Support and Treatment

Until recently, work on trauma-related issues was considered outside the scope of the substance use counsellor's practice, and substance use issues were considered to be beyond the scope of the trauma counsellor's work. The rationale for that separate or sequential approach was the belief that addressing issues related to trauma in early recovery from substance use problems could precipitate relapse. Similarly, it was believed that people with substance use problems could not reasonably make progress on trauma-related issues when they were still using. More recently, an integrated approach has emerged that acknowledges the links between trauma and substance use problems and embraces some aspects of trauma treatment. For example, Najavits (2002) has designed an integrated treatment model that focuses on developing skills to mitigate trauma-related symptoms, understanding the connections between trauma and substance use and connecting to community services in order to decrease the risk of relapse.

Recovery from substance use problems and recovery from trauma are similar processes, particularly in the first stage. Many of the concrete strategies long employed in substance use treatment help clients achieve safety, develop other coping skills and understand the motivational shifts that accompany the change process. The early stages of trauma treatment, like early treatment for substance use problems, involve establishing safety, developing skills to manage symptoms and understanding how the adaptations initially developed to survive may now be negatively affecting relationships and other aspects of one's life.

In fact, service providers working with people who have mental health, substance use and violence concerns in substance use services, housing shelters, children's mental health programs and many other settings increasingly identify the need to work in "trauma-informed" ways if they are to be helpful to their clients (Poole & Greaves, 2012).

Harris and Fallot (2001) first coined the term "trauma informed" to describe services that consider trauma in all aspects of service delivery and place priority on trauma survivors' safety, choice and control. Others continue to build on Harris and Fallot's work. (e.g., Bloom & Yanosy Sreedhar, 2008; Elliot et al., 2005; Hopper et al., 2010; Prescott et al., 2008). With trauma-informed services, staff attends to issues of safety and empowerment through policies, practices and ways of relating to clients. Safety is considered in every interaction, and confrontational approaches are avoided. Working in a trauma-informed way does not require disclosure of trauma; rather, a trauma-informed approach is taken as a universal precaution, given how pervasive trauma is among people coming for substance use and related health and social services.

Many substance use services also incorporate "trauma-specific" approaches, which directly address the need for healing from traumatic life experiences and facilitate trauma recovery through counselling and other clinical interventions. In the following section, we describe how trauma-informed and trauma-specific work is being achieved in substance use treatment settings to address the needs of clients such as Magda, whose story began this chapter.

Practice Implications

Trauma-Informed Practice

Researchers and clinicians have identified principles of trauma-informed practice, which share similarities with principles underlying evidence-based practices in the mental health and substance use fields. The Canadian Network of Substance Abuse and Allied Professionals (2012) describes the following four principles of trauma-informed practice:

- trauma awareness
- emphasis on safety and trustworthiness
- opportunity for choice, collaboration and connection
- strengths-based and skill building.

Agencies need to consider these principles and ensure an integrated understanding of trauma throughout their programs, as well as incorporating these principles in practice and policy (Klinic Community Health Centre, 2008).

Implementing trauma-informed practice involves a sweeping examination of such factors as policies, procedures, environment, language and program design. In effect, the transformation to a trauma-informed practice takes a change management approach leading to a culture shift. Within this culture, it is automatically assumed that clients have experienced trauma. All practices, therefore, emanate from this assumption. Being trauma informed is not about becoming a trauma counsellor, but about being aware of the impact of trauma and viewing clients and their challenges through a trauma-informed lens.

This section describes how agencies can become more trauma informed to address the needs of clients like Magda for whom a sense of safety and trust is integral to healing and benefiting from treatment.

Magda's experience is fairly typical of clients who attend inpatient addiction treatment programs. With growing understanding of the link between trauma and addiction and from the results of client satisfaction surveys, it is clear that a shift to trauma-informed care addresses the impact of trauma in clients' lives. This requires that agencies examine all aspects of their operations, staffing and physical environment. The next section outlines factors agencies would need to consider in becoming trauma informed.

Information and training

Awareness of trauma and its effects, and a commitment to incorporate this understanding into an agency's practices, would require an ongoing infusion of information, discussion and support at all levels of the organization, rather than limiting this training to static events.

Board awareness and commitment

The board or governing body's awareness and commitment are essential. The governing body could be presented with an "expert panel" outlining best practice principles and relevant sector data, along with client profiles or testimonials. A member of the board could be nominated to champion the change, and trauma survivors could be appointed to the board.

Agency leadership

Administrative and clinical leadership implications need to be considered and included in a strategic planning process, and all leaders need to be trained. Clinical and administrative management personnel with a trauma lens could review all policies and procedures. Trauma-informed policies would need to address such areas as hiring practices, data collection, health and safety, privacy, performance appraisals, supervision model, staff training and development, crisis intervention, client exclusion/inclusion criteria for programs, diversity, property (e.g., layout, decor, safety features) and food services (considering factors such as disordered eating, culture, religion, traditions).

The clinical management team would need intensive training in both trauma-informed care and clinical supervision skills.

Support staff

Integral to the process of becoming trauma informed is providing training for all employees, including support staff, and ensuring consistent understanding and care of clients and a common language regarding care. Support staff includes anyone who may have contact with clients in a non-clinical capacity, such as people working in maintenance, food services, housekeeping and administration. They need to be trained at a level appropriate to their responsibilities, so they do not feel responsible for providing clinical care, but do feel competent and confident in their interactions with clients. Topics discussed could include ensuring a safe physical environment, effective engagement practices, behavioural tolerance, boundaries, handling disclosures, determining the need for clinical assistance, recognizing when they are being personally affected and using supervision and self-care techniques.

Direct service clinical staff

Clinical staff plays a pivotal role in providing trauma-informed care. In addition to receiving the training provided for non-clinical staff, clinical staff also needs intensive training in first-stage trauma treatment and practicum experience for both group and individual counselling. Areas of focus could include strength-based intervention and awareness of transference, personal attitudes, and beliefs and biases.

A key component of clinician training is regularly scheduled clinical supervision. Trauma and related issues and skills need to become standing items on staff meetings, program planning meetings and supervision sessions. Clinical supervision participation could be built in to primary responsibilities and include both supervisor-led and peer supervision.

Individual training plans could be developed and implemented to include cultural competency, concurrent disorders and client-centred modalities such as motivational interviewing, Seeking Safety and mindfulness. Training is planned to create team competence, with specialties represented in individual team members.

The agency would need to explore the effects of vicarious trauma, compassion fatigue and other issues related to working with people with trauma in order to identify information and resources for personal/confidential supports (e.g., an employee assistance program).

The agency would need to use effective supervision processes (e.g., case studies, role plays, observation, peer supervision) for ongoing assessment of staff attributes—recognizing that in a trauma-informed environment, strong provider/client relationships are the foundation for positive outcomes. Assessment should look for development in the following areas: empathy, effective expression of compassion, self-awareness, flexibility, emotional regulation, seeing the client as a teacher and equal participant, and willingness to access supervision.

Clients

Therapists cannot assume that clients who have experienced trauma will necessarily understand or identify their experiences as trauma, or that they will always be compassionate toward the behaviours of others who have experienced trauma. A client education program is part of the design of a trauma-informed service.

The agency could provide pamphlets and other resources, and display posters that provide information about trauma, which demonstrate an understanding of the relationship between trauma and addiction. Information sessions and orientations could include discussions of individual and group safety and tolerance and compassion for fellow program participants. Group norms should be established with client input, regularly reviewed in groups and posted. Therapists can be provided with further client-friendly information to give clients as needed.

Agency environment

People affected by trauma are often hypervigilant and have increased sensitivity and awareness of the physical environment and its impact on their safety and comfort. The agency could conduct an environmental scan and identify areas that would enhance trauma-informed care.

Issues to consider include choice of colours (softer tones), comfort items (e.g., stress balls, pillows), quiet/reflection rooms, posters/messages (about safe space, anti-oppression, LGBTTQ positive), security cameras, exits/entrances (clearly marked), hallways, lighting (no dark corners), emergency instructions/procedures (clearly marked), office set-ups (safe escape route for client) and group room set-ups. The agency could also develop a checklist to be included in monthly health and safety inspections.

Program design

To ensure that program design is in keeping with trauma-informed practice, map a client's journey through the agency using a trauma lens. The major stages would include:

First contact

The agency can identify all "first contact" points, including website, written materials (brochures, publications), voice mail messages, telephone contact and reception.

Written materials and the website should use trauma-informed language.

To make your agency welcoming to clients, write a script for both the voice mail message and for the receptionist who answers the phone. Emphasize ways the receptionist can talk "with," not "at," the (prospective) client on the phone and in person. Include information about what to expect, how to get to the agency, how long the visit will take and who the client will see. Allow for the client to voice concerns and ask questions.

Assessment

Rather than relying on a formal diagnosis of trauma, the assessment process should *assume* trauma. This moves the nature of the questions from "Do you have . . ." probing for symptoms to "What helps you with . . .," which focuses on coping and strengths.

A one-session assessment may not be enough. Staff should explore the client's comfort level with the process and check in to see how the client is feeling during the assessment. Provide information both orally and in writing: keep the written portion short and include the therapist's name and contact information.

Expand the assessment beyond information gathering to provide information that can allay anxiety or stress. Introduce the client to agency staff; discuss confidentiality protocols; and explore the client's comfort with visitors and family contact and involvement. Discuss physical, emotional and psychological safety, including the need for crisis or safety plans and withdrawal management services.

Pre-treatment and wait-lists

Following an assessment, there is often a period of "limbo" in which contact with the client is limited as he or she awaits entry into the treatment program. This wait time is potentially a source of fear and anxiety for clients. The agency could start up a drop-in pre-treatment group and initiate weekly telephone check-in calls to the client to provide some continuity of care between initial contact and the start of treatment.

Treatment and therapeutic interventions

Perhaps the greatest impact of the shift to trauma-informed practice is on the intensive treatment phase in residential settings. Residential programs are traditionally "rich" in rules and restrictions and are often designed with the comfort of the group, rather than of the individual, as the primary concern. Important components of trauma-informed practice such as flexibility become a challenge in residential settings because individual flexibility requires an increase in the skill level of staff to manage group resistance to what may be seen as favouritism. In addition, there is the challenge of nurturing staff's understanding, tolerance and acceptance of clients. The fact that clients "live" at residential facilities means that trauma-informed practices must be in place 24/7, over several shift changes and often with staff with varying skill levels.

On the flip side, aspects of residential programs can actually help clients with trauma by providing 24-hour support, and having certain safety features in place, such as limiting access to the public and screening telephone calls. As an example, women should be served in an all-women environment, where possible; where this is not possible, they should be served by female staff and given gender-specific options (Currie, 2001).

The following list outlines some changes agencies can make to become more trauma informed. Even small changes can make big differences. The first two points relate specifically to residential settings, while the remainder are applicable to all treatment settings.

- Alter the process through which residential facilities search clients' belongings. Although a search for drugs and other paraphernalia may still be necessary for safety reasons, it can be made easier for the client: explain the process and the reason for it to the client; let the client know ahead of time it will happen; ensure that the space where the search is conducted is private; and allow the client to be an active participant by, for example, opening his or her bags.
- Adjust the "rules" in residential programs to allow more flexibility, while still maintaining an environment that is safe and equitable for everyone. Although some rules are non-negotiable (e.g., violence), most rules can be considered guidelines. Part of being less rigid may include taking down posters that contain "do not," "must not" and "cannot" messages. Update handbooks to replace the word "rules" with "rights and responsibilities," whenever possible. For example, instead of "Don't gossip," you could say "You have the right to confidentiality and you have the responsibility to maintain confidentiality on behalf of your fellow clients." Replace "Clean your room" with "You have the right to a clean and comfortable space and you have the responsibility to contribute to the cleanliness and comfort of this shared space."
- Implement a buddy system so that clients do not feel they are navigating the new environment alone.
- Institute a therapist/client matching process.
- Rewrite relapse/lapse policies to consider lapses without negative consequences, recognizing that reducing substance use may result in an increase of PTSD/trauma symptoms. Pay attention to language around lapses and relapses (i.e., refer to urine as "positive" or "negative" for substances, rather than "dirty" or "clean").
- Develop crisis/safety plans with all clients at the beginning of their treatment cycle and give them a copy of their plans, inviting them to touch base with any changes.
- Include in the program such components as grounding and mindfulness, trauma education and a general discussion of trauma as part of clients' lives and journeys. Where possible, give clients a menu of program component options.

Discharge planning

Trauma-informed practices extend from first engagement to beyond completion of the program. Clients may learn to trust a therapist or treatment provider; however, it may still be difficult for clients to transition to the community when they finish treatment.

Starting discharge planning at the beginning of treatment can help ease the transition. Clients' short- and long-term goals can drive this planning. Agencies can institute continuing care programs with discharge planning guided by a "transfer of trust"; for example, a client may be given the name of the service provider at the service to which he or she is referred, the client and therapist could visit agencies together and meetings could be held with the next service provider before treatment ends.

Trauma-Specific Practice

These "change of culture" components require intentional leadership, patience and perseverance. While the process may at times seem arduous, the result will be an environment in which trauma-informed practices become the norm: not something an organization *does*, but rather, something it *becomes*. Trauma-informed practices will be reflected in both direct and indirect client interactions—in case notes, staff discussions and direct interactions with clients.

While clients will be more effectively engaged and stabilized in trauma-informed environments (Morrissey et al., 2005), trauma-specific treatment may be important for many (Hien et al., 2009). Trauma-specific support needs to be seamlessly and effectively linked to services using a trauma-informed approach. According to Haskell (2003), different tasks and therapeutic strategies in phase-oriented trauma treatment are associated with the various phases of therapy.

Building on the groundbreaking work of Herman (1992), Haskell (2009) describes three distinct phases of treatment for complex posttraumatic stress responses:

Phase 1: Therapy focuses on helping clients understand and manage their responses and develop safety and coping skills.

Phase 2: Therapy focuses on helping clients modify and process their memories of the traumatic events.

Phase 3: The final phase of trauma treatment involves going beyond the actual experiences of trauma to address other life issues, such as relationships, work, family, and spiritual and recreational activities (p. 64).

As trauma treatment is a specialized field, most addiction treatment programs will not be mandated to address Phase 2 or 3; however, first-stage trauma approaches can be integrated into the existing design and content of treatment programs. Staff needs to be thoroughly trained and equipped to facilitate first-phase evidence-based interventions.

Haskell (2003) lists the essential components of Phase 1 trauma treatment:

- establishing a therapeutic alliance

- promoting client safety
- addressing the client's immediate needs
- normalizing and validating the client's experiences
- educating the client about posttraumatic stress and treatment
- using a gender-sensitive approach so the damaging ways in which traditional social-ization and gender inequality affect women's lives are recognized
- nurturing hope and emphasizing the client's strengths
- collaboratively generating treatment goals
- teaching coping skills and managing posttraumatic stress responses (intrusive ide-ation, hyperarousal, avoidance, dissociation) (pp. 65–66).

Integrated treatment models and trauma-informed approaches are more effective than treatment as usual, and do not cost more, according to the Women, Co-occurring Disorders and Violence Study (Cusack et al., 2008; Domino et al., 2005; Morrissey et al., 2005). Examples of integrated treatment models in the study include Seeking Safety (Najavits, 2002), the Triad model (Clark et al., 2005) and the Trauma Recovery and Empowerment model (Harris, 1998).

Work with Specific Populations Affected by Trauma

Trauma-informed and trauma-specific practices are being tailored to the needs of dif-ferent populations, spanning gender, race, culture, migration status, disability, sexual orientation, gender identity, age and other differences. As counsellors work in specific contexts, they will need to consider how these differences operate and interact for clients, so they can tailor their approaches. The next section provides one example of adapting practice in a particular context.

Women Who Have Lost Custody of Their Children

Many women whose children are taken into the custody of child welfare suffer a devastating sense of grief and loss. This loss is complicated by feelings of shame, help-lessness, anger and emotional numbness. The fact that the grief is rarely acknowledged as "legitimate" or met with compassion further freezes the experience of these women and heightens their isolation. The apprehension of a child, while it may be necessary, alters a woman's sense of self and can result in many of the symptoms we have come to recognize as trauma and posttraumatic stress.

Unresolved grief as trauma is a newer concept in clinical practice. Bringing a trauma-informed perspective to services for women who have lost custody of their children should start with a more formal acknowledgment that the woman may be struggling with parallel manifestations of both grief and trauma. It is also important to recognize that women with trauma histories are more likely to experience subsequent grief as complex trauma (Cantwell-Bartl, n.d.). This is particularly relevant, since a high proportion of women in substance use treatment have experienced trauma, including physical and sexual abuse (Finkelstein et al., 1997; Health Canada, 2001; Najavits, 2002; Women's Service Strategy Work Group, 2005).

Revisiting the Case Study

Two years have passed since Magda was discharged from the residential treatment program. She continues to use alcohol, benzodiazepines and opiates and has tried repeatedly to regain custody of her children without success. Magda feels that, even though she was discharged from the program, she has made some positive connections and would like to give the program another try.

Magda went on the agency's website and was intrigued by its section on the connection between trauma and addiction, which caused her to wonder about her own circumstances. When Magda reconnected with the agency, the receptionist introduced herself, gave her an assessment appointment and asked her if there was anything she needed to support her in getting there.

Prior to the assessment appointment, staff reviewed Magda's file and discussed how they could better support her through the treatment process. In the assessment, Magda was not asked about her trauma; rather, she was asked what helps her cope with her insomnia and night terrors. She was relieved that the therapist recognized that sharing a bedroom and a washroom could be difficult and discussed strategies to cope with this arrangement. Magda was given an admission date, along with a telephone number for questions, concerns or crisis. Privacy and safety were discussed with her, as were her rights and responsibilities. She was given an opportunity to talk about her concerns and was told that it would be okay if she had questions later. She was also given the name and number of a primary contact person. Magda asked for the same therapist she had the last time. She was informed that her previous therapist was no longer at the agency, but was asked what qualities and style would work best for her, and was assured that her preferences would be considered when assigning her a therapist.

When Magda arrived for her residential stay, she was introduced to staff and taken to a private space and asked if she would help the therapist go through her belongings to make sure there were no items that were unsafe for her or others. She was given a tour of the facility, and was shown the safety measures in place. In Magda's first group, the therapist began the group with a grounding exercise that, to Magda's surprise, helped to lessen her anxiety.

She noticed on the program schedule that there was an optional relaxation/ mindfulness group and a yoga class. Several days into the program, Magda became quite anxious, reminding her of how she had felt two years before. She was becoming agitated with other clients, and arrived late for individual appointments. Her therapist had arranged a meeting with her to check in. Magda was nervous that she would be discharged again. In preparation for the meeting, staff met to discuss how they could better support Magda to ensure that they maximized the benefit of the program to her. They decided to offer Magda a more flexible schedule. Magda's fears were quickly alleviated when she discovered that she was not going to be discharged. She described the experience later as "the first time I felt someone truly understood me."

Conclusion

This chapter discussed efforts to integrate support on trauma-related experiences into work with clients who have substance use and mental health concerns, as well as other issues that affect their health and recovery. We advocate a trauma-informed approach applied as a universal precaution, and which, at the organizational level, is linked closely to trauma-specific treatments. There is no "one-size-fits-all" formula for our work in the substance use field. But given the pervasiveness of trauma and violence among clients, bringing a trauma-informed lens to practice is an important step forward for our field.

Practice Tips

- As a universal precaution, assume a history of trauma for people accessing substance use treatment.
- Identify trauma as having no cultural, racial, gender, age or geographical boundaries.
- Recognize that trauma symptoms are complex and can "masquerade" as inappropriate or unexplained behaviours.
- Integrate trauma-informed principles into all aspects of a service or agency, so they are reflected in the organizational culture.
- Integrate broad trauma-informed agency practices and first-stage trauma approaches into all existing substance use treatment programs.
- Incorporate trauma-informed care as an integral part of substance use treatment.

Resources

Publications

Covington, S.S. (2003). *Beyond Trauma: A Healing Journey for Women*. Center City, MN: Hazelden.

Haskell, L. (2001). *Bridging Responses: A Front-Line Worker's Guide to Supporting Women Who Have Post-Traumatic Stress*. Toronto: Centre for Addiction and Mental Health. Retrieved from http://knowledgex.camh.net/amhspecialists/specialized_treatment/trauma_treatment/bridging_responses/Pages/default.aspx

Haskell, L. (2003). *First Stage Trauma Treatment: A Guide for Mental Health Professionals Working with Women*. Toronto: Centre for Addiction and Mental Health.

Hien, D., Litt, L.C., Cohen, L.R., Meile, G.M. & Campbell, A. (2009). *Trauma Services for Women in Substance Abuse Treatment: An Integrated Approach*. Washington, DC: American Psychological Association.

Najavits, L.M. (2002). *Seeking Safety: A Treatment Manual for PTSD and Substance Abuse*. New York: Guilford Press.

Poole, N. (2012). *Essentials of . . . Trauma-Informed Care*. Ottawa: Canadian Network of Substance Abuse and Allied Professionals. Retrieved from www.cnsaap.ca/SiteCollectionDocuments/PT-Trauma-informed-Care-2012-01-en.pdf

Poole, N. & Greaves, L. (Eds.). (2012). *Becoming Trauma Informed*. Toronto: Centre for Addiction and Mental Health.

Internet

Centre for Addiction and Mental Health Knowledge Exchange portal for professionals—overview of trauma treatment
https://knowledgex.camh.net/amhspecialists/specialized_treatment/trauma_treatment/Pages/default.aspx

Coalescing on Women and Substance Use—trauma-informed online tool
www.coalescing-vc.org/virtualLearning/section1/default.htm

SAMHSA National Center for Trauma-Informed Care
www.samhsa.gov/nctic/

References

American Psychiatric Association. (2000). *Diagnostic and Statistical Manual of Mental Disorders* (4th ed., text rev.). Washington, DC: Author.

American Psychiatric Association (APA). (2013). *Diagnostic and Statistical Manual of Mental Disorders* (5th ed.). Washington, DC: Author.

Ballon, B.C., Courbasson, C.M.A. & Smith, P.D. (2001). Physical and sexual abuse issues among youths with substance use problems. *Canadian Journal of Psychiatry, 46,* 617–621.

Bloom, S.L. & Yanosy Sreedhar, S. (2008). The Sanctuary model of trauma-informed organizational change. *Reclaiming Children & Youth, 17* (3), 48–53.

Bonin, M.F., Norton, G.R., Asmundson, G.J., Dicurzio, S. & Pidlubney, S. (2000). Drinking away the hurt: The nature and prevalence of PTSD in substance abuse patients attending a community-based treatment program. *Journal of Behavior Therapy and Experimental Psychiatry, 31,* 55–66.

Canadian Network of Substance Abuse and Allied Professionals. (2012). *Essentials of . . . Trauma-Informed Care.* Ottawa: Author. Retrieved from www.cnsaap.ca/SiteCollectionDocuments/PT-Trauma-informed-Care-2012-01-en.pdf

Cantwell-Bartl, A. (n.d.). *Is This Person Suffering Grief or Trauma or Traumatic Grief?* Retrieved from www.nevdgp.org.au/files/latestnews/Grief%20Trauma%20or%20Traumatic%20Grief.pdf

Clark, C., Giard, J., Fleisher-Bond, M., Slavin, S., Becker, M. & Cox, A. (2005). Creating alcohol and other drug, trauma, and mental health services for women in rural Florida: The Triad Women's Project. *Alcoholism Treatment Quarterly, 22* (3), 41–61.

Covington, S.S. (2003). *Beyond Trauma: A Healing Journey for Women.* Center City, MN: Hazelden.

Currie, J.C. (2001). *Best Practices: Treatment and Rehabilitation for Women with Substance Use Problems.* Ottawa: Health Canada. Retrieved from www.hc-sc.gc.ca/hc-ps/pubs/adp-apd/bp_women-mp_femmes/report-eng.php

Cusack, K.J., Morrissey, J.P. & Ellis, A.R. (2008). Targeting trauma-related interventions and improving outcomes for women with co-occurring disorders. *Administration and Policy in Mental Health and Mental Health Services Research, 35,* 147–158.

Domino, M., Morrissey, J.P., Nadlicki-Patterson, T. & Chung, S. (2005). Service costs for women with co-occurring disorders and trauma. *Journal of Substance Abuse Treatment, 28,* 135–143.

Elliot, D.E., Bjelajac, P., Fallot, R., Markoff, L.S. & Glover Reed, B. (2005). Trauma-informed or trauma-denied: Principles and implementation of trauma-informed services for women. *Journal of Community Psychology, 33,* 461–477.

Finkelstein, N., Kennedy, C., Thomas, K. & Kearns, M. (1997). *Gender-Specific Substance Abuse Treatment.* Alexandria, VA: National Women's Resource Centre for the Prevention and Treatment of Alcohol, Tobacco, and Other Drug Abuse and Mental Illness.

Harris, M. (1998). *Trauma Recovery and Empowerment: A Clinician's Guide for Working with Women in Groups.* New York: Free Press.

Harris, M. & Fallot, R.D. (2001). *Using Trauma Theory to Design Service Systems.* San Francisco: Jossey-Bass.

Haskell, L. (2003). *First Stage Trauma Treatment: A Guide for Mental Health Professionals Working with Women.* Toronto: Centre for Addiction and Mental Health.

Haskell, L. & Randall, M. (2009). Disrupted attachments: A social context complex trauma framework and the lives of Aboriginal Peoples in Canada. *Journal of Aboriginal Health, 5* (3), 48–99.

Health Canada. (2001). *Best Practices: Treatment and Rehabilitation for Women with Substance Use Problems.* Ottawa: Author.

Herman, J. (1992). *Trauma and Recovery.* New York: HarperCollins.

Hien, D., Litt, L.C., Cohen, L.R., Miele, G.M. & Campbell, A. (2009). *Trauma Services for Women in Substance Abuse Treatment: An Integrated Approach.* Washington, DC: American Psychological Association.

Hopper, E.K., Bassuk, E.L. & Olivet, J. (2010). Shelter from the storm: Trauma-informed care in homelessness services settings. *Open Health Services and Policy Journal, 3,* 80–100.

Kessler, R.C., Sonnega, A., Bromet, E. & Hughes, M. (1995). Posttraumatic stress disorder in the National Comorbidity Survey. *Archives of General Psychiatry, 52,* 1048–1060.

Klinic Community Health Centre. (2008). *Trauma–Informed: The Trauma Toolkit: A Resource for Service Organizations and Providers to Deliver Services That Are Trauma-Informed.* Retrieved from www.trauma-informed.ca

MacMillan, H.L., Fleming, J.E., Streiner, D.L., Lin, E., Boyle, M.H., Jamieson, E. et al. (2001). Childhood abuse and lifetime psychopathology in a community sample. *American Journal of Psychiatry, 158,* 1878–1883.

Mills, K.L., Lynskey, M., Teesson, M., Ross, J. & Darke, S. (2005). Post-traumatic stress disorder among people with heroin dependence in the Australian treatment outcome study (ATOS): Prevalence and correlates. *Drug & Alcohol Dependence, 77,* 243–249.

Morrissey, J.P., Ellis, A.R., Gatz, M., Amaro, H., Reed, B.G., Savage, A. et al. (2005). Outcomes for women with co-occurring disorders and trauma: Program and person-level effects. *Journal of Substance Abuse Treatment, 28,* 121–133.

Najavits, L.M. (2002). *Seeking Safety: A Treatment Manual for PTSD and Substance Abuse.* New York: Guilford Press.

Najavits, L.M., Runkel, R., Neuner, C., Frank, A.F., Thase, M.E., Crits-Christoph, P. & Blaine, J. (2003). Rates and symptoms of PTSD among cocaine-dependent patients. *Journal of Studies on Alcohol and Drugs, 64,* 601–606.

Ouimette, P.C. & Brown, P.J. (Eds.). (2002). *Trauma and Substance Abuse: Causes, Consequences and Treatment of Comorbid Disorders.* Washington, DC: American Psychological Association.

Ouimette, P.C., Kimerling, R., Shaw, J. & Moos, R.H. (2000). Physical and sexual abuse among women and men with substance use disorders. *Alcoholism Treatment Quarterly, 18,* 7–17.

Poole, N. (2007). Interconnections among women's health, violence and substance use: Findings from the Aurora Centre. In N. Poole & L. Greaves (Eds.), *Highs & Lows: Canadian Perspectives on Women and Substance Use* (pp. 211–212). Toronto: Centre for Addiction and Mental Health.

Poole, N. & Greaves, L. (Eds.). (2012). *Becoming Trauma Informed.* Toronto: Centre for Addiction and Mental Health.

Prescott, L., Soares, P., Konnath, K. & Bassuk, E. (2008). *A Long Journey Home: A Guide for Generating Trauma-Informed Services for Mothers and Children Experiencing Homelessness.* Rockville, MD: Substance Abuse and Mental Health Services Administration, The Daniels Fund, National Child Traumatic Stress Network & W.K. Kellogg Foundation.

Savage, A. Quiros, L., Dodd, S. & Bonavota, D. (2007). Building trauma informed practice: Appreciating the impact of trauma in the lives of women with substance abuse and mental health problems. *Journal of Social Work Practice in the Addictions, 7,* 91–116.

Women's Service Strategy Work Group. (2005). *Best Practices in Action: Guidelines and Criteria for Women's Substance Abuse Treatment Services.* Toronto: Ministry of Health and Long-Term Care, Ontario.

Wu, N.S., Schairer, L.C., Dellor, E. & Grella, C. (2010). Childhood trauma and health outcomes in adults with comorbid substance abuse and mental health disorders. *Addictive Behaviors, 35* (1), 68–71.

Chapter 18

Acquired Brain Injury and Fetal Alcohol Spectrum Disorder: Implications for Treatment

Carolyn Lemsky and Tim Godden

Daniel is a 48-year-old married plumber from Toronto who has been convicted twice for impaired driving. Probation referred Daniel to a community-based addiction agency for treatment following the second conviction. The referral form includes the statement: "Client is mandated to attend treatment for alcohol abuse," but provides little more background information. In extending a welcome to Daniel in the waiting room, Olena, a staff member at the addiction agency, says: "How are you doing today?" Daniel replies: "This is a big misunderstanding. Let's get this over with." Daniel is accompanied to the appointment by Dana, his spouse of 20 years, who asks to be included in the assessment interview because "Daniel sometimes forgets important details." Daniel's body language seems to indicate that he's not entirely comfortable with this prospect.

This chapter provides an introduction to acquired brain injury (ABI) and fetal alcohol spectrum disorder (FASD). Although the causes, natural history and outcome of each are very different, they are addressed together because people with these conditions share some important characteristics when it comes to treatment for substance use problems. ABI and FASD are very common comorbidities in people seeking help for substance use problems. But both are in some sense "invisible disabilities" that may go undiagnosed in their milder forms. And their cognitive and behavioural presentations are often construed as a lack of motivation for treatment.

FASD and ABI may be difficult to confirm based on history alone. When signs of cognitive impairment are evident, the clinician should expect that the client's history may contain elements of ABI, FASD or both. It is less critical to understand the source of the neurocognitive impairment than it is to recognize when the impairment may influence an intervention's effectiveness, and to accommodate accordingly.

We begin with overviews of ABI and FASD. Implications for intervention are addressed in the last part of the chapter. We also provide information about "disability etiquette," which can be applied to any person with a disability.

The case study of Daniel is used throughout the chapter to illustrate how clinicians can address neurological impairment in care planning, regardless of its cause. As with many neurological impairments, memory problems are just one of the difficulties the client and family will be forced to cope with after a brain injury. The question of whether there are other sources of impairment that should be explored—including FASD—can only be answered through detailed inquiry.

Acquired Brain Injury

ABI is generally defined as an insult to the brain due to trauma, infection or disease. In most cases, it excludes genetic or congenital conditions, or progressive conditions such as multiple sclerosis or dementia. The impact of brain injury can be subtle or quite dramatic, affecting emotional regulation, self-management and cognition. Traumatic brain injury (TBI) refers to that subset of injuries that is the direct result of trauma, such as a fall or motor vehicle accident. Non-traumatic injuries include medical conditions such as stroke, anoxia (loss of oxygen to the brain) and neurotoxic injuries (e.g., the damage caused by drugs or other toxic agents) and infection.

Variables That Affect the Outcome of ABI

The outcome of an ABI depends on a number of factors, including the cause of the injury, its severity, the part of the brain affected, the age at which the injury was sustained, and the person's pre-injury status and life circumstances.

Traumatic brain injury

The severity of TBI is generally associated with the length of time the person loses consciousness and/or how long he or she remains in an altered mental state. Injuries may range from mild (momentary or no loss of consciousness) to severe (up to several months in coma). Concussions are mild TBIs that result in brief loss of consciousness and rapid return to a non-confused state. Depending on the severity of the concussion, the person may experience lingering symptoms that include fatigue, irritability, headache, changes in balance, ringing in the ears and reduced attention, concentration and memory. However, in the vast majority of cases, these symptoms will also clear within months.

More severe TBIs may result in disturbances of any brain-related function, including memory, executive functioning, physical mobility, visual perception, self-regulation and the ability to process information associated with emotion. About 75 per cent of TBIs that come to the attention of medical professionals are mild, and people recover within months to their usual state of functioning (National Center for Injury Prevention and Control, 2003). However, in recent years we have become aware that even apparently mild traumatic injuries (those with a relatively brief loss of consciousness or period of posttraumatic confusion) can result in subtle, but significant changes in personality, self-awareness and self-management—even when there are no obvious changes in intelligence, language and memory (Iverson, 2010).

Non-traumatic brain injury

Some non-traumatic acquired injuries, such as stroke, may not be associated with coma, but have very serious cognitive consequences. Strokes, which may be the result of blood clotting or bleeding in the brain, vary widely in severity. The larger the area of the brain affected, the more cognitive problems will be evident. Transient ischemic attacks (TIA), sometimes called "mini strokes," are brief events in which stroke-like symptoms occur, but last less than 24 hours. However, symptoms lasting longer generally indicate permanent damage. Natural recovery after a stroke does occur, and the period of rehabilitation and recovery may last from months to years, depending on the severity of the stroke.

Anoxic injuries, and those associated with infection, also vary greatly in severity. With the most severe injuries, the person may go into a coma, followed by a period of recovery, the length of which is determined by the severity of the anoxic event or infection. Milder cases may result in an initial period of confusion, followed by rapidly improving mental function. People with more severe cases require a longer recovery and may never recover completely.

What ABI Looks Like

The impairments that arise from an ABI can be categorized as sensory, physical, communication, cognitive and behavioural. Difficulties in any of these categories may range in severity from very subtle to very severe, and may occur in any combination. Examples of sensory, physical and communication problems are provided in Table 18-1.

TABLE 18-1

ABI-Related Sensory, Physical and Communication Problems

TYPE OF IMPAIRMENT	COMMON CLINICAL PRESENTATION
Sensory	Vision changes, including double vision and neglect of visual information (usually on the left side)
	Hearing loss
	Changes in, or loss of, sense of smell and taste
	Body temperature disturbance
	Chronic pain

TYPE OF IMPAIRMENT	COMMON CLINICAL PRESENTATION
Physical	Total or partial paralysis, with partial usually affecting one side
	Fatigue
	Poor visual–motor co-ordination
	Tremor
	Headaches
	Seizures
	Balance disturbance
Communication	Slurred speech
	Reading or writing difficulties
	Expressive disorder
	Word-finding difficulties
	Difficulty understanding

While problems with sensory, physical and communication functioning may be apparent and very difficult to live with after a brain injury, it is often the behavioural or "personality" changes that pose the greatest threat to productive living. Because ABI survivors may retain most of their intellectual abilities, and may demonstrate only minimal or no physical impairment, ABI can be an invisible disability. It is our clinical experience that people with severe traumatic injuries or medical conditions that result in overt changes in motor functioning and cognition are most likely to be recognized by professionals as having specialized needs. By contrast, the needs of people with relatively subtle difficulties are least likely to be recognized and accommodated. We therefore focus on the most common cognitive and behavioural difficulties encountered in a sub-stance use treatment setting.

Cognitive functioning post-injury

Specific examples of cognitive impairments among people with ABI are listed in Table 18-2. Screening for cognitive impairments is discussed later in the Practice Implications section, along with suggestions for managing them. When someone seems to be having trouble attending appointments, living by program guidelines and following straightfor-ward instructions or advice, cognitive impairment should be suspected.

TABLE 18-2
ABI-Related Cognitive Impairment

TYPE OF COGNITIVE IMPAIRMENT	COMMON CLINICAL PRESENTATION
Mental fatigue	Yawning and increased inattention after a relatively short period of work
Impaired attention and concentration	Tangential speech Easily distracted
Memory loss	Poor retention of information across settings Repeating stories and questions Paranoid behaviour (belief that others are taking objects or being untruthful about events)
Planning difficulties	Missed appointments Poor follow-through
Cognitive rigidity	Difficulty changing topics Inability to interpret metaphors Stubborn adherence to ideas

Subtle changes in the brain's capacity to recognize social cues, connect emotional information to thought processes and perform complex executive functions may result in devastating changes in social behaviour and decision-making (Damasio, 1994; Koenigs et al., 2007). Some of these changes are listed in Table 18-3.

TABLE 18-3
ABI-Related Impairments in Emotional and Behavioural Functioning

BEHAVIOURAL DIFFICULTY	COMMON CLINICAL PRESENTATION
Impaired capacity to process reward and consequences	Demonstrates greater than average disparity between stated intentions and actual behaviour, based on pronounced difficulty delaying gratification
Reduced sensitivity to social cues	Dominates discussion and interrupts others Seems to lack empathy Asks intrusive questions Is overly personal

BEHAVIOURAL DIFFICULTY	COMMON CLINICAL PRESENTATION
Reduced initiation	Reports difficulty in getting started Spends days in passive activities, such as watching TV, despite stated goals
Irritability or aggression	Angers quickly over trivial matters Is verbally abusive
Emotional lability	Laughs or cries in a manner that seems out of proportion to the situation
Lack of awareness	Seems unaware of a difficulty or seems unconcerned about problems he or she is able to name (difficult to differentiate from denial)
Disinhibition	Behaves in a way that seems childish or out of place Bluntly expresses opinions, makes sexually inappropriate remarks or behaviours

In the healthy human brain, the connections between the frontal lobes and other brain structures, such as the limbic system deep in the temporal lobe responsible for processing memory, emotion and pleasure, ensure co-ordination of all the brain's activities, and result in behaviour that is appropriately responsive to the environment. Simply put, the ability to think things through before acting, determine which behaviours will produce a desired long-term payoff, inhibit less productive behaviours and ignore distractions requires a frontal lobe that is in good working order and connected to the rest of the brain.

The frontal and temporal lobes are particularly vulnerable to traumatic injury because they are situated over sharp bony structures in the skull. When the brain is shaken, neural connections may be damaged, resulting in injuries referred to as diffuse axonal shearing (e.g., Alexander, 1995). These injuries disrupt the connections among brain structures and may result in subtle but widespread changes in cognitive and behavioural functioning, such as those listed in Tables 18-1 and 18-2. Direct injury to the frontal and temporal lobes, and diffuse axonal injury affecting structures deep in the brain, can result in changes in the ability to organize and regulate behaviour, while sparing basic abilities, such as speech, movement and visual-spatial abilities (Stuss & Levine, 2002). The pattern of damage resulting from non-traumatic injury varies from person to person, and disease to disease. For example, some infections may have widespread effects on functioning, while others may only affect structures responsible for memory. Strokes tend to affect one side of the brain and usually include physical as well as cognitive problems.

Psychiatric symptoms post-injury

The most common psychiatric symptoms to develop after brain injury, affecting as many as half of survivors, are anxiety and depression (Draper et al., 2007). However, some of the behavioural symptoms typically associated with depressed mood, such as reduced initiation and flat affect, may be directly related to damage to the frontal and temporal lobes, and can occur without depressed or anxious mood. Other cognitive and behavioural difficulties, such as inattention, impulsivity, changes in sleep/wake cycles and irritability, can also mimic psychiatric symptoms but be directly caused by damage to structures deep in the brain. For example, suspiciousness resulting from impairments of memory and reasoning is common and can easily be mistaken for paranoia associated with psychosis. It is also common for people with neurocognitive impairments to express unusual beliefs or even hallucinations that have their origin in altered sensory functioning. Confabulation (filling in gaps in knowledge without awareness of doing so) often occurs, and can have the appearance of delusional thinking or intentional deception. Some of the personality changes common after brain injury (e.g., tendencies to be egocentric and non-empathic) may easily be mistaken for a personality disorder. When there is a history of brain injury, the client may not respond in the expected way to standard care, and specialized consultation is warranted.

Awareness of disability after brain injury

Since cognitive impairments are the result of brain damage, and it is the brain that we use to evaluate our own abilities, it is not surprising that difficulties with self-awareness are common after ABI. Certainly that is true of Daniel from our case study. In their most extreme forms, problems with awareness may cause people with ABI to entirely deny having any difficulties with physical or mental functioning. More often, problems with awareness are subtler. For example, it is not unusual for a person to have difficulty recognizing the extent to which changes in attention and memory affect day-to-day functioning, even if the person reports having problems in this area. Some difficulties associated with awareness are directly related to brain functioning. This is because having full awareness of a cognitive difficulty requires recollection of the problems caused and integration of that memory into a person's self-concept. These are among the most complex and delicate cognitive functions.

Psychological factors can also affect awareness of disability. The emotional losses that result from injury cannot be ignored. It often takes many years to learn how to live with the impact of disability in a way that allows the person to accept support, have a positive self-image and set realistic goals. People often cope with their losses by avoiding problematic situations or denying a problem exists.

The most difficult types of cognitive problems to become aware of and compensate for appropriately are those that affect social functioning, long-term planning and initiation. Providing feedback and demonstrating how to use compensation strategies will often improve performance, and should be considered the best initial strategy.

However, when the person seems to be unaware of neurocognitive impairment and will not discuss ways to compensate for it, consultation with a brain injury expert is often necessary. In general, a person with little awareness of the disability needs more help from others. For example, instead of expecting a client to make in-session notes, the therapist may need to begin sessions by reviewing what was discussed in previous sessions, and provide notes for the client to review between sessions. Other strategies are discussed later in this chapter.

At a minimum, it is important to realize that changes in cognitive and emotional regulation are common after brain injury and that their subtle presentation can easily be mistaken for problems in personality, adjustment and motivation. In many cases, what separates the brain injury survivor from others served in addiction programs is more a matter of severity than of the nature of the problem. For example, survivors of brain injury often have difficulty reading facial expressions, and may appear egocentric due to problems attending to subtle social cues. Although being insensitive to cues may be common, the person may appear to entirely ignore or grossly overreact to feedback. Some seem to have difficulty weighing the relative importance of a particular circumstance and respond with equal intensity (or apathy) to everything they encounter. The most damaging aspect of emotional dysregulation, however, may be increased sensitivity to immediate rewards, which makes it very difficult for the person to attend to the long-term consequences of behaviour, and may even prevent him or her from doing so. When this is the case, people with brain injury (and, as described below, those whose brains have been injured by substance use) depend much more on environmental cues compared to the average person (see reviews in Feeney, 2010, and Stuss, 2011).

The Link between Brain Injury and Substance Use Problems

The link between brain injury and substance use is undeniable, with evidence suggesting that each may contribute to the other.

Brain Injury in People Seeking Treatment for Substance Use Problems

North American studies have found that 38 to 63 per cent of clients in addiction programs report a history of brain injury (see review in Corrigan et al., 2005). In the largest of these studies, Walker and colleagues (2007) found that 32 per cent of their rural sample of 7,784 adults seeking addiction treatment reported one or more head injuries resulting in loss of consciousness. According to the Addiction Severity Index, people reporting two or more injuries were more likely to have serious mental health problems and to have used substances longer. In a follow-up study of 51 people admitted to a program for comorbid substance use and serious mental illness, Corrigan and Deutschle (2008) found that 72 per cent had a history of TBI. Admission criteria included a history of repeated inpatient admissions and/or legal involvement. The authors found that participants with a history of TBI had more severe and complex psychiatric symptoms and an increased likelihood of being diagnosed with an Axis II personality disorder. A history of TBI was also associated with earlier onset of problematic substance use. Having more injuries and experiencing the first injury at an earlier age were also associated with more severe symptoms.

Substance Use History in People with a Brain Injury

A recent systematic review found that between 30 to 51 per cent of adolescents and adults with brain injuries requiring hospitalization have a pre-injury history of substance use problems (Parry-Jones et al., 2006). Given the impact of intoxication on judgment, cognition and motor co-ordination, it isn't surprising that people with substance use problems are at an increased risk of brain injury, resulting in reduced cognitive functioning.

Alcohol

American and Australian research reveals that alcohol use declines for the first year or two after substantial brain injury (Ponsford et al., 2007; Taylor et al., 2003)—during a period of active rehabilitation and recovery. For those who receive medical treatment after brain injury, a period of abstinence from alcohol use—traditionally one year—is recommended. Reduced alcohol use may be related to clients' adherence to professional recommendations and their reduced overall abilities in the early days following injury. Studies that prospectively followed survivors of brain injury for more than the traditional six months to one year post-injury found gradually increasing rates of alcohol use and alcohol use problems, although their reported use of substances other than alcohol did not return to pre-injury levels (Ponsford et al., 2007; Taylor et al., 2003).

Bombardier and colleagues (2003) found that, overall, people hospitalized for ABI decreased their alcohol intake in the first post-injury year. They also reported that those with a pre-injury history of drinking problems were more than 10 times more likely than the general population to exhibit problematic alcohol use during the first post-injury year. Alcohol use problems after brain injury have been associated with re-injury, poorer psychosocial outcomes and unemployment (Parry-Jones et al., 2006; Taylor et al., 2003).

Other substances

The substance use literature on epidemiology and treatment for survivors of brain injury has focused primarily on alcohol use. Little is known about the use of marijuana and other street drugs. Stimulants, opioids and benzodiazepines are often prescribed after brain injury to address fatigue, chronic pain, anxiety and difficulty sleeping. While survivors of brain injury may be particularly vulnerable, the risks of addiction, misuse or abuse of prescribed medications in this group have not been studied (Graham & Cardon, 2008). Although strong evidence is lacking, it is generally recognized that clinicians should be aware of the potential for increased sensitivity to prescribed medications and other drugs, in addition to the risks associated with mixing alcohol with prescribed medications.

Risk factors for developing substance use problems

There is consensus in the literature that a pre-injury history of moderate to heavy alcohol use, higher functional status post-injury and long-term unemployment (Graham & Cardon, 2008) are risk factors for substance use problems after brain injury.

While we lack direct evidence for why and how some people develop new problems with substance use after brain injury, there are two possible mechanisms for increased risk of substance addiction or misuse. First, it has been speculated that difficulties with self-regulation resulting from injury are a direct cause of vulnerability to substance use problems (Corrigan et al., 2010). There is some evidence that changes in the functioning of brain centres known to affect executive functioning, including behavioural regulation, decision-making, judgment, working memory and processing rewards and punishment (prefrontal and orbital-frontal cortex) are associated with the development of substance misuse. For example, impulsivity and difficulties with self-monitoring social behaviour and anticipating consequences when sober may be amplified when the person is intoxicated.

It has also been suggested that the increased psychosocial stressors that accompany long-term disability in combination with cognitive changes increase risk for problematic substance use (Graham & Cardon, 2008; Walker et al., 2007). Changes in emotional regulation and cognitive problems often limit flexible and productive options for coping with negative mood. The increased incidence of strong, uncontrolled affect after brain injury may then set the stage for a greater incidence of substance use. Supporting this hypothesis, Walker and colleagues (2007) found that brain injury survivors are more likely than the general population to use substances to dull unwanted emotional responses such as grief and anger.

Age is another risk factor for substance use problems. Most traumatic brain injuries occur in adolescence and young adulthood (National Center for Injury Prevention and Control, 2003). This is a period of development when binge drinking is a very common social practice. It may be that sustaining a brain injury at this young age makes it less likely that the person will move away from binge drinking. The physical and psychosocial changes that come with brain injury may also be a predisposing factor. Depressed mood, loss of important relationships and unemployment are common after brain injury.

Post-injury vulnerability to substance use problems may occur regardless of the age at which the injury happened. Therefore, it is important to ask about and pay attention to injuries that occurred early in life. Children who appeared to have made a reasonably good recovery from an early injury often develop problems associated with self-regulation and judgment that only become apparent when they fail to develop age-appropriate behaviour (Anderson & Catroppa, 2005). The capacity for self-regulation usually develops gradually, and nears completion in early adulthood, but can be interrupted by a brain injury in adolescence. The end result may be an adult who continues to demonstrate the impulsivity, risk taking and social skills of an adolescent.

Combined with psychosocial difficulties, even a mild brain injury may predispose a person to substance use problems (Bjork & Grant, 2009). The effects of brain injuries are additive; the data suggests that people presenting for addiction treatment who have a history of more than one brain injury are more likely to have serious symptoms of mental illness and difficulty managing violent behaviour and cognitive symptoms (Walker et al., 2007). They also have the longest histories of substance use problems.

While most substance use after brain injury seems to be a resumption of a previous pattern of problematic substance use, an estimated 20 per cent of brain injury survivors develop a new substance use problem (see review in Corrigan & Cole, 2008). Daniel from our case study would appear to fall under this latter category. His spouse, Dana, reports that up until about three years ago, Daniel was a "light social drinker," consuming four or five beer in a typical week, generally on the weekend while socializing. After the accident, Daniel began drinking nearly every day, generally three to five drinks—more on the weekend. Even a small amount of alcohol seems to have a pronounced effect on his behaviour. A pattern has developed where Daniel goes to a bar with colleagues after work, stays after they leave, has a second beer and then buys more beer on the way home to continue drinking. He reports that drinking helps him cope with the fact that he is no longer a supervisor at work, and cannot do what he used to do. He admits to occasionally having an open beer in the car. Dana describes Daniel as "an angry drunk." She says his verbal abuse while intoxicated has brought her to the point of considering leaving the marriage.

Substance Use–Related Brain Impairment

Even when there is no specific history of ABI, injury to the brain as the direct result of substance use is common.

Alcohol

Imaging studies of people with substance use disorders have consistently demonstrated cerebral atrophy (e.g., see review in Bates et al., 2002). This damage seems to be worse for up to 80 per cent of people with chronic alcohol problems who are deficient in thiamine (Bates et al., 2002), but can also occur in people without nutritional deficiencies or liver damage (Harper, 2009). An acute form of cognitive impairment associated with thiamine deficiency can result in Wernicke's encephalopathy, a condition that includes confusion, changes in muscle functioning around the eye and generally disturbed muscle co-ordination. The condition is to some extent reversible with abstinence and improved nutrition. In its more severe form, the Wernicke's encephalopathy can lead to Korsakoff's psychosis, an irreversible condition in which the person has profound difficulty creating new memories and with motor co-ordination.

In outpatient settings, the milder form of alcohol-related brain dysfunction typically encountered has a much more subtle presentation with an insidious onset. Studies of older adults (age 45 and older) with daily, heavy alcohol use suggest that the regions of the brain that seem to be most susceptible to damage are the areas of the brain responsible for higher-order executive functions (pre-frontal cortex) and memory and emotional functioning (temporal cortex), as well as areas responsible for co-ordination and sensory integration (Bates et al., 2002; Harper, 2009; Hermens et al., 2013). A smaller number of studies with younger people with alcohol use disorders show similar patterns of brain changes in both binge drinkers and those with daily use patterns (Hermens et al., 2013).

The cognitive functions most affected by chronic alcohol use are those that require conscious effort in order to process novel information, as well as the ability to focus attention and to divide or shift attention in a flexible way (Green et al., 2010; Hermens et al., 2013). For example, the tendency to ignore long-term risk for immediate gain as measured by simulated gambling tasks has been found to be impaired in studies of alcohol-using adolescents (Hermens et al., 2013) and alcohol-using adults (Loeber et al., 2009). Cognitive impairments associated with chronic alcohol use are typically found alongside intellectual ability that is in the broad range of average. The ability to perform automatic or over-learned cognitive processes also seems to be relatively unaffected by alcohol use (Bates, 2002).

Cognitive functions affected by chronic alcohol use include:
- learning new information for immediate recall
- recalling newly learned information after a delay
- problem solving using non-verbal materials
- working memory (using information held in mind)
- abstract reasoning
- evaluation of risk versus reward
- cognitive control (shifting attention, selective attention).

There is a significant overlap between the symptoms of mild TBI and chronic alcohol use. Two studies found that these clinical groups cannot be reliably distinguished from one another on the basis of cognitive testing (Iverson et al., 2005; Lange et al., 2008). As described above, substance use is a risk factor for sustaining a brain injury resulting in a high number of people who have a history of both the milder forms of brain injury and of heavy substance use, which may account for some of the observed similarities between these two groups. However, the impairments listed above are known to occur in those without a reported history of brain injury (Bates et al., 2013).

There is no clear answer to how much alcohol must be consumed to result in brain injury. There appears to be an interaction between a person's overall health and pre-existing characteristics. However, the studies reviewed above were all conducted among people seeking treatment for substance use problems. While there is some conflicting evidence, most research has found a dose-response relationship, in which the longer the substance use problem has existed, the greater the neurological changes (Harper, 2009). Evidence suggests that alcohol may also have a particularly damaging impact on developing brains: damage may occur at a lower threshold of use in adolescents and may establish a pattern of cognitive impairment with lasting psychosocial and neurocognitive problems (Hermens et al., 2013).

Recovery from alcohol-related brain impairment does seem to occur, particularly in the first two years of abstinence. The early months of abstinence are a period of rapid recovery with noticeable improvements; however, slower ongoing improvements may be observed for several years after abstinence begins (Bates et al., 2002). The ability to evaluate risks and benefits as measured by a gambling task (Loeber et al., 2009) and verbal learning are among the first issues to resolve, while changes in perceptual-motor skills (visual-spatial problem solving) and abstract reasoning may persist (Bates et al., 2002).

Other substances

Evidence suggests that some substances may actually create impairments in executive functions of the brain. As with alcohol use, the tendency to ignore long-term risk for immediate gain, as measured by simulated gambling tasks, is associated with cocaine (Cunha et al., 2011) and methamphetamine (Walker et al., 2007) in the absence of a known history of brain injury. Using single photon emission computed tomography, researchers have found that compared to healthy controls, people with cocaine addiction showed reduced activity in the orbital-frontal cortex, which is responsible for the integration of decision-making and social behaviour (Adinoff, 2004). Studies conducted over the past 20 years have suggested that the lasting cognitive effects of marijuana include reduced cognitive speed, and impaired attention, concentration, short-term memory and executive functioning (see review in Sofuoglu et al., 2010).

Whether as a direct result of brain injury or substance use, or a combination of the two, some degree of cognitive inefficiency or impairment is found in most people seeking treatment for alcohol use problems (Bates et al., 2002; Green et al., 2010; Harper, 2009). If we consider chronic alcohol and other substance use as a brain insult, then people who use substances while recovering from a brain injury can be, quite literally, adding insult to injury.

Fetal Alcohol Spectrum Disorder

The effects of alcohol on a developing fetus seem largely to depend on the extent and timing of the exposure, but other factors, such as the mother's diet and age, are thought to be important as well. The lifelong symptoms of FASD range in type and severity from mild learning disabilities and abnormalities in social behaviour to severe physical and mental disabilities (Riley et al., 2011). FASD is not a medical diagnosis, but an umbrella term used to refer to the group of disorders that result from prenatal exposure to alcohol (see Table 18-4). FASD includes fetal alcohol syndrome (FAS), alcohol-related birth defects (ARBD) and alcohol-related neurodevelopmental disorders (ARND).

FAS, the most often recognized and diagnosed form of FASD, is associated with growth retardation; characteristic facial features, including reduction of the ridges under the nose and above the lips (philtrum), broad forehead, smaller chin, small head, folds extending from the eyelids to the nose; and changes in the central nervous system (Chudley et al., 2005). Partial FAS may be diagnosed when some of the facial features are not present but other symptoms are observed. ARBD can include congenital malformations, such as heart defects, skeletal abnormalities, renal dysfunction, eye problems and hearing impairment. It is diagnosed when a complex of behavioural and cognitive abnormalities consistent with fetal alcohol exposure is present. Fetal alcohol effects (FAE) is a less common term used to refer to children for whom there is a confirmed or suspected history of maternal prenatal alcohol use, but who do not have the physical characteristics of FASD or obvious ARND. These children are generally of average intellectual ability, but exhibit some of the social and behavioural difficulties associated with FASD.

TABLE 18-4

FASD Diagnostic Categories and Related Features

CATEGORY	FEATURES
Fetal alcohol syndrome (FAS)	Confirmed maternal exposure Evidence of facial anomalies Growth retardation Neurodevelopmental abnormalities (evidence of alcohol-related birth defects)
Alcohol-related birth defects (ARBD)	Congenital anomalies, including malformations and dysplasias affecting the heart, skeletal system, kidneys, vision and hearing
Alcohol-related neurodevelopmental disorder (ARND)	Central nervous system development abnormalities, including small head size, brain abnormalities and neurological signs, including poor co-ordination and poor fine-motor skills Learning and behavioural impairments, such as poor school performance and poor impulse control

The true prevalence of FASD is difficult to estimate. When there is a known history of prenatal exposure to alcohol and significant mental disability, and the common facial characteristics of FASD are present, early diagnosis is much more likely. However, in adolescence and adulthood, and in milder cases of neurobehavioural impairment, FASD may go undiagnosed (Public Health Agency of Canada, 2011). Health Canada has estimated that as many as nine in 1,000 babies experience some long-term impact from prenatal alcohol use. It is widely believed that a much larger group of children (likely three times as many) with unknown histories, and only cognitive and behavioural difficulties, go undiagnosed and uncounted. Diagnosed FASD has been identified as a leading cause of non-genetic intellectual disability worldwide (May et al., 2009).

FASD is not associated with any specific ethnocultural background, and relative risk factors are not easily determined because risks are highly interrelated and likely vary from population to population (see review in Chudley et al., 2005). However, Chudley and colleagues suggest that higher maternal age, lower socioeconomic status, smoking, cocaine use, reduced access to medical care, inadequate nutrition and poor developmental environment (e.g., neglect, abuse stress) are associated with the development of FASD.

Like ABI, FASD can be an invisible disability. Addiction counsellors are most likely to encounter the more subtle forms of FASD in their practice, which present as a range of intellectual and behavioural difficulties quite similar to those observed after ABI. As with brain injury, problems with judgment and self-regulation often appear without outward signs of disability. One big difference between FASD and ABI is that with FASD some degree of intellectual or behavioural difficulty is generally observed in childhood. The first indication of FASD may be delayed achievement of developmental milestones, or behavioural or attentional impairments when the child enters school. When the main cognitive issues are related to executive and emotional functioning, children with FASD, like those who sustained their brain injury in childhood, will grow into their disability. They fail to develop age-appropriate self-management, judgment and social skills when they enter school, or later in adolescence when even more independence is expected.

Although the entire brain may be affected by alcohol, it is impairments of executive functioning and emotional regulation that result in poor social judgment and that often prove to be the most disabling aspects of neurocognitive impairment associated with FASD (Fast & Conry, 2009; Streissguth et al., 2004). When FASD is moderate to severe, the most common findings from magnetic resonance imaging are a reduction in the overall size of the brain (cerebral atrophy), as well as reduced volume of the corpus collosum (a brain structure responsible for transmitting information between the brain's hemispheres) and cerebellum (responsible for co-ordinating movement and complex cognitive processing; see review in Lebel et al., 2011). Intellectual and behavioural problems can be characterized as a failure of the brain systems to work in co-ordination—attention is disordered, judgment is lacking and social skills are poorly developed. Abstract thinking and problem solving are often affected (e.g., Mattson et al., 2011).

As in the case of many people with ABI, the reward system may not properly process events and emotions. People with FASD often have a very limited capacity to learn from the consequences of their behaviour, to plan for the future or to manage their emotions. Socially, they are often described as gullible—tending to be easily led and exploited. Behaviourally, they perform best in situations that directly promote productive behaviour. In the absence of these supports, they often respond to situations impulsively—doing whatever is foremost in their mind at the moment (see reviews in Kodituwakku, 2007; Mattson et al., 2011).

Long-Term Outcomes of FASD

The problems associated with FASD last into adulthood. As with ABI, the brain regions associated with cognitive and social behaviour are altered in FASD, making people with the disorder more dependent on their environment to function well. Those with physical traits associated with FASD and severe cognitive impairment may be recognized earlier and provided with care and support. When they are taught about their disability and given appropriate supports and coping strategies, they often function quite well—but the need for environmental supports is ongoing. Those without obvious signs of disability often go undiagnosed. As they age, their disordered social behaviour and intellectual impairment may interrupt their education and result in trouble with the law, sexual exploitation or substance use problems. Paradoxically, the highly structured and rule-governed nature of the penal system may allow them to function at their best—but they are often exploited by other inmates. FASD is estimated to be 10 times more prevalent among the prison population than in the general population. (See reviews in Fast & Conry, 2009; Nash et al., 2008; Paley & O'Connor, 2009.)

Substance use in adolescents and adults with FASD

Data suggests that 50 per cent of females and 70 per cent of males age 21 to 51 with FASD have alcohol and other drug problems (Streissguth et al., 2004). Some of this substance use may be the result of being overly susceptible to environmental cues and difficulty in self-monitoring. It is also possible that people with FASD use substances as a way to self-medicate in response to repeated failures and psychosocial difficulties.

Substance Use Intervention Outcomes for People with ABI or FASD

Mainstream addiction services are often ill suited to meet the needs of people with ABI. And as we have discussed, many people who have substance use problems but no identified brain injuries or FASD may have some degree of cognitive impairment. In reviewing the literature on treatment outcome and cognitive impairment, Corrigan and Bogner (2007) and Bates and colleagues (2002) note that cognitive impairment is negatively associated with treatment retention and that staying in treatment is positively associated with treatment outcome. These authors also note that most addiction programs do not specifically address cognitive impairments.

Brain injury itself has not been well examined as a predictor of substance use treatment outcome. Abundant research suggests that people with comorbid mental health issues and cognitive impairment are the least likely to benefit from treatment for substance use problems (see review in Corrigan & Bogner, 2007). There is evidence that as many as 70 per cent of people seeking services in concurrent disorders programs have a history of brain injury with loss of consciousness (Walker et al., 2007).

> In starting to formulate what type of treatment plan she could recommend to Daniel, his assessment therapist, Olena, could attempt to tease out whether Daniel's history indicates ABI, FASD or both as the source of his cognitive impairment. Given the marked difference in Daniel's social functioning pre- and post-injury, ABI seems to be an important factor. If exploration of his history reveals a maternal history of heavy alcohol use, along with difficulties in childhood and adolescence (e.g., trouble in school), Olena might also consider whether FASD is a contributing factor. In either case, it would be important for Olena to consider how changes in Daniel's behaviour and cognition might affect the course of intervention.

Models of Addiction Care for People with Neurological Impairment

The attributes of ABI and FASD that are particularly pertinent to treatment planning and case management are summarized in Table 18-5. These difficulties necessitate intervention strategies that help compensate for intellectual impairments and that emphasize environmental supports. Given the paucity of literature on treating substance use problems for people with FASD, we focus on models that have been developed for people with brain injury.

TABLE 18-5
Common Elements of ABI and FASD

ATTRIBUTE	ABI	FASD
Often invisible	May or may not be associated with physical disability	More severe forms associated with facial anomalies
Intellectual impairment	Tendency toward a pattern of distinct strengths and weaknesses	Tendency toward consistent level of impairment across cognitive domains

ATTRIBUTE	ABI	FASD
Altered response to reward and punishment resulting in impulsivity and difficulty learning from mistakes	Common	Common
Difficulty with planning and problem solving	Common	Common
Difficulty interpreting social cues	Common	Common
Impaired awareness and insight	Common	Common

One significant difference between FASD and brain injury acquired in adulthood is that a person who acquired an injury as an adult will have had a period of impairment-free functioning prior to developing neurocognitive impairment. In some cases, the client's pre-existing self-image, skills and habits constitute a strength to be exploited in treatment. In others cases, a client's focus on returning to pre-injury roles and activities may hinder realistic planning. In cases of childhood brain injury and FASD, the clinician should be sensitive to the fact that the client may not have had the opportunity to develop a well-functioning adult self-image on which to build recovery. For this reason, treatment may need to focus initially on helping the person develop a positive self-image and gain functional skills and habits in the context of the neurocognitive impairment.

Over the past 15 years, brain injury rehabilitation providers have conducted fewer than 20 studies of intervention specifically designed for people with moderate to severe brain injury. (See reviews in Graham & Cardon, 2008; Parry-Jones et al., 2006; Taylor et al., 2003.) The vast majority of work around FASD interventions is related to education and prevention efforts with women who might consume alcohol before knowing they are pregnant, as well as women who have an alcohol use problem and are at risk for continuing to drink throughout pregnancy (Burd, 2006; Public Health Agency of Canada, 2005). The literature related to adults with FASD is limited to care recommendations, such as those provided by the National Organization for Fetal Alcohol Spectrum Disorder and the Substance Abuse and Mental Health Services Administration. To our knowledge, no studies have evaluated the impact of providing accommodation for brain injury and FASD in screening and brief interventions (Corrigan et al., 2010) and mainstream programs, and no studies have considered neurocognitive impairment in treatment matching (Graham & Cardon, 2008).

Secondary Prevention

In terms of secondary prevention (limiting further injury or disability once the person has had an injury), the first issue is determining how much of a substance is too much when living with neurological impairment. Most people with a moderate to severe brain injury or cognitive impairment are advised to refrain from all non-prescribed substance use for one to two years. Because substances may affect the injured brain differently, substance use, even in small amounts, may have adverse effects after the first couple of years. With FASD or any other condition resulting in neurocognitive impairment, the effects of alcohol or other substances may also be more pronounced, although this con-clusion is based on clinical observation rather than empirical evidence.

The Ohio Valley Center for Brain Injury Prevention and Rehabilitation has been a recognized world leader in the field of substance use and brain injury for its work in primary research and clinical intervention. Through a combination of focus groups and professional consultation, it has developed a set of secondary prevention messages that provide a summary of the good reasons to avoid substance use after brain injury (Ohio Valley Center, 2009a):

- Substance use may limit recovery from the brain injury.
- Problems in balance and speech may be made worse by intoxication.
- The disinhibiting effect of alcohol and other drugs may be particularly problematic for someone who has limited self-control.
- After brain injury, drugs may have a more powerful effect.
- Substance use may worsen cognitive symptoms, such as memory impairment and difficulty concentrating.
- People who have a brain injury are at a significantly greater risk for depression—many substances have depressant effects.
- People who use substances after injury are more likely to suffer a second injury.
- Alcohol or other drug use may increase the risk of seizure after brain injury.

It is often useful for clients to consider their current substance use in the context of these additional risks after brain injury. Logically, these risks would also be topics of discussion relevant to others with neurocognitive impairment. The Ohio Valley Center has created client materials that deliver these messages in a non-confrontational way.[1]

Intervention for people with neurological impairment

When cognition, self-awareness and self-regulation are impaired, special approaches to treatment are needed. Talk therapies that emphasize developing self-control without providing adequate environmental supports seem to be less effective for people with executive functioning impairments. A person with limited awareness of his or her cog-nitive deficits may not be able to ask for help, take in information or cope well with the

---

[1] Resources for clients about substance use after brain injury can be found on the website of the Ohio Valley Center for Brain Injury Prevention and Rehabilitation. Visit http://ohiovalley.org/informationeducation/materials/.

inevitable stress of making major life changes. Flexible programming may be needed to accommodate required rest periods, limited attention and slowed cognitive processing.

A number of interventions may be useful with ABI clients, but only four main types have been systematically evaluated as specialized treatments for people with TBI in individual, group and long- and short-term formats (see reviews in Graham & Cardon, 2008; Parry-Jones et al., 2006; Taylor et al., 2003). These interventions are:

1. strategies for treatment retention
2. intensive case management
3. skills training with peer support
4. motivational interviewing and counselling.

Strategies for treatment retention

Corrigan and colleagues (2005) compared a motivational interviewing–based approach to two other methods for increasing participation in substance use treatment for clients with TBI. One group received support to reduce logistical barriers to attendance and members of another group received a $20 gift certificate as an incentive to complete their treatment plan within one month. This study was designed to test which of the three approaches would be most effective in keeping clients in treatment. All three approaches were administered through structured, brief telephone interventions. Of the 175 participants, those randomly assigned to the barrier reduction and financial incentive groups were more likely to sign the service plan within 30 days—74 per cent and 83 per cent respectively—compared to the motivational interviewing group (45 per cent). Although therapeutic alliance was not directly related to outcomes, participants who received a financial reward were less likely to leave treatment prematurely and more likely to meet their treatment goals (33 per cent for financial incentive, 23 per cent for barrier reduction, 17 per cent for attention control and motivational interviewing).

In discussing their findings, Corrigan and Bogner (2007) grappled with the unexpected success of the incentive and barrier reduction interventions. People in the financial incentive condition scheduled more appointments, attended the appointments and had better outcomes, even though the reinforcement they received was both modest and delayed. This is counterintuitive when we consider that both substance use problems and brain injury are associated with more impulsive (immediate reward–driven) behaviour. Corrigan and Bogner (2007) propose that the type of learning required in the financial incentive condition (rule-governed learning) is more accessible after brain injury than contingency-based learning (natural feedback from the environment). In rule-governed learning, the outcome a person is working toward, and the steps required to achieve it, are much more clear and unambiguous compared with feedback from the natural environment. Offering financial incentives may not be possible in many Canadian treatment programs. However, these findings highlight the importance of promoting early attendance in treatment, and the need to design interventions that provide clear and unambiguous feedback and alter a person's environment.

Intensive case management

Intensive case management provides support to meet people's rehabilitation and substance use–related treatment goals in a holistic fashion, by creating community-based teams of providers and ensuring the availability of appropriate services. Bogner and colleagues (1997) evaluated an intensive case management model designed around participation in a vocational re-entry program. They found that this model of care resulted in increased rates of abstinence and employment in the 72 survivors of TBI they monitored for one year. Intensive case management may include an emphasis on harm reduction while working toward a client's life goals.

Skills training

In the first study of its kind, Vungkhanching and colleagues (2007) reported on a program that specifically trained participants in communication, problem solving and self-management skills in a group setting. The intervention included repetition and role-playing, as well as specific goal setting and self-monitoring. The authors found that this type of treatment was well accepted by participants, and resulted in a trend toward using less alcohol and other drugs. Other clinical program evaluations have also suggested that approaches that include behavioural rehearsal and skill training show promise. While the literature describes different program models, specific adaptations of programming for people with impaired executive functioning are not readily found in the literature.

There are also a few reports of long-term residential rehabilitation programs for people with ABI that included modules designed to address substance use problems. While these programs showed promising results, there are only a handful of them in North America, and they are not typically available in Canada (see review in Graham & Cardon, 2008).

Motivational interviewing

For more than three decades, motivational interviewing (MI) has provided a practical framework for working with clients who have mixed feelings about making changes (Miller & Rollnick, 2013). Client-centred but therapist-guided, this model has been repeatedly shown to address ambivalence and encourage behaviour change in varied populations. Research has demonstrated that the more statements clients make about their rationale for change, the more likely they are to make a change. Too much questioning, confrontation and direct advice are likely to backfire, diminishing the chances that clients will consider and work toward changing their behaviour. Using MI strategies enables the therapist and client to move forward in a therapeutic conversation, even when significant ambivalence about change remains.

In recent years, more attention has been paid to using MI with clients with cognitive difficulties. However, the literature remains scant on how MI can be adapted for use with clients who have ABI. At least six articles have explored this topic and, in all cases, the authors have concluded that MI principles and strategies have potential usefulness but remain largely untested in the ABI population. We have found MI principles and skills to be very helpful in our work with clients who have cognitive impairments. We are not aware of any published investigations of the use of MI with FASD.

Practice Implications

Screening for Cognitive Impairment

Recognizing a client who is struggling with cognitive impairments is not necessarily straightforward. As clinicians, we can have a sense that something is getting in the way of achieving optimal engagement, but may attribute the barrier to something other than a brain injury or illness (e.g., unresolved ambivalence to change). However, if we consider the high co-occurrence of substance use problems and cognitive impairment (from a variety of sources), our job can be made much simpler by subscribing to the "high index of suspicion" (Mueser et al., 2003) approach from the concurrent disorders literature. This approach is based on the default assumption that if one issue is present (i.e., substance use disorder), then our best tack is to screen for the presence of the other—cognitive impairment from some other source, such as ABI or FASD. The process of screening can only be effective if we recognize the need to do it.

Part of the challenge in recognizing the problems with thinking, learning, behaviour and self-awareness that occur after a brain injury is that they sometimes overlap with the problems that are caused by substance use. As we will continue to emphasize, the reason for the impairment is not the central issue.

The client, family and other significant people in the client's life are important sources of information about a history of FASD, brain injury or other events that produce cognitive impairment. Clinicians need to judge for themselves how accurate an historian a client is and whether they need to obtain a collateral history.

Screening for brain injury

Screening measures for brain injury can range from a few simple questions to detailed interview protocols with many questions (e.g., Bogner & Corrigan, 2009).[2] One example is the TBI screener summarized in Table 18-6.

---

[2] For a more comprehensive look at screening for brain injury and cognitive impairment, read the *Substance Use Brain Injury Provider Manual*, which is available by registering through the Substance Use / Brain Injury Bridging Project at www.subi.ca.

TABLE 18-6

TBI Screener Summary

ISSUES TO SCREEN FOR	SCREENING QUESTION EXAMPLES
Trauma	Have you ever had an accident or injury that included a blow to your head?
Behaviour	Were you knocked out, dazed or confused? Did you get treatment at a clinic or hospital?
Impact on everyday functioning	Did any of these problems persist for more than several weeks after the injury? • headaches • dizziness or balance problems • tiredness or fatigue • problems paying attention or concentrating • sensitivity to bright lights or loud noises? In the months after your injury did you: • have new problems at work or school, or lose a job? • notice changes in your relationships with your family (wife, husband, parents, friends)? • have trouble remembering things or solving problems? • feel depressed or anxious more than before the injury? • have trouble controlling your temper?

Adapted from Ohio Valley Center for Brain Injury Prevention and Rehabilitation (2009b).

When evaluating the clinical implications of the information gathered during screening, it is important to consider how severe the injury is, when the injury occurred and how much evidence there is of current difficulties.

In general, more severe injuries are associated with more pronounced and longer alterations in cognitive processes. Momentary loss of consciousness signals a milder injury, whereas prolonged confusion or coma suggests a more severe injury. More severe injuries also tend to be associated with greater and more persistent effects on day-to-day functioning.

The Ohio Valley Center for Brain Injury Prevention and Rehabilitation (2009b) suggests that clinicians consider the following:

• More recent TBI will be associated with greater problems in attention and new learning, and greater likelihood of depression.
• Early developmental TBI (before age 10) may be associated with less adept interpersonal functioning, and with attention deficit, learning problems, conduct disorder or adolescent onset of substance use problems.

- TBI in early adolescence may arrest emotional and behavioural development and/or trigger the development of a substance use problem (p. 2).

Diagnosing FASD and identifying risk factors

Diagnosing FASD in adults is complicated by the fact that facial anomalies may resolve and the slowed growth evident in childhood is caught up by the time the person reaches adulthood. To help determine diagnosis, the clinician should review the client's history for the following FASD risk factors:

- FASD diagnosis in a sibling
- raised in foster care or adopted
- history of child protection
- history of developmental delay
- history of slow growth as a child
- diagnosis of ADHD
- diagnosed with varied mental health conditions
- behavioural symptoms, including distractibility, hyperactivity, impulsivity
- behavioural fluctuations or instability
- involvement in criminal activity
- ability to identify correct behaviour or a rule, but difficulty following the rule
- repeated errors or mistakes
- unstable job history
- mother was diagnosed with and/or received treatment for substance use problems
- mother died due to complications from substance use
- history of removal from home due to substance-related problems
- mother died due to complications from substance use problems
- other high-risk behaviours, such as employment or legal problems related to drinking
- presence of substance at birth, as indicated by medical records.

Sample screening interview questions

In order to implement a relatively brief screening system, a good starting point is to ask the client's permission to gather historical information that will provide a solid foundation for the treatment plan. In her meeting with Daniel from our case study, Olena may have used the following opening statements:

> *"I'm hoping it's okay for me to ask you if there's anything we should know about that will make things easier for you while you're in the program."*
> or
> *"We want to do everything possible to make this program fit your needs. So I'd like to take a few minutes to ask you some questions about how we could adapt things so they work well for you."*

Operating from such a platform, the clinician can ask questions designed to uncover a history of a head injury, or the existence of FASD or illness that may be at the root of cognitive impairments. Following is a list of sample questions.

History:

- How would you describe your childhood? What was it like for you growing up?
- What do you know about your development? Did you reach milestones on time?
- Have you ever been hospitalized?
- Have you ever experienced a stroke, heart attack, tumour, encephalitis or other infection, HIV or drug overdose?
- Have you ever lost consciousness? What was your recovery like?
- Was that the only injury?
- How did you get that injury?
- Please tell me about yourself as a child. Did you walk, talk, develop skills on time (as far as you know)?
- How was school for you?
- Did you ever receive special education supports?

Functional difficulties. Have you ever had difficulties with:

- getting your point across to others?
- sitting still?
- focusing your attention?
- understanding what others are saying?
- communicating your thoughts and feelings?
- managing anger?
- remembering things?
- following instructions (e.g., directions on how to get somewhere)?
- becoming tired easily?
- getting along with others?
- being impulsive—doing before thinking?
- getting thoughts out of your head?
- making up your mind?
- getting started on something you need or want to do?

Once the clinician has established the nature and extent of the reported functional difficulties, it is a good time to consider how the clinician's approach can be adapted to take these issues into account. As we discussed earlier, a substantial number of people in concurrent disorders programs have a history of ABI, and problems with mental health are common after brain injury. Some symptoms of ABI can even mimic mood and thought disorders. A clinician may face the challenge of trying to sort out the complex interplay of psychiatric symptoms, substance use and the effects of ABI or FASD. In the shadow of such complexity, it makes sense to request a consultation when in doubt about how to adapt an intervention.

However, there is a final step that can be useful before the clinician attempts to tailor the treatment plan; namely, asking the client directly about strategies he or she may already have implemented to compensate for cognitive difficulties. The take-home message is that practitioners should be alert for all of these possibilities, and that referral to services designed for people with neurological impairment may be necessary. Even when the origins of the disability you are observing remain a mystery, adapting your intervention is possible.

Following is a list of questions clinicians can ask clients about the strategies they have used to compensate for cognitive difficulties:

General question:
- What do you do in particular to get around the problems you mentioned?

Probing questions:
- Do you have a datebook?
- Do you make notes?
- What helps you pay attention?

Functional questions:
- I would be interested in seeing how you use your book to remember appointments. How would you feel about showing me?
- What is your system for remembering things to do?
- Does finding a quiet place help?
- Do you schedule important appointments for early in the day?

Here-and-now questions:
- How will you remember our next appointment?
- Would it help if I make notes as we talk?
- Should I close the curtains?

Treatment

It is beyond the scope of this chapter to provide a comprehensive picture of all the ways clinicians can adapt substance use treatment plans to address significant cognitive impairments. Readers who are interested in a more comprehensive look at this issue should access the *Substance Use Brain Injury Providers Manual* listed in the Resources section. Here we provide a summary of strategies for dealing with interpersonal and cognitive difficulties that clients may experience.

Addressing Interpersonal Difficulties

Clients with brain injury or FASD are often not aware when their behaviour is inappropriate for the situation. Clinicians can help clients with interpersonal difficulties in various ways:
- create plans and signals that can be used in difficult situations

- review information and repeat key messages
- rehearse coping strategies.

How to Compensate for Cognitive Difficulties

In general, when working with clients who experience cognitive and behavioural effects of brain injury or FASD, it is a good idea to:
- use concrete examples
- simplify written material to emphasize basic points
- use written schedules and reminders
- present information in both visual and verbal formats
- orient the client to the goals of a session and review information afterwards, whether you are doing individual counselling or running a group. When in doubt, talk with the client directly about what you are seeing and problem solve with the person.

Specific strategies for addressing difficulties

Clinicians can use the following strategies to address various problem areas people with brain injury or FASD may experience.

Problems with attention:
- **filtering out distractions:** ensure you have the client's attention before providing information; begin each session by pointing out and then removing potential distractions; clear your desk so items on it don't distract the client; acknowledge a distraction when it occurs and make a direct statement to get back on track; ask the client to repeat what he or she has understood.
- **staying on topic:** ensure the session agenda includes a clear goal; acknowledge what the client has said and bring the discussion back on topic, using visual aids (e.g., agenda) as needed.
- **easing client fatigue:** build in breaks or shorten sessions, and build in some physical activity to increase alertness.

Problems with memory:
- **recalling information between sessions:** provide cues, such as, "Daniel, have you made any notes about important events this week? I think I remember that last week you had an important specialist's appointment coming up." Taping sessions, and providing written notes and handouts can help as reminders.
- **remembering to do something:** encourage the client to select and use reminders, notes and alarms; attribute failures to follow through to memory gaps rather than to a lack of motivation; build on routines by matching therapeutic tasks with activities that regularly take place (e.g., practise relaxation after setting the alarm clock).

- **dealing with selective memory:** repeat information and ask the client to discuss what he or she understood; make information more personal and memorable (e.g., "Daniel, maybe we could capitalize on your interest in bands. What song can you think of that will remind you to think before you act?").
- **addressing confabulation:** treat misinformation as a confabulation rather than a lie; avoid repeating confabulated information and instead just provide the correct information; include others who can provide correct information; try to avoid too many open-ended questions.

Problems with executive functioning:
- **getting started:** consider whether a support person should be present during the planning discussion and whether alarms would help cue the client begin an activity.
- **learning from mistakes:** use a motivational interviewing approach in working toward the client accepting structure in the environment (e.g., someone who can provide cues or manage money).
- **making plans:** help the client brainstorm ideas and create a step-by-step plan.
- **thinking before acting:** minimize exposure to high-risk situations until a productive response is developed and rehearsed; encourage the client to use a catchphrase such as "Stop, think and act," and enlist a caregiver to deliver direct cues to the client.

Problems with communication:
- **understanding the client's speech:** try having a frank discussion about communication and ask the client about the use of communication aids; let the client know that you will ask for repetition if you don't understand; plan for sessions to last longer to allow for a slower pace of communication. In some cases, a familiar person may be able to help the client demonstrate the best modes of communication or may facilitate interaction.
- **addressing aphasia (difficulty using some aspect of language):** consult with a rehabilitation professional about the best communication techniques to use and encourage the client to talk around the word he or she is having difficulty grasping.
- **reading social cues:** prepare and rehearse before joining a group; lay out some ground rules for communication; set up obvious signals to cue the client when it is time to listen and time to talk; make a habit of providing verbal summaries and ask the client to do the same; always let the client know when you need clarification.

Promoting Engagement in Treatment

To benefit from treatment, the client has to attend sessions and stick with the therapy. Research and clinical experience has demonstrated that one of the most important factors in treatment success is the duration of treatment (Simpson, 1981; Simpson et al., 1997). People who are not yet expressing a willingness to make changes in their lives tend to quit treatment before they reap its benefits, unless special measures are taken to help them feel comfortable about getting help. In addition, research about optimal support for people with cognitive issues suggests it is especially important that the first sessions a client attends be as positive as possible to increase the chances that they will come back and benefit from therapy. The other important consideration is removing barriers to treatment.

Clients often have difficulty managing the day-to-day logistics of their lives. In some cases, active problem solving with the client to eliminate barriers to treatment is helpful in improving attendance. When you make the first appointment, it is a good practice to ask the client to identify what might keep him or her from attending. A list of possible difficulties can be reviewed with clients who have trouble coming up with their own ideas. For example, a client may find it difficult to arrange transportation, child care or lunch money, or to remember the appointment. When possible, it may be useful to offer accommodations, such as transportation fare, child care or reminder calls.

Positive engagement with clients requires that clinicians are respectful and sensitive to their needs. If you have not had much contact with people who have disabilities, you may sometimes experience awkward moments. Get to know your client as a person. By using common sense and courtesy, and by asking questions and requesting permission when in doubt, you can easily address most issues. For "disability etiquette," see this chapter's appendix.

Including caregivers in therapy

It is often very useful to have someone in the client's life participate in counselling sessions. Unfortunately, many clients feel a loss of control after brain injury, which may negatively affect their relationship with caregivers. With careful planning, including directly addressing client confidentiality concerns, involving a caregiver can be useful. Here are some important points to remember:

- It is usually best to develop rapport with a client before inviting someone to attend the session. This guideline may be set aside when clients ask to have others involved from the start.
- Guidelines for having caregivers involved should be reviewed with all parties. They may cover topics such as how information will be shared, how decisions will be made, how contacts outside the therapy sessions will be handled, how the caregiver will know when his or her presence is welcome, and when the client is to have private time with the treatment provider.

When a caregiver cannot attend a session, a therapy notebook can be a good way to transmit information. Clients should understand how the notebook is used and play a role in formulating the information recorded. The caregiver can be asked to review the information with the client between sessions. The caregiver's assistance can be requested in following up with action plans. In Daniel's scenario, his counsellor, Olena, noticed that Daniel seemed to be uncomfortable with his wife, Dana, joining the session right away. Olena gave Daniel three options:

1. Daniel and Olena meet for the session and bring Dana in for a briefing on the outcome of the assessment.
2. Dana joins the assessment interview only for the first few minutes to provide a bit of background.
3. Dana joins the interview for the first few minutes and the concluding few minutes.

Daniel tells Olena that he isn't sure which option he prefers, so Olena suggests she meet with Daniel alone to sort out how he wants to proceed. She also suggests checking back with Dana as soon as possible.

The importance of the community team

If you work in a substance use program, it is important to understand that rehabilitation after brain injury often involves a team of professionals; this may also be the case in working with clients who have FASD. Your goal should be to become an active member of your client's rehabilitation team. Although the number of professionals involved tends to diminish with time, it is possible to have teams involved decades after a brain injury occurred. Continuing support largely depends on the nature of the injury, when it occurred and the client's financial resources. There may be many people involved, or just you.

When a client requires support to manage activities of daily living, there will usually be someone available to collaborate with you in conducting a comprehensive assessment and constructing and implementing a treatment plan. Support people may be family members or paid professionals. Taking some simple steps early in the assessment process will ensure that the relationships established with your client's support team will be productive and acceptable to everyone involved, and meet the requisite ethical standards. Here are some steps to follow:

- Get a complete picture of who is currently providing treatment and think through how they might be included in plans for intervention. Obtain necessary consents for disclosure or sharing information.
- Review with the client who will have access to his or her information and the limits of confidentiality.
- Establish who the client is willing to have participate in treatment. It is not unusual for clients to request that an external clinician or family member be present to help them provide information.
- Establish when and with whom information will be shared.
- Establish who holds decision-making capacity. Very often clients will have someone making financial decisions for them, but be aware that personal decision-making is assessed separately, and a financial trustee is not necessarily the person who makes personal or treatment decisions.

A Framework for Guiding Work with Clients Who Have Cognitive Difficulties

"Whatever It Takes" (WIT) is a set of principles developed by Willer and Corrigan (1994) to help service providers assess and address the needs of people living long term with the effects of ABI. The authors' clinical experience has demonstrated that these principles are also useful in working with clients who have cognitive difficulties for other reasons. The principles are based on the idea that providers do "whatever it takes" to help clients be successful.

WIT (Willer & Corrigan, 1994) operates on the assumption that no two people are alike—and no two brain injuries are either. No matter what the cause (e.g., stroke, injury, illness), living with cognitive and behavioural impairment is an enormous challenge—one that requires creativity, persistence and optimism. This is particularly true because the person may not be fully aware of the changes resulting from the injury. Although the availability of services is improving, people who leave rehabilitation centres with ongoing difficulties may find that services that fit their unique needs are not available. Here are the six most relevant WIT principles for working with clients in substance use programs who have cognitive difficulties:

1. No two people with ABI are alike.

The brain can be thought of as a set of highly interconnected structures. When one or more structures are affected by brain injury, the whole system can be disrupted in ways that are not easy to predict. As discussed earlier, a wide array of problems can result from brain injury and can be present in very different forms in each person. Now consider the fact that a person's pre-injury characteristics most certainly have an effect on the outcome of the injury. To be successful, programming needs to be adapted and individualized to suit each client's needs.

2. Skills are more likely to generalize when they are taught in the environment where they will be used.

Generalization means transferring a skill from one setting to another. Because of changes in reasoning, memory and initiation, teaching a client something in a counselling session often doesn't get used in real life. The more complex the skill, the less likely it is to generalize. In teaching a client how to refuse the offer of alcohol or other drugs, it may not be possible to visit together the place where the offers are most likely to originate (i.e., a bar). However, the next best activity is—within a counselling session—to simulate a high-risk scenario and have the client rehearse the skills needed to negotiate the scenario successfully.

3. Environments are easier to change than people.

Self-management is tough for all of us, and the challenge increases after brain injury. Difficulties with self-awareness, impulsivity and memory can make it very hard to change habits. Sometimes the easiest, most robust plans for change involve altering some part of the environment. For example, it's probably easier to change roommates than it is to teach a client not to drink when housemates are partying.

4. Life is a place-and-train venture.

People generally work better when the link between meaningful goals and their own efforts are clear. It is more motivating to get right down to the real thing than spend more time in training on a simulated task. In vocational rehabilitation, this means finding a job placement and providing training on the job. Because of problems with generalizing skills, this model is recommended with this client group. The same approach is also useful in learning other life skills, such as navigating the community or attending to domestic chores or finances. Often clients will not accept the principles of using a datebook, but if their job requires making notes and using a calendar (and others on the job do the same), this compensation strategy is more likely to be accepted.

5. Natural supports last longer than professionals.

Social interactions often change after brain injury. Friends before the injury may not remain involved in the person's life. Intervention should seek to involve natural supports and help the client to identify new social opportunities that will be available in the long run. In general, encourage unpaid supports over paid supports.

6. Interventions must not do more harm than good.

The goals of intervention should be clearly defined, and interventions considered for their potential effects. For example, when colleagues are the most available social contacts in the client's environment, the client may not develop other relationships. And too much functional support can reduce the client's actual capacity. For example, a group home that provides for all of a client's needs, such as meals and recreation, may foster dependence unless the client is directly engaged in developing skills to increase functional capacities in these areas (see Willer & Corrigan, 1994).

Daniel's First Session

After the therapist Olena provides a brief overview of the agency, and Daniel discusses how he feels about coming to therapy, Olena asks if Daniel's wife, Dana, can join in the session to discuss some historical details that Daniel is having difficulty remembering. Dana begins by reporting that about five years ago, while on his way to a job, Daniel was in a motor vehicle accident. It took Daniel about three months to heal from the orthopedic injuries from his accident, but he continued to have headaches and problems with memory. Neuropsychological tests at the time showed that he retained most of his intellectual abilities, but that he was still having some problems with attention recalling new information. Everyone thought he should be able to go back to work and he felt okay so he returned almost immediately, with the advice to take it easy in the early going.

When asked directly, Daniel admits that it is hard for him these days to tell when he has had too much to drink. He also recognizes some of the downsides of drinking too much, such as loss of balance and relationship conflict. However, he is ambivalent about quitting, mainly because he enjoys having a beer or two to wind down after work. And he doesn't see the connection between his drinking and the impaired driving incidents, even though the second one resulted in the loss of his driver's licence. Olena employs the MI strategy of emphasizing personal choice and control by saying: "For any plan to go forward it has to make sense to you and go at the pace that works for you. My approach to supporting people is to really work in partnership. Your ideas about the way forward are really important."

CONSIDERATIONS FOR TREATMENT PLANNING

Daniel seems to be an opportunistic drinker. When it's available, he overdoes it. despite being more sensitive to the effects of the alcohol since his injury. On his own, he doesn't go through extraordinary efforts to get alcohol. Like many people after brain injury, he is now more dependent on his environment in general. He doesn't initiate ideas or activities—needing cues from others or from routines. He no longer self-monitors well. He doesn't fully appreciate the problems associated with his use of alcohol—and he isn't fully aware of the neurobehavioural changes he's had since his injury. Even without alcohol, his judgment is reduced, but he manages in most social situations. With even modest amounts of alcohol on board, his behaviour deteriorates. Both his neurobehavioural changes and substance use need to be addressed together.

The following treatment plan is generated:
- With Daniel's permission, Olena will provide education about the particular risks associated with substance use after injury. They discuss how these risks apply to him.
- Daniel accepts referral to an outpatient substance use group, based on harm reduction principles, endorsing a goal of continuing his abstinence of alcohol in the short term, potentially returning to moderate drinking (with some behavioural supports) at some point in the future.
- Olena and Daniel agree that if the group does not work out for any reason, that Olena would facilitate a referral to individual counselling, with an addictions clinician trained in working with clients with ABI.
- A referral is made for assessment regarding Daniel's eligibility for ABI community supports.

Conclusion

Adapting substance use counselling approaches to the needs of people with neurocognitive impairments is challenging but possible. The necessary precursor to program adaptation is identifying which clients require a tailored treatment plan. To this end, screening is important and can be relatively straightforward, especially when it involves a few simple questions. The "Whatever it takes" principles provide a framework that will likely facilitate counsellors' success in engaging and retaining clients with cognitive difficulties in substance use programs. Close collaboration between the substance use counsellor and the care team in the community can also optimize outcomes.

Practice Tips

- Establish screening for ABI and FASD in your practice. Even simple screening protocols can yield critical information for care planning.
- Be aware that cognitive impairment may masquerade as limited motivation for change and a lack of willingness or interest in participating in treatment.
- If a client screens positively for ABI or FASD, you can increase the likelihood of a better outcome by addressing cognitive impairment in the treatment plan.
- Find the ABI and FASD agencies in your area. In the absence of specialized, integrated programs, meet client needs by forming partnerships with other treatment providers.
- Use concrete visual aids to do session activities. For example, use flipchart paper in a group to create colourful illustrations of conceptual material. For individual sessions, keep a piece of paper on the desk between you and your client for notes, illustrations and reminders.
- Whenever possible, support the client to participate in meaningful "real-life" activities.
- Encourage your client to preserve existing natural supports while developing new social opportunities.
- Remember that changing some aspect of a client's environment (e.g., going home by a different route) can greatly reduce risks and increase the chances of a positive outcome.
- Start and end every counselling session with a summary. Include in the starting summary an overview of the purpose of the session.
- Assume that the client likely won't get content on the first or second run-through, but may get it the third time around.

- Always end the session on a positive note. The client may not remember the content of what you've talked about, but most likely will remember how he or she felt after the session (a client who felt good is more likely to return).
- Normalize the fact that for people with ABI, short-term memory is adversely affected, so self-monitoring tends to be an important strategy.
- Expect a higher-than-average number of no-shows, but build in appointment reminder strategies whenever possible that involve members of the client's informal or formal support network.
- If the client has a community ABI worker or an informal support person, think of a plan to include ABI workers or informal support people in some sessions or parts of sessions, especially when it comes to implementing cognitive compensation strategies. Also, if your client is in a relationship, consider referring the partner to family support services.

Resources

Publications

Public Health Agency of Canada. (2011). *Assessment and Diagnosis of FASD among Adults: A National and International Systematic Review.* Ottawa: Author. Retrieved from www.phac-aspc.gc.ca

Internet

Brainline.org
    www.brainline.org
Canadian Association of Pediatric Health Centres, Knowledge Exchange Network
    http://ken.caphc.org/xwiki/bin/view/Main/WebHome
FASD Center for Excellence
    www.fasdcenter.samhsa.gov
National Organization on Fetal Alcohol Syndrome
    www.nofas.org
Ohio Valley Center for Brain Injury Prevention and Rehabilitation
    http://ohiovalley.org/informationeducation/materials/
Substance Use / Brain Injury Bridging Project (*Substance Use Brain Injury Providers Manual*)
    www.subi.ca
The Brain from Top to Bottom
    www.thebrain.mcgill.ca

References

Adinoff, B. (2004). Neurobiologic processes in drug reward and addiction. *Harvard Review of Psychiatry, 12*, 305–320.

Alexander, M. (1995). Mild traumatic brain injury: Pathophysiology, natural history, and clinical management, *Neurology, 45*, 1253–1260.

Anderson, V. & Catroppa, C. (2005). Recovery of executive skills following paediatric traumatic brain injury (TBI): A 2 year follow-up. *Brain Injury, 19*, 459–470.

Bates, M.E., Bowden, S.C. & Barry D. (2002). Neurocognitive impairment associated with alcohol use disorders: Implications for treatment. *Experimental and Clinical Psychopharmacology, 10*, 193–212.

Bates, M.E., Buckman, J.F. & Nguyen, T.T. (2013). A role for cognitive rehabilitation in increasing the effectiveness of treatment for alcohol use disorders. *Neuropsychological Review, 23*, 27–47.

Bjork, J.M. & Grant, S.J. (2009). Does traumatic brain injury increase risk for substance abuse? *Journal of Neurotrauma, 26*, 1077–1082.

Bogner J. & Corrigan, J.D. (2009). Reliability and predictive validity of the Ohio State University TBI identification method with Prisoners. *Journal of Head Trauma and Rehabilitation, 24*, 279–291.

Bogner, J.A., Corrigan, J.D., Spafford, D.E. & Lamb-Hart, G.L. (1997). Integrating substance abuse treatment and vocational rehabilitation following traumatic brain injury. *Journal of Head Trauma Rehabilitation, 12*, 57–71.

Bombardier, C., Temkin, N., Machamer, J. & Dikmen, S. (2003). The natural history of drinking and alcohol related problems after traumatic brain injury. *Archives of Physical Medicine and Rehabilitation, 84*, 185–191.

Burd, L.J. (2006). Intervention in FASD: We must do better. *Child Care, Health and Development, 33*, 398–400.

Chudley, A.E., Conry, J., Cook, J.L., Loock, C., Rosales, T., LeBlanc, N. & Public Health Agency of Canada's National Advisory Committee on Fetal Alcohol Spectrum Disorder. (2005). Fetal alcohol spectrum disorder: Canadian guidelines for diagnosis. *Canadian Medical Association Journal, 172* (Suppl. 5), 1–21.

Corrigan, J.D. & Bogner, J. (2007). Interventions to promote retention in substance abuse treatment. *Brain Injury, 21*, 343–356.

Corrigan, J.D., Bogner, J., Hungerford, D.W. & Schomer, K. (2010). Screening and brief intervention for substance misuse among patients with traumatic brain injury. *Journal of Trauma Injury, Infection, and Critical Care, 69*, 722–726.

Corrigan, J.D., Bogner, J., Lamb-Hart, G., Heinemann, A.W. & Moore, D. (2005). Increasing substance abuse treatment compliance for persons with traumatic brain injury. *Psychology of Addictive Behaviors, 19*, 131–139.

Corrigan, J.D. & Cole, T.B. (2008). Substance use disorders and clinical management of traumatic brain injury and posttraumatic stress disorder. *Journal of the American Medical Association, 46*, 67–76.

Corrigan, J.D. & Deutschle, J.J. (2008). The presence and impact of traumatic brain injury among clients in treatment for co-occurring mental illness and substance abuse. *Brain Injury, 22*, 223–231.

Cunha, P.J., Bechara, A., de Andrade, A.G. & Nicastri, S. (2011). Decision-making deficits linked to real-life social dysfunction in crack cocaine-dependent individuals. *American Journal of Addiction, 20*, 78–86.

Damasio, A.R. (1994). *Descartes' Error: Emotion, Reason, and the Human Brain.* New York: Penguin.

Draper, K., Ponsford, J. & Schonberger, M. (2007). Psychosocial and emotional outcomes 10 years following traumatic brain injury. *Journal of Head Trauma Rehabilitation, 22*, 278–287.

Fast, D.K. & Conry, J. (2009). Fetal alcohol spectrum disorders and the criminal justice system. *Developmental Disabilities Research Reviews, 15*, 250–257.

Feeney, T.J. (2010). There's always something that works: Principles and practices of positive support for individuals with traumatic brain injury and problem behaviors. *Seminars in Speech and Language, 31*, 145–161.

Graham, D.P. & Cardon, A.L. (2008). An update on substance use and treatment following traumatic brain injury. *Annals of the New York Academy of Sciences, 1141*, 148–162.

Green, A., Garrick, T., Sheedy, D., Blake, H., Shores, E. & Harper, C. (2010). The effect of moderate to heavy alcohol consumption on neuropsychological performance as measured by the repeatable battery for the assessment of neuropsychological status, *Alcoholism and Clinical and Experimental Research, 34*, 443–450.

Harper, C. (2009). The neuropathology of alcohol-related brain damage. *Alcohol & Alcoholism, 44*, 136–140.

Hermens, D.F., Lagopoulos, J., Tobias-Webb, J., De Regt, T., Dore, G., Juckes, L. et al. (2013). Pathways to alcohol-induced brain impairment in young people: A review. *Cortex, 49*, 3–17.

Iverson, G.L. (2010). Mild traumatic brain injury meta-analyses can obscure individual differences. *Brain Injury, 24*, 1246–1255.

Iverson, G.L., Lange, R.T. & Frazen, M.D. (2005). Effects of mild traumatic brain injury cannot be differentiated from substance abuse, *Brain Injury, 10*, 29–46.

Kodituwakku, P.W. (2007). Defining the behavioral phenotype in children with fetal alcohol spectrum disorders: A review. *Neuroscience and Biobehavioral Reviews, 31*, 192–201.

Koenigs, M., Young, L., Adolphs, R., Tranel, D., Cushman, F., Hauser, M. & Damasio, A. (2007). Damage to the prefrontal cortex increases utilitarian moral judgements. *Nature, 19*, 908–911.

Lange, R.T, Iverson, G.L. & Franzen, M.D. (2008). Comparability of neuropsychological test profiles in patients with chronic substance abuse and mild traumatic brain injury. *Clinical Neuropsychologist, 22*, 209–227.

Lebel, C., Roussotte, F. & Sowell, E.R. (2011). Imaging the impact of prenatal alcohol exposure on the structure of the developing brain. *Neuropsychology Review, 21*, 102–118.

Loeber, S., Duka, T., Welzel, H., Nakovics, H., Heinz, A., Flor, H. & Mann, K. (2009). Impairment of cognitive abilities and decision making after chronic use of alcohol: The impact of multiple detoxifications. *Alcohol & Alcoholism, 44*, 372–381.

Mattson, S.M., Crocker, N. & Nguyen, T.T. (2011). Fetal alcohol spectrum disorders: Neuropsychological behaviours and features. *Neuropsychology Review, 21*, 81–101.

May, P.A., Gossage, P.J., Kalberg, W.O., Roninson, L.K., Buckley, D. Manning, M. & Hoyme, H.E. (2009). *Developmental Disabilities Research Reviews, 15*, 176–192.

Miller, W.R. & Rollnick, S. (2013). *Motivational Interviewing: Helping People Change* (3rd ed.). New York: Guilford Press.

Mueser, K., Noordsy, D.L., Drake, R.E. & Fox, L. (2003). *Integrated Treatment for Dual Disorders: A Guide to Effective Practice* (pp. 49–64). New York: Guilford Press.

Nash, K., Sheard, E., Rovet, J. & Koren, G. (2008). Understanding fetal alcohol spectrum disorders (FASDs): Toward identification of a behavioral phenotype. *Scientific World Journal, 8*, 873–882.

National Center for Injury Prevention and Control. (2003). *Report to Congress on Mild Traumatic Brain Injury in the United States: Steps to Prevent a Serious Public Health Problem*. Atlanta, GA: Centers for Disease Control and Prevention. Retrieved from www.cdc.gov/ncipc/pub-res/mtbi/mtbireport.pdf

Ohio Valley Center for Brain Injury Prevention and Rehabilitation. (2009a). *User's Manual for Faster . . . More Reliable Operation of a Brain after Injury*. Columbus, OH: Author. Retrieved from http://ohiovalley.org/informationeducation/materials/users-manual

Ohio Valley Center for Brain Injury Prevention and Rehabilitation. (2009b). *T-B-I Screening*. Columbus, OH: Author. Retrieved from www.brainline.org/downloads/PDFs/TBI-Screening_v2.pdf

Paley, B. & O'Connor, M.J. (2009). Intervention for individuals with fetal alcohol spectrum disorders: Treatment approaches and case management. *Development Disabilities Research Reviews, 15*, 258–267.

Parry-Jones, B.L., Vaughan, F.L. & Cox, W.M. (2006). Traumatic brain injury and substance misuse: A systematic review of prevalence and outcomes research (1994–2004). *Neuropsychological Rehabilitation, 16*, 537–560.

Ponsford, J., Whelan-Goodinson, R. & Bahar-Fuchs, A. (2007). Alcohol and drug use following traumatic brain injury: A prospective study. *Brain Injury, 21*, 1385–1392.

Public Health Agency of Canada. (2005). *Fetal Alcohol Spectrum Disorder (FASD): A Framework for Action*. Ottawa: Author. Retrieved from www.phac-aspc.gc.ca

Public Health Agency of Canada. (2011). *Assessment and Diagnosis of FASD among Adults: A National and International Systematic Review*. Ottawa: Author. Retrieved from www.phac-aspc.gc.ca

Riley, E.P., Infante, M.A. & Warren, K.R. (2011). Fetal alcohol spectrum disorders: An overview. *Neuropsychology Review, 21*, 73–80.

Simpson, D.D. (1981). Treatment for drug abuse: Follow-up outcomes and length of time spent. *Archives of General Psychiatry, 38*, 875–880.

Simpson, D.D., Joe, G.W. & Rowan-Szal, G.A. (1997). Drug abuse treatment retention and process effects on follow-up outcomes. *Drug and Alcohol Dependence, 47*, 227–235.

Sofuoglu, M., Sugarman, D.E. & Carroll, K.M. (2010). Cognitive function as an emerging treatment target for marijuana addiction. *Experimental and Clinical Psychopharmacology, 18*, 109–119.

Streissguth, A.P., Bookstein, F.L., Barr, H.M., Sampson, P.D., O'Malley, K. & Young, J.K. (2004). Risk factors for adverse life outcomes in fetal alcohol syndrome and fetal alcohol effects. *Journal of Developmental and Behavioral Pediatrics, 25*, 228–238.

Stuss, D.T. (2011). Functions of the frontal lobes: Relation to executive functions. *Journal of the International Neuropsychological Society, 17*, 759–765.

Stuss, D.T. & Levine, B. (2002). Adult clinical neuropsychology: Lessons from studies of the frontal lobes. *Annual Review of Psychology, 53*, 401–433.

Taylor, L.A., Kreutzer, J.S., Demm, S.R. & Meade, M.A. (2003). Traumatic brain injury and substance abuse: A review and analysis of the literature, *Neuropsychological Rehabilitation, 13*, 165–188.

Vungkhanching, M., Heinemann, A.W., Langley, M.J., Ridgely, M. & Kramer, K.M. (2007). Feasibility of a skills-based substance abuse prevention program following traumatic brain injury. *Journal of Head Trauma Rehabilitation, 22*, 167–176.

Walker, R., Cole, J.E., Logan, T.K. & Corrigan, J.D. (2007). Screening substance abuse treatment clients for traumatic brain injury: Prevalence and characteristics. *Journal of Head Trauma Rehabilitation, 22*, 360–367.

Willer, B. & Corrigan, J.D. (1994). Whatever It Takes: A model for community-based services. *Brain Injury, 8*, 647–659.

Appendix

Disability Etiquette

Don't use terminology that defines someone by their disability. The current way of referring to disabilities emphasizes that clients are people first. Accepted terminology is "person with brain injury" rather than "brain-injured person." Most people would not like to be referred to as the "victim" of a disability or disease.

Ensure physical accessibility. Be sure that whatever room you use for meetings can accommodate the person's mode of mobility. Even when a facility is generally accessible, furniture may have been arranged in a way that makes doorways impassable. A person who uses a wheelchair will feel most welcome if furniture has been arranged before-hand. People who use a wheelchair or scooter may prefer to transfer to a chair once in the room. It is polite to offer them the opportunity to transfer with a simple statement, such as, "Would you like to stay in your chair or transfer to one here?" Know where the accessible washrooms are. Take note of the location of stairs—even one or two (or a ramp that is too short and steep) can be barriers.

Ask before helping. What may seem like a hassle to you may be a normal activity for someone else. Sometimes help may be appreciated—other times it may feel like an intrusion. But watching someone struggle with a door or curb is also awkward. Asking whether or not the person needs help or support and what they would prefer is generally the best tactic.

Don't touch assistive devices unless you've been given permission. People often consider their wheelchair, walker or cane as an extension of themselves.

If you don't understand something the client has said, ask. You may feel awkward asking a person whose speech is difficult to understand to repeat themselves. However, it is generally considered polite to work at understanding the person's message. Honest attempts at understanding communicate respect and build trust.

Don't be afraid to ask questions. Clients may have assistive devices that are new to you. They may use terms in describing their situation that are unfamiliar. It is better to ask for clarification than to feign knowledge of facts you think you should have known.

Don't tell people with disabilities about all of the other people with disabilities you know. Most people would like to be seen as individuals first, regardless of whether or not they belong to any particular group.

Some disabilities are invisible. Clients with ABI often have no obvious impairments. It is appropriate to ask them directly about how they feel their injury has affected them.

Avoid false reassurance. Most people with disabilities you meet have had the experience of people saying everything will be fine, when they know their world has been radically altered. It is usually better to acknowledge and validate a client's perspectives on living with a disability.

Make sure to address the client directly. Some clients will come with helpers of various kinds. Be sure to honour the client's status by speaking directly to him or her (even if interpretation is needed).

It isn't necessary to change the way you use words. There are many sayings that, in the context of various disabilities, might make the speaker feel awkward; for example, saying "I see" to a person with a visual disability, or asking a person in a wheelchair to "stand up for yourself." Most people are familiar with these common phrases and do not resent their use.

Be careful not to make assumptions about the nature and extent of a person's difficulties. The presence of one disability does not suggest the existence of others. For example, some people who have visual impairments complain that when someone finds out they have low or no vision, they often speak loudly, as if their hearing is impaired as well.

Chapter 19

Treating Addictions in Correctional Settings

Andrea E. Moser, Flora I. Matheson, Brian A. Grant and John R. Weekes

Peter, 37, is a first-time offender who is serving a three-year sentence for a series of fraud convictions. He is married with three children, and, at the time of his arrest, was employed full time as the sales representative for a large hardware supply company. He was convicted of defrauding his employer of $13,200 by submitting phony sales invoices. Although he and his wife have been married for 12 years, their marriage has been strained in recent years due to financial difficulties, challenges raising their children and the fact that Peter is frequently out of town on business.

Peter began drinking at age 13, and used marijuana recreationally until he got his first full-time job at 19, and quit. As an adult, he continues to drink—somewhat heavily when he is on the road and bored. About nine years ago, Peter was diagnosed with depression and was prescribed antidepressants to deal with this condition.

Richard, 26, is an Aboriginal man from an isolated reserve in northern Alberta who is serving a five-year sentence for aggravated assault. At the time of the offence, Richard had just arrived in Edmonton to look for work. After drinking eight beers at a downtown bar, he got involved in an argument that quickly escalated into a physical fight in which Richard broke the other man's nose and jaw. The bar manager called the police and Richard was arrested. The other man was taken by ambulance to the hospital where he was treated for his injuries and released two days later.

Richard has a long history of involvement with the police. He has been incarcerated in the provincial jail system in Alberta and Saskatchewan four times—all involving violence while intoxicated. He has also served a 40-month sentence in a federal correctional institution for assault causing bodily harm. Richard has a history of alcohol and other drug use that started when he was a teenager. In addition to drinking beer and liquor, he occasionally uses cocaine and has tried methamphetamine several times.

✦

Renée, 31, makes her living as a sex trade worker in downtown Montreal. She grew up in an abusive family just outside Quebec City. Her mother's live-in boyfriend repeatedly physically and sexually abused her from age 11 until she ran away from home at 15. Renée began using alcohol and smoking marijuana when she was 12 to help her cope with the trauma. Her alcohol use continued to increase in her teen years and she began using more serious drugs, including crack and heroin. For the last six years, she has been injecting a number of opiate-based pain relief medications daily. When Renée was 22, she tested positive for hepatitis C (HCV). She has had thousands of sexual partners over the years. Although she uses condoms regularly, she is not sure if she has infected her clients with hepatitis C. Renée has been in and out of withdrawal management and treatment centres many times but has been unable to stop her drug use. Her life as a sex trade worker has brought her into repeated contact with the police, and she has been incarcerated numerous times for drug possession and prostitution. Renée and her pimp were recently convicted of assaulting one of her clients for not paying her for sex. She received a two-year sentence.

Most people entering the correctional system have multiple issues that either contribute to or result from substance use problems. Specifically, many have emotional difficulties and mental health problems (Fazel et al., 2006; Grant & Gileno, 2008; Grant et al., 2008) and often struggle with issues around employment, education and community functioning (Babooram, 2008). In addition, involvement in the drug trade is common, with up to 25 per cent of offenders having been convicted for drug offences (Motiuk & Vuong, 2006). This complexity presents unique challenges in providing treatment services to this group.

Statistics Canada reports that 95 per cent of people sentenced to custody in Saskatchewan and 81 per cent admitted to federal penitentiaries had moderate or severe substance use problems (Babooram, 2008). Data from Nova Scotia indicates that 77 per cent of inmates have substance use problems requiring treatment (Kitchin, 2006). It is believed that offenders serving their sentence in the community have a similar rate of substance use issues. For example, in a sample of federal offenders, 84 per cent reported drug use in the community and 42 per cent reported injection drug use (Zakaria et al., 2010).

This chapter describes evidence-informed best practices for substance use interventions for offenders. The focus is on the key elements of effective interventions—specifically assessment, treatment and aftercare. We briefly discuss unique offender groups that require additional considerations, such as women, Aboriginal people and people with concurrent mental health and substance use problems. The three case vignettes that opened this chapter are used to illustrate the practical implications of the practices outlined in each section.

Assessment

As with non-correctional populations, the principal role of assessment is to inform and shape the development of a relatively individualized treatment plan, regardless of whether treatment will be delivered on an individual or group basis. In addition, information elicited during the assessment process can be usefully incorporated into different phases of treatment. At a minimum, areas that should be targeted in assessment with offenders include:

- severity of alcohol use
- severity of drug use
- possible "poly" (i.e., multiple) use and abuse
- previous treatment history
- client motivation and treatment readiness (Weekes et al., 1999).

Within the criminal justice and corrections context, another very important component of assessment is the link between an offender's substance use problems and criminal behaviour (direct or indirect).

In addition to a clinical interview, standardized instruments, such as the Michigan Alcohol Screening Test ([MAST]; Selzer, 1971); the Alcohol Dependence Scale ([ADS]; Skinner & Horn, 1984); the Drug Abuse Screening Test ([DAST]; Skinner, 1982); and the Severity of Dependence Scale ([SDS]; Gossop et al., 1995), are appropriate for use with a criminal justice population. Not only are these instruments short and easy to administer (either in paper-and-pencil or electronic formats, or administered verbally); they have also been used extensively with criminal justice and corrections clients, as well as clients in a wide variety of other settings.

Like other clinical populations, offenders vary in intellectual or cognitive ability, language ability and usage, reading ability, gender, ethnicity and many other dimensions—differences that must be considered in the assessment process.

Finally, referrals for mental and physical health assessments are key for identifying issues such as concurrent mental health disorders and exposure to infectious diseases caused by high-risk behaviours such as needle sharing that will influence the offender's treatment plan.

> Upon arriving at the penitentiary, Peter participated in a standardized substance use assessment that included administering the Alcohol Dependence Scale (ADS) and the Drug Abuse Screening Test (DAST). The results of this assessment indicated that he has a mild problem with alcohol and no problem with illicit drugs. The fact that Peter has taken antidepressants to manage depression suggests that he may have a concurrent substance use and mental health disorder. He was referred for a mental health assessment to explore this possibility more thoroughly.

◆

Richard was administered a battery of screening measures that included the ADS, DAST and Severity of Dependence Scale (SDS). This assessment confirmed that he has a moderately severe problem with alcohol and a low-severity problem with other drugs.

✦

The results of Renée's DAST and SDS indicated that she has a severe substance use problem, including addiction to opiate pain-relief medications and alcohol. Because of this addiction to opiates, her history of needle sharing and her HCV positive status, Renée was referred to a health care centre at her placement penitentiary to assess whether she met the criteria for opiate substitution therapy (OST) and to develop a treatment plan for her health care needs related to the hepatitis C. A health assessment for her HCV infection determined that she was currently asymptomatic, but that she would be monitored regularly to identify if her health status changed. Renée was also referred for a mental health assessment due to the trauma she had suffered from her childhood physical and sexual abuse.

Treatment

Despite the challenges of working with correctional clients, treatment can have a positive impact. Numerous studies have demonstrated that treatment programs can reduce readmissions to custody that are often associated with a return to substance use (Grant et. al., 2003; Kunic & Varis, 2010; Matheson et al., 2011). While the primary objective of substance use treatment may be the reduction or cessation of substance use, a secondary benefit for correctional clients is the associated reduction in new crimes. Research has shown that many crimes are committed under the influence of alcohol and other drugs, in the pursuit of money for drugs or as a result of the drug trade (Pernanen et al., 2002). The more severe the substance use problem, the stronger the association is with criminal behaviour (Brochu et al., 2001; Kunic & Grant, 2007; Weekes et al., 1999).

For community treatment, clients may be mandated to undergo treatment by a court through a probation sentence or as part of a parole condition, or they may receive services through a drug treatment court, depending on the crime. Some research has shown that, while community-based treatments can be highly effective (Lattimore et al., 2005; Matheson et al., 2011), barriers may exist to accessing treatment services in rural centres (Oser et al., 2012). Some correctional clients may be serving a short sentence—less than two years and often less than 30 days—in a provincial jail. In this situation, interventions need to be modular and brief in order to ensure that clear treatment objectives are met. Other people may be serving longer sentences—two years or more—in a federal penitentiary. The type and length of the sentence will affect the type of programming that can be offered (e.g., brief or intensive interventions vs. an extended treatment program), but the sentence and setting do not alter the principles under which effective treatment should be delivered.

A large body of research exists indicating what general approaches to correctional intervention are best suited for this population (Lipsey & Cullen, 2007; Smith et al., 2009), as well as identifying the features of effective substance use programs in general (McMurran, 2007; Moos, 2003). From this research, seven key components of effective substance use programs for a correctional clientele have emerged.

1. Match the Intensity of Treatment to Problem Severity

A key component to consider when assessing a person's substance use history is the severity of the problem. Some writers have criticized a "one-size-fits-all" approach to substance use treatment for applying the same rigorous standards of treatment for people with both mild and serious problems, such as putting a client with a mild addiction through several weeks of residential treatment (Weekes et al., 1999). Aside from the obvious inefficiencies in cost and access to treatment posed by such an approach, research on correctional populations has demonstrated that putting low-need offenders in high-intensity programs may have negative effects, perhaps by interfering with positive factors in the person's life, such as good family relationships, positive supports, pro-social attitudes and steady employment (Lowenkamp & Latessa, 2005).

Based on such research, certain correctional jurisdictions, including the Correctional Service of Canada (CSC), have begun providing correctional programs based on an assessment of offender risk for reoffending and problem severity. Treatment options range from community-based low-intensity interventions (if required) for people assessed as having a low-intensity problem to intensive prison-based programs for those with substantial and severe substance use histories. Research on these programs has demonstrated their effectiveness, particularly in reducing recidivism (Grant et al., 2003; Kunic & Varis, 2010).

2. Adopt a Social Learning and Cognitive-Behavioural Approach

From a social learning and overlapping cognitive-behavioural perspective, addiction is largely a learned, maladaptive behaviour that can be addressed by teaching and modelling pro-social behaviour (Pearce & Holbrook, 2002). According to this view, offenders initially develop antisocial thoughts and behaviours, including substance use problems, as coping mechanisms. These thoughts and behaviours are then maintained by immediate internal reinforcers, such as feelings of excitement and pleasure, which are more powerful than delayed negative consequences, such as arrest and incarceration.

Treatment approaches based on these interrelated theories attempt to modify the person's behavioural coping skills and cognitive processes to change the target behaviour (Parks & Marlatt, 1999). The rationale behind this approach is that if substance use is initiated and maintained by past learning experiences—including peer modelling, reinforcement contingencies and cognitive beliefs (Donovan & Marlatt, 2005)—then these same processes can be used to help the person learn more adaptive cognitive, behavioural and interpersonal coping responses (Andrews & Bonta, 2010; Parks & Marlatt, 1999). Typically, this approach emphasizes acquiring skills through techniques such as role play, cognitive restructuring (i.e., identifying and correcting thinking patterns that support the maladaptive behaviour) and behavioural rehearsal (Smith et al., 2009).

Research has strongly and consistently supported the effectiveness of interventions based on social learning and cognitive-behavioural interventions over other non-behavioural treatment modalities for offenders to target behaviours including substance abuse (Antonowicz & Ross, 1994; Smith et al., 2009).

3. Adhere to the "Risk-Need-Responsivity" Model

According to this model, originally articulated by Andrews and Bonta (2010), three conditions must be met for effective intervention with offenders:

1. The risk principle: Treatment is prioritized so that it is delivered to the highest-risk offenders first. These offenders are the most appropriate targets for intensive services because they typically represent a higher risk to reoffend and also have more room for change compared to people who pose a lower risk (Smith et al., 2009).
2. The need principle: Dynamic or changeable risk factors should be the targets of change in order to reduce recidivism. Alcohol and other drug abuse are clearly identified in correctional research literature as one of the predominant need areas for offenders (Andrews & Bonta, 2010).
3. The responsivity principle: General responsivity supports the notion that the most effective interventions for offenders are those based on cognitive, behavioural and social learning theories (Gendreau, 1996). Specific responsivity, on the other hand, refers to the need for treatment providers to match offenders to interventions according to key offender characteristics, including factors such as motivation and cognitive functioning (Gendreau, 1996), as well as gender and ethnicity (Hubbard, 2007). Literature reviews since the early 1990s have provided clear empirical support for the efficacy of programs, including those that target substance use problems, based on the risk-need-responsivity model in reducing recidivism among offenders (Smith et al., 2009).

4. Use Motivational Enhancement Techniques

While research clearly shows that appropriate treatment interventions with offenders who have substance use problems can have a significant impact on outcomes, studies have also indicated that people who complete a program and remain engaged in aftercare following the intensive phase of an intervention reap the best results. In a meta-analysis of cognitive-behavioural treatment outcome studies, McMurran and Theodosi (2007) found that non-completers of both institutional and community programs were more likely to be reconvicted than offenders in untreated comparison groups, with this effect being more marked for offenders in the community. The authors note that the findings on recidivism rates indicate that it is critical to address recruitment and retention in treatment.

Motivational interviewing, originally developed by Miller and Rollnick (2002), is one important technique for motivating people with substance use problems to commit to engaging in the treatment process. The key element of the approach is to elicit "change talk" by using specific techniques, such as expressing empathy and working on ambivalence, to strengthen the commitment to change (Miller, 2011). Motivational enhancement techniques, such as allowing clients to establish their own treatment goals and complete exercises (e.g., a "decisional balance," which helps clients evaluate the pros and cons of their substance use), can be incorporated into group treatments.

Research demonstrates the effectiveness of motivational interviewing as both a stand-alone intervention and a prelude to more intensive interventions (Burke et al., 2003; Vasilaki et al., 2006). The approach should therefore be viewed as an important element of any comprehensive and inclusive approach to addressing engagement and retention in substance use treatment.

5. Apply Therapeutic Integrity

Beyond highlighting the importance of having a research-based theoretical framework in correctional programs, studies have also demonstrated the key role of "therapeutic integrity" for program success (Gendreau, 1996; Gendreau et al., 2006). Therapeutic integrity refers to such factors as adequately selecting, training and supervising therapists and delivering the program consistently and in a standardized way. Studies using the Correctional Program Assessment Inventory, an assessment tool that evaluates eight domains of therapeutic integrity for correctional programs (Gendreau & Andrews, 2001), have demonstrated a positive correlation between principles of therapeutic integrity and treatment effectiveness (Lowenkamp et al., 2006).

6. Opioid Substitution Therapy

Opioid substitution therapy is one of the most widely used and effective interventions for addiction to heroin and other opiates. Research indicates that it has multiple benefits for people with an opiate addiction, including:

- reduction in use of illicitly obtained opioids
- reduction in use of other substances
- reduction in injection drug use behaviour
- less time involved in criminal activities
- less time incarcerated
- much lower death rates compared to people not receiving treatment
- lower risk of acquiring HIV/AIDS, hepatitis C or other blood-borne pathogens
- improvement in physical and mental health
- increased likelihood of gaining full-time employment
- improved overall quality of life (Health Canada, 2002, pp. 17–18).

By reducing risk behaviours in people with opiate addiction, opioid substitution therapy also benefits society by decreasing criminal activity and improving public health (Health Canada, 2002; Stallwitz & Stöver, 2007).

7. Treatment Maintenance

In many addiction treatment settings, the focus of program resources is often on the "intensive" phase of a program, which typically consists of frequent sessions over a specified period in either an inpatient or outpatient treatment setting. However, research has demonstrated the critical role of ongoing, longer-term engagement (often referred to as maintenance or continuing care) beyond the intensive phase of treatment. In fact, several studies have shown that the duration of care is more important than the amount of care (Crits-Christoph & Siqueland, 1996; Moos et al., 2000). Moos (2003) states that this finding "is consistent with the fact that the enduring aspects of individuals' life contexts are associated with the recurrent course of remission and relapse" (p. 4). The importance of treatment maintenance in the context of continuity of care is discussed in the next section.

> Peter was referred to a community-based, low-intensity substance use program, which he would participate in once released. He was also referred for a mental health assessment, which indicated the presence of moderate clinical depression with no current risk of suicide. Peter was prescribed antidepressants and was referred to an institutional psychologist for cognitive-behavioural therapy.

Richard was referred to an institutionally based moderate-intensity substance use program for Aboriginal men that blended social learning, cognitive-behavioural and motivational techniques with traditional Aboriginal healing approaches. Through the program, Richard increased his engagement in Aboriginal culture and began to participate in cultural activities outside of the program, including regular sessions with an Aboriginal Elder.

Renée was referred for an institutionally based high-intensity substance use program for women that incorporated social learning, cognitive-behavioural and motivational techniques. She also began methadone maintenance treatment. Once she had stabilized on a maintenance dose of methadone, she started the intensive phase of the substance use program. Ongoing consultation between heath services and programs staff ensured that the methadone maintenance and substance use treatment worked in concert to address Renée's treatment needs.

Continuity of Care

To be most effective, substance use interventions should continue to be provided once the person has left prison. Continuity of care refers to the continued provision of therapeutic activities to support positive behaviours learned during treatment, rather than procedures that promote new treatment goals (Harmon et al., 1982). In this way, lessons learned in prison are reinforced for offenders released into the community. Such programs allow offenders to continue to develop and maintain the skills they learned in institutional programs and apply them to situations in the community.

Offenders released from prison have a better chance to remain prison free if they have participated in aftercare programs in the community, particularly given that 66 per cent of all relapses occur within the first 90 days after treatment (Marlatt & Gordon, 1985). If we accept that slips and relapses naturally follow substance use treatment, then service providers must commit to providing support to offenders once they have completed their initial treatment, and help prevent recidivism.

According to Turnbull and McSweeney (2000), 19 countries worldwide have policies on aftercare pre- and post-release, with the length of time for services varying from 12 weeks to two years. The primary objectives of these aftercare policies are to provide information, continue treatment, enhance social reintegration, prevent drug use and connect prisoners with community-based drug services. Spain, the Czech Republic, Latvia, Malta, Portugal and Sweden have policies recommending at least six months of aftercare, while 21 countries report providing pre-release assistance within six months of release.

The types of services provided include relapse prevention; information on drug treatment, helping services and counselling; and assistance with arranging new or continued treatment. Approaches to aftercare vary in both frequency of contact and theoretical approach. Not surprisingly, the aftercare component of a treatment intervention is almost always based on the same model of intervention as the more intensive treatment phase. For example, aftercare programs developed by CSC, the federal department responsible for the supervision of adults sentenced to two or more years of imprisonment, focus on offenders maintaining skills that reduce the risk of drug relapse and return to prison. Cognitive-behavioural strategies, experiential exercises and coping-skills practice are essential aspects of these aftercare programs.

Self-help groups focus on helping people develop and maintain skills, such as problem solving and identifying high-risk situations. In correctional facilities, they play a crucial role in providing positive countercultural alternatives to gangs and to social isolation by offering fellowship and an ethic of abstinence and recovery. Alcoholics Anonymous, Narcotics Anonymous and Cocaine Anonymous are the most well-known self-help groups and, theoretically grounded in the disease model of addiction, encourage the practice of sobriety. These groups can also provide an additional layer of community social support for offenders after they leave prison and can help them achieve and maintain abstinence through social support and a healthy lifestyle (Emrick et al., 1993; Hanninen & Koski-Jannes, 1999; Peyrot, 1985; Snow et al., 1994; Weiss et al., 1996; Wells, 1987).

Challenges in Providing Continuity of Care

Multiple challenges exist in providing continuity of care from prison to the community. Programming is more difficult to implement in less-populated urban and rural areas; fewer offenders live in these areas, and staff and program resources are scarce. Employment (for men and women) and child care responsibilities (primarily among women) often supersede program attendance. Reliable and affordable sources of transportation may also be a challenge. Retention in treatment programs requires co-ordination and integration of services for newly released offenders. With the overall goal of reducing crime and substance use among offenders, factors such as the nature of relationships between service providers and correctional agencies, current capacity among service providers (including community corrections) to engage and retain men and women, and the degree to which linkages between services are facilitated all need to be considered.

> Health services staff are concerned for Peter because his depression, while under control through medication, persists. Before Peter left prison, staff referred him to a community mental health program, where he will be able to access a psychiatrist to monitor his condition and his medication.

✦

Richard has completed his sentence and has returned to his community in northern Alberta. There are no traditional treatment programs there, so before Richard's release, prison staff worked with Aboriginal Elders in the facility to identify a community-based Elder who will work with Richard to continue his relapse prevention plan upon his return home.

Reneé is apprehensive about her imminent departure from prison. She has worked with health services and programs staff to develop a relapse prevention plan. Renée is concerned that she will slip back into opiate use once she returns to her old haunts. Treatment has helped her recognize that pressure from her former drug-using friends and old sights and sounds may trigger an incredible urge to use. However, Renée has learned a range of skills to cope with these situations when they arise. She admits that she often used drugs in the past to avoid "sad feelings" that relate to her history of childhood sexual abuse. She is hoping that treatment and support in the community will help her maintain the progress she has made in prison.

Unique Client Groups

Women Offenders

Women offenders experience social and emotional problems, including unstable housing; mental and physical health problems that stem in part from childhood and adult physical and sexual abuse; poly- and injection drug use; poor employment prospects; low education; poverty and unhealthy living conditions (Bloom et al., 2002; Dowden & Blanchette, 1999; Erickson et al., 2000; Langan & Pelissier, 2001; Sanders et al., 1997). Women in prison are up to 10 times more likely to have a drug addiction than women in the general population (Fazel et al., 2006; Henderson, 1998). Eight out of 10 women offenders have a substance use problem (Grant & Gileno, 2008). Up to 60 per cent of women entering the prison system report non-injection drug use, and 29 per cent report injection drug use (Zakaria et al., 2010).

Offenders who are mothers are often estranged from their children or risk losing access to their children because of their continued substance use problems, posing an additional layer of complexity to their drug treatment. Women offenders traditionally make up only seven per cent of the prison population, with the result that women-specific program models have only recently been introduced to the prison environment: gender-responsive programs were introduced in the United States in the late 1980s and in Canada in 1995. For these reasons, evidenced-based practice around drug treatments for women offenders is not well established; however, some principles do exist. Summarizing the theoretical literature, Bloom and colleagues (2002) suggest considering the following six principles when developing and delivering gender-specific correctional programming to women and girls:

1. Gender: Acknowledge that gender makes a difference.
2. Environment: Create an environment based on safety, respect and dignity.
3. Relationships: Develop policies, practices and programs that are relational and promote healthy connections to children, family, significant others and the community.
4. Services and supervision: Address substance use, trauma and mental health issues through comprehensive, integrated and culturally relevant services and appropriate community supervision.
5. Socio-economic status: Provide women with opportunities to improve their socio-economic conditions.
6. Community: Establish a system of community supervision and re-entry with comprehensive, collaborative services.

Aboriginal Offenders

Aboriginal offenders—First Nations, Inuit and Métis—make up a large percentage of correctional populations relative to their representation in the Canadian population. They represent 20 per cent of offenders in custody in federal penitentiaries (CSC, 2009), but only three per cent of the Canadian population (Statistics Canada, 2010). The high number of Aboriginal offenders in Canadian prisons presents special challenges to people who are providing substance use treatment in this environment. Not only are Aboriginal people overrepresented, but most also have substance use problems associated with their criminal behaviour. The prevalence of substance use problems in this population is staggering: 93 per cent of First Nations and Inuit, and 91 per cent of Métis offenders are assessed on intake as having a high need for intervention for substance use problems (Motiuk & Nafekh, 2000).

Some correctional jurisdictions have responded to these complex health and social needs by developing programs tailored specifically for Aboriginal people that incorporate cultural traditions and healing and engage Elders in the healing process (see Kunic & Varis, 2010, for a review). The highly successful Aboriginal Offender Substance Abuse Program developed by CSC teaches Aboriginal offenders about their culture and history to help them understand the issues that may have led to their use of alcohol and other drugs. The program then relies on Aboriginal cultural teachings to show how to overcome the challenges and create a positive future. Using cognitive-behavioural approaches, the program teaches the skills and attitudes needed to reduce the likelihood of a return to problematic substance use. The program and its results demonstrate the need to include cultural and historical issues in the treatment of correctional clients who may not see themselves as part of the mainstream society.

Offenders with Concurrent Mental Health and Substance Use Problems

The comorbidity of substance use and mental health issues, particularly among people with the most severe psychiatric disorders, such as schizophrenia, is of increasing concern to correctional jurisdictions (DiClemente et al., 2008). Although data from several countries, including Canada, the United States and the United Kingdom, suggest that rates of mental health problems among offenders have been increasing over the last decade, estimates of current substance use problems among offenders with mental health problems are difficult to attain due to inconsistencies in screening and assessment processes, the inaccuracy of records and variations in diagnostic criteria (Weldon & Ritchie, 2010).

However, studies do indicate that many people in forensic settings have concurrent substance use and mental health disorders. Wheatley (1998) found that 62 per cent of patients in a secure unit who were diagnosed with schizophrenia had a concurrent substance abuse disorder. Fifty-one per cent had a forensic history. And in a study that examined four groups of offenders—with concurrent disorders, a substance use problem only, a mental health disorder only or no problem—the concurrent disorders group had the highest risk and need ratings and more extensive criminal histories than the other groups. Controlling for other factors associated with reoffending, the concurrent disorders group was also nearly two times more likely to reoffend than the no problem group (Wilton & Stewart, 2012).

Key to interventions for offenders is the integration of long-term ongoing mental health and substance use treatment services. Psychosocial interventions that incorporate cognitive-behavioural therapy and motivational interviewing principles in addition to coping and social skills training also show promising results with this group (Weldon & Ritchie, 2010).

Conclusion

People entering the criminal justice system typically present with multiple issues, including substance use problems, which contribute to their involvement in crime. In many cases, coming before the courts or under the jurisdiction of a correctional system may provide these people with an opportunity to participate in treatment, sometimes for the first time. A great deal of evidence demonstrates that substance use treatment that aligns to certain principles is effective in reducing both substance use and reoffending. Canadian correctional jurisdictions, most specifically the CSC, have been at the forefront of developing evidence-based substance use interventions for offenders, including specific subgroups of offenders, such as Aboriginal people and women, who require specialized treatment approaches.

Practice Tips

- Complete a comprehensive assessment and use the assessment results to inform treatment assignment and clinical decision-making.
- Have multiple levels of treatment available and assign treatment based on the severity of the substance use problem.
- Use substance abuse treatment programs based on best practices identified in the research literature on "what works" with a correctional population. Specifically, this refers to programs using a cognitive-behavioural and social learning approach that incorporate motivational enhancement techniques.
- Provide services beyond the initial intensive treatment phase, and continue to provide support to the client once he or she has been released from prison.
- Consider the needs of unique client groups such as women, Aboriginal people and people with mental health and cognitive functioning issues.
- Incorporate evidence-based techniques such as motivational interviewing to enhance treatment engagement and build effective therapeutic relationships.

Resources

Publications

Blanchette, K. (2006). *The Assessment and Treatment of Women Offenders: An Integrative Perspective.* Hoboken, NJ: Wiley & Sons.

Center for Substance Abuse Treatment. (2005). *Substance Abuse Treatment for Adults in the Criminal Justice System.* Treatment Improvement Protocol (TIP) series 44. Rockville, MD: Author. Retrieved from www.ncbi.nlm.nih.gov/books/NBK64137/

Couture, J.E. (2001). Programming for Aboriginal offenders. In L.L. Motiuk & R.C. Serin (Eds.), *Compendium 2000 on Effective Correctional Programming* (pp. 158–159). Ottawa: Ministry of Supply and Services Canada.

National Institute on Drug Abuse. (2011, May). Treating offenders with drug problems: Integrating public health and public safety. *NIDA Topics in Brief.* Rockville, MD: Author. Retrieved from www.drugabuse.gov/sites/default/files/drugs_crime.pdf

Springer, D.W., McNeece, C.A. & Arnold, E.M. (2003). *Substance Abuse Treatment for Criminal Offenders: An Evidence-Based Guide for Practitioners.* Washington, DC: American Psychological Association.

Walters, S.T., Clark, M.D., Gingerich, R. & Meitzer, M.L. (2007). *A Guide for Probation and Parole: Motivating Offenders to Change.* Washington, DC: National Institute of Corrections. Retrieved from http://static.nicic.gov/Library/022253.pdf

Internet

Correctional Service of Canada—Aboriginal corrections
   www.csc-scc.gc.ca/text/pblcsbjct-eng.shtml#aboriginal

References

Andrews, D.A. & Bonta, J. (2010). *The Psychology of Criminal Conduct* (5th ed.). New Providence, NJ: LexisNexis Group.

Antonowicz, D.H. & Ross, R.R. (1994). Essential components of successful rehabilitation programs for offenders. *International Journal of Offender and Comparative Criminology, 38*, 97–194.

Babooram, A. (2008, December). The changing profile of adults in custody, 2006–2007. *Juristat, 28* (10). Ottawa: Statistics Canada. Retrieved from www.statcan.gc.ca/pub/85-002-x/2008010/article/10732-eng.htm

Bloom, B.E., Owen, B. & Covington, S.S. (2002). *Gender Responsive Strategies: Research, Practice, and Guiding Principles for Women Offenders.* Washington, DC: National Institute of Corrections. Retrieved from http://static.nicic.gov/Library/018017.pdf

Brochu, S., Cousineau, M.-M., Gillet, M., Cournoyer, L.-G., Pernanen, K. & Motiuk, L. (2001). Drugs, alcohol and criminal behaviour: A profile of inmates in Canadian federal institutions. *Forum on Corrections Research, 13*, 20–24.

Burke, B.L., Arkowitz, H. & Menchola, M. (2003). The efficacy of motivational interviewing: A meta-analysis of controlled clinical trials. *Journal of Consulting and Clinical Psychology, 71*, 843–861.

Correctional Service of Canada (CSC). (2009). *The Changing Federal Offender Population: Aboriginal Offender Highlights 2009.* Ottawa: Author. Retrieved from www.csc-scc.gc.ca/text/rsrch/special_reports/ah2009/Aboriginal_Highlights-2009-eng.pdf

Crits-Christoph, P. & Siqueland, L. (1996). Psychosocial treatment for drug abuse: Selected review and recommendations for national health care. *Archives of General Psychiatry, 53*, 749–756.

DiClemente, C.C., Nidecker, M. & Bellack, A.S. (2008). Motivation and stages of change among individuals with severe mental illness and substance abuse disorders. *Journal of Substance Abuse Treatment, 34*, 25–35.

Donovan, D.M. & Marlatt, G.A. (Eds.). (2005). *Assessment of Addictive Behaviors* (2nd ed.). New York: Guilford Press.

Dowden, C. & Blanchette, K. (1999). *An Investigation into the Characteristics of Substance-Abusing Women Offenders: Risk, Need and Post-release Outcome.* Ottawa: Correctional Service of Canada. Retrieved from www.csc-scc.gc.ca/text/rsrch/reports/r81/r81_e.pdf

Emrick, C.D., Tonigan, J.S., Montgomery, H. & Little, L. (1993). Alcoholics Anonymous: What is currently known? In B.S. McCrady & W.R. Miller (Eds.), *Research on Alcoholics Anonymous: Opportunities and Alternatives* (pp. 41–76). Piscataway, NJ: Rutgers Center of Alcohol Studies.

Erickson, P.G., Butters, J., McGillicuddy, P. & Hallgren, A. (2000). Crack and prostitution: Gender, myths, and experiences. *Journal of Drug Issues, 30,* 767–788.

Fazel, S., Bains, P. & Doll, H. (2006). Substance abuse and dependence in prisoners: A systematic review. *Addiction, 101,* 181–191.

Gendreau, P. (1996). The principles of effective intervention with offenders. In A.T. Harland (Ed.), *Choosing Correctional Options That Work: Defining the Demand and Evaluating the Supply* (pp. 117–130). Thousand Oaks, CA: Sage.

Gendreau, P. & Andrews, D.A. (2001). Correctional Program Assessment Inventory (CPAI-2000). Saint John, NB: University of New Brunswick.

Gendreau, P., Goggin, C., French, S. & Smith, P. (2006). Practicing psychology in correctional settings: "What works" in reducing criminal behavior. In I.B. Weiner & A.K. Hess (Eds.), *Handbook of Forensic Psychology* (3rd ed., pp. 722–750). New York: John Wiley & Sons.

Gossop, M., Darke, S., Griffiths, P., Hando, J., Powis, B., Hall, W. & Strang, J. (1995). The Severity of Dependence Scale (SDS): Psychometric properties of the SDS in English and Australian samples of heroin, cocaine and amphetamine users. *Addiction, 90,* 607–614.

Grant, B.A., Furlong, A., Hume, L, White, T. & Doherty, S. (2008). *The Women Offender Substance Abuse Programming: Interim Research Report.* Ottawa: Correctional Service of Canada. Retrieved from www.csc-scc.gc.ca/text/rsrch/reports/r171/r171-eng.pdf

Grant, B.A. & Gileno, J. (2008). *The Changing Federal Offender Population.* Ottawa: Correctional Service of Canada.

Grant, B.A., Kunic, D., MacPherson, P., McKeown, C. & Hansen, E. (2003). *The High Intensity Substance Abuse Program (HISAP): Results from the Pilot Programs.* Ottawa: Correctional Service of Canada. Retrieved from www.csc-scc.gc.ca/text/rsrch/reports/r140/r140_e.pdf

Hanninen, V. & Koski-Jannes, A. (1999). Narratives of recovery from addictive behaviours. *Addiction, 94,* 1837–1848.

Harmon, S.K., Lantinga, L.J. & Costello, R.M. (1982). Aftercare in chemical dependence treatment. *Bulletin of the Society of Psychologists in Substance Abuse, 1,* 107–109.

Health Canada. (2002). *Best Practices—Methadone Maintenance Treatment.* Ottawa: Health Canada. Retrieved from www.hc-sc.gc.ca

Henderson, D.J. (1998). Drug abuse and incarcerated women: A research review. *Journal of Substance Abuse Treatment, 15,* 579–587.

Hubbard, D. (2007). Getting the most out of correctional treatment: Testing the responsivity principle on male and female offenders. *Federal Probation, 71* (1): 2–8.

Kitchin, H. (2006). Addictions programming: A perspective on corrections in Nova Scotia. *Forum on Corrections Research, 18* (1), 9–11.

Kunic, D. & Grant, B.A. (2007). *The Computerized Assessment of Substance Abuse (CASA): Results from the Demonstration Project.* Ottawa: Correctional Service of Canada. Retrieved from www.csc-scc.gc.ca

Kunic, D. & Varis, D.D. (2010). *The Aboriginal Offender Substance Abuse Program (AOSAP): Examining the Effects of Successful Completion on Post-Release Outcomes.* Ottawa: Correctional Service of Canada. Retrieved from www.csc-scc.gc.ca

Langan, N.P. & Pelissier, B.M. (2001). Gender differences among prisoners in drug treatment. *Journal of Substance Abuse, 13,* 291–301.

Lattimore, P., Krebs, C., Koetse, W., Lindquist, C. & Cowell, A. (2005). Predicting the effect of substance abuse treatment on probationer recidivism. *Journal of Experimental Criminology, 1,* 159–189.

Lipsey, M.W. & Cullen, F.T. (2007). The effectiveness of correctional rehabilitation: A review of systematic reviews. *Annual Review of Law and Social Science, 3,* 297–320.

Lowenkamp, C.T. & Latessa, E.J. (2005). Increasing the effectiveness of correctional programming through the risk principle: Identifying offenders for residential placement. *Criminology and Public Policy, 4,* 263–289.

Lowenkamp, C.T., Latessa, E.J. & Smith, P. (2006). Does correctional program quality really matter? The importance of adhering to the principles of effective intervention. *Criminology and Public Policy, 5,* 210–220.

Marlatt, G.A. & Gordon, J.R. (1985*). Relapse Prevention: Maintenance Strategies in the Treatment of Addictive Behaviors.* New York: Guilford Press.

Matheson, F., Doherty, S. & Grant, B.A. (2011). Community-based aftercare and return to custody in a national sample of substance-abusing women offenders. *American Journal of Public Health, 101,* 1126–1132.

McMurran, M. (2007). What works in substance misuse treatment for offenders? *Criminal Behaviour and Mental Health, 17,* 225–233.

McMurran, M. & Theodosi, E. (2007). Is offender treatment non-completion associated with increased reconviction over no treatment? *Psychology, Crime and Law, 13,* 333–343.

Miller, W.R. (2011). Motivational interviewing: Research, practice, and puzzles. *Addictive Behaviors, 21,* 835–842.

Miller, W.R. & Rollnick, S. (2002). *Motivational Interviewing: Preparing People for Change* (2nd ed.). New York: Guilford Press.

Moos, R.H. (2003). Addictive disorders in context: Principles and puzzles of effective treatment and recovery. *Psychology of Addictive Behaviors, 17,* 3–12.

Moos, R., Finney, J.W., Federman, B. & Suchinsky, R. (2000). Specialty mental health care improves patients' outcomes: Findings from a nationwide program to monitor the quality of care for patients with substance use disorders. *Journal of Studies on Alcohol, 61,* 704–713.

Motiuk, L.L. & Nafekh, M. (2000). Aboriginal offenders in federal corrections: A profile. *Forum on Corrections Research, 12* (1), 10–15.

Motiuk L.L. & Vuong, B. (2006). Re-profiling the drug offender population in Canadian federal corrections. *Forum on Corrections Research, 18* (1), 24–29.

Oser, C., Harp, K., O'Connell, D., Martin, S. & Leukefeld, C. (2012). Correlates of participation in peer recovery support groups as well as voluntary and mandated substance abuse treatment among rural and urban probationers. *Journal of Substance Abuse Treatment, 42,* 95–101.

Parks, G.A. & Marlatt, G.A. (1999). Keeping "what works" working: Cognitive-behavioral relapse prevention therapy with substance abusing offenders. In E.J. Latessa (Ed.), *Strategic Solutions: The International Community Corrections Association Examines Substance Abuse* (pp. 161–233). Lanham, MD: American Correctional Association Press.

Pearce, S.C. & Holbrook, D. (2002). *Research Findings and Best Practices in Substance Abuse Treatment of Offenders: A Review of the Literature.* Report prepared for the North Carolina Department of Corrections Substance Abuse Advisory Council.

Pernanen, K., Cousineau, M.M., Brochu, S. & Sun, F. (2002). *Proportions of Crimes Associated with Alcohol and Other Drugs in Canada.* Ottawa: Canadian Centre on Substance Abuse. Retrieved from www.ccsa.ca

Peyrot, M. (1985). Narcotics Anonymous: Its history, structure, and approach. *Substance Use & Misuse, 20,* 1509–1522.

Sanders, J.F., McNeill, K.F., Rienzi, B.M. & DeLouth, T.N. (1997). The incarcerated female felon and substance abuse: Demographics, needs assessment, and program planning for a neglected population. *Journal of Addictions & Offender Counseling, 18,* 41–51.

Selzer, M.L. (1971). The Michigan Alcohol Screening Test (MAST): The quest for a new diagnostic instrument. *American Journal of Psychiatry, 127,* 1653–1658.

Skinner, H.A. (1982). The Drug Abuse Screening Test. *Addictive Behaviors, 7,* 363–371.

Skinner, H.A. & Horn, J.L. (1984). *Alcohol Dependence Scale: Users Guide.* Toronto: Addiction Research Foundation.

Smith, P., Gendreau, P. & Swartz, K. (2009). Validating the principles of effective intervention: A systematic review of the contributions of meta-analysis in the field of corrections. *Victims and Offenders, 4,* 148–169.

Snow, M.G., Prochaska, J.O. & Rossi, J.S. (1994). Processes of change in Alcoholics Anonymous: Maintenance factors in long-term sobriety. *Journal of Studies on Alcohol, 55,* 362–371.

Stallwitz, A. & Stöver, H. (2007). Impact of substitution treatment in prisons: A literature review. *International Journal of Drug Policy, 18,* 464–474.

Statistics Canada. (2010). *Aboriginal Statistics at a Glance.* Ottawa: Author.

Turnbull, P.J. & McSweeney, T. (2000). *Drug Treatment in Prison and Aftercare: A Literature Review and Results of a Survey of European Countries.* Brussels, Belgium: Council of Europe Publishing.

Vasilaki, E., Hosier, S.G. & Cox, W.M. (2006). The efficacy of motivational interviewing as a brief intervention for excessive drinking: A meta-analytic review. *Alcohol and Alcoholism, 41,* 328–335.

Weekes, J.R., Moser, A. & Langevin, C.M. (1999). Assessing substance abusing offenders for treatment. In E.J. Latessa (Ed.), *Strategic Solutions: The International Community Corrections Association Examines Substance Abuse* (pp. 1–41). Lanham, MD: American Correctional Association Press.

Weiss, R.D., Griffin, M.L., Najavits, L.M., Hufford, C., Kogan, J., Thompson, H.J. et al. (1996). Self-help activities in cocaine dependent patients entering treatment: Results from the NIDA Collaborative Cocaine Treatment Study. *Drug and Alcohol Dependence, 43,* 79–86.

Weldon, S. & Ritchie, G. (2010). Treatment of dual diagnosis in mentally disordered offenders: Application of evidence in the mainstream. *Advances in Dual Diagnosis, 3,* 18–23.

Wells, B. (1987). Narcotics Anonymous (NA): The phenomenal growth of an important resource. *British Journal of Addiction, 82,* 581–582.

Wheatley, M. (1998). The prevalence and relevance of substance use in detained schizophrenic patients. *Journal of Forensic Psychiatry, 9,* 114–129.

Wilton, G. & Stewart, L.A. (2012). *Outcomes for Offenders with Concurrent Substance Abuse and Mental Health Disorders.* Ottawa: Correctional Service of Canada.

Zakaria, D., Thompson, J.M., Jarvis, A. & Borgatta, F. (2010). *Summary of Emerging Findings from the 2007 National Inmate Infectious Diseases and Risk-Behaviours Survey.* Ottawa: Correctional Service of Canada. Retrieved from www.csc-scc.gc.ca

Chapter 20

What if it's Not About a Drug? Addiction as Problematic Behaviour

Nina Littman-Sharp, Kathryn Weiser, Lisa Pont, Janis Wolfe and Bruce Ballon*

PROBLEM GAMBLING

Joanne is a 45-year-old married woman with three teenaged children. She has worked for a small printing company for 16 years. Her husband, Tim, is a foreman in a manufacturing firm. Joanne's company was taken over by new owners five years ago, and since then most of the office staff has gradually been laid off, without any reduction in workload. As a dedicated and conscientious employee, Joanne rose to the challenge, working long hours and taking on many extra responsibilities. As the pressure has continued, Joanne has become very stressed and increasingly resentful. Friends have suggested she look for a new job, but for many reasons Joanne feels stuck where she is.

On top of work stress, Joanne is often at odds with Tim about two of their children, who are having difficulties in school and acting out at home. As well, Tim's widowed mother is having health problems and needs frequent assistance with errands, a job that mainly falls on Joanne due to Tim's shift work.

Joanne was introduced to casino slot machines in her mid-30s at a "girls' night out." She returned to gamble from time to time with friends. About four years ago, leaving work after a 12-hour day, she went to the casino on her own and spent three straight hours at a machine. Since then she has gambled more and more often. Sitting at a slot machine, Joanne finds that her stress and worries fall away. She also likes that no one knows where she is or can demand anything of her, and that this time is "just for me." But this stress release is temporary: the extra time away from home increases the pressure to get her many tasks done. Her children are rarely available when she tries to talk to them. Notes from their school are becoming alarming.

The money for gambling has come from the family finances, which Joanne manages. She has used up their savings, unbeknownst to Tim. A year ago, caught short, Joanne took some cash from work, replacing it the next day.

* With special thanks to Martin Zack for reviewing this chapter and providing helpful material.

On the next occasion she was unable to replace it, and began to increase her bets, looking for a win to pay back the money and have some left for more gambling. The more she has tried to win, the more her losses have mounted, and the more she has gambled in order to avoid thinking about the looming consequences. In her position of trust at work she has been able to manipulate accounts to hide the theft of more than $20,000. On some level she has distanced herself from and rationalized what she is doing. At first she thought of herself as "borrowing" the money; then she told herself that her employers in a sense owed it to her. But now auditors have discovered her misappropriations, and Joanne is devastated at what she has perpetrated and inflicted on her family, and the consequences she now faces.

✦

ONLINE GAMING

Chen, a 22-year-old university student, presents in treatment with concerns about the amount of time he spends online. Chen lives with his younger brother and his parents, who support him and give him spending money. He has not held a summer job successfully in two years. His family often expresses concern about the amount of time Chen spends on the computer. He admits that he often misses meals, and that he is not interested in spending time with family or friends the way he used to. Chen's parents have high academic expectations of him and are not aware that he is failing his courses. Although Chen intends to study, as soon as he sits down at the computer he logs into the online multi-player fantasy game World of Warcraft. He tells himself he will do so only for an hour and then get down to work, but instead he plays for hours, and often through the night.

Chen has created some powerful characters in the game and is part of an online group that goes on "raids" together. Images of the game frequently intrude on his thoughts when he is at school. Chen is reluctant to let his online team down by absenting himself. Once engaged in the game, he loses track of time and any real-life concerns.

In the therapist's office, Chen appears somewhat anxious, with a low mood. He says he felt depressed off and on through primary and middle school, because he was often the target of bullying. Chen changed districts for high school in order to escape this pattern, and his mood improved somewhat, but he has continued to feel isolated and has few friends. His mood is now very low, which he relates to his course failures.

At this point, Chen finds relief, satisfaction and a sense of competence only by playing World of Warcraft. There he has a wide group of friends and a reputation as a skilled and aggressive player. Conversations during the game are easy and comfortable for him. The one "real-world" friend he still has contact with is another Warcraft player; most of their conversations are online.

PROBLEM SPENDING

Marta is a 27-year-old single woman who works in public relations. She presents for help with excessive spending problems after she is charged with theft for failing to return a car she rented for a weekend trip. Marta delayed returning the car because she had no cash or credit to pay the fees.

Most of Marta's overspending is on clothes, accessories and makeup. Her closets are packed with clothes and handbags, some of which she has never worn or used. She has eight credit cards and two lines of credit, all of which are maxed out. Her debt is approximately $120,000. She uses shopping to cope with negative moods, including stress over the money she owes.

Marta had bulimia in her teens, and still thinks a lot about her weight and what she eats. She is a perfectionist in terms of her appearance; any perceived fault in her clothes, hair or makeup can lead her to leave a situation. Marta describes her family as undemonstrative and distant. Both parents are high-level professionals, one in medicine, the other in finance. They do not approve of Marta's career. Marta has appeased them by saying she is just taking time to decide on a "better" career, even though she enjoys her work and feels it suits her well.

PROBLEMATIC SEXUAL BEHAVIOUR

Hassan is a 23-year-old single man who works as a sales clerk and lives alone in a rented apartment. His parents were born in Pakistan, but he and his two sisters were born in Canada. A year ago Hassan sought help for a gambling problem, and was successful in achieving and maintaining abstinence. Recently he has returned to therapy because of concerns about masturbation, which he engages in five or six times a day, using online pornography. Hassan also describes having frequent sex with a variety of women, saying he often feels lonely and doesn't want to stay home alone. As a religious Muslim, he is self-condemnatory about his sexual behaviour, and about his use of porn in particular. He feels disgusted by it, which only feeds into his negative self-image.

Hassan describes his mother as having been physically and emotionally abusive toward him and his sisters when they were children. This history has never been discussed in the family. His mother is still sometimes verbally abusive to her grown children, in person or by phone. Hassan has experienced flashbacks, hyperarousal and anxiety symptoms, and during his treatment for problem gambling was diagnosed with posttraumatic stress disorder (PTSD). He refused medications or treatment for the PTSD.

Relating or opening up to women is not easy for Hassan, and most of his relationships are very brief. He admits that there have been occasions when he engaged in risky sexual practices.

If addiction is something that happens because a person puts powerful psychoactive substances in their body, how can behaviours be considered addictive? Why are problems with gambling, gaming, Internet use, sex, shopping and other behaviours sometimes described as "addictions?" Is the term just a handy metaphor, or is there science and clinical experience to support its use? Can this broader view of addiction expand our understanding and inform our approach to age-old challenges in addressing substance use and other behaviours?

This chapter examines the implications of applying a wider meaning to the term addiction for so-called "process" or "behavioural" addictions. We look not only at the behaviours themselves and their treatment, but also at the question of whether an addiction lens is useful for problematic behaviours other than substance use. Will that lens assist us in bringing together biopsychosocial and systemic factors that help with identification and response?

For an overview of five common behavioural addictions—gambling, the Internet, sex, shopping and video gaming—see this chapter's appendix.

Excessive Behaviours: Evolving Perspectives

The concept of addiction to psychoactive substances has a long history in the medical, research and therapeutic literature. Physiological impacts of drugs on the brain and body are particularly well documented, and for many years the term addiction has been identified with the influence of powerful chemicals acting on the central nervous system. Addiction to a behaviour is a less familiar concept, although one that is receiving increasing attention. Gambling, shopping, Internet use, video gaming and sexual activities are examples of behaviours where excessive engagement is now being described as an addiction.

Stanton Peele (1978) was an early proponent of this wider concept of addiction:

Psychoactive chemicals are perhaps the most direct means for affecting a person's consciousness and state of being. But any activity that can absorb a person in such a way as to detract from the ability to carry through other involvements is potentially addictive. It is addictive when the experience eradicates a person's awareness; when it provides predictable gratification; when it is used not to gain pleasure but to avoid pain and unpleasantness; when it damages self-esteem; and when it destroys other involvements. When these conditions hold, the involvement will take over a person's life in an increasingly destructive cycle. (p. 67)

Orford (2001) emphasizes the instructive importance of non-chemical addictions within his "excessive appetites" model. In this model, addictions are described as enjoyable or pleasant behaviours that have become excessive enough to cause harm: "There exists a range of objects and activities which are particularly risky for humans, who are liable to develop such strong attachment to them that they then find their ability to moderate their behaviour significantly diminished" (pp. 15–16).

Despite these efforts to expand the definition of addiction, standard classifications have only recently begun to categorize excessive behaviours as addictions. The fourth edition of the *Diagnostic and Statistical Manual of Mental Health Disorders* ([DSM-IV-TR], American Psychiatric Association, 2000) classified several behaviours discussed in this chapter as impulse control disorders, along with trichotillomania (hair pulling), pyromania and kleptomania. An impulse control disorder is defined as a failure or extreme difficulty in controlling impulses despite negative consequences. While this definition may seem appropriate for excessive behaviours, impulsivity is associated with a wide range of mental health disorders, and thus could be seen more as a symptom than as a disorder in itself. Also, grouping these disparate behaviours together creates a number of conceptual difficulties.

The newly released DSM-5 (APA, 2013) introduces a new category called "Addiction and Related Disorders." What was previously called "pathological gambling" is now "gambling disorder." It is the only behavioural addiction specified in DSM-5, which does recognize the category of behavioural addictions but feels that only disordered gambling has the research base required to be explicitly included. A report (First, 2010) about one of the DSM-5 diagnosis-related research planning conferences states:

> The core components of addictive behavior include continuing the behavior despite adverse consequences, diminished control or compulsive engagement in the behavior, and a craving or appetitive urge to engage in the behavior, opening up the construct to behaviors beyond substance use, like gambling, sex, shopping, eating, and computer use. Whether to classify these disorders as addictions, compulsive disorders or impulse control disorders is a matter of ongoing scientific debate. (p. 14)

These behavioural issues are described in the literature, using terms that vary according to the paradigm the author uses to understand them. Some terminology is descriptive rather than diagnostic: behaviour disorders, overused behaviours, excessive behaviours. These reflect a cognitive-behavioural paradigm. Other terminology suggests a theoretical association with substance addictions: process addictions, behavioural addictions.

Another theory on the source of excessive behaviours focuses on the experience of obsession or compulsion, and makes the association with obsessive-compulsive disorder (OCD). This theory is reflected in popular, as well as clinical, terminology for excessive behaviours (e.g., "compulsive sexual behaviour," "compulsive gambling," "obsessive shopping," "obsessive gaming disorder"). However, people with OCD experience their obsessive thoughts as unpleasant and intrusive, and compulsive behaviours are engaged in to reduce anxiety rather than for enjoyment, whereas behaviours described as addictive are generally experienced, at least initially, as strongly pleasurable.

It is true that an accumulation of negative consequences can eventually make continuing a behaviour disturbing or unpleasant. At that point, the person may experience his or her involvement as a lack of personal control so strong that it feels like a compulsion. Substances may also be used simply for symptom relief or to avoid withdrawal. Some similarities do appear to exist between, for example, problem gambling and OCD. However, research has found that OCD occurs in people with gambling problems at a rate no higher than that in the general population (Grant & Potenza, 2006). This suggests that the similarities are no more than superficial.

Classification of disorders has implications for assessment and treatment, and reflects current knowledge and research on how these disorders develop. However, what is known about most of these excessive behaviours is restricted by limited research, small sample sizes and a good deal of variability in definitions. The problem gambling field has garnered more attention than others due to the rapid recent expansion of legalized gambling and its impacts (and perhaps because of its inclusion in the DSM). In some jurisdictions, increases in gambling revenue have been invested in treatment, prevention and research, and thus there is more evidence in this area to draw upon. The expanding evidence base on problem gambling has resulted in a shift toward an addiction paradigm for this particular disorder. It may be that in the future, for the sake of consistency, other behavioural addictions will follow suit.

A Broader Concept of Addiction

Parallels at the Psychological, Social and Systemic Levels

As different as substance use issues and disorders such as problem gambling may appear to be, might there be common ground on which a more fundamental understanding of addiction can be developed? According to Grant and colleagues (2010), "Growing evidence suggests that behavioural addictions resemble substance addictions in many domains, including natural history, phenomenology, tolerance, comorbidity, overlapping genetic contribution, neurobiological mechanisms, and response to treatment" (p. 233).

While we acknowledge that most of these ideas are contestable and not fully proven, for the purposes of this chapter, we use the term "behavioural addictions" so we can explore how this concept helps us understand and address excessive behaviours of all kinds. (Note, however, that the use of this concept on a theoretical level does not mean the terminology is required for work with clients. For clinical purposes, it is often better to avoid labels, an issue that we discuss in the section on clinical applications.)

All addictions as behavioural

The existence of non-chemical addictions invites us to rethink our conception of addiction in general, as well as the behavioural aspect of substance use problems. Addiction in all of its forms is not just about personal vulnerability or about the compelling effects of a drug or an activity; it is always something that is enacted, performed, "behaved." Successfully addressing these problems requires not just stopping or reshaping these behaviours, but also developing alternative activities to replace them. In this sense, all addictions are behavioural addictions.

Addictive behaviours, including ones involving substances, are those that are engaged in repeatedly, in maladaptive patterns, despite the consequences of disruption or harm to the person's physical or emotional health; relationships; and ability to function and to meet responsibilities at work, school or home, or in the community. These behaviours may be enjoyable and even healthy when they are engaged in at moderate levels, and when they are balanced with other activities. However, when a person becomes increasingly absorbed by and dependent on a behaviour to the extent that it crowds out other involvements, a negative cycle can be initiated. Other areas of life are neglected, and the person's functioning and relationships come under pressure. Rather than being sources of satisfaction, support or pleasure, these life areas become associated with conflict, stress, unhappiness, fear or a sense of failure. A person who does not pull out of the pattern will tend to become more and more dependent on the one thing in his or her life that, as Peele (1978) describes, provides "predictable gratification." Problems addressed by avoidance rather than healthy coping tend to multiply; confidence is weakened; and the excessive behaviour intensifies in response.

JOANNE'S CASE (PROBLEM GAMBLING)

Here we describe a classic addiction cycle as applied to the case of Joanne, the woman with a gambling problem presented in one of this chapter's opening vignettes.

Joanne is suffering from chronic stress and overwork, which she feels helpless to resolve. She is angry at her employers, but continues to perform heroically at work with little complaint. She is also overloaded at home. Long hours and time pressures mean the ordinary rewards of life are rarely available to her. Aspects of personality or family history may prevent Joanne from addressing these issues or expressing her anger in healthy ways. For example, she may be overly conscientious and self-denying based on a dysfunctional family of origin, or perhaps based simply on a strong cultural message about the role of women as caregivers.

In any case, the relief offered by gambling is such a welcome contrast to Joanne's daily life that she comes to rely on this activity. As a result, she has less time for her family, sees increasing problems at home and is experiencing suppressed but mounting stress, guilt and dread over her financial losses. Joanne copes, avoids thinking about her problems and maintains hope of fending off approaching disaster by gambling more. The longer the pattern continues, the fewer alternatives appear to be available.

Generally speaking, addictive behaviour narrows coping options and exacerbates whatever problems it is being used to address, soothe or avoid. The cycle in the case of gambling is intensified by money losses and attempts to win back lost money, and it is often a financial crisis that brings someone with a gambling problem into treatment. Shopping addiction may bring financial crises, but has no potential for replacing lost funds; the cycle in this case includes fear over mounting debt, the loss of alternative activities and the loss of self-respect. In the case of video gaming, isolation and loss of "real-world" social skills and networks are common elements of the addiction cycle. Problematic sexual behaviours tend to damage or prevent committed partner relationships, and thus reduce the options for healthier validation and support.

The addictive cycle may intensify a problem to severe levels. Addictive behaviours, whether substance based or not, exist on a continuum, with behavioural health at one end and severe addictive behaviour at the other. There is no unambiguous point at which "normal" levels of the behaviour end and problem levels begin. At-risk and moderate levels not only exist, but in some cases can continue for years, and many people resolve their problematic behaviour patterns without treatment. Progression is by no means inevitable.

A behaviour's perceived location on the continuum is also influenced by social and cultural factors. For example, what is regarded as normative—as opposed to excessive or problematic—sexual behaviour is changing over time, and varies widely from one social or cultural group to another. A client-centred approach will consider clients' concerns about negative impacts of the behaviour, as well as an assessment of actual harm, and will avoid judgment of a behaviour based on personal or cultural bias.

Apart from the addiction cycle and continuum, on what basis can we compare excessive or problematic behaviours to substance addictions? For the individual, the experiences of preoccupation, craving, tolerance and a sense of loss of control are common to both. Many of the same purposes are served, such as pleasure, excitement, socialization, self-soothing and escape. Vulnerabilities and risk factors are similar (e.g., concurrent mental health disorders, trauma history, stress or poor coping skills). Adolescent experimentation and risk taking are common factors when it comes to early potentially addictive behaviour such as substance use and gambling.

There are parallels as well in the interaction between behavioural addictions and family functioning. Many people with behavioural addictions have family histories of addiction or mental health problems. Peer and family influences are powerful when it comes to the development of excessive behaviours, just as they are with substance use problems. As with substance addictions, people with behavioural addictions tend to become the focus of conflict, concern and attention in their family system. Another similarity is the damage to relationships and family functioning. For example, excessive gambling and excessive sexual behaviour both lead to a loss of trust, and the effects on family relationships are potentially even more severe and lasting than in the case of substance use problems.

Parallels also exist at the broader systemic level. For example, lack of support, as well as pressures to succeed, which might leave an immigrant vulnerable to substance use problems, can also make that person vulnerable to problem gambling. Poverty may similarly increase vulnerability. The Internet is now at least as ubiquitous in our society as alcohol, and peer pressure to engage in social networking is particularly intense for young people. Just as with alcohol, some cultures normalize gambling, while others frown on it.

The existence of so many parallels and shared features between substance and behavioural addictions suggests that these addictions should not be conceptualized as distinct categories. Rather, within each category, the biopsychosocial dynamics both vary and are often similar. Clinicians need to understand not only overarching features and features specific to certain problem behaviours, but also how these manifest and become meaningful for individual clients.

The next section discusses some characteristics more specific to behavioural addictions.

Differences Between Behavioural and Substance Addictions

Behavioural addictions differ from substance addictions in a few ways that are more or less unique to the specific behavioural problems. For example, gambling addiction often involves mistaken beliefs about odds, luck and the value of persistence and of betting "systems." An early big win is a frequent precursor to excessive gambling. Financial problems are generally far more severe than they are for substance use problems. Both gambling and gaming include a fantasy aspect, as well as powerful game elements that are exploited intensively by marketers in the interest of increasing revenue, with very little attention to the impact on consumers' health or safety, whereas the marketing of alcohol and tobacco have been strictly regulated for some time. Excessive shopping is also engendered and continuously triggered by the marketing and consumerism that are so ubiquitous in our society.

Internet use has also become ubiquitous. The amount of time people spend online has increased rapidly with the advent of new technologies. What used to be seen as excessive is now normative behaviour, particularly since the Internet has become so integrated with our day-to-day lives. Internet use is integral to many other behavioural addictions, including online gaming, online gambling, social networking, porn surfing and online sexual behaviour. Rapid advances in hardware (e.g., smartphones) and software applications are making engagement in such behaviours easier and easier. For those engaged in excessive use, Internet use is increasingly difficult to avoid.

Parallels in Neurobiology

The most obvious distinction between behavioural and substance addictions is, of course, the method by which the brain is affected. As we know, psychoactive drugs are exogenous substances that overwhelm the brain's internal neurological processes. However, behavioural addictions have the uncanny power to evoke and condition the brain's processes to produce addiction without the necessity of an exogenous substance. In attempting to understand the nature of addiction, such addictive behavioural processes could be seen as more eloquent and pure, and thus more instructive, than those processes that require powerful chemicals to have an impact.

One obvious difference between chemical and behavioural addictions is that chronic use of substances has marked physical impacts, both immediate and long term. Behavioural addictions carry some physical risks, particularly when taken to extremes (e.g., lack of exercise, sleep loss and poor nutrition for those who gamble or game excessively; risk of sexually transmitted infections or violence for those who have multiple sexual encounters), but these behaviours rarely act as destructively on the body and brain as substances often do. People with behavioural addictions thus tend to be physically healthier and higher functioning, and may be more likely to be employed. Unfortunately, this can also mean that the problem is easier to conceal, or may continue longer without reaching a crisis point that brings the person into treatment.

Research has identified a variety of complex relationships between substance addiction and genetic and neurological factors (see Chapter 6). Genetic, biochemical and structural variations in the brain have an impact on several factors related to addiction, including reward and pleasure seeking, decision making, impulsivity, stress coping and vulnerability to cravings.

There has also been research on the neurobiology of non-chemical addictive behaviours. Chakraborty and colleagues (2010) discuss the neural pathways involved in behavioural addictions. Schmitz (2005) attributes behavioural addictions to dysfunctional neurocircuits that link craving and withdrawal behaviours to pleasure centres. Another "reward-deficiency hypothesis" links chemical and non-chemical addictions by proposing that some people derive less satisfaction from natural rewards (e.g., food, sex) as a result of genetically based malfunctions in the transmission of dopamine. To achieve reward-pathway stimulation, they turn to more powerful substances or activities (Blum et al., 1996; Comings & Blum, 2000; Esch & Stefano, 2004; Vetulani, 2001). There is some evidence from neuroimaging studies that behavioural addictions and substance use disorders share the same neural circuitry (Brewer & Potenza, 2008).

The brain's mesocorticolimbic tract (a combination of dopamine pathways in the brain involved in motivational and emotional responses) has been identified as an important pathway for moderating pleasure responses. The release of dopamine in the brain has been shown to affect the reinforcing properties of substances such as alcohol and cocaine; similar processes appear to occur with gambling, computer gaming and other risk-taking and highly repetitive behaviours (Becker, 1999; Blum et al., 1996;

Comings & Blum, 2000; Esch & Stefano, 2004; Schmitz, 2005; Vetulani, 2001; Zack & Poulos, 2009).

Pharmacological interventions that have been shown to reduce urges for substances (e.g., naltrexone, and medications that alter glutamatergic activity in the brain) have also had some success in trials with behavioural addictions, including gambling, Internet, sexual and shopping addictions (Grant et al., 2010). This suggests the existence of shared neurobiological mechanisms for substance and behavioural addictions.

What are these shared mechanisms? The key point is that repeated exposure to an "addictive" reinforcer changes the brain to shift priorities in motivation that will bias future behaviour toward the addictive reinforcer (Olsen, 2011). Whereas drugs of abuse accomplish this neural restructuring by inducing supra-physiological levels of dopamine release, the stimuli that mediate behavioural addictions may accomplish this by the frequency rather than the magnitude of dopamine release they are capable of causing. Non-drug reinforcers lose their ability to elicit dopamine release as they become more familiar. However, certain non-drug reinforcers, such as gambling and gaming, offer the opportunity for indefinite dopamine release because the delivery of rewards is never entirely predictable (Fiorillo et al., 2003).

Delivery of unpredicted rewards is a natural event that instigates dopamine release (Schultz, 1998). Gambling or gaming enables ongoing, virtually unlimited opportunities for dopamine release by the delivery of rewards that, although hoped for, are never fully predicted. Sex and shopping can become addictive in the age of the Internet and multiple sources of credit because of unlimited access to novelty. In males, the ability to activate dopamine is reinstated by a new sexual partner even during the sexual refractory period (the so-called "Coolidge effect;" see Beach & Jordan, 1956). With the Internet, one can have "encounters" (sexual gratification) with multiple partners in the space of minutes. With each new partner, dopamine fires again, reinforcing the behaviour that would otherwise satiate or extinguish over time. Similarly, Internet shopping and malls permit virtually limitless opportunities to encounter novel ways to adorn oneself or to feather one's nest. Thus, speed and ease of access permit ongoing, frequent exposure to novel rewards, each of which is capable of causing dopamine release, not by directly engaging dopamine neurons (like drugs), but by engaging the natural process designed to activate dopamine, that is, novel reward delivery. Behavioural addictions are fundamentally similar to substance addictions at the neurophysiological level because these activities permit ongoing, indefinite activation of dopamine via novelty. This reconfigures the brain in ways that bias the person to return to the activity again and again—just like drugs of abuse.

Addictive behaviour and neurobiology are strongly interactive, in that brain structures, chemistry and neural pathways influence not only behaviour, but also change in response to experience. So it is in some cases difficult to say whether differences in brain structure and functioning are a cause or a result of addictive behaviour. This dynamic interactivity is one aspect of the complexity of this addiction model, which integrates the neurological level with the psychological and social systems in which each person is embedded.

In sum, the evidence strongly supports an expansion of the concept of addiction beyond substance use to a more extensive range of problem behaviours. This broadening scope brings new light to familiar issues, and gives us a head start in our approach to new problems.

TABLE 20-1

Prevalence of Addictive Behaviours by Population*

PROBLEM BEHAVIOUR	PREVALENCE RANGE	POPULATION
Gambling	2% 1.2%–3.4% (moderate to severe) 0.2%–5.3%	Ontario students (grades 7–12)[1] Ontario adults[2,3] Adults worldwide[4]
Internet use	0.9%–38% 2%* 4%–13%	Youth (age not specified)[5] U.S. adults[6] U.S. adults[7]
Video gaming	12% Unknown	Ontario students (grades 7–12)[1] Adults
Shopping	3.5% 6%*	U.S. high-school students (age 14–18)[8] U.S. adults[6]
Sexual behaviours	10.3% 3%**	Canadian college students (age 19)[6] U.S. adults[6]

*Due to limited uniformity of the sampling and assessment methods used, widely varying prevalence rates have been reported worldwide. As such, until more vigorous prevalence studies are conducted, these data should be interpreted with caution.

**All U.S. adult statistics are estimates of prevalence in the general U.S. adult population in a 12-month period.

1. Paglia-Boak, A., Adlaf, E.M., Hamilton, H.A., Beitchman, J.H., Wolfe, D. & Mann, R.E. (2012). *The Mental Health and Well-Being of Ontario Students, 1991–2011: OSDUHS Highlights*. Toronto: Centre for Addiction and Mental Health.

2. Williams, R.J., Volberg, R.A. & Stevens, R.M.G. (2012). *The Population Prevalence of Problem Gambling: Methodological Influences, Standardized Rates, Jurisdictional Differences, and Worldwide Trends*. Report prepared for the Ontario Problem Gambling Research Centre and the Ontario Ministry of Health and Long-Term Care.

3. Wiebe, J., Mun, P. & Kauffman, N. (2006). *Gambling and Problem Gambling in Ontario 2005*. Toronto: Responsible Gambling Council.

4. Hodgins, D., Stea, J.N. & Grant, J.E. (2011). Gambling disorders. *The Lancet, 378*, 1874–1884.

5. Shaw, M. & Black, D.W. (2008). Internet addiction: Definition, assessment, epidemiology and clinical management. *CNS Drugs, 22*, 353–365.

6. Sussman, S., Lisha, N. & Griffiths, M. (2011). Prevalence of the addictions: A problem of the majority or the minority? *Evaluation & the Health Professions, 34* (1), 3–56.

7. Aboujaoude, E., Koran, L.M., Gamel, N. & Serne, R.T. (2006). Potential markers for problematic Internet use: A telephone survey of 2,513 adults. *CNS Spectrum, 11*, 750–755.

8. Grant, J.E., Potenza, M.N., Krishnan-Sarin, S., Cavallo, D.A. & Desai, R.A. (2011). Shopping problems among high school students. *Comprehensive Psychiatry, 52*, 247–252.

Concurrent Mental Health Issues

Both clinical experience and research indicate a strong co-occurrence between mental disorders and behavioural addictions. For example, data from the *2009 Ontario Student Drug Use and Health Survey* ([OSDUHS], Cook et al., 2010) indicates that young people who are gambling problematically are also at higher risk for depressive symptoms, low self-esteem, psychological distress and suicide attempts. The prevalence of drug use, truancy, gang involvement and delinquency are also markedly elevated in this group. The OSDUHS examined co-occurrence and not causality; thus research has not made it clear whether, for example, depression causes behavioural addiction or vice versa, or whether both are caused by other factors. What is clear is that in youth, excessive gambling tends to be associated with multiple problems. Such problems tend to exacerbate one another. However, a good assessment will often clarify causality in individual cases, and is an important consideration in clinical work.

There is particularly strong evidence of co-occurring trauma and mental health and addiction disorders among women. In a sample of 365 women with untreated gambling problems, Boughton and Brewster (2002) found histories of co-occurring disorders and trauma as follows:

- sought treatment for mental health concerns: 71 per cent
- suicide attempts: 29 per cent
- physical abuse: 46 per cent
- sexual abuse: 38 per cent
- binge eating: 27 per cent
- shopping addiction: 24 per cent.

Garcia and Thibaut (2010) identify mood and anxiety disorders and substance use disorders as most commonly co-occurring with sexual addictions. Kaplan and Krueger (2010) found correlations between personality disorders and paraphilias (abnormal sexual fantasies, urges or behaviours). Kuzma and Black (2006) found that shopping addiction tends to co-occur with mood, substance use and eating disorders.

Evidence suggests that both genetic and environmental factors induce brain alterations that increase susceptibility to behavioural addictions. For example, impulsivity is a risk factor, as is the disturbance of early attachments (Vazquez et al., 2005).

Addictive behaviours frequently act as coping strategies for underlying mental health and stress-related problems. Clinical experience suggests, for example, that excessive Internet use may be a strategy related to many disorders. For example:

- Asperger's syndrome (previously a separate diagnosis, but now subsumed under autism spectrum disorders in DSM-5 [APA, 2013]) may create a drive to learn everything about a topic by constantly researching it online.
- People with social anxiety may feel more able to socialize in chat rooms and role-play gaming worlds than in real life.
- People may use the Internet to enhance their mood when depressed.

- People with OCD may use the Internet to deal with contamination fears by limiting real-world involvement.
- Sexual addiction may involve long hours seeking and downloading pornography.
- Self-harm behaviours can be supported in online chat rooms where people share thoughts and techniques on suicide and other self-harm behaviours, such as cutting, burning and disordered eating.
- Internet use may enable online extramarital affairs and thus exacerbate relationship issues.

In other words, Internet overuse and other excessive behaviours can serve many purposes, and have complex relationships with other concurrent issues. Patterns of concurrence may be seen more or less frequently, but there are no simple causes to point to for any specific problem behaviour.

Practice Implications

The behavioural addiction health continuum is a very useful model at a theoretical level. However, an addiction label (e.g., "sex addiction" or "gambling addiction") is often neither useful nor necessary when providing treatment. Such labels may not only lead the client to reject the services; labels may limit how the clinician identifies the nature of the problem during screening and assessment. On the other hand, clients may already self-identify as being addicts, and may belong to one of the many recovery fellowships that apply the 12 steps or other mutual aid models to what they self-describe as eating, sex, shopping, gambling or other behavioural addictions. Being client-centred in this new terrain can actually have a grounding value, given the lack of an evidence base to firmly guide practice.

Since any excessive behaviour can serve many purposes, at the clinical level, the therapist must explore the meanings and functions of the behaviour for each client, and understand how these relate to other issues and disorders. For clients with complex issues, this exploration may take some time and patience. The importance of engagement and relationship building cannot be overstated, particularly if, as noted above, early attachment experiences are disturbed, in which case the person will be physiologically more susceptible to forming a "relationship" with a potent (i.e., dopamine-activating) reinforcing behaviour. Treatment is likely to include interventions that help such clients find rewards through interpersonal interaction.

Although each client's motivations are unique, most clients can benefit from group therapy that addresses common issues. Programming is most helpful when it is specific to particular behavioural addictions, as each problem behaviour has some more or less unique precursors, issues and triggers, and clients in such groups are more able to identify with and support one another. Training is recommended for clinicians on the particular characteristics of various behavioural addictions.

Screening

As mentioned, behavioural addictions typically have fewer physical symptoms than does addiction to substances, and they often go unidentified. Clients may or may not admit to excessive behaviours during assessments for other problems. Exploring the time they spend on leisure activities can lead to discoveries about gambling, Internet and gaming behaviour. Financial issues may reveal gambling and shopping addictions. Sexual addictions may come to light through discussions about relationships and sexual behaviour.

Available screening tools for behavioural addictions are listed in the appendix. Apart from these tools, any validated addiction screen (with some wording changes) may provide useful information. These tools include questions about frequency and impacts of the behaviour, as well as whether others have expressed concern about it. The answers may be explored to reveal the salience the behaviour has in the person's life, as well as the impact it has on functioning. Screening for co-occurring addiction and mental health issues is also recommended. Screening and subsequent discussion can offer valuable information about motivations for behaviour, as well as creating an effective and informed treatment plan. For example, in this chapter's opening vignette about online gaming, Chen screened positive for both anxiety and depression, and these became early focuses in the assessment phase.

Assessment

The assessment for all behavioural addictions should include:
- history, frequency, patterns and impacts of the problem behaviour
- previous attempts to stop or cut down
- family history, circumstances, engagement in the problem and its consequences
- education, employment and legal history
- physical and mental health issues
- coping skills and social supports
- goals and motivation, and stage of change.

Ideally, the family would be involved in at least some portion of the assessment, in order to look at the person's issues in the context of the family system, and to facilitate a systemic approach to treatment. A family approach is particularly crucial when working with youth, given their dependent relationship with parents. However, clients at any age are generally embedded in family systems, which can be powerfully affected by the behavioural addiction, and which can also be instrumental in the process of change.

Information culled from the assessment, as well as the results of a reliable and valid screening tool, if available, are typically used to devise a client- and family-centred treatment plan.

CHEN'S CASE (ONLINE GAMING)

Chen's depressive symptoms began in childhood when he was targeted by other children at school. His mood improved somewhat in high school when he was more isolated than bullied, but his recent failing grades have deepened his depression and led to increasing anxiety.

Antecedents to and consequences of the problem behaviour should be explored, as well as the complexities and nuances of its meaning to the client. For Chen, who had few friends, online gaming was entertainment that he could engage in on his own. As time went on, he developed game skills and an online reputation, which he found much more satisfying than his experiences elsewhere. Chen felt awkward at school, and felt that he was still seen as "a geek and a loser." He excelled in online games, and experienced himself as skilled, powerful and respected.

When asked about the point at which his online behaviour began interfering with his day-to-day life, Chen identified the period eight months earlier when he lost a summer job in his first week. Unwilling to search for other employment, he spent the rest of the summer alone in his room playing online games. Exploring the meaning of this job loss was important, as Chen attached a lot of negative significance to the event, seeing it as confirmation of his inadequacy and a sign that attempts to succeed were hopeless.

A thorough assessment will clarify motivations around the problem behaviour, as well as impacts and interactions. Chen's long hours of gaming, combined with the loss of positive expectations, quickly affected his school performance, an area where he had previously done well. Chen described the pressure he felt from his family to achieve high grades; his increasing anxiety, depression and isolation as he concealed his failures; and his escape into gaming, the only place in his life where he felt safe from the stress of unreachable expectations. Assessment of the family revealed some entrenched issues about material success, particularly for eldest sons, as well as a family history of anxiety and depression, which had been largely concealed from the younger generation.

Assessments, always an ongoing process, should cover co-occurring mental health and addiction issues past and present, including trauma, substance use and other excessive behaviours. It is not unusual for people with behavioural addictions to engage in more than one behavioural addiction, or to substitute one behaviour for another.

In Chen's case, treatment planning prioritized addressing his mood disorders and issues with socialization, and included a referral for psychiatric assessment. Family issues were also given priority, given the need for the parents' support in addressing Chen's urgent school problems.

Treatment

As noted earlier, potentially problematic behaviours exist on a continuum of severity, from healthy to severely disordered. For this reason, appropriate interventions also range in intensity, and may include anything from bibliotherapy to brief interventions to more involved treatments that address co-occurring disorders. Clients with a behavioural addiction who are otherwise functioning well usually have the resources and support to make effective use of briefer interventions. Those with multiple issues underlying their behavioural problem will need longer-term and more comprehensive treatment. Cases where the problem behaviour is entangled with complex issues (e.g., a gambling client with severe financial losses leading to family breakdown, loss of job and housing, extreme stress, emotional crisis) require a good deal of support during the process of recovery.

Assessment and treatment are not entirely distinct processes, as assessment in itself can create change, and will also continue throughout the course of therapy. Motivational interviewing is recommended as a framework for both assessment and treatment. Behavioural addictions and co-occurring issues are often deeply entrenched, and—as with substance addictions—change is not easy. Motivational interviewing can greatly enhance the client's commitment to the process (see Chapter 5 on motivational interviewing).

Treatment should address the behaviour problem and co-occurring issues as simultaneously as possible. Some issues may take precedence over others, depending on their severity or immediacy. But whatever the concurrent issues, it is important to keep a focus on addressing the behaviour itself. Problem behaviours may be used chiefly as coping mechanisms, but their effects can be serious in themselves, particularly when the consequences are part of a negative spiral. Even when the original antecedent has been dealt with, the outcomes can live with a person for years.

Cognitive-behavioural therapy (CBT) is a well-supported modality for addressing addictive behaviours. CBT can be used to explore and address triggers to the behaviour, such as detrimental cognitions and related affect (e.g., "No one likes me except in the game"). Because cognitive distortions often shape how the person is involved in the addictive behaviour, CBT works to expose and contest these distortions so the person can develop a more balanced perception and awareness. The therapist helps the client to explore positive as well as negative aspects of the behaviour in order to develop alternative ways of getting needs met, and to build more effective coping and problem-solving skills. CBT also helps with longer-term relapse prevention, anticipating future triggers and building healthy coping skills in advance. Developing alternative activities will help to deter relapse by establishing a new default to compete with the addictive behaviour.

Techniques from dialectical behaviour therapy (DBT) may be used to help a client recognize and regulate emotions. The treatment plan can include psychotherapy, trauma counselling, mindfulness or other modalities, depending on the issues involved.

Clinical trials of medications for behavioural addictions have shown some promise (Grant et al., 2010). Naltrexone, which is currently used to reduce urges in alcohol and opioid addictions, has had some efficacy for gambling, Internet, sexual and shopping addictions. Medications such as topiramate that alter glutamatergic activity in the brain have been effective in reducing urges in both behavioural and substance use problems (Grant et al., 2010). However, these medications are likely only to be useful for certain subsets of individuals. For example, recent evidence suggests that naltrexone works best in people with a family history of substance abuse problems (Grant et al., 2008). Interventions aimed at reducing urges are likely to be most helpful for people whose urges are powerful and who have problems controlling their impulses. Such medications will not be effective with people who engage in their problem behaviours to ameliorate depression, anxiety or social isolation. Some medications may be best in particular phases and stages of care, such as early on when urges are high and cravings for the behaviour are highest, and when client resilience and social support are most compromised. Note that many medications have side-effects and potential hazards, so caution is necessary.

The best case for using medication to address excessive behaviours is when there is a clearly indicated co-occurring mental health problem, such as anxiety, depression or attention-deficit/hyperactivity disorder (ADHD). In general, improvements in the addictive behaviour can be expected once untreated mental health problems are addressed through therapy and/or medication if indicated. Relief from depression, for example, will give a client more energy to try alternatives to the problematic behaviours. Clients with ADHD will find it easier both to resist impulses and to engage successfully in more everyday activities.

Treatment may occur in various contexts, including individually, or within a group, couple or family. Depending on the issues and behaviours, group support can be normalizing, and an effective way to develop coping skills. For example, in our clinic for youth with behavioural addictions, we treat many young people with gaming addiction who also have Asperger's syndrome and/or mood disorders, as well as difficulties engaging socially. Teaching social skills to these clients in a group setting can be particularly helpful.

Involving the Family and Significant Others

Best practice in treatment includes involving family or significant others. Focusing only on the identified client means that many key perspectives may be overlooked. Certainly a chance is missed to help the whole family unit, which can be both profoundly affected by the problem and instrumental in its resolution. In problem gambling cases, for example, relationship counselling is often crucial to the entire family's recovery, given the impact on trust caused by concealing the gambling, lying and misusing family funds.

Issues in the family also frequently predate the behaviour that brings a person into treatment. On a systemic level, the family dynamics may in fact support the problem behaviour. For example, parents who are invested in avoiding an empty nest may not address their child's gambling or video gaming problems if it is keeping the young adult at home and dependent on the parents. In such a case, working with the person in isolation will be less effective and involving the family is strongly recommended. It is not unusual at a collateral session to uncover mental health issues that have affected several generations, such as the anxiety that ran through Chen's family.

Significant others may need help to align with and support the goals of the therapy, particularly when they are wary of interventions that seem to threaten entrenched dynamics. Some clients will not want their families involved. It is important to explore this and to encourage leaving the door open for a later time. When issues emerge that point to relationship problems, clients will sometimes be more open to including their family in treatment. Some fears can be addressed by assigning significant others to a different therapist, with full respect for confidentiality. This is recommended in any case when conflict levels are high. Issues for families where a member engages in problem gambling can be so intense that the other family members will often benefit from receiving their own support.

In rare cases, trauma histories or toxic environments will mean that helping a client distance from significant others is more therapeutic than inviting them into treatment. However, most families do care about their loved ones, and want to help.

Families need to have their own concerns and needs heard. The door should be open to welcome them on their own, or in parallel to the client receiving care individually where it is not possible to take an integrated family-focused approach to treatment. Families need information about the behavioural problem and any mental health issues, so they can put what they see in context and respond to it appropriately. Just educating family members or helping them adapt their style of helping can sometimes greatly enhance the treatment outcome.

Healthy communication should be facilitated and promoted, so that family members can express feelings, thoughts and needs effectively. Other interventions depend to some extent on the nature of the presenting problem. In families where problem gambling occurs, trust and respect are often serious issues, as they are in families where there has been problematic sexual behaviour. Emotionally focused therapy is a good model for longer-term work with couples in such cases, as it addresses the attachment injuries inflicted by the problem behaviour. Video gaming problems in youth often relate to parents' difficulties with boundaries and setting limits, so effective parenting should be a focus when treating these families. Developmental change can be supported by contracting around specific action plans, such as the steps involved in preparing to send a child away to university.

Special Populations

Certain concurrent issues or histories may create vulnerabilities to specific behavioural addictions. For example, people who have experienced childhood sexual abuse can be at greater risk for problematic sexual behaviour, as they may have learned to see this behaviour as the only way they can receive affection. With excessive shopping, the literature suggests that a history of emotional deprivation is often a precursor. As mentioned earlier, clinical experience suggests that milder severity autism spectrum disorder (formerly called Asperger's syndrome in the DSM-IV-TR) is particularly common in youth with gaming and Internet addictions.

The problem gambling field has identified a number of groups that require specialized services and care. For example, First Nations communities have higher rates of problem gambling than the general population. This vulnerability is related to the loss of culture and language, and the disruption in parenting caused by the residential school experience. Gambling and concepts around luck and fortune are integral to some Asian cultures, leading to higher participation rates and thus more vulnerability to problem gambling. Recent immigrants can be at risk due to dislocation, isolation, financial pressures and threats to identity. Trauma victims may use repetitive gambling behaviour (e.g., on slot machines) to dissociate from painful emotions. People with ADHD are at higher risk of addiction due to impulsivity, and also because substances and activities such as gambling and video gaming provide the stimulation that is at too low a level in certain areas of the brain.

Older adults are statistically less likely than other adults to develop a problem with gambling, but when they do, the impact is often more devastating, because older adults have little opportunity to earn back money they have gambled away. Health issues, limited recreational options, serious personal losses and isolation are all risk factors for excessive gambling behaviour in older adults, as is the casino industry's targeted marketing to this age group, which includes providing free transportation to gambling venues. Any effective treatment intervention will need to address these specific factors.

Conclusion

This chapter has summarized what is known about a few disorders that are considered behavioural addictions. For more detailed descriptions of specific disorders, see the appendix.

We have examined problematic behaviours that share many characteristics with chemical addiction, but which do not involve ingesting a substance. Applying the concept of addiction to these behaviours allows us to use our previously acquired knowledge to address a much wider range of disorders, most of which are currently poorly studied and poorly resourced. This expansion also sheds a new light on addiction to alcohol and other drugs. If the ingestion of substances is not necessary to develop an addiction, then what is? The answers are multifaceted and complex, including a full range of biological, psychological, social and systemic factors that influence people to engage in potentially problematic behaviours at levels that are on a continuum from healthy to extremely harmful.

The field of behavioural addictions is at a relatively early stage of development, although the problem gambling literature has expanded rapidly in recent years, and has paved the way for the exploration of Internet and gaming addictions. Prevalence estimates make clear the serious need for treatment resources for these disorders, but focused, evidence-based treatments are rare. Behavioural addictions can have very serious impacts on the person involved, as well as on his or her family and community. With the explosion of online technologies, legal gambling opportunities and the pressure from marketers to buy and consume, vulnerable people are at even more risk of developing behavioural addictions, without the requisite help available to reduce the harm.

Practice Tips

- Explore the presence of behavioural addictions when assessing for other issues.
- Educate yourself about the behaviour itself, including its positive and negative outcomes.
- Include in a behavioural addiction assessment:
  - an exploration of the meaning of the behaviour for the client—avoid assumptions
  - context and pattern of the behaviour—how it fits within the client's life, beliefs and plans for the future
  - comprehensive history, including co-occurring issues
- Use tools from substance addiction treatment, such as motivational interviewing, CBT, relapse prevention and harm reduction.
- Be aware of how behavioural addictions differ from substance addictions and mental health problems; for example, in terms of:
  - impacts, areas of life affected (e.g., finances, relationships)
  - supports for the behaviour (e.g., social demand for online technologies, easy credit, consumerism)
  - vulnerabilities among populations
- Address co-occurring disorders.
- Consider medications for co-occurring disorders before those for the behavioural problems themselves.

Resources

Publications

Dell'Osso, B., Altamura, C., Allen, A., Marazziti, D. & Hollander, E. (2006). Epidemiologic and clinical updates on impulse control disorders: A critical review. *European Archives of Psychiatry and Clinical Neuroscience, 256*, 464–475.

Grant, J.E. (2008). *Impulse Control Disorders: A Clinician's Guide to Understanding and Treating Behavioral Addictions.* New York: W.W. Norton.

Grant, J.E., Potenza, M.N., Weinstein, A. & Gorelick, D.A. (2010). Introduction to behavioral addictions. *American Journal of Drug and Alcohol Abuse, 36*, 233–241.

Hollander, E. & Stein, D.J. (2006). *Clinical Manual of Impulse Control Disorders.* Arlington, VA: American Psychiatric Publishing.

Sussman, S., Lisha, N. & Griffiths, M. (2011). Prevalence of the addictions: A problem of the majority or the minority? *Evaluation & the Health Professions, 34* (1): 3–56.

Internet

Problem gambling

Ontario Problem Gambling Research Centre
www.gamblingresearch.org

Problem Gambling Institute of Ontario
www.problemgambling.ca (search for "Introduction to process addictions")

Responsible Gambling Council
www.responsiblegambling.org

Internet addiction

Centre for Online Addiction
www.netaddiction.com

TechAddiction: Internet & Video Game Addiction Treatment Centre
www.techaddiction.ca

Sex addiction

Sex Help
www.sexhelp.com

Society for the Advancement of Sexual Health
www.sash.net

Shopping addiction

Shopaholic No More
www.shopaholicnomore.com

Shopaholics Anonymous
www.shopaholicsanonymous.org

References

American Psychiatric Association (APA). (2000). *Diagnostic and Statistical Manual of Mental Disorders* (text rev.). Washington, DC: Author.

American Psychiatric Association (APA). (2013). *Diagnostic and Statistical Manual of Mental Disorders* (5th ed.). Washington, DC: Author.

Beach, F.A. & Jordan, L. (1956). Sexual exhaustion and recovery in the male rat. *Quarterly Journal of Experimental Psychology, 8,* 121–133.

Becker, H.C. (1999). Alcohol withdrawal: Neuroadaptation and sensitization. *CNS Spectrums, 4* (1), 38–65.

Blum, K., Cull, J.G. & Comings, E.D. (1996). Biogenetics of reward deficiency syndrome. *Scientific American, 84,* 132–145.

Boughton, R. & Brewster, J. (2002). *Voices of Women Who Gamble in Ontario: A Survey
of Women's Gambling—Barriers to Treatment and Treatment Service Needs.* Toronto:
Ministry of Health and Long-Term Care, Ontario.

Brewer, J.A. & Potenza, M.N. (2008). The neurobiology and genetics of impulse
control disorders: Relationships to drug addictions. *Biochemical Pharmacology, 75,*
63–75.

Chakraborty, K., Basu, D. & Kumar, K.G.V. (2010). Internet addiction: Consensus, con-
troversies, and the way ahead. *East Asian Archives of Psychiatry, 20,* 123–132.

Comings, D.E. & Blum, K. (2000). Reward deficiency syndrome: Genetic aspects of
behavioral disorders. *Progress in Brain Research, 126,* 325–341.

Cook, S., Turner, N., Paglia-Boak, A., Adlaf, E.M. & Mann, R.E. (2010). *Ontario Youth
Gambling Report: Data from the 2009 Ontario Student Drug Use and Health Survey.*
Retrieved from www.problemgambling.ca

Esch, T. & Stefano, G.B. (2004). The neurobiology of pleasure, reward processes,
addiction and their health implications. *Neuroendocrinology, 4,* 235–251.

Fiorillo, C.D., Tobler, P.N. & Schultz, W. (2003). Discrete coding of reward probability
and uncertainty by dopamine neurons. *Science, 299,* 1898–1902.

First, M.B. (2010). Obsessive Compulsive Spectrum Disorders Conference (June
20–22, 2006). Retrieved from www.dsm5.org/research/pages/
obsessivecompulsivespectrumdisordersconference(june20-22,2006).aspx

Garcia, F.D. & Thibaut, F. (2010). Sexual addictions. *American Journal of Drug and
Alcohol Abuse, 36,* 254–260.

Grant, J.E., Kim, S.W., Hollander, E. & Potenza, M.N. (2008). Predicting response
to opiate antagonists and placebo in the treatment of pathological gambling.
Psychopharmacology (Berl), 200, 521–527.

Grant, J.E. & Potenza, M.N. (2006). Compulsive aspects of impulse-control disorders.
Psychiatric Clinics of North America, 29, 539–551.

Grant, J.E., Potenza, M.N., Weinstein, A. & Gorelick, D.A. (2010). Introduction to
behavioral addictions. *American Journal of Drug and Alcohol Abuse, 36,* 233–241.

Kaplan, M.S. & Krueger, R.B. (2010). Diagnosis, assessment, and treatment of hypersexuality. *Journal of Sex Research, 47,* 181–198.

Kuzma, J. & Black, D.W. (2006). Compulsive shopping: When spending begins to consume the consumer. *Current Psychiatry, 7,* 27–40.

Olsen, C.M. (2011). Natural rewards, neuroplasticity, and non-drug addictions.
Neuropharmacology, 61, 1109–1122.

Orford, J. (2001). Addiction as excessive appetite. *Addiction, 96,* 15–31.

Peele, S. (1978, September). Addiction: The analgesic experience. *Human Nature,*
61–67. Retrieved from http://peele.net/lib/analgesic.html

Schmitz, J.M. (2005). The interface between impulse-control disorders and addictions: Are pleasure pathway responses shared neurobiological substrates? *Sexual Addiction & Compulsivity, 12,* 149–168.

Schultz, W. (1998). Predictive reward signal of dopamine neurons. *Journal of Neurophysiology, 80* (1), 1–27.

Vazquez, V., Penit-Soria, J., Durand, C., Besson, M.J., Giros, B. & Daugé, V. (2005). Maternal deprivation increases vulnerability to morphine dependence and disturbs the enkephalinergic system in adulthood. *Journal of Neuroscience, 25,* 4453–4462.

Vetulani, J. (2001). Drug addiction. Part II: Neurobiology of addiction. *Polish Journal of Pharmacology, 53,* 303–317.

Zack, M. & Poulos, C.X. (2009). Parallel roles for dopamine in pathological gambling and psychostimulant addiction. *Current Drug Abuse Reviews, 2,* 11–25.

Appendix

Behavioural Addictions

This section provides an overview of five common behavioural addictions: gambling, Internet, sex, shopping and video gaming. Except for problem gambling, these disorders have not been included in the DSM (APA, 2000, 2013). The newly released DSM-5 (APA, 2013) replaces pathological gambling, a unique phrase, with language that is more consistent with DSM nomenclature, so that it is now referred to as "gambling disorder" (with mild, moderate and severe levels). Other behavioural addictions are acknowledged but not specified in the DSM-5, because the DSM-5 panel felt the evidence base was not sufficient to justify their inclusion, unlike gambling and substance use disorders.

Due to limited uniformity of sampling and assessment methods, widely varying prevalence rates for these behavioural addictions have been reported across different cultures and countries. Thus, the rates cited in this section should not be used for making final epidemiological statements. Furthermore, the screening tools we list are for description purposes only. We would like readers to refer to the original references for more information on the reliability and validity of these scales and whether they are used for clinical or prevalence rating purposes.

Assessment of the various behavioural addictions is fairly consistent and involves taking a detailed medical and psychological history, as well as using screening tools. Since many of the screening tools for these addictions have not been rigorously tested, we advise gathering a detailed client history in addition to using these tools, rather than using only the tools. As well, for all of the listed behavioural addictions, it is important to treat the co-occurring disorder simultaneously. Other symptoms can be a risk factor for the addiction, as well as for an accompanying or interdependent condition. Although treatment may vary, new technologies, such as brain single photon emission computed tomography (SPECT), have the potential to add clinical information vital to client care. SPECT can, for example, evaluate underlying brain systems pathology and assess the impact of treatment using a post-treatment scan (Amen et al., 2012).

The next section begins with a brief look at common co-occurring disorders seen among clients at a clinic for youth between age 18 and 25 who have behavioural addictions, and what treatment typically entails in this program at the Centre for Addiction and Mental Health (CAMH).

Problem Behaviours among Youth in the Advanced Clinical and Educational Services Clinic

The Advanced Clinical and Educational Services clinic (ACES) at CAMH works with youth between age 18 and 25 who have behavioural addictions. Some of these young people have co-occurring disorders. The main co-occurring disorders are:

- social anxiety
- depression
- trauma-related conditions
- autistic spectrum disorders
- attention-deficit disorders
- learning disorders
- personality disorders
- substance use disorders
- psychosis (rare).

At ACES, treatment for behavioural addictions typically involves matching clients to treatments on the basis of client characteristics, known as treatment matching. This includes individual therapy, which usually consists of a combination of motivational interviewing, CBT, interpersonal therapy and family therapy. Medication management for co-occurring conditions (e.g., antidepressants for depression) is standard. It is also common for clients to participate in group therapy, such as social skills groups, motivational interviewing groups and DBT-like groups. Standard client psychoeducational assessments help to identify certain issues for tailoring treatment protocols.

Problem Gambling

Definition

A pattern of gambling behaviour that may compromise, disrupt or damage family, personal or vocational pursuits. Problem gambling:
- interferes with work, school or other activities
- leads to emotional or physical health problems
- causes financial problems
- harms the family or other relationships (CAMH, 2008).

Common terms

- gambling addiction
- pathological gambling
- compulsive gambling
- gambling disorder.

Prevalence

- Among Ontario students in grades 7–12, 3 per cent have a gambling problem (about 29,000 students). Males are more likely than females to report a gambling problem (about 4 per cent compared to 1 per cent) (Paglia-Boak et al., 2010).

- Among Ontario adults, 1.2–3.4 per cent are moderately to severely affected by problem gambling (Wiebe et al., 2006; Williams et al., 2012).
- In Ontario, 2.1 per cent of older adults (60+) are moderately to severely affected by problem gambling (Wiebe et al., 2004).
- 0.2 per cent to 5.3 per cent of adults worldwide are affected by problem gambling (Hodgins et al., 2011).
- In the last 12 months of a survey, prevalence of gambling addiction was an estimated 2 per cent in the general U.S. adult population (Sussman et al., 2011).

Risk factors

- a big win early in the gambling history
- boredom susceptibility and poor impulse control (e.g., ADHD)
- a poor understanding of randomness
- a tendency to rely on escape as a way of coping with stress
- a stressful life with a lack of support and direction around the time gambling began
- a history of overspending
- a history of addiction or mental health problems, particularly depression or anxiety
- a trauma or abuse history
- a family history of addiction or mental health issues (CAMH, 2008; Turner et al., 2006).

Vulnerable groups

- Youth have higher prevalence rates than adults, especially young males.
- Older adults have lower prevalence rates but are more vulnerable to losses.
- New immigrants may be vulnerable due to dislocation, isolation and financial stresses.
- Low-income people are vulnerable to developing a gambling problem.
- Aboriginal people may be at increased risk due to factors associated with isolation, poverty, racism, oppression and the loss of culture and language (CAMH, 2008).

Types and subtypes

Blaszczynski's pathway model combines biological, personality, developmental, cognitive, learning theory and ecological determinants of problem and pathological gambling into the following three pathways, which are helpful for directing treatment:
- behaviourally conditioned problem gamblers
- emotionally vulnerable problem gamblers
- antisocial, impulsive problem gamblers (Blaszczynski & Nower, 2002).

Common negative impacts

- employment, relationships and physical and mental health
- individual and family finances, far more than with other addictive behaviours

- chronic poor levels of functioning, bankruptcy, job loss, loss of housing, illegal behaviour, family breakups and child neglect
- a widening circle of stress and loss experienced by those whom the problem gambler affects (CAMH, 2008).

Co-occurring disorders

- Among Ontario students in grades 7 to 12, co-occurring disorders include substance-related problems, mental health problems (specifically suicidality) and delinquencies, such as theft and selling drugs (Cook et al., 2010).
- It is estimated that 50 per cent, 30 per cent and 20 per cent of problem gamblers are also addicted to smoking, alcohol and illicit drugs, in that order (Sussman et al., 2011).
- Common co-occurring disorders among CAMH clients in treatment for problem gambling are major depressive disorder, PTSD, substance abuse/dependence, bipolar disorder, anxiety disorders, personality disorders and ADHD.

Screening tools

- CAMH Gambling Screen (Turner & Horbay, 2000)
- Canadian Problem Gambling Index (Ferris & Wynne, 2001)
- Check Your Gambling (Cunningham et al., 2009)
- GA 20 Questions (Gamblers Anonymous, n.d.)
- South Oaks Gambling Screen—RA (SOGS-RA) (Lesieur & Blume, 1987)
- Canadian Adolescent Gambling Inventory (Tremblay et al., 2010).

Treatment

Treatment can entail individual, group, couple or family counselling. CBT and motivational interviewing are frequently used, as are financial counselling and online self-help/support tools. Mutual aid associations, including Gamblers Anonymous, provide peer-based social support that supplements formal treatment and provide a structured model to recovery, especially for people who self-identify as being addicted to gambling. (See Chapter 14 on mutual help groups.)

In review studies, various drugs, opioid antagonists, glutamatergic agents, antidepressants and mood stabilizers were found to be more effective than a placebo as treatment for problem gambling. At this time, no drug has received regulatory approval for problem gambling treatment worldwide (Hodgins et al., 2011).

Problem Internet Use

Definition

- Problematic use of online technology that is time-consuming and causes distress or impairs one's functioning in important life domains (Shaw & Black, 2008).

Common terms

- compulsive computer use
- Internet dependency
- Internet addiction
- Internet addiction disorder
- pathological Internet use.

Prevalence

- Problem Internet use affects between 0.9 and 38 per cent of youth (Shaw & Black, 2008).
- One review article estimated that 2 per cent of U.S. adults are affected in a 12-month period (Sussman et al., 2011). Another study estimated that 4 to 13 per cent of U.S. adults are affected (Aboujaoude et al., 2006).

Risk factors and vulnerable groups

- Research points to a male predominance, with onset in the late 20s or early 30s. Problem Internet use affects people worldwide but is more prevalent in countries where computer access is more widespread (Shaw & Black, 2008).

Common negative impacts

- personal: marriages, parent-child relationships and friendships
- social: isolation, neglecting family and friends
- occupational: work-related problems and poor academic performance
- psychological: loneliness, frustration and depression
- physical: sleep deprivation, lack of exercise, increased risk for carpal tunnel syndrome and back and eye strain
- financial: spending and losing money gambling online or shopping online.

Types and subtypes

Subtypes are related to the specific activities engaged in that may overlap or interact and include: social networking (e.g., Twitter, Facebook), cybersex (e.g., porn, sex-related chat), shopping and auction sites, gambling, online video gaming (Kuss & Griffiths, 2012) and web surfing.

Co-occurring disorders

- An estimated 10 per cent have an addiction to one of the following: sex, love, shopping, video gaming, gambling, exercise, smoking, drugs or work (Sussman et al., 2011).
- Other co-occurring disorders can include mood, anxiety, substance use, affective disorders, other addictive disorders, impulse control disorders and personality disorders (Kuss & Griffiths, 2012; Shaw & Black, 2008).

Screening tools

- Internet Addiction Test (Young, 1998)
- Griffith's diagnostic criteria (Griffiths, 1998)
- Beard and Wolf's diagnostic criteria (Beard & Wolf, 2001)
- Generalized Problematic Internet Use Scale (Caplan, 2002)
- Internet Consequences Scale (Clark et al., 2004)
- Morahan-Martin & Schumacher's 13-item scale and the Internet Behavior and Attitude Scale (Morahan-Martin & Schumacher, 2000).

Treatment

Although no medications are currently approved for treating behavioural addictions such as this one (Grant et al., 2010), psychopharmacological treatments have proven effective for treating Internet gaming addiction, which demonstrates the biochemical components of this problem (Huang & Tau, 2010; Kuss & Griffiths, 2012).

CBT, self-help books and tapes, support groups, financial counselling, marriage or couple counselling and family therapy may be helpful (Shaw & Black, 2008).

Problem Sexual Behaviours

Definition

This definition focuses on non-paraphilic behaviours, as described in the fourth bullet:
- Sex addictions are categorized as either paraphilias or paraphilia-related disorders (sometimes called non-paraphilic sexual addictions).
- Paraphilias, such as pedophilia, are classified in the DSM (APA, 2000, 2013) and consist of socially deviant sexual cognitions, urges or behaviours that are typically strong and continual and either involve non-consenting persons or lead to distress or impairment in functioning (Allen & Hollander, 2006).
- Paraphilia-related disorder (non-paraphilic sexual addictions), such as phone sex dependency, are typified by a loss of control over sexual fantasies, urges and behaviours, which are accompanied by negative consequences and/or personal distress (Allen & Hollander, 2006).

- Non-paraphilic sexual addictions are behaviours that are viewed as normative but are engaged in with a frequency or intensity that leads to distress or greatly interferes with functioning (Allen & Hollander, 2006).
- There is lack of consensus as to whether problem sexual behaviours fall under compulsive, impulsive or addictive disorders (Allen & Hollander, 2006; Kaplan & Krueger, 2010).

Common terms

- hypersexuality
- sexual compulsivity
- compulsive sexual behaviour
- impulsive-compulsive sexual behaviour.

Prevalence

- 10.3 per cent of 19-year-old Canadian college students have a sexual addiction, and 3 per cent of U.S. adults have a sexual addiction (Sussman et al., 2011).
- Among U.S. adults, an estimated 3 to 6 per cent have a sexual addiction, with males more likely to be affected than females (Garcia & Thibaut, 2010; Kaplan & Krueger, 2010).

Risk factors and vulnerable groups

- Risk factors include a history of dysfunctional family of origin; and physical, traumatic, sexual or emotional abuse (Coleman-Kennedy & Pendley, 2002).
- Some research points to neurobiological causes of sex addiction, including among people with certain medical conditions, such as dementia, Tourette's syndrome, brain injury and stroke (Kaplan & Krueger, 2010).

Types and subtypes

Subtypes include sexual behaviour with consenting adults (e.g., anonymous sex, multiple sex partners, affairs, use of prostitutes); compulsive masturbation; and dependency on pornography, phone sex, cybersex (e.g., sexual chat rooms) or strip clubs (Kaplan & Krueger, 2010).

Common negative impacts

- personal distress
- problems in relationships
- risk to reputation
- increased risk of sexually transmitted diseases
- unwanted pregnancy

- excessive financial expenses
- work or educational role impairment (Kafka, 2010).

Co-occurring disorders

- Mood disorders, anxiety disorders and substance use disorders are the most common (Garcia & Thibaut, 2010).
- Co-occurring disorders often include affective disorders, substance use disorders, anxiety disorders, personality disorders and paraphilic disorders (Kaplan & Krueger, 2010).
- Comorbidities of Internet sex addiction include affective disorders, substance-related addictions, behavioural addictions, PTSD and eating disorders (Griffiths, 2012).

Screening tools

- Sexual Addiction Screening Test (SAST) (Carnes, 1989)
- Gay and Bisexual Male Sexual Addiction Screening Test (G-SAST) (adapted by Carnes from the SAST)
- Women's Sexual Addiction Screening Test (W-SAST) (Carnes & O'Hara, 1994)
- Sexual Dependency Inventory Revised (SDI-R) (Delmonico et al., 1998)
- Compulsive Sexual Behaviour Inventory (CSBI) (Miner et al., 2007)
- Sexual Compulsivity Scale (SCS) (Kalichman & Rompa, 2001)
- Sexual Inhibition Scales (SIS) and Sexual Excitation Scale (SES) (Janssen et al., 2002).
- Of these, the CSBI, SCS and SES have the strongest empirical reliability and validity.

Treatment

Although no medications have been approved for treating behavioural addictions (Grant et al., 2010), some have shown to be effective, such as selective serotonin uptake inhibitors, anti-androgens (Garcia & Thibaut, 2010) and naltrexone (Kaplan & Krueger, 2010).

A multi-faceted treatment approach includes CBT (relapse prevention therapy and behaviour therapy), psychotherapy, couples therapy and psychopharmacological medications. Twelve-step programs such as Sex and Love Addicts Anonymous and Sexaholics Anonymous offer peer-based recovery fellowships that are valued particularly by people who self-identify as having a sex addiction (Kaplan & Krueger, 2010).

Problem Shopping

Definition

- Characterized by excessive shopping preoccupation and buying behaviour that leads to distress or impairment. It involves four typical phases: anticipation, preparation, shopping and spending (Black, 2007).

Common terms

- compulsive shopping
- compulsive buying
- addictive buying
- uncontrolled buying
- excessive buying.

Prevalence

- 3.5 per cent of U.S. high-school students between age 14 and 18 (Grant et al., 2011)
- 6 per cent of U.S. adults (Sussman et al., 2011).

Risk factors and vulnerable groups

- being female
- having a history of depression, bipolar disorder, substance use disorders, impulse control disorders or eating disorders (Black, 2007; Lejoyeux & Weinstein, 2010).

Types and subtypes

Shopping addiction over the Internet is a subtype of problem shopping, where people can avoid face-to-face social contact and keep their transactions private; continuous Internet advertising feeds the addiction (Lejoyeux & Weinstein, 2010).

Other people have a shopping addiction in a retail environment.

Common negative impacts

- financial problems (e.g., bankruptcy, debt)
- legal problems (e.g., writing bad cheques)
- psychological distress (e.g., feeling guilty or remorseful)
- interpersonal and marital conflict (e.g., family issues and divorce) (Lejoyeux & Weinstein, 2010).

Co-occurring disorders

- Other co-occurring disorders include mood disorders (depression and bipolar disorder), OCD, eating disorders, substance use disorders, impulse control disorders and personality disorders (Dell'Osso et al., 2008; Lejoyeux & Weinstein, 2010).
- About 20 per cent of people with a shopping addiction have a co-occurring sex or love addiction, gambling addiction, Internet addiction, eating addiction, substance use addiction, exercise addiction or work addiction (Sussman et al., 2011).

Screening tools

- Compulsive Buying Scale (Faber & O'Guinn, 1992)
- Yale-Brown Obsessive Compulsive Scale—Shopping version (Monahan et al., 1996)
- Canadian Compulsive Buying Measurement Scale (Valence et al., 1988)
- Edwards Compulsive Buying Scale (Edwards, 1993)
- Minnesota Impulsive Disorder Interview (Christenson et al., 1994)
- Ridgway's Compulsive Buying Scale (Ridgway et al., 2008)
- Preliminary operational criteria for the diagnosis of compulsive buying (Murali et al., 2012).

Treatment

There is no standard treatment for problem shopping, but self-help books, Debtors Anonymous, marriage or couple counselling, CBT and financial counselling may be helpful (Black, 2007). No medication has shown to be effective in controlled trials (Lejoyeux & Weinstein, 2010) despite case studies identifying antidepressants as effective (Murali et al., 2012).

Problem Video Gaming

Definition

- Video game playing becomes dysfunctional when it harms the person's social, occupational, family, school and psychological well-being (Gentile et al., 2011).

Common terms

- video game addiction
- excessive video gaming
- dependent video gaming
- pathological video gaming
- video game dependency
- technological addictions.

Prevalence

- In 2009, 10.3 per cent of Ontario students (97,000) reported having a video gaming problem: 16 per cent were male and 4 per cent were female) (Paglia-Boak et al., 2010).
- Among U.S. youth between age 8 and 18, 8 per cent exhibit pathological patterns of play, with higher rates among males (Gentile, 2009).
- A recent review points to the variability of prevalence, which ranges from 0.3 percent to 12 percent, due to, for example, using dissimilar assessment tools and ages (Kuss & Griffiths, 2012).

Risk factors and vulnerable groups

- single males from mid-adolescence to their late 20s with computing experience (King et al., 2010)
- youth who are impulsive, have low social competence skills, low empathy skills and poor emotional regulation skills (Gentile et al., 2011)
- youth who have attention problems, such as ADHD (Gentile, 2009).

Personality traits have been found to be significantly related to problem Internet gaming. These traits include loneliness and introversion, social inhibition, sensation seeking, boredom inclination, narcissistic personality traits, low self-esteem, state and trait anxiety and low emotional intelligence (Kuss & Griffiths, 2012).

Types and subtypes

- Online gaming is more likely to be addictive than offline, stand-alone gaming, because online games never pause or end (Griffiths & Meredith, 2009).
- Multiple routes may exist to problem video gaming, in much the same way as they exist for problem gambling (identified in Blaszczynski & Nower's [2002] pathways model), but no such subtypes have been examined empirically (King et al., 2010).

Common negative impacts

- psychosocial problems (i.e., no real-life relationships)
- inattention
- aggressive or oppositional behaviour and hostility
- maladaptive coping, stress
- decreased academic achievement
- sacrificing hobbies, sleep, work, education, socializing, time with partner/family
- lower psychosocial well-being and loneliness and increased thoughts of suicide
- psychosomatic problems (found to be consequences of Internet gaming addiction and include psychosomatic challenges, seizures and sleep abnormalities)
- interpersonal, academic and social problems (Derevensky, 2012)
- primer for problem gambling among youth (Kuss & Griffiths, 2012).

Co-occurring disorders

In a review study, Internet gaming was found to be associated with symptoms of generalized anxiety disorder, depression, social phobia, school phobia, ADHD and psychosomatic symptoms (Kuss & Griffiths, 2012).

Screening and assessment tools

Assessment tools (King et al., 2010)

- Brown's components model of addiction: addiction is defined by six features (salience, tolerance, withdrawal, relapse, mood modification and harm); a person who meets some of the criteria is seen as a "problem" user, while a person who meets all criteria is considered to be addicted.
- The DSM (APA, 2000, 2013) classification for problem gambling.

Self-reporting tools (King et al., 2010)

None of the following tools has been clinically validated:

- Problem Video Game Playing Test (PVGT)
- Video Game Addiction Inventory (VGAI) modelled after the Exercise Addiction Inventory
- Computer-Related Addictive Behavior Inventory (CRABI) modelled on Young's Internet Addiction Test—the word "Internet" is replaced with "video game"
- Game Addiction Scale (GAS).

Treatment

Prevention strategies that parents can implement include:

- monitoring choice of games and play behaviour
- keeping computers in the family area to enable supervision
- maintaining time limits on use
- discouraging solitary game playing
- providing multiple alternative activities (Griffiths & Meredith, 2009).

Treatment may include online support forums, CBT and motivational interviewing. Some clinical research results point to the efficacy of psychopharmacological treatments (Griffiths & Meredith, 2009). Online Gamers Anonymous, based on a 12-step model, is available for people who want to participate in peer-based social support with an addiction focus.

References

Aboujaoude, E., Koran, L.M., Gamel, N., Large, M.D. & Serpe, R.T. (2006). Potential markers for problematic Internet use: A telephone survey of 2,513 adults. *CNS Spectrums, 11*, 750–755.

Allen, A. & Hollander, E. (2006). Sexual compulsions. In E. Hollander & D.J. Stein (Eds.), *Clinical Manual of Impulse Control Disorders* (pp. 87–114). Arlington, VA: American Psychiatric Publishing.

Amen, D.G., Willeumier, K. & Johnson, R. (2012). The clinical utility of brain SPECT imaging in process addictions. *Journal of Psychoactive Drugs, 44* (1), 18–26.

American Psychiatric Association (APA). (2000). *Diagnostic and Statistical Manual of Mental Disorders* (4th ed., text rev.). Washington, DC: Author.

American Psychiatric Association (APA). (2013). *Diagnostic and Statistical Manual of Mental Disorders* (5th ed.). Washington, DC: Author.

Beard, K.W. & Wolf, E.M. (2001). Modification of the proposed diagnostic criteria for Internet addiction. *CyberPsychology & Behavior, 4,* 377–383.

Black, D.W. (2007). A review of compulsive buying disorder. *World Psychiatry, 6* (1), 14–18.

Blaszczynski, A. & Nower, L. (2002). A pathways model of problem and pathological gambling. *Addiction, 97,* 487–499.

Caplan, S.E. (2002). Problematic Internet use and psychosocial wellbeing: Development of a theory-based cognitive-behavioral measurement instrument. *Computers in Human Behavior, 3,* 377–383.

Carnes, P. (1989). *Contrary to Love.* Minneapolis, MN: CompCare.

Carnes, P. & O'Hara, S. (1994). Women's Sexual Addiction Screening Test. Retrieved from www.insideoutlivinginc.org

Centre for Addiction and Mental Health (CAMH). (2008). *Problem Gambling: A Guide for Helping Professionals.* Toronto: Author.

Christenson, G., Faber, R.J., DeZwaan, M., Raymond, N.C., Specker, S.M., Ekern, M.D. et al. (1994). Compulsive buying: Descriptive characteristics and psychiatric comorbidity. *Journal of Clinical Psychiatry, 55,* 5–11.

Clark, D.J., Frith, K.H. & Demi, S.A. (2004). The physical, behavioral, and psychosocial consequences of Internet use in college students. *CIN: Computers, Informatics, Nursing, 22,* 153–161.

Coleman-Kennedy, C. & Pendley, A. (2002). Assessment and diagnosis of sexual addiction. *Journal of the American Psychiatric Nurses Association, 8* (5), 143–151.

Cook, S., Turner, N., Paglia-Boak, A., Adlaf, E.M. & Mann, R.E. (2010). *Ontario Youth Gambling Report: Data from the 2009 Ontario Student Drug Use and Health Survey.* Retrieved from www.problemgambling.ca

Cunningham, J.A., Hodgins, D.C., Toneatto, T., Rai, A. & Cordingley, J. (2009). Pilot study of a personalized feedback intervention for problem gamblers. *Behavior Therapy, 40,* 219–224.

Delmonico, D.L., Bubenzer, D.L. & West, J.D. (1998). Assessing sexual addiction with the sexual dependency inventory-revised. *Sexual Addiction & Compulsivity, 5,* 179–187.

Dell'Osso, B., Allen, A.A., Altamura, C., Buoli, B. & Hollander, E. (2008). Impulsive-compulsive buying disorder: Clinical overview. *Australia and New Zealand Journal of Psychiatry, 42,* 259–266.

Derevensky, J.L. (2012). *Teen Gambling: Understanding a Growing Epidemic.* Lanham, MD: Rowman & Littlefield.

Edwards, E.A. (1993). Development of a new scale for measuring compulsive buying behavior. *Financial Counseling and Planning, 4*, 67–84.

Faber, R.J. & O'Guinn, T.C. (1992). A clinical screener for compulsive buying. *Journal of Consumer Research, 19*, 459–469.

Ferris, J. & Wynne, H. (February, 2001). *The Canadian Problem Gambling Index: Final Report*. Retrieved from www.cclat.ca/Eng/Priorities/Gambling/CPGI/Pages/default. aspx

Gamblers Anonymous. (n.d.). 20 Questions. Los Angeles: Author. Retrieved from www.gamblersanonymous.org/ga/content/20-questions

Garcia, F.D. & Thibaut, F. (2010). Sexual addictions. *American Journal of Drug and Alcohol Abuse, 36*, 254–260.

Gentile, D.A. (2009). Pathological video game use among youth 8 to 18: A national study. *Psychological Science, 20*, 594–602.

Gentile, A.D., Choo, H., Liau, A., Sim, T., Li, D., Fung, D. & Khoo, A. (2011). Pathological video game use among youths: A two-year longitudinal study. *Pediatrics*. doi: 10.1542/peds.2010-1353

Grant, J.E., Potenza, M.N., Krishnan-Sarin, S., Cavallo, D.A. & Desai, R.A. (2011). Shopping problems among high school students. *Comprehensive Psychiatry, 52*, 247–252.

Grant, J.E., Potenza, M.N., Weinstein, A. & Gorelick, D.A. (2010). Introduction to behavioural addictions. *American Journal of Drug and Alcohol Abuse, 36*, 233–241.

Griffiths, M. D. (1998). Internet addiction: Does it really exist? In J. Gackenbach (Ed.), *Psychology and the Internet: Intrapersonal, Interpersonal, and Transpersonal Implications* (pp. 61–75). San Diego, CA: Academic Press.

Griffiths, M.D. (2012). Internet sex addiction: A review of empirical research. *Addiction Research and Theory, 20*, 111–124.

Griffiths, M.D. & Meredith, A. (2009). Videogame addiction and its treatment. *Journal of Contemporary Psychotherapy, 39*, 247–253.

Hodgins, D., Stea, J.N. & Grant, J.E. (2011). Gambling disorders. *The Lancet, 26*, 1874–1884.

Huang, X. & Tau, M.L. (2010). Treatment of Internet addiction. *Current Psychiatry Reports, 12*, 462–470.

Janssen, E., Vorst, H., Finn, P. & Bancroft, J. (2002). The Sexual Inhibition (SIS) and the Sexual Excitation (SES) scales: I. Measuring sexual inhibition and excitation proneness in men. *Journal of Sex Research, 39*, 114–126.

Kafka, M.P. (2010). Hypersexual disorder: A proposed diagnosis for DSM-V. *Archives of Sexual Behaviour, 39*, 377–400.

Kalichman, S.C. & Rompa, D. (2001). The Sexual Compulsivity Scale: Further development and use with HIV-positive persons. *Journal of Personality Assessment, 76*, 379–395.

Kaplan, M.S. & Krueger, R.B. (2010). Diagnosis, assessment, and treatment of hypersexuality. *Journal of Sex Research, 47*, 181–198.

King, D.L., Delfabbro, P.H. & Griffiths, M.D. (2010). Cognitive behavioral therapy for problematic video game players: Conceptual considerations and practice issues. *Journal of Cybertherapy & Rehabilitation, 3*, 261–273.

Kuss, D.J. & Griffiths, M.D. (2012). Internet gaming: A systematic review of empirical research. *International Journal of Mental Health Addictions, 10*, 278–296.

Lejoyeux, M. & Weinstein, A. (2010). Compulsive buying. *American Journal of Drug and Alcohol Abuse, 36*, 248–253.

Lesieur, H. & Blume, S.B. (1987). The South Oaks Gambling Screen (SOGS): A new instrument for the identification of pathological gamblers. *American Journal of Psychiatry, 144*, 1184–1188.

Miner, M.H., Coleman, E., Center, B.A., Ross. M. & Rosser, B.R.S. (2007). The Compulsive Sexual Behavior Inventory: Psychometric properties. *Archives of Sexual Behavior, 36*, 579–587.

Monahan, P., Black, D.W. & Gabel, J. (1996). Reliability and validity of a scale to measure change in persons with compulsive buying. *Psychiatry Research, 64*, 59–67.

Morahan-Martin, J. & Schumacher, P. (2000). Incidence and correlates of pathological Internet use among college students. *Computers in Human Behavior, 16*, 13–29.

Murali, V., Ray, R. & Shaffiullha, M. (2012). Shopping addiction. *Advances in Psychiatric Treatment, 18*, 263–269.

Paglia-Boak, A., Mann, R.E., Adlaf, E.M., Beitchman, J.H., Wolfe, D. & Rehm, J. (2010). *The Mental Health and Well-Being of Ontario Students, 1991–2009: Detailed OSDUHS Findings.* CAMH Research Document series no. 29. Toronto: Centre for Addiction and Mental Health.

Ridgway, N.M., Kukar-Kinney, M. & Monroe, K.B. (2008). An expanded conceptualization and a new measure of compulsive buying. *Journal of Consumer Research, 35*, 622–639.

Shaw, M. & Black, D.W. (2008). Internet addiction: Definition, assessment, epidemiology and clinical management. *CNS Drugs, 22*, 353–365.

Sussman, S., Lisha, N. & Griffiths, M. (2011). Prevalence of the addictions: A problem of the majority or the minority? *Evaluation & the Health Professions, 34*, 3–56.

Tremblay, J., Stinchfield, R., Wiebe, J. & Wynne, H. (2010). *Canadian Adolescent Gambling Inventory (CAGI) Phase III Final Report.* Retrieved from www.ccsa.ca

Turner, N.E. & Horbay, R. (2000). CAMH gambling screen. Unpublished screening tool.

Turner, N., Littman-Sharp, N. & Zangeneh, M. (2006). The experience of gambling and its role in problem gambling. *International Gambling Studies, 6*, 237–266.

Valence G., d'Astous, A. & Fortier L. (1988). Compulsive buying: Concept and measurement. *Journal of Consumer Policy, 11*, 419–433.

Wiebe, J., Mun, P. & Kauffman, N. (2006, September). *Gambling and Problem Gambling in Ontario 2005.* Toronto: Responsible Gambling Council. Retrieved from www.responsiblegambling.org/docs/research-reports/gambling-and-problem-gambling-in-ontario-2005.pdf?sfvrsn=12

Wiebe, J., Single, E., Falkowski-Ham, A. & Mun, P. (2004). *Gambling and Problem Gambling among Older Adults in Ontario.* Retrieved from www.responsiblegambling. org/docs/research-reports/
gambling-and-problem-gambling-among-older-adults-in-ontario.pdf?sfvrsn=10

Williams, R.J., Volberg, R.A. & Stevens, R.M.G. (2012). *The Population Prevalence of Problem Gambling: Methodological Influences, Standardized Rates, Jurisdictional Differences, and Worldwide Trends.* Retrieved from http://hdl.handle.net/10133/3068

Young, K.S. (1998). *Caught in the Net: How to Recognize the Signs of Internet Addiction—and a Winning Strategy for Recovery.* New York: John Wiley & Sons.

SECTION 4

SPECIFIC POPULATIONS

Chapter 21

Working with Women

Nancy Poole, Susan Harrison and Eva Ingber

A 20-year-old Caucasian woman with no fixed address is engaging in survival sex to pay for food and crack cocaine for herself and her pimp.

✦

A 30-year-old mother with two preschool-aged children has been living in a transition house to escape an abusive partner. While she has been trying to reduce her drinking, one night she returned to the house drunk, and has been asked to leave.

✦

A 50-year-old Asian woman who is working as a senior civil servant takes antidepressant and anti-anxiety medications and drinks heavily to manage symptoms of posttraumatic stress disorder.

✦

A 12-year-old Métis girl took up smoking cigarettes and drinking alcohol when she was 10 years old.

✦

A 20-year-old Caucasian woman who is eight months pregnant is afraid to go to her prenatal appointments for fear her doctor will find out she is using cocaine, diet pills and alcohol and will report her to child welfare authorities.

✦

A 45-year-old single black woman who works as a nurse and who comes from a family with alcohol problems drinks following her shifts to cope with stress and isolation.

These vignettes exemplify key realities—and great variance—in the circumstances influencing girls' and women's substance use, and how prevention, harm reduction and treatment responses need to take these gendered influences into account. In health research, policy and practice, there is increasing recognition of the importance of attending to sex and gender differences in the experience of health problems (Clow et al., 2009).

Sex differences—biological characteristics that distinguish males and females, such as differences in how alcohol is metabolized—are often overlooked in substance use treatment. Gender differences (in roles, traits, attitudes, values and relative power that society ascribes to women and men) in the experience of substance use are also important to understand, challenge and address in our treatment responses; this includes the harsh stigma experienced by pregnant women who use substances.

This chapter focuses on sex and gender differences in substance use and addiction, as they apply to girls and women. We provide a short overview of research on sex, gender and substance use, and then discuss the practical implications of this research for our treatment interactions with individual women, and for improving the overall systemic response. We also make reference to the diverse needs of girls and women with substance use problems, as illustrated in the introductory vignettes, demonstrating how age, different types of substance use and varying stressors can be addressed.

Literature on Girls, Women and Substance Use

This brief overview of sex and gender differences in the experience of substance use touches on four key issues: mothering, experiences of trauma and violence, mental health challenges and physiological vulnerabilities. The findings illustrate how important it is to bring a sex and gender lens to our work as treatment providers. As experts at the Substance Abuse and Mental Health Services Administration have noted, "When women's specific needs are addressed from the outset, improved treatment engagement, retention and outcomes are the result" (Center for Substance Abuse Treatment [CSAT)], 2009, p. xvii). In Canada, we have stated it simply as "gender matters" (Zbogar, 2007).

Pregnancy, Mothering and Substance Use

Attention to women's substance use during pregnancy and in the childbearing years is central to a gender-informed treatment response. While this is not a new issue, we have growing evidence of the health impacts of substance use for mothers and children; gendered barriers to treatment and support; effective outreach, engagement and treatment strategies; and successful cross-system collaborative efforts.

Fetal alcohol spectrum disorder (FASD) is now recognized by health care and addiction service providers as related to heavy alcohol use by women before and during pregnancy (Chudley et al., 2004). Alcohol use in pregnancy is also linked to violence, mental health problems, isolation, lack of prenatal care, poor nutrition and other determinants of girls' and women's health (Astley et al., 2000; Best Start, 2002). Multi-layered programming, with strong outreach and engagement components that respectfully reach women with substance use problems and these related health concerns, has been identified as critical to preventing FASD and improving the health of women facing these multiple burdens (Hume & Bradley, 2007; Poole, 2008; Watkins & Chovanec, 2006). Such programming has benefits for both women's and children's health. For example, Breaking the Cycle, a Toronto-based early identification, prevention and treatment program for pregnant and parenting women who have substance use problems, has demonstrated the importance of modelling supportive relationships to help mothers increase their capacity for healthy and satisfying relationships, leading to positive mother-child interactions (Motz et al., 2007).

Women and girls who use substances are often judged harshly in the media and by families, communities and service providers, particularly when they are pregnant or mothering (Greaves et al., 2002). This stigma and the fear of losing custody of their children create significant barriers to accessing needed treatment (Poole & Isaac, 2001). Not surprisingly, women report that the assistance of an accepting and empathic service provider who supports them in addressing shame and guilt and their mistrust of systems is pivotal to their engagement and willingness to remain in treatment (Boyd & Marcellus, 2007; Network Action Team on FASD Prevention, 2010).

When mothers use substances, children are often seen as being automatically at risk (Rutman et al., 2007). Fathers' substance use may not be as closely observed or judged, particularly when a mother is present. Cross-system collaboration, involving substance use treatment providers and social workers, shows promise for improving the health and parenting capacity of substance-using mothers, and providing integrated support for mothers and children (Chaim & Practice Guidelines Working Group, 2005; Drabble & Poole, 2011).

Interconnections between Trauma and Substance Use for Girls and Women

The most prominent gendered pathway to substance use by girls and women, identified in the literature and from service provision contexts, is the experience of early childhood abuse, sexual assault and intimate partner violence, all of which are more commonly experienced by girls and women (Gutierres & Van Puymbroeck, 2006). Yet girls and women who seek help for these interconnected issues are at risk of being turned away from support and treatment, misdiagnosed, overprescribed anti-anxiety and antidepressant medication, and even retraumatized by their encounters with health care and treatment providers who are insensitive to these links or dismiss their claims of abuse (Currie, 2003; Poole & Pearce, 2005; Veysey & Clark, 2004).

Evidence-based models exist for the delivery of integrated support for women with substance use, mental health and trauma/violence issues. For example, the Women, Co-occurring Disorders and Violence Study (WCDVS) found that:

- women with trauma, substance use and mental health problems were able to reduce these problems when integrated models that were "trauma informed" and financially accessible were provided
- integrated counselling in a trauma-informed policy and service context was more effective than services as usual
- collaborative approaches involving consumers, providers and system planners in all aspects of the policy design, implementation and evaluation of services are foundational to the effectiveness of this work (Moses et al., 2004; Veysey & Clark, 2004).

In Canada, some community-based addiction services and women-serving agencies have built on the WCDVS findings to develop, evaluate and refine programming on integrated trauma and substance use issues for women (Gose & Jennings, 2007; Hiebert-Murphy & Woytkiw, 2000; Van Wyck & Bradley, 2007). Evidence-based, integrated models such as Seeking Safety (Najavits, 2002) and Beyond Trauma (Covington, 2003) are being used and adapted for particular Canadian contexts.

Co-occurring Mental Health Concerns

Research has found that mental health problems and substance use disorders often co-occur (Myrick & Brady, 2003; Watkins et al., 2004). What is often not apparent to or addressed by treatment providers is the fact that women are almost twice as likely as men to be diagnosed with depression and anxiety, and have a greater risk of co-occurring anxiety and substance use problems (Health Canada, 1996; Kang, 2007; Koehn & Hardy, 2007). Women are also more likely than men to be diagnosed with seasonal affective disorder, eating disorders, panic disorders and phobias, and to make more suicide attempts (Harrop & Marlatt, 2010; McCarty et al., 2009; Morrow, 2007). All of these mental health problems are shown to co-occur with substance use, create barriers to treatment access and have implications for integrated treatment.

Particularly notable is the vulnerability of young women: service providers in the Youth Addiction and Concurrent Disorders Service at the Centre for Addiction and Mental Health (CAMH) in Toronto have found significant gender differences in types of mental health concerns, abuse histories and substances used by clients between age 16 and 24 years (Chaim & Henderson, 2009). For example, young women with substance use problems were more likely than their male counterparts to have posttraumatic stress disorder (24.6 per cent vs. 13.5 per cent) and major depressive disorder (38.5 per cent vs. 16.6 per cent). Young women were also more likely to use cocaine (71.4 per cent vs. 60.9 per cent) and benzodiazepines (42.9 per cent vs. 12.5 per cent). These differences in the experience of mental health concerns and substance use problems, and the evidence for addressing them in gendered and culturally relevant ways, should guide our treatment and ongoing support of women with co-occurring mental health and substance use problems (Gil-Rivas et al., 2009; Greenfield et al., 2008; MacMillan et al., 2008).

Physical Health Concerns

The differing physical responses to substances and the greater susceptibility to health problems associated with all substances for girls and women, while known, have not adequately informed our approach to treatment. In general, females are more vulnerable than males to alcohol-related liver and other organ damage, cardiac-related conditions, reproductive consequences, breast and other cancers and osteoporosis (CSAT, 2009). Recent evidence has emerged related to sex differences, For example:

- The gender gap in the prevalence of alcohol use is closing, especially in the case of heavy drinking by girls and young women (Keyes et al., 2008; Zilberman et al., 2003). This finding is of particular concern given that the health risks of alcohol use, which include liver damage, brain damage and heart disease, are greater for girls and women (National Institute on Alcohol Abuse and Alcoholism, 2002).

- Women report higher rates of use in most categories of prescription drugs, including painkillers, sleeping pills, tranquillizers, antidepressants and diet pills (Ritter et al., 2004; Therapeutics Initiative, 2004). Health care providers and women are often unaware of the range of withdrawal symptoms associated with stopping tranquillizer use when withdrawal is not managed, and treatment programs have often excluded people using benzodiazepines from care (Currie, 2003).

- Women represent an increasing proportion of adult HIV/AIDS cases attributable to intravenous drug use in Canada, and Aboriginal women are particularly at risk (Spittal et al., 2002).

- Tobacco use among girls and women is a serious problem in Canada and worldwide (Greaves et al., 2006). In Canada, 12 per cent of young men and women smoked in 2010 (Health Canada, 2010), and the health impacts on girls and women are more serious (Office of the Surgeon General, 2001). Despite tobacco use being the most deadly of all addictions, it is often not considered as urgent to treat as other substance use problems (Poole et al., 2003).

This short summary of research in the four key areas we identified earlier has not allowed us to adequately acknowledge the role of socio-economic issues, cultural diversity and many other determinants of health that intersect with gender. Space limitations also preclude exploration of gender differences in processes related to treatment initiation, retention, completion and outcomes (Grella et al., 2008). The rest of this chapter discusses the practice implications of the four key issues—mothering, experience of trauma and violence, mental health challenges and physiological vulnerabilities—and illustrates how important it is to bring a sex and gender lens to our work as treatment providers.

Practice Implications

Mothers and Pregnant Women with Substance Use Problems

Acknowledging and reducing barriers to treatment

In one of the vignettes that open this chapter, we describe a young woman who is eight months pregnant and afraid to go to prenatal appointments because she fears that her doctor will discover she is using substances and will report her to child welfare authorities. A Canadian study (Poole & Isaac, 2001) revealed that this situation is common. The biggest barriers to treatment for mothers or pregnant women dealing with substance use issues were:
- shame (cited by 66 per cent of study participants)
- fear of losing children if they identified a need for treatment (62 per cent)
- fear of prejudicial treatment on the basis of their motherhood or pregnancy status (60 per cent)
- feelings of depression and low self-esteem (60 per cent)
- belief that they could handle the problem without treatment (55 per cent)
- lack of information about what treatment was available (55 per cent)
- waiting lists for treatment services (53 per cent) (Poole & Isaac, 2001, p. 12).

Many women postpone treatment for months, even years, in order to avoid losing custody, or to minimize the disruption to their children's lives. When they do come for help, they may face strict service policies and rules, such as those that dictate the length of abstinence required prior to admission and that demand punctuality without exception. These rules may be challenging for a woman trying to seek support while arranging child care, or having to drop off her children at school. It is important to consider how such rules can create more hurdles for women with substance use problems who are challenged by child care responsibilities, depression or poor self-esteem when seeking help.

Welcoming mothers to treatment and support

When working with mothers, service providers need to provide child care (or help mothers find it), address parenting and provide services to children who may also require support. Breaking the Cycle is a collaborative program in Toronto for women who are pregnant and/or parenting, which was developed with seven partnering agencies to provide substance use, mental health, parenting, child development and outreach services. Its philosophy is based on acceptance, empathic understanding, honour, respect and empowerment, caring, love and hope (Leslie, 2007).

Women need to know that they will be heard, and that their children will not be instantly apprehended if they acknowledge that they require support to make changes. Nishimoto and Roberts (2001) found that women who have custody of their children stay in treatment longer than women who do not have custody. According to the Women's Service Strategy Work Group (2005):

To support the relationships of mothers and their children, treatment environments must be welcoming of pregnant women and women with children. Dedicated spaces for visits with children, childcare, children's assessments, children's programming, and mother-child programming are needed in both residential and non-residential services. Numerous research studies have established the effectiveness of services that provide residential programming for mothers and children together. (p. 31)

Although many treatment providers do not offer this array of programming and services, they can still create an atmosphere that acknowledges women's various needs, help refer women to services that can be accommodating and incorporate models of care based on relational models. Women require choice about local options and a collaborative approach to planning their treatment program. Individual differences need to be considered: while some women may want to bring their children to child care at the treatment centre, others may prefer financial support to hire a child care provider they know and with whom their children are comfortable.

Exploring our judgments of mothers and pregnant women

As counsellors and people working in health care, we have the dual responsibility of helping women and children get the care they need and assessing the safety of children and mothers. We may carry judgments and fears and need to explore these feelings, values and biases when working with mothers who are using substances, and how our beliefs influence our connection with women. It is our responsibility to work collaboratively with women, letting them know our responsibilities and our goal to work in partnership with them through the stages of making change. This includes being supportive and understanding during challenging conversations with women about their ability to care for their children while using.

Women generally try hard to provide care for their children to the best of their ability, even when using substances (Richter & Bammer, 2000). When working with women, counsellors hear mothers say they try to minimize the effects of their substance use on their children by using only when the children are at school, or by sending children away to family when they are relapsing. People in recovery, including mothers, are expected to have slips. It is important that we see the woman in terms of her strengths, goals and values, helping her to let go of the labels she may have learned to carry about herself.

Supporting family: A woman's focus on others

When a woman has a family member (adult child, spouse/partner, parent) with a substance use problem, she often struggles with what her roles, rights and responsibilities are. Does she help a spouse through recovery? Does she set boundaries with an adult or adolescent who continues to use in her home? Does she provide financial support to protect the user? Women may seek support to figure out how to take care of themselves while sorting through their responsibilities to the person using substances, to themselves and to other family members. A woman typically has many questions—around how to cope with ongoing relapses, find treatment services that are a fit and deal with stigma and shame, and about what recovery means.

Women who have a history of problematic substance use and mental health issues often speak about their fear that their children will have substance use problems as a result of learned behaviour, genetics or both. A woman may blame herself and feel guilty for family problems. Concerns about judgment from family members, friends and colleagues, and financial dependency on partners may cause a woman to try to figure out these issues on her own. She may not know what counselling and support are available.

Treatment programs do not always welcome family members, and issues of confidentiality can make the woman feel disconnected when her loved one is seeking help. In many systems, being a family member trying to find resources puts that person into the role of client. As a family member, a woman may be ignored and silenced. Many women may need help to navigate the treatment system and find resources that are a fit for themselves and their loved ones.

When supporting women, service providers need to explore common issues women confront, such as how a loved one's substance use is affecting the woman financially, emotionally and physically, and whether she feels safe. Women can experience exhaustion and burnout caring for others, while letting go of their own self-care, daily routines and goals. These women may be at risk for neglecting their own health issues, using substances and food to cope with the isolation and struggles of family members who relapse. When partners are using, there may be an expectation that the woman also continues to use substances. As a woman decreases or stops using, she may feel pressure and anger from her partner for making changes.

Many women like the sense of connection they get from self-help groups such as Al-Anon, where they can join together to deal with a similar situation. *A Family Guide to Concurrent Disorders* (O'Grady & Skinner, 2007) addresses recovery, relapse, understanding and negotiating the treatment system, and stigma. This program is facilitated using an in-person group format, as well as an online group. Online groups may allow women the anonymity they are looking for, as well as the option to seek help from home, at a time that fits their schedule without needing to travel or pay for child care.

A Trauma-Informed Approach

One of the opening vignettes of this chapter involves a 50-year-old Asian woman who takes antidepressant and anti-anxiety medications, and drinks heavily to manage symptoms of posttraumatic stress disorder. We also introduced a 30-year-old mother with two preschool-aged children who is trying to leave an abusive partner and reduce her drinking, and who has been asked to leave a transition house because she did not comply with its rules about abstinence. These are but two examples of how trauma and gender-based violence affect the lives of women, and are connected to their use of substances.

Many women in substance abuse treatment have experienced trauma, including physical and sexual abuse (Finkelstein et al., 1997; Health Canada, 2001; Najavits, 2002; Women's Service Strategy Work Group, 2005). Women who use substances need to know that it is common for women with a trauma/violence history to cope with feelings related to trauma by using substances. When women are *not* helped to understand the connections, further secrecy, shame and substance use can result. There are opportunities to support making these connections between experiences of violence, trauma and substance use at all stages of treatment. This is the essence of "trauma-informed" practice: we assist women with safety, building trust and developing new coping skills and compassion for their past choices, without forcing disclosure or retraumatizing them.

In an assessment, the counsellor (and system) needs to consider the purpose of asking questions about a woman's history of trauma. Retelling stories of past and current violence can be retraumatizing, leaving the woman feeling raw and at risk for substance use, and possibly self-harming thoughts and behaviours. The assessment phase of treatment can be a time to help women feel safe and respected, without having them tell stories of past trauma. At the same time, safety plans need to be developed if a woman is living in a situation that is harmful to herself and her children. The service provider needs to work in partnership with the woman to determine what supports she is ready and willing to engage.

Best practice in trauma treatment is to provide treatment and support in stages (Herman, 1997). In first-stage trauma work, counsellors work with women on establishing safety and developing coping skills and grounding techniques (Haskell, 2003). At this stage, women may focus on learning self-care to cope with flashbacks and cravings to use when memories arise, as well as to nurture feelings and practise self-compassion without any self-harming behaviours. Women need to know that when they stop substance use, traumatic thoughts and feelings may arise, which may cause them to feel worse emotionally and physically. As a counsellor, you may hear women in early stages of recovery say they feel like they are "going crazy." Women may be losing their most familiar way of numbing these painful thoughts and feelings. Herman (1997) explains that when a woman is prepared for the symptoms of hyperarousal, intrusion and numbing, she will be far less frightened when they occur (p. 157).

Creating a safe environment for recovery

Counsellors need to learn about trauma-informed care, including knowing how to help women develop skills related to emotion regulation and distress tolerance and to understand how their present difficulties with emotions, relationships and substance use may be related to trauma. Trauma-informed care is about creating safety and choice for survivors, and working collaboratively and supportively with them, rather than providing trauma-specific treatment, where counsellors more directly address the trauma with the client (Harris & Fallot, 2001). Manuals such as *Seeking Safety* (Najavits, 2002) provide practical techniques for working with women in this way. These manuals can support counsellor learning and also provide useful client handouts. Such trauma-informed practice is discussed in more detail in Chapter 17.

Addiction counsellors need to incorporate trauma-informed approaches in their practice, given the high number of women with histories of trauma and violence who access services. When working in a trauma-informed way, it is also important to know about resources and services to which you can refer women for trauma-specific support. Being part of a community-based network of service providers will enable you together to build a system of care that assists women at all stages of readiness to heal from trauma and substance use problems.

Mental Health and Substance Use: Making the Connections

Two of this chapter's opening vignettes introduced a young homeless woman who uses cocaine and is engaged in sex work, and a middle-aged woman working in government who takes antidepressant medication. Both women may have mental health issues, as well as substance use problems. Wherever women come for treatment (e.g., mental health, substance use counselling or outreach services), it is critical to provide support for both concerns.

As with concurrent trauma and substance use problems, it is important to acknowledge how common it is for mental health and substance use concerns to coexist for women. As substance use counsellors, we need to be well informed about mental health symptoms, medications and treatments if we are to help women determine which services may best address their needs and goals. (See Chapter 16 for a discussion of concurrent disorders.) Symptoms of anxiety and depression may not only interfere with optimum outcomes from substance use treatment; they are often also triggers for relapse (Health Canada, 2001).

In integrated treatment programs, the same clinician (or team of clinicians) provides treatment for mental health and substance use disorders concurrently. Although some staff may not feel confident to address mental health and addiction issues, the interconnectedness of these issues needs to be explored. Our job as counsellors is to discuss the connections between substance use, mental health problems and trauma with women, and to let them know that these issues are likely influencing their life and their recovery process. By acknowledging the connections, we decrease stigma and women's fear of sharing their experiences. This means working collaboratively with a woman to explore how these issues are interdependent in her recovery; for example, how her feelings of depression trigger thoughts to drink and binge on food. The Women's Service Strategy Work Group (2005) describes the connections:

> Depression and anxiety can be rational responses to environmental and life situations but may be pathologized clinically. Limiting treatment to pharmaceutical intervention is likely to discount the context of women's lives. Underlying issues such as loss and grief or the effects of trauma may be dismissed or remain unaddressed. (p. 51)

Addressing Physical Health Concerns within Substance Use Services

One of this chapter's opening vignettes described an adolescent girl of Métis descent who took up smoking cigarettes and drinking alcohol when she was 10 years old. Another vignette involved a pregnant woman who uses cocaine, diet pills and alcohol. As these examples illustrate, it is common for girls and women to use multiple substances and not understand their health impacts. It is important to discuss the sex-specific physical health impacts of substances with women coming to treatment, as this can be important information for their relapse prevention, harm reduction and recovery plans.

Given that girls, Aboriginal girls in particular, have the highest rates of smoking in Canada, we need to be concerned about the short- and long-term implications of smoking on their health. Often as substance use counsellors, we do not stress enough the serious health impacts of smoking for women (Office of the Surgeon General, 2001). Women's hormones and reproductive systems are affected, leading to problems with fertility and menstruation, increased risk of cervical cancer and early menopause. Smoking also greatly increases a woman's risk of stroke and heart attack. A number of web-based resources are now available that can help girls understand and reduce or stop their tobacco use.[1]

There are also many ways we can support girls and women to understand the sex- and gender-specific impacts of alcohol; for example, we can discuss how women metabolize alcohol differently. Given the same amount of alcohol, women get more intoxicated, faster and for longer than their male counterparts. This difference is due to factors such as:
• percentage of body fat: women have a higher percentage and therefore have less body water to dilute the alcohol (Romach & Sellers, 1998)
• hormonal differences
• metabolism, including differing activity of the stomach enzyme that breaks down alcohol (Frezza et al., 1990).

We can also provide education on how the long-term effects of drinking differ for women. Women, as compared to men, experience serious health problems after a shorter period of drinking, often referred to as "telescoped" effects. These health problems include liver disease; cancer (particularly of the breast, tongue, pharynx and esophagus); heart disease; and brain damage. Knowing that it is not a level playing field can help motivate women to reduce their drinking.

We also need to stay up to date with and convey information about the health effects of alcohol that may be of particular interest to women; for example, about the impact of heavy episodic drinking on belly fat. At the 2009 meeting of the European Society of Cardiology, Martin Bobak of University College London reported that this type of binge drinking (large amounts consumed in a single session—a bottle of wine, six

[1] One example of a web-based resource to help girls understand and reduce or stop their tobacco use is www.expectingtoquit.ca.

beers or six 1.5 oz shots of spirits) results in increased abdominal fat independent of the amount of alcohol consumed over a year. The health consequences of abdominal fat are increased risk of heart disease and diabetes (Schenck-Gustafsson, 2009).

Substance use counsellors can also play an important role in educating women about the withdrawal effects of certain medications, particularly given the fact that treatment programs often make abstinence a requirement for admission: as a result, women may decide to go off benzodiazepines, opioids or antidepressants, not realizing the medical and psychological risks of withdrawal (Currie, 2007). Women need expert medical support for tapering when trying to stop using these medications, and we need to support them in finding this assistance.

Gender-informed treatment programs are now delivering interventions that specifically address the health impacts of substances for women. For example, programs are including discussions of sex differences in the impact of substance use to help women make informed choices and develop goals for themselves. They are supporting girls and women in getting thorough medical assessments by physicians who specialize in addiction medicine, arranging for nutritional assessments with dietitians and teaching positive health practices such as walking, tailored aerobic exercise, introductory yoga and making low-budget, nutritional meals.

Gender-informed programs also devote significant attention to mothers to ensure they have accurate, non-stigmatizing information about the impact of substance use in pregnancy, and help them work through guilt and shame about the effects of their substance use on their children. The Effects series, produced by the former Alberta Alcohol and Drug Abuse Commission (2003), is a helpful resource that explains how various drugs affect women, with special focus on how drug use may affect pregnancy, birth and child development.[2]

Substance use counsellors are also working closely with primary care providers, who may not be effectively screening women for excessive substance use. Given all the health consequences of alcohol and other drugs for girls and women, as well as the increased risk of blood-borne diseases, particularly from intravenous drug use and unprotected sex, a thorough health assessment should routinely be offered as a component of beginning treatment. Liaising with primary care providers means that counsellors—on their own or in partnership with health care providers—are better equipped to recommend and ensure linkages to other interventions that will support recovery, for example, physical activity programs, nutritional counselling, stress management programs such as yoga and meditation, and massage.

---

2 Fact sheets from the Effects series are available from the Alberta Health Services website at www.albertahealthservices.ca. Under "Health Information," see "Addiction & Substance Abuse," then go to "Information for Women" and "Fact Sheets."

Assessment and Treatment Models

Assessment

An effective treatment plan begins with a comprehensive assessment. Assessment instruments should be chosen for their proven appropriateness with women, and with consideration for the diverse populations of women with whom they will be used. To know what services a client will need, the assessor will need to attend to the realities of women's lives by exploring the following factors that may make her substance use problems unique, more serious or based on gendered risks:

- health status and sex-specific medical problems, and any mental health concerns
- current safety issues for all women, and history of abuse and other forms of violence when safety and readiness are present (disclosure of past violence/abuse is not required to receive trauma-informed services)
- self-harming behaviours, including disordered eating
- substance use by the woman's partner, including the partner's support or lack of support for the woman making change around her substance use
- whether she shares needles with or lives with someone who injects drugs
- what, if any, social supports she already has in place
- whether she has children or other dependents (including pets) for whom she will need care arrangements
- financial needs, including money for transportation
- the woman's current and past coping and self-care strategies, with an emphasis on her strengths.

Treatment

This section discusses evidence-based intervention models that may be particularly well suited to address the treatment needs of women.

Recovery model

In recent years, the recovery model has taken on new meaning and significance in the addiction and mental health fields. It has come to signify empowerment as a guiding principle for an individual's journey of healing and transformation. This philosophy or framework is particularly relevant to women in recovery, as it counterbalances the negative journeys of stigma, barriers and inflexibility in programming that women have often experienced. Mary Ellen Copeland and Shery Mead (2004) write about peer support in their book *Wellness Recovery Action Plan and Peer Support*. Through peer support, people in recovery learn from one another in a non-hierarchical relationship and are responsible for their own recovery. Mutual learning is part of the process of sharing strengths and resources, and shedding labels like "addict."

Motivational interviewing

Many women have been silenced, or told what to do to "recover." By contrast, the motivational interviewing approach helps the counsellor attend to the client's readiness and her reasons for wanting change. The counsellor helps the woman assess the level of importance of and confidence about making change. Acting as a guide, the counsellor draws out the woman's unique pathway to change. Consider the 20-year-old woman in our opening vignettes who engages in survival sex to pay for food and crack cocaine for herself and her pimp. For her, a motivational interviewing approach is likely to be experienced as non-threatening when space is created for her to realistically consider what is feasible for her, exploring her ambivalence, examining her values and eliciting her ideas about moving toward her goals. Research shows the effectiveness of motivational interviewing for women who use substances in a range of life circumstances. For example, several U.S. studies have found this approach to be effective in helping female college students reduce their alcohol consumption and the negative consequences of drinking (Ingersoll et al., 2005; LaBrie et al., 2007). (Motivational interviewing is discussed in Chapter 5.)

Cognitive-behavioural therapy

Cognitive-behavioural therapy is designed to help women explore the function of the substance use, understand their thoughts and feelings leading to triggers and focus on developing alternative coping strategies. According to Covington (2002), women's treatment needs to be based on the premise of the whole person, incorporating the holistic model of addiction and emphasizing affective, cognitive and behavioral change in various areas, not simply substance use. The affective aspect is especially important for women, who often see their substance use in the context of their emotional lives.

Mindfulness

Jon Kabat-Zinn (1994) defines mindfulness as paying attention in a particular way: on purpose, in the present moment and non-judgmentally. Women who use substances have often had their thoughts and feelings invalidated by others, and thus have learned to invalidate themselves. The practice of mindfulness teaches acceptance of one's thoughts and feelings, helping women to let go of judgments, and listen with compassion to their needs. "This practice may help one to become more aware of the emotion that drives the cravings, such as fear and loneliness, and have compassion for one's own suffering rather than a reactive need to fix or escape it" (Bowen et al., 2011).

Women-specific groups

Women-specific groups can allow women to explore personal, behavioural and attitudinal changes, as well as express difficult feelings such as anger and shame; discuss the social determinants of their problems such as poverty, experience of violence and lack of social support networks; and learn to trust and value women. For many women, these groups also provide the safety they need to take risks (an exception may be women who have been abused by their mothers or lesbian partners). While the findings are mixed, some studies point to the benefits of same-sex counsellors and gender-specific programming (Greenfield et al., 2008; Koch & Rubin, 1997; Wintersteen et al., 2005).

Mutual aid groups

Mutual aid groups are very important for women, both during and following more intensive treatment. A U.S. study of gender differences in factors predicting the transition from using to recovery found that attending self-help sessions was more significant for women than for men as a pathway to recovery (Grella et al., 2008). In many communities, women can access all-women Alcoholics Anonymous (AA), Women for Sobriety or 16 Steps for Discovery and Empowerment groups. A naturalistic study that followed men and women problem drinkers over eight years found that women experienced more benefit from ongoing participation in AA than men (Timko et al., 2002). Witbrodt (2010) found that having a network of trusted friends to talk to about personal problems was positively associated with attendance in mutual aid groups for women but not for men. Linking women to volunteers associated with mutual aid groups and encouraging participation in these groups may therefore work well for women with substance use problems who need treatment and support, especially those who face barriers to accessing treatment. These groups are free and accessible, have no waiting period and are available on different days and at different times. Resources such as *A Woman's Way through the Twelve Steps* (Covington, 1994) can help women navigate traditional (not gender-specific) mutual aid programs.

Technology-supported interventions

Given the barriers women often confront in accessing treatment services, technology-supported substance abuse interventions may be an important support. Many years ago, Sanchez-Craig and colleagues (1996) showed the effectiveness of telephone intervention for rural clients, particularly females. Now studies of gender-specific web-based treatment are showing comparable benefits to standard treatment for women (Finfgeld-Connett & Madsen, 2008). A recent exploratory study showed promise in expanding access to treatment, particularly for women and parents, through technology-assisted interventions (VanDeMark et al., 2010). Recent studies by Schinke and colleagues (2009) lend support to the potential of gender-specific, parent-involved and computerized approaches to preventing substance use among adolescent girls.

System-Level Change to Improve Our Response to Women

Changing Our Attitudes as Service Providers

Women with substance use problems have historically been perceived as sicker and harder to treat; yet studies published over the past 15 years demonstrate that this is not the case. When women come for treatment, they are likely to be experiencing more problems as a result of their substance use, but they recover as well as, if not better than, men when provided with appropriate treatment. Sometimes they struggle because of environmental factors and barriers, such as pregnancy, child or elder care responsibilities, a spouse who uses substances heavily or is abusive, or posttraumatic stress symptoms.

Any provider within the helping system may unconsciously stigmatize women. We are affected by the society in which we live. We need to begin by asking ourselves: Do I have a positive regard for women, or have I internalized negative societal attitudes toward them? We need to ask ourselves specific questions related to situations we will likely face in working with women. Could you work effectively with a woman who:
- told you she had abused her children, either physically or verbally?
- revealed heavy drinking and/or other drug use during pregnancy?
- wishes to end her marriage and has school-aged children?
- insists on staying in an abusive relationship?
- talks about the difficulties in her relationship with her same-sex partner?
- tells you she has had or is contemplating an abortion?
- makes sexual advances toward you?
- earns money as a sex-trade worker?
- is often angry in interviews?
- is obese?

Visualize yourself working with a woman in one of these situations. Could you be supportive and create a therapeutic environment conducive to her growth? Or do you recognize personal values or biases that would affect your work with her? Explore these issues or judgments in clinical consultation or supervision so they do not get played out with your clients and cause them harm. Attitudes and empathy are the two key ingredients for effective recovery when working with women who have substance use problems—they lay the foundation for all other knowledge and skills.

System-Level Change

Front-line workers can be informed advocates for change, but often do not have the authority to make and implement decisions about policy development or program delivery. For example, a counsellor may well recognize the problems endemic to an agency policy requiring a woman to get help for her substance use problem and become absti-nent before she can get treatment for a co-occurring mental health problem. However, the decisions to change policy and to try innovative service delivery, like partnering between addiction and mental health service providers or integrating these aspects of treatment, can only be made by people with the authority and mandate to do so.

Groups such as the Ad Hoc Working Group on Women, Mental Health, Mental Illness and Addictions (2006), convened by the Canadian Women's Health Network and the Centres of Excellence for Women's Health, serve as role models for continued vigi-lance to improve women's health by bringing research on sex and gender differences in health into the policy realm. Everyone must work toward sex- and gender-based analysis of research, programs and policies in order to best address the needs of women and men, boys and girls.

Conclusion

Research is demonstrating key gender differences in the physical effects of substance use for women, their pathways to treatment and support, and how interconnected issues such as parenting, experience of violence and mental health concerns interact with sub-stance use. In this chapter we have highlighted some of this research, considered the practice implications and pointed to the need for supportive systems of care.

Practitioners in Canada are achieving promising work in individual programs. Yet we still have much to do to integrate support on issues that affect women (and sub-groups of women) disproportionately. For example, programming that addresses the needs of mothers and pregnant women is shockingly scarce. Integrating our support on trauma, mental health and substance use problems will attract more women who need treatment to treatment, and ensure positive outcomes once they are there. We still have much to do to bring the evidence for gender-informed practice into intensive treatment settings and to link treatment with other tiers of treatment and support.

We have come a long way toward better understanding the needs of women with substance use problems, and there is tremendous potential for practitioners to apply this understanding in individual practice and system-wide collaborations.

Practice Tips

- Consider the way mothers and pregnant women with substance use problems are treated within the health and social service systems. It is important to pay attention to our own values, thoughts and feelings, and how our judgments may affect the way we work with individual women.
- Consider your program, practice and policies from the perspective of a mother with a substance use problem. We need to think about how our programs welcome mothers and pregnant women. When difficult decisions are being considered, include mothers in decision making as much as possible.
- Notice the links among women's experience of violence/trauma, mood "disorders" and substance use problems. Learn about the connections and share information about the connections as a universal practice. By sharing how common these connections are, we help normalize symptoms and acknowledge coping strategies.
- Assume that violence has played a role in female clients' lives, even if they haven't immediately identified this as a source of difficulty. Support women in examining their safety and help them make safety plans. Offer tools, strategies and support for reducing stress and increasing safety and self-determination.
- Make linkages with other agencies that support women's health and reduce harms related to substance use. Encourage women to learn about resources in their community and how to access them. Women need to know they have the right to interview potential health care providers and choose for themselves about what services meet their needs.
- Involve women in program planning specific to your service. Women who are making changes or are in recovery can play a key role in providing feedback, being involved in program development, acting as mentors and guiding service improvement as alumni.
- Consider how your service works to address the stigma and barriers women face in accessing services. Explore the physical environment of your agency. It is important to think about confidentiality when entering the building, the physical environment (do the pictures on the walls reflect the diversity of the women who are seeking support?) and feelings of safety. Discuss with your colleagues how stigma and discrimination are acknowledged to the women seeking help. Explore whether the services are inviting for diverse women—such as those who are pregnant, women in conflict with the law, older women, lesbian and bisexual women and women caring for others who are coping with concurrent disorders.

Resources

Publications

Poole, N. & Greaves, L. (2007). *Highs & Lows: Canadian Perspectives on Women and Substance Use.* Toronto: Centre for Addiction and Mental Health.

Substance Abuse and Mental Health Services Administration. (2009). *Substance Abuse Treatment: Addressing the Specific Needs of Women.* Treatment Improvement Protocol (TIP) series 51. Rockville, MD: Author. Retrieved from http://kap.samhsa.gov/products/manuals/tips/pdf/TIP51.pdf

Curriculum resources by Stephanie Covington
www.stephaniecovington.com/books.php
A Woman's Way through the Twelve Steps (1994, 2009)
Beyond Trauma: A Healing Journey for Women (2003)
Helping Women Recover: A Program for Treating Addiction (2002)
Voices: A Program of Self-Discovery and Empowerment for Girls (2005)
Women and Addiction: A Gender Responsive Approach (2007)

Internet

Canadian Centre on Substance Abuse—women's topic section
www.ccsa.ca/Eng/Topics/Populations/Women/Pages/default.aspx

Centre for Addiction and Mental Health Knowledge Exchange website—working with women section
http://knowledgex.camh.net/amhspecialists/specialized_treatment/women/Pages/default.aspx

Coalescing on Women and Substance Use
www.coalescing-vc.org

References

Ad Hoc Working Group on Women, Mental Health, Mental Illness and Addictions. (2006). *Women, Mental Health and Mental Illness and Addiction in Canada: An Overview.* Winnipeg, MB: Canadian Women's Health Network & Centres of Excellence for Women's Health.

Astley, S.J., Bailey, D., Talbot, C. & Clarren, S.K. (2000). Fetal alcohol syndrome (FAS) primary prevention through FASD diagnosis II: A comprehensive profile of 80 birth mothers of children with FAS. *Alcohol and Alcoholism, 35,* 509–519.

Best Start. (2002). *Reducing the Impact: Working with Pregnant Women Who Live in Difficult Life Situations.* Toronto: Best Start—Ontario's Maternal, Newborn and Early Child Development Resource Centre.

Bowen, S., Chawla, N. & Marlatt, A. (2011). Mindfulness-Based Relapse Prevention for Addictive Behaviours: A Clinician's Guide. New York: Guilford Press.

Boyd, S.C. & Marcellus, L. (2007). *With Child: Substance Use during Pregnancy. A Woman-Centred Approach.* Halifax: Fernwood.

Center for Substance Abuse Treatment (CSAT). (2009). *Substance Abuse Treatment: Addressing the Specific Needs of Women.* Treatment Improvement Protocol (TIP) series 51. Rockville, MD: Substance Abuse and Mental Health Services Administration. Retrieved from www.ncbi.nlm.nih.gov/books/NBK83252/pdf/TOC.pdf

Chaim, G. & Henderson, J. (2009, March). *From data to the right services.* Paper presented at the Looking Back, Thinking Ahead Conference, Halifax.

Chaim, G. & Practice Guidelines Working Group. (2005). *Practice Guidelines between Toronto Substance Abuse Treatment Agencies and Children's Aid Societies.* Toronto.

Chudley, A.E., Conry, J., Cook, J.L., Loock, C., Rosales, T. & LeBlanc, N. (2004). Fetal alcohol spectrum disorder: Canadian guidelines for diagnosis. *Canadian Family Physician, 172* (Suppl. 5), 1–21.

Clow, B., Pederson, A., Haworth-Brockman, M. & Bernier, J. (2009). *Rising to the Challenge: Sex and Gender-Based Analysis for Health Planning, Policy and Research in Canada.* Halifax: Atlantic Centre of Excellence for Women's Health.

Copeland, M.E. & Mead, S. (2004). *Wellness Recovery Action Plan and Peer Support.* West Dummerston, VT: Peach Press.

Covington, S.S. (1994). *A Woman's Way through the Twelve Steps.* Centre City, MN: Hazelden.

Covington, S.S. (2002). Helping women recover: Creating gender-responsive treatment. In A.L.S. Straussner & S. Brown (Eds.), *Handbook of Addiction Treatment for Women* (pp. 52–72). San Francisco: Jossey-Bass.

Covington, S.S. (2003). *Beyond Trauma: A Healing Journey for Women.* Center City, MN: Hazelden.

Currie, J.C. (2003). *Manufacturing Addiction: The Over-Prescription of Benzodiazepines and Sleeping Pills to Women in Canada.* Vancouver: British Columbia Centre of Excellence for Women's Health.

Currie, J.C. (2007). The silent addiction: Women and prescribed psychotropic drugs. In N. Poole & L. Greaves (Eds.), *Highs & Lows: Canadian Perspectives on Women and Substance Use* (pp. 449–464). Toronto: Centre for Addiction and Mental Health.

Drabble, L. & Poole, N. (2011). Collaboration between addiction treatment and child welfare fields: Opportunities in a Canadian context. *Journal of Social Work Practice in the Addictions, 11,* 124–149.

Finfgeld-Connett, D. & Madsen, R. (2008). Web-based treatment of alcohol problems among rural women. *Journal of Psychosocial Nursing and Mental Health Services, 46,* 46–53.

Finkelstein, N., Kennedy, C., Thomas, K. & Kearns, M. (1997). *Gender-Specific Substance Abuse Treatment.* Alexandria, VA: National Women's Resource Centre for the Prevention and Treatment of Alcohol, Tobacco, and Other Drug Abuse and Mental Illness.

Frezza, M., di Padova, C., Pozzato, G., Terpin, M., Baraona, E. & Lieber, C.S. (1990). High blood alcohol levels in women: The role of decreased gastric alcohol dehydrogenase activity and first-pass metabolism. *New England Journal of Medicine, 322,* 95–99.

Gil-Rivas, V., Prause, J. & Grella, C.E. (2009). Substance use after residential treatment among individuals with co-occurring disorders: The role of anxiety/depressive symptoms and trauma exposure. *Psychology of Addictive Behaviors, 23,* 303–314.

Gose, S. & Jennings, L. (2007). Seeking Safety: Integrating substance use programming at a sexual assault centre. In N. Poole & L. Greaves (Eds.), *Highs & Lows: Canadian Perspectives on Women and Substance Use* (pp. 373–380). Toronto: Centre for Addiction and Mental Health.

Greaves, L., Jategaonkar, N. & Sanchez, S. (2006). *Turning a New Leaf: Women, Tobacco and the Future.* Vancouver: British Columbia Centre of Excellence for Women's Health & International Network of Women Against Tobacco.

Greaves, L., Varcoe, C., Poole, N., Morrow, M., Johnson, J.L., Pederson, A. & Irwin, L. (2002). *A Motherhood Issue: Discourses on Mothering under Duress.* Ottawa: Status of Women Canada.

Greenfield, S.F., Potter, J.S., Lincoln, M.F., Popuch, R.E., Kuper, L. & Gallop, R.J. (2008). High psychiatric symptom severity is a moderator of substance abuse treatment outcomes among women in single vs. mixed gender group treatment. *American Journal of Drug & Alcohol Abuse, 34,* 594–602.

Grella, C.E., Scott, C.K., Foss, M.A. & Dennis, M.L. (2008). Gender similarities and differences in the treatment, relapse, and recovery cycle. *Evaluation Review, 32* (1), 113–137.

Gutierres, S. & Van Puymbroeck, C. (2006). Childhood and adult violence in the lives of women who misuse substances. *Aggression and Violent Behavior, 11,* 497–513.

Harris, M. & Fallot, R.D. (2001). *Using Trauma Theory to Design Service Systems.* San Francisco: Jossey-Bass.

Harrop, E.N. & Marlatt, G.A. (2010). The comorbidity of substance use disorders and eating disorders in women: Prevalence, etiology, and treatment. *Addictive Behaviors, 35,* 392–398.

Haskell, L. (2003). *First Stage Trauma Treatment: A Guide for Mental Health Professionals Working with Women.* Toronto: Centre for Addiction and Mental Health.

Health Canada. (1996). *Women and Mental Health.* Ottawa: Author.

Health Canada. (2001). *Best Practices: Treatment and Rehabilitation for Women with Substance Use Problems.* Ottawa: Health Canada. Retrieved from www.hc-sc.gc.ca/hc-ps/pubs/adp-apd/bp_women-mp_femmes/index-eng.php

Health Canada. (2010). *Summary of Annual Results for 2010—Canadian Tobacco Use Monitoring Survey (CTUMS).* Ottawa: Author. Retrieved from www.hc-sc.gc.ca/hc-ps/tobac-tabac/research-recherche/stat/_ctums-esutc_2010/ann_summary-sommaire-eng.php

Herman, J.L. (1997). *Trauma and Recovery: The Aftermath of Violence—from Domestic Abuse to Political Terror.* New York: Basic Books.

Hiebert-Murphy, D. & Woytkiw, L. (2000). A model for working with women dealing with child sexual abuse and addictions: The Laurel Centre, Winnipeg, Manitoba, Canada. *Journal of Substance Abuse Treatment, 18*, 387–394.

Hume, L. & Bradley, N. (2007). Reaching mothers and children affected by substance use. In N. Poole & L. Greaves (Eds.), *Highs & Lows: Canadian Perspectives on Women and Substance Use* (pp. 257–262). Toronto: Centre for Addiction and Mental Health.

Ingersoll, K.S., Ceperich, S.D., Nettleman, M.D., Karanda, K., Brocksen, S. & Johnson, B.A. (2005). Reducing alcohol-exposed pregnancy risk in college women: Initial outcomes of a clinical trial of a motivational intervention. *Journal of Substance Abuse Treatment, 29*, 173–180.

Kabat-Zinn, J. (1994). *Wherever You Go, There You Are: Mindfulness Meditation in Everyday Life.* New York: Hyperion.

Kang, S. (2007). Anxiety spectrum disorders and substance use interconnections in women. In N. Poole & L. Greaves (Eds.), *Highs & Lows: Canadian Perspectives on Women and Substance Use* (pp. 147–154). Toronto: Centre for Addiction and Mental Health.

Keyes, K.M., Grant, B.F. & Hasin, D.S. (2008). Evidence for a closing gender gap in alcohol use, abuse, and dependence in the United States population. *Drug & Alcohol Dependence, 93* (1/2), 21–29.

Koch, D.S. & Rubin, S.E. (1997). Challenges faced by rehabilitation counselors working with alcohol and other drug abuse in a "one size fits all" treatment tradition. *Journal of Applied Rehabilitation Counseling, 28* (1), 31–35.

Koehn, C.V. & Hardy, C. (2007). Depression and problem substance use in women. In N. Poole & L. Greaves (Eds.), *Highs & Lows: Canadian Perspectives on Women and Substance Use* (pp. 129–141). Toronto: Centre for Addiction and Mental Health.

LaBrie, J.W., Thompson, A.D., Huchting, K., Lac, A. & Buckley, K. (2007). A group motivational interviewing intervention reduces drinking and alcohol-related negative consequences in adjudicated college women. *Addictive Behaviors, 32*, 2549–2562.

Leslie, M. (Ed.). (2007). *BTC Compendium: Volume 1. The Roots of Relationship.* Toronto: Mothercraft & Breaking the Cycle.

MacMillan, H.L., Jamieson, E., Walsh, C.A, Wong, M.Y., Faries, E., McCue, H. et al. (2008). First Nations women's mental health: Results from an Ontario survey. *Archives of Women's Mental Health, 11* (2), 109–115.

McCarty, C.A., Kosterman, R., Mason, W.A., McCauley, E., Hawkins, J.D., Herrenkohl, T.I. & Lengua, L.J. (2009). Longitudinal associations among depression, obesity and alcohol use disorders in young adulthood. *General Hospital Psychiatry, 31*, 442–450.

Morrow, M. (2007). Women's voices matter: Creating women-centred mental health policy. In M. Morrow, O. Hankivsky & C. Varcoe (Eds.), *Women's Health in Canada: Critical Perspectives on Theory and Policy* (pp. 355–379). Toronto: University of Toronto Press.

Moses, D.J., Huntington, N. & D'Ambrosio, B. (2004). *Developing Integrated Services for Women with Co-occurring Disorders and Trauma Histories: Lessons from the SAMSHA Women with Alcohol, Drug Abuse and Mental Health Disorders Who Have Histories of Violence Study.* Washington, DC: National Center on Family Homelessness. Retrieved from www.nationaltraumaconsortium.org/documents/Lessons_Final.pdf

Motz, M., Leslie, M. & DeMarchi, G. (2007). Breaking the cycle: Using a relational approach to address the impact of maternal substance use on regulation and attachment in children. *Zero to Three, 27* (4), 19–25.

Myrick, H. & Brady, K. (2003). Current review of the comorbidity of affective, anxiety, and substance use disorders. *Current Opinion in Psychiatry, 16,* 261–270.

Najavits, L.M. (2002). *Seeking Safety: A Treatment Manual for PSTD and Substance Abuse.* New York: Guilford Press.

National Institute on Alcohol Abuse and Alcoholism. (2002). Women and Alcohol: An Update. *Alcohol Research & Health, 26* (4). Retrieved from http://pubs.niaaa.nih.gov/publications/arh26-4/toc26-4.htm

Network Action Team on FASD Prevention. (2010). *Taking a Relational Approach: The Importance of Timely and Supportive Connections for Women.* Vancouver: Canada Northwest FASD Research Network. Retrieved from www.canfasd.ca/files/PDF/RelationalApproach_March_2010.pdf

Nishimoto, R.H. & Roberts, A.C. (2001). Coercion and drug treatment for postpartum women. *American Journal of Drug and Alcohol Abuse, 27,* 161–181.

Office of the Surgeon General. (2001). *Women and Smoking: A Report of the Surgeon General.* Washington, DC: Department of Health and Human Services.

O'Grady, C.P. & Skinner, W.J. (2007). *A Family Guide to Concurrent Disorders.* Toronto: Centre for Addiction and Mental Health.

Poole, N. (2008). *Fetal Alcohol Spectrum Disorder (FASD) Prevention: Canadian Perspectives.* Ottawa: Public Health Agency of Canada.

Poole, N., Greaves, L. & Cormier, R. (2003). Integrating treatment for tobacco and other drugs: The work of the Aurora Centre at BC Women's Hospital. *Journal of Nursing Research, 35* (1), 95–102.

Poole, N. & Isaac, B. (2001). *Apprehensions: Barriers to Treatment for Substance-Using Mothers.* Vancouver: British Columbia Centre of Excellence for Women's Health.

Poole, N. & Pearce, D. (2005). *Seeking Safety, An Integrated Model for Women Experiencing Post Traumatic Stress Disorder and Substance Abuse: A Pilot Project of the Victoria Women's Sexual Assault Centre, Evaluation Report.* Victoria, BC: Victoria Women's Sexual Assault Centre.

Richter, K.P. & Bammer, G. (2000). A hierarchy of strategies heroin-using mothers employ to reduce harm to their children. *Journal of Substance Abuse Treatment, 19,* 403–413.

Ritter, G., Strickler, G. & Simoni-Wastila, L. (2004). Gender and other factors associated with the non-medical use of abusable prescription drugs. *Substance Use & Misuse, 39,* 1–23.

Romach, M.K. & Sellers, E.M. (1998). Alcohol dependence: Women, biology, and pharmacotherapy. In E.F. McCance-Katz & T.R. Kosten (Eds.), *New Treatments for Chemical Addictions* (pp. 35–73). Washington, DC: American Psychiatric Press.

Rutman, D., Callahan, M. & Swift, K. (2007). Risk assessment and mothers who use substances. In N. Poole & L. Greaves (Eds.), *Highs & Lows: Canadian Perspectives on Women and Substance Use* (pp. 269–282). Toronto: Centre for Addiction and Mental Health.

Sanchez-Craig, M., Davila, F. & Cooper, G. (1996). A self-help approach for high-risk drinking: Effects of an initial assessment. *Journal of Consulting and Clinical Psychology, 64,* 694–700.

Schenck-Gustafsson, K. (2009). Risk factors for cardiovascular disease in women. *Maturitas, 63,* 186–190.

Schinke, S.P., Fang, L. & Cole, K.C. (2009). Preventing substance use among adolescent girls: 1-year outcomes of a computerized, mother-daughter program. *Addictive Behaviors, 34,* 1060–1064.

Spittal, P.M., Craib, K.J., Wood, E., Laliberte, N., Li, K., Tyndall, M.W. et al. (2002). Risk factors for elevated HIV incidence rates among female injection drug users in Vancouver. *Canadian Medical Association Journal, 166,* 894–899.

Therapeutics Initiative. (2004). Use of benzodiazepines in BC: Is it consistent with recommendations? *University of British Columbia Therapeutics Letter, 54,* 1–2.

Timko, C., Moos, R.H., Finney, J.W. & Connell, E.G. (2002). Gender differences in help-utilization and the 8-year course of alcohol abuse. *Addiction, 97,* 877–889.

Van Wyck, L. & Bradley, N. (2007). A braided recovery: Integrating trauma programming at a women's substance use treatment centre. In N. Poole & L. Greaves (Eds.), *Highs & Lows: Canadian Perspectives on Women and Substance Use* (pp. 365–372). Toronto: Centre for Addiction and Mental Health.

VanDeMark, N., Burrell, N., LaMendola, W., Hoich, C., Berg, N. & Medina, E. (2010). An exploratory study of engagement in a technology-supported substance abuse intervention. *Substance Abuse Treatment, Prevention, and Policy, 5.* doi: 10.1186/1747-597X-5-10

Veysey, B. M. & Clark, C. (Eds.). (2004). *Responding to Physical and Sexual Abuse in Women with Alcohol and Other Drug and Mental Disorders.* Binghamton, NY: Haworth Press.

Watkins, K., Hunter, S., Wenzel, S., Wenli, T., Paddock, S., Griffin, A. & Ebener, P. (2004). Prevalence and characteristics of clients with co-occurring disorders in outpatient substance abuse treatment. *American Journal of Drug & Alcohol Abuse, 30,* 749–764.

Watkins, M. & Chovanec, D. (2006). *Women Working toward Their Goals through AADAC Enhanced Services for Women.* Edmonton, AB: Alberta Alcohol and Drug Abuse Commission.

Wintersteen, M.B., Mensinger, J.L. & Diamond, G.S. (2005). Do gender and racial differences between patient and therapist affect therapeutic alliance and treatment retention in adolescents? *Professional Psychology: Research & Practice, 36*, 400–408.

Witbrodt, J. (2010). Gender differences in mutual-help attendance one year after treatment: Swedish and U.S. samples. *Journal of Studies on Alcohol and Drugs, 71*, 125–135.

Women's Service Strategy Work Group. (2005). *Best Practices in Action: Guidelines and Criteria for Women's Substance Abuse Treatment Services.* Toronto: Ministry of Health and Long-Term Care, Ontario.

Zbogar, H. (Ed.). (2007). Gender Matters: Taking Action on Women and Substance Use. *CrossCurrents: The Journal of Addiction and Mental Health, 10* (3).

Zilberman, M., Tavares, H. & el-Guebaly, N. (2003). Gender similarities and differences: The prevalence and course of alcohol- and other substance-related disorders. *Journal of Addictive Diseases, 22* (4), 61–74.

Chapter 22

Working with Youth and Their Families

Gloria Chaim and Joanne Shenfeld

Anja is a 17-year-old teen who has grown up in a small town with her parents and two younger sisters, age 12 and 14. Her parents have had a long-standing conflictual relationship and a couple of brief separations, mainly related to her father's drinking and related job losses. Anja's mother works evenings at a local diner as a waitress. She is always tired and stressed, but does her best to keep the family together and feed and clothe the girls. With little time to watch out for the younger children, she has tried to count on Anja, as the oldest, to supervise her sisters.

Anja had her first drink at age 10, taken from her father's supply, and started using cannabis at 13. Since then, she has also been experimenting with "whatever is in town," available at "pill parties" or in the family medicine cabinet.

Anja has a history of skipping school, not doing homework and getting poor grades. When she was much younger, the school advised her parents to have her tested, as she was inattentive and her school performance was inconsistent. Anja was put on a wait-list but never did get tested. Over the past couple of years, she has been hanging out with a group of older youth and has been brought home several times by the police. The resulting conflicts at home between Anja and her parents, and between her parents about her, have become "unbearable." Anja's mother wants her to go into a residential treatment program where she could "be taken care of." Her mother imagines that this will "change" Anja and that when she returns home, their lives will be different.

The Age of Change

The emergence of substance use and mental health problems is not uncommon for someone like Anja—an adolescent living in a difficult family situation, with a parent who has a substance use problem, her own school difficulties and the natural risk taking and turbulence of adolescence. Heightened family conflict and the view that all problems rest with the troubled teen are also not unusual.

Youth, including adolescents age 12 to 17 and transitional-aged youth (or "emerging" adults) age 18 to 24, are in a process of cognitive, emotional and biological change and transition. Although we may expect youth to be "grown up" and to be proficient in problem solving and decision making, it is now known that physiological change, including brain development, continues well into a person's twenties. These changes account for behaviour that may appear impulsive and erratic and demonstrate ongoing "adolescent experimentation," but that can also be mitigated by resilience, learning and change.

As youth strive to discover who they are and define themselves along their developmental path, they are more likely to experiment with various roles and ways of coping and interacting, sometimes before they have mastered self-regulation strategies to manage the situations they encounter. As a result, they are more likely than people at other life stages to engage in risk-taking behaviours. Prevalence of traffic accidents, homicides and sexually transmitted infections is highest among youth (Statistics Canada, 2008, 2012). They are more likely to initiate substance use and to experience the emergence of mental health concerns; however, behaviours and trajectories for young men and young women may vary, and gender needs to be considered when assessing risk and resiliency (Arrington & Wilson, 2000; Bava & Tapert, 2010; Schulenberg et al., 2001; White et al., 2005). Young women report higher levels of physical and sexual abuse, and are therefore more likely to require intervention that addresses substance use and trauma (Najavits et al., 2006).

Historically, youth substance use was addressed with the same principles, tools and approaches used with adults. Although there is still much work to be done in understanding the unique needs of youth and developing effective youth-specific interventions, it is clear that the same patterns of use and behaviour do have different consequences and meanings for youth than they do for adults. This chapter provides an overview of youth-specific strategies and considerations in engaging, assessing and treating youth with substance use issues, as well as youth with co-occurring mental health and other concerns. A "harm reduction" perspective provides the overarching framework. The aim is to engage youth in a process of change that minimizes the consequences of risk-taking behaviours and conceptualizes change as an evolving journey, with ups and downs and changes of direction along the way.

Engaging Youth

Working with Youth in Context

Substance use is rooted in a biological, psychological, social, cultural and political context. To engage and assess youth, it is essential to understand each youth's substance use problem within his or her unique context. As populations, particularly in urban areas, become increasingly diverse, the counsellor must be sensitive to issues related to gender and sexual identity and culture, among other determinants of health.

The counsellor must be aware of his or her own biases, beliefs and values and how they interface with those of individual youth. Youth need to feel accepted and safe in order to trust enough to engage in the assessment and treatment process. Power is inherent in the counsellor's role, and this must also be considered. Open and honest sharing of what the counsellor knows, and genuine interest in and curiosity about what he or she does not know, can help engage youth in a process of investigation and potential change.

A Developmental Perspective

It is important to engage youth in a manner appropriate to their developmental stage and to consider their chronological age, as substance use and mental health concerns often have an impact on navigating developmental tasks and milestones. Schulenberg and colleagues (2001) offer a "developmental-contextual framework" that emphasizes "stability and change occurring as a function of the dynamic interaction between individuals and their contexts" (p. 19). They identify the following developmental transitions and opportunities of adolescence:

- puberty
- cognitive development
- emotional development: increased self-regulation
- affiliation transitions: changes in relationships with parents, peers, romantic partners
- achievement transitions: school and work changes
- identity transitions: changes in self-definition.

Certain factors can help youth navigate this life stage. Some factors may naturally be part of the context that youth encounter; others may be facilitated by parents, teachers or treatment providers. These factors include:

- opportunities to develop coping strategies and life skills
- minimal transitions (school changes, moves)
- balance between parents and schools nurturing and monitoring youth, and providing them with opportunities to seek independence and self-expression
- developmentally appropriate challenges and experiences
- social networks that discourage risky behaviour.

Despite stereotypes, jokes and lore to the contrary, most youth navigate the stage between adolescence and adulthood without undue conflict and upheaval. They experiment, develop skills, use the challenges of this period of transition as opportunities, and are able to successfully take on adult roles and responsibilities. Youth are resilient; they are often able to navigate developmental challenges by having significant "protective factors" in their lives, starting with healthy infant-caregiver attachment and growing up with a strong bond with a parent or other adult. It is important for youth to have caregivers who provide pro-social role modelling and who set and monitor limits and expectations that are age appropriate. Protective factors also include success in school or work; involvement in appropriate community, recreational and leisure activities; delayed experimentation with substances and other risky behaviours; and of course, throughout the life span, having basic needs met (i.e., food security, safe housing, access to health care).

On the other hand, exposure to risk factors is associated with substance use and related problems in youth. Simply being male is a primary risk factor. More male youth become involved in problematic substance use than any other population group; they represent more than half of the total treatment population. Parental substance use, a history of physical or sexual abuse and observing violence are also risk factors. The younger the age of first substance use, the more likely a youth is to develop problematic use. Identity issues, self-esteem, socio-economic factors, family stress and poor coping skills are other risk factors (Health Canada, 2001). Youth with mental health problems are also at higher risk for substance use problems. Later in this chapter, we discuss the interaction of substance use and mental health, known as concurrent disorders.

Prevalence and Patterns of Substance Use among Youth

A certain amount of risk taking in youth can be considered a normative part of successfully negotiating the transition between adolescence and adulthood. Smoking, drinking and experimenting with other drugs are a way to test social and family limits, as well as personal boundaries. Young people often engage in risk-taking behaviour or experimentation as a way to gain autonomy from parents, explore alternative identities and ultimately form a new adult identity. It is therefore important to thoroughly assess and address these behaviours: while substance use may have a minimal or transitory impact on the lives of youth, it may also have tragic results in the short term or result in ongoing, chronic concerns.

It is helpful to understand the trends and patterns of youth substance use and to review the most current data available in your locale so you have a sense of what to expect and what to ask about. Data specific to population groups, such as young men and young women and urban or rural youth can be useful. A Canadian Centre on Substance Abuse (n.d.) report summarizes provincial and national studies of youth substance use, including studies of substance use patterns among youth in school, as well as among street-involved youth (although there is limited data on the latter).

Substance use trends among youth in Canada

The Canadian Centre on Substance Abuse (n.d.) reports that youth substance use, excluding alcohol and tobacco, is currently at levels near the historic highs found in the late 1970s. However, on average, one-third to one-quarter of Canadian high-school students (age 12–19) reported abstinence from all substances in the past year. The most commonly used substances continue to be alcohol, cannabis (marijuana, hash, hash oil) and tobacco; about two-thirds report alcohol use; approximately one-third used cannabis and one-quarter used tobacco in the past year. The fourth most commonly used drug class is hallucinogens (e.g., LSD, psilocybin, mescaline). Fewer Canadian students (5–10 per cent) use other substances, such as inhalants and stimulants (both medical and non-medical), and fewer than five per cent report using cocaine, methamphetamine, heroin and PCP, and non-medical use of other medications. There is less information on "club drugs" such as ecstasy, Rohypnol, GHB and ketamine. Injection drug use by students is rare, reported by two to 2.5 per cent.

It is important to note that prevalence of substance use increases with age, and is usually higher among males. For example, in the 2009 *Ontario Student Drug Use and Health Survey* (Paglia-Boak et al., 2010), binge drinking increased from 25 per cent to 50 per cent of students by Grade 12. The age at which students first use alcohol, tobacco and cannabis has either remained the same or has increased. However, attitudes toward use have generally become more tolerant than was the case about 10 years ago, with fewer students expressing moral disapproval or perceiving a risk of harm in experimenting with various substances. Reports of problem use among students (e.g., current use of more than one substance, high number of heavy drinking episodes, more frequent drinking or cannabis use) have risen in recent years.

Prevalence and patterns of substance use by urban street youth in Canada vary from city to city, but according to the limited information available, rates of use are much higher than among students. Various studies have found that at least one in five street youth, including Aboriginal youth, have injected drugs. Street youth continue to be at risk for an array of health problems, particularly HIV and hepatitis B and C, as a result of injection drug use and needle sharing (Public Health Agency of Canada, 2006).

A Harm Reduction Approach

Harm reduction has been described as "reduction and/or elimination of the harms to individuals and communities . . . associated with the use and/or distribution of illicit drugs" (Toronto Harm Reduction Task Force, n.d.).

Harm reduction strategies provide an excellent framework for working with youth at all stages along the substance use continuum.

Harm reduction is an accepting, youth-centred approach that fits well with the Stages of Change model (see Chapter 4) and with a motivational enhancement approach using motivational interviewing strategies (see Chapter 5). Many of the youth who come to a clinical setting are in the pre-contemplative or contemplative stage, and are under pressure from school, parents or even a legal mandate. Working with youth to set goals that are appropriate to their stage of change within a harm reduction framework can help keep them in treatment. For youth in the early stages of change, an initial goal may simply be to engage them in dialogue about their use, and to explore the possibility that such use may have negative consequences, whereas initiating change may have some benefits. Over time, as trust builds or the problem worsens, the young person may be willing to engage in further treatment and goal setting.

Youth generally present for treatment with multiple, complex concerns. Those in the early stages of change are often not willing to set any type of substance use goal at first. Using a harm reduction approach sets the stage for empowering youth to identify their concerns and priorities for change. This holistic approach to engaging youth can help to establish an alliance and facilitate work with them on a goal they define as important. For example, youth may be unhappy about the pressure they are receiving at school or at home regarding their substance use behaviour or other issues. They may be willing to get support on ways to reduce this pressure, and may then be more open to seeing links between their use and other problematic areas. Youth who use several substances, which is common, may be willing to set a goal of abstaining from or reducing use of one of the substances, but not others. They may also be willing to consider change in certain areas of their lives, such as abstaining while at school or during the week. Or they may choose to work on a separate but related goal, such as improving school attendance that may be incompatible with their current substance-using pattern. The potential reluctance around setting a goal that is too far outside the norm for their peer group should be considered when working on goal setting. Once youth have experienced success in an initial or harm-reducing goal, they may be more willing to go further in reducing or even abstaining from use.

Strengths-Based and Holistic Perspective

When engaging and assessing young people, a holistic approach that incorporates a strengths-based perspective is the most helpful. A holistic approach looks at all aspects of the young person's life; a strengths-based perspective highlights his or her strengths, skills and personal assets, unlike traditional approaches, which focus on and highlight problems. Strengths-based assessments help counsellors identify protective factors and build a hopeful view, even if numerous risk factors exist.

Motivational, solution-focused and narrative strategies also help to engage young people; build positive expectancies, hope and strength; and move youth in a positive direction (Breslin et al., 1999). These strategies acknowledge young people's need to experiment and learn from experience, and allow them to perform developmental tasks at their own pace.

Inviting Context

On a more practical level, it is important to ensure that the agency setting is youth and family "friendly." Flexible hours and an accessible location can be helpful. Ease of communication, including e-mail, texting and prompt phone response can also be important. For staff, a flexible mandate that includes family work, co-therapy, peer and formal supervision, team support and consultation can all be useful. A staffing complement that allows for separate workers for the young person and the family is ideal, but not always possible. As with any ongoing clinical work, training and education are critical.

Screening and Assessment

Youth may enter the service system through various doors, including community-based drop-ins, health centres, school-based services, justice settings, primary care services and formal substance use and mental health services. Early identification and intervention have been shown to improve outcomes. Current evidence supports screening youth seeking services for substance use and mental health concerns, regardless of the point of entry. "Every door is the right door" is a recurring theme in a number of substance use and mental health policy frameworks, suggesting that regardless of the point of entry, processes need to be in place to help people determine and access the most appropriate services and resources given their needs (National Treatment Strategy Working Group, 2008).

As we embark on a discussion of screening tools, it should be noted that the emphasis shifts to problem identification. It is important to maintain a strengths-based and holistic view during this process; this requires attending to and highlighting the positives, as well as identifying challenges. Strengths provide a hopeful context and a base and building blocks for change.

Screening

Start with a valid and reliable screener and screening process. The Center for Substance Abuse Treatment (CSAT) defines screening as a "formal process of testing to determine whether a client does or does not warrant further attention at the current time in regard to a particular disorder" (CSAT, 2005, p. 66). Ideally, such processes provide an opportunity for youth to talk about their concerns with an engaging service provider, as well as to identify their concerns by completing relevant questionnaires. Rush and colleagues (2009) recommend a two-stage screening process that uses standardized measures, followed by further assessment if required. A first-stage screener is generally a very sensitive tool that identifies red flags across a range of possible disorders. These red flags suggest there may be a concern, without specifying exactly what the concern might be, and indicate the need for more in-depth screening or assessment. A second-stage screener provides more in-depth screening to identify the likelihood of a specific substance use or mental health disorder. A full assessment is required to confirm the existence of the problem and to understand its nature and extent (i.e., impact and severity, as well as the broader context in which the problem occurs).

A number of valid, reliable youth-specific measures have been developed (CSAT, 2005; Rush et al., 2009). When choosing a screening tool, consider:
- validity and reliability
- cost
- qualifications and training required for administration and scoring
- time required to administer the screener
- fit with agency mandate
- suitability for population served (i.e., age, gender, cultural factors).

Screening tools for youth

The Global Appraisal of Individual Needs—Short Screener (GAIN-SS) is an excellent example of a first-stage screening tool. It meets the criteria of having demonstrated validity and reliability across a wide range of settings and population groups (age 10 to senior adulthood). This validation across age ranges distinguishes the GAIN-SS from most other tools, which are either for children *or* adolescents *or* adults. The screener is also inexpensive, easy to access, user friendly for both service providers and youth and easily implemented across a wide range of agencies. Service providers who work in settings that serve a range of populations can use the same tool for adolescents, transitional-aged youth and adults.[1]

The Problem-Oriented Screening Instrument for Teenagers (POSIT) is another excellent example of a second-stage screening tool, validated for youth age 12 to 19.[2] POSIT examines substance use, mental health and nine other areas of functioning. GAIN-SS and POSIT are available in English and Spanish; in Canada, the GAIN-SS has recently been validated in French, and the POSIT is available in Portuguese.

---

1 Information and licensure for the Global Appraisal of Individual Needs—Short Screener can be found at www.chestnut.org/li/gain.
2 The Problem-Oriented Screening Instrument for Teenagers can be found at http://eib.emcdda.europa.eu/html.cfm/index4439EN.htm.

Assessment

A comprehensive assessment may include information gathered through informal discussions, standardized interviews and questionnaires, and by using tools designed and validated for assessing youth. Collateral information from family members or other significant people in the young person's life can be extremely important for treatment planning (Smith & Chaim, 2000). Research supports family-based treatment as the most effective approach with youth, and including family as part of the assessment is critical (Bender et al., 2006; Liddle, 2002).

Assessments in settings that address issues related directly or indirectly to substance use generally cover the same standard categories, regardless of the person's age. These categories include:

- substance use history
- family history
- education
- vocational/leisure activities
- legal history
- medical concerns.

Over the years, the category of medical concerns has expanded to include mental health and trauma history. More recently, many settings have added questions about ethnicity, cultural identification and spirituality. In Ontario, addiction treatment agencies are required to gather minimal data on gambling and behaviours such as injection drug use and safer sexual practices (e.g., condom use). Some agencies ask questions designed to encourage disclosure of gender identity and sexual orientation (Barbara et al., 2002). Although agency mandate, service provider training and interests, and the young person's presentation may focus attention on specific or limited areas, a thorough assessment should be comprehensive and explore all domains of functioning to ensure nothing is missed.

With youth, the questions in each area of assessment need to be adapted and considered through the lens of "developmental tasks" or the concept of "age-appropriate" behaviour. Counsellors need to be aware of normative developmental tasks and expectations, know what to look for in each area of assessment and understand how all the information fits together in order to develop a helpful service or treatment plan. In addition, the questions and approach should be tailored as much as possible to address the unique issues of adolescents and transitional-aged youth. For immigrant or newcomer youth, counsellors should make sure the young person understands the process and questions; ideally, they also would be able to access an interpreter if needed.

Substance use history

As with adults, obtaining a thorough substance use history with young clients is necessary to identify problems and plan treatment. Although youth under a certain age (usually between 19 and 21, depending on the jurisdiction) are legally prohibited from drinking, and substances commonly used by adolescents (e.g., cannabis, club drugs, cocaine) are illegal, some level of use is to be expected. It is helpful to place youth substance use along a continuum from non-use to dependent use (see Table 22-1). Although "harmful use" appears at the end of the continuum, keep in mind that harm can occur at any point on the continuum, other than non-use, depending on individual circumstances and context. For example, one episode of binge drinking may result in death due to risky behaviour, such as driving under the influence or diving into an empty swimming pool. It is essential for the counsellor to assess the potential and actual harm related to the young person's level of use.

TABLE 22-1

Substance Use Continuum

STAGE	DESCRIPTION	GOAL	COURSE OF ACTION
Non-use	Has never used a particular substance	Prevent initiation of substance use	Reinforce Education & prevention Monitoring
Experimental use	Has tried a substance once or several times. Use is motivated by curiosity about the substance's effect	Enhance motivation for change Prevent further involvement in substance use Reverse involvement in substance use Reduce harm from substance use	Education & prevention Harm reduction Monitoring
Irregular use	Use is infrequent and irregular, usually confined to special occasions or when opportunities present themselves directly	Prevent further involvement Reverse involvement	Education & prevention Monitoring

STAGE	DESCRIPTION	GOAL	COURSE OF ACTION
Regular use	Use has a predictable pattern, which may entail frequent or infrequent use. The user actively seeks to experience the substance effect, or to participate in the substance-using activities of the peer group. Usually feels in control of the substance use	Prevent further involvement Reverse involvement Reduce harm from substance use	Education & prevention Harm reduction Monitoring Assessment
Dependent use	Use is regular and predictable and usually frequent. The user experiences a physiological and/or psychological need for the substance. Feels out of control with use, and will continue to use despite adverse consequences	Enhance motivation for change Reverse involvement Reduce harm from substance use	Harm reduction Assessment Treatment
Harmful use	Use has resulted in harmful consequences. Use has resulted in high-risk behaviours	Enhance motivation for change Reverse involvement Reduce involvement Reduce harm	Harm reduction Assessment Treatment

Source: Adapted from Centre for Addiction and Mental Health (2004), pp. 59–60.

Youth between age 16 and 21 are most likely to use substances experimentally and recreationally, and may be more likely to binge at parties and on weekends. Polysubstance use is common. Youth who use substances may experiment with whatever is available, whether in their family's medicine cabinet or at a party, often using several substances at once or a variety of substances at different times. Young people tend to experience fewer withdrawal symptoms than adults and tolerate them more comfortably; as a result, they may develop tolerance to substances over a shorter time.

Earlier onset substance use—under age 15—may be more common in youth where there is a family history of substance addiction, or substance addiction and comorbid mental health problems. These young people may seek out peers who engage in risky behaviours and will likely demonstrate problems in many other areas of their lives: these problems are usually most evident in school performance, peer relationships and family functioning. Beginning to use substances before age 18, coupled with regular or dependent patterns of use, usually interferes with successfully completing developmental tasks and prolongs the stage of adolescence. When onset is over age 18, the person may be considered an adult for both assessment and treatment purposes, depending on how far along he or she may be in the completion of developmental tasks, and where he or she would best fit (particularly if group treatment is being considered).

Legal, social and family limits and expectations shift through the period of adolescence, so that the context and meaning of the behaviour changes. Drinking can be seen by the adolescent as a rebellious behaviour at age 13 or 14, more within the norm at 15 to 17, and as a right of passage into adulthood by 19 or 20. Of course, specific ethnocultural or religious group norms create different contexts, limits and expectations.

Concurrent Mental Health Concerns

Because adolescence can be a turbulent period, it is often difficult to determine whether certain presentations are "typical" adolescent behaviour or the result of a mental health problem or substance use. As adolescence is also the time when some mental health disorders begin to emerge, many of which can trigger or be triggered by substance use, mental health is an essential area to assess when a young person presents with a substance use concern. It is also necessary to assess suicidality because substance use and mental health disorders have been associated with increased suicidality and completed suicide (Hershberger & d'Augelli, 2000). Suicide rates among adolescents have quadrupled over the last 50 years; 12 per cent of youth die by suicide (Connor, 2002). The mental health concerns most commonly seen among youth in substance use treatment are explored later in this chapter.

In the past, young people who presented for substance use treatment were often not assessed for mental health problems, so these problems remained undiagnosed and untreated. Substance use and mental health problems were seen as separate problems to be treated in separate specialized treatment settings. If both concerns were identified, substance use and mental health treatment providers were often in conflict as to which concern should be treated first. As a result, clients were often sent back and forth between facilities as symptoms of either the mental health or substance use problem became manifest. Over time, both types of problems were exacerbated, or one would appear to resolve as the other became more prominent.

Studies have shown a high prevalence of concurrent disorders. In a large U.S. study (CSAT, 2005), 75 per cent of youth in substance use treatment facilities were diagnosed with a concurrent mental health disorder. In a Toronto cross-sectoral youth network screening study, more than 70 per cent of young people seeking service from hospitals and outreach, housing and support agencies had co-occurring substance use and mental health issues; approximately 50 per cent of youth seeking service at community-based agencies had concurrent issues. Transitional-aged youth—between 17 and 21 years—reported the highest rate of concurrent issues (Chaim & Henderson, 2009).

Since there is such high prevalence of concurrent issues, it is important to identify them and understand how they may interact in order to develop an effective treatment plan. Trupin & Boesky (2001) explain how substance use and mental health problems may affect one another:

Create: Substance use can create psychiatric symptoms (e.g., using crystal meth may result in a psychotic episode).

Trigger: Substance use can trigger the emergence of some mental health disorders if a youth is predisposed to mental illness (e.g., cannabis use may trigger earlier onset of schizophrenia).

Exacerbate: Symptoms of mental illness may get worse when a young person uses alcohol or other drugs (i.e., alcohol may increase symptoms of depression).

Mimic: Substance use can look like symptoms of a psychiatric disorder (e.g., a young person's behaviour while using ecstasy may look like a manic episode).

Mask: Symptoms of mental illness may be hidden by alcohol or other drug use (e.g., cocaine may improve concentration in a young person with attention-deficit/hyperactivity disorder).

Independent: Substance use and mental health problems may have a common underlying cause that has created vulnerability, such as experiencing trauma or witnessing violence.

While the causality and links between substance use and mental health disorders may not be fully understood, the evidence points to a need for a comprehensive approach to concurrent problems. Youth is a time of crucial developmental transitions, risks and opportunities. Treatment providers need to identify and address issues affecting development, such as mental health and substance use problems; when they cannot provide the interventions required, they must make appropriate, timely referrals. Depending on the problems, interventions may be sequential or concurrent.

Assessment considerations

In addition to addressing both substance use and mental health, a comprehensive assessment may cover a variety of areas. Table 22-2 summarizes some of these areas and looks at the issues from the perspective of younger teens and older youth.

The assessment should also identify potential safety concerns for each client before treatment is recommended, particularly group and family modalities.

TABLE 22-2

Youth Assessment Domains

ASSESSMENT AREA	ISSUES TO CONSIDER	DEVELOPMENTAL PERSPECTIVE
Family (as defined by the young person)	Substance use and mental health issues in other family members are a risk factor for youth. Collateral information may be critical to the assessment process and can broaden understanding of the young person's situation. Family may be an important support and factor for treatment planning. Impact of substance use on siblings, including increased risk for use themselves.	Family involvement may be particularly critical for younger clients who are living with their family of origin. Older youth may be struggling with individuation from family, whose support may still be very important.
Peer relationships	Peers are particularly important in adolescence. Use may be related to social skills: youth may tend to use alone to manage poor social skills or social anxiety, or may use with others as a way to belong to a group. Concerns about peers may be a barrier to change or seeking treatment.	Younger teens are beginning to shift their focus away from family toward peers, and may be vulnerable to using substances to belong to a group. Older youth may have substance use patterns related to peers and/or socializing that are quite set.
Gender identity and sexual orientation	LGBT youth may face additional challenges around identity in adolescence. Fear of stigma, discrimination and concern over acceptance by peers and family may be present and may increase vulnerability to problematic substance use. Feeling safe in assessment and treatment may be particularly important.	Younger teens may face growing awareness of their sexual orientation and/or gender identity and may struggle with this. Youth may face issues related to acceptance as they "come out" (Barbara et al., 2002; Hershberger & d'Augelli, 2000).

ASSESSMENT AREA	ISSUES TO CONSIDER	DEVELOPMENTAL PERSPECTIVE
Education	School behaviour and performance are often affected by use; they are often seen as a barometer of youth functioning. Academic ability can be a protective factor. Learning disabilities or school difficulties may be a risk factor for substance use or mental health problems.	Younger teens may begin to have problems with school functioning, behaviour or attendance. Older youth may have dropped out of school or may begin to have problems in post-secondary. Binge drinking can be associated with post-secondary social environments.
Vocation	Transition from school to work may be difficult for many youth; stress over selecting and obtaining work may contribute to substance use and/or mental health problems. Acquiring job skills may be delayed due to substance use and/or mental health problems.	Issues related to vocation may be more prominent for older teens and transitional-aged youth.
Leisure and recreation	It is important to assess how much leisure and recreation is focused on substance use. Developing non-using leisure activities may be challenging. Involvement in positive non-using activities can be a protective factor.	Younger teens may need support to develop and maintain non-using activities. Older youth may have abandoned or dropped out of activities due to use and may need support to reconnect or develop new interests.

ASSESSMENT AREA	ISSUES TO CONSIDER	DEVELOPMENTAL PERSPECTIVE
Financial situation	Financial impact of use may lead to other high-risk behaviour or legal difficulties. Parents may need to miss work for appointments for youth or to deal with behaviour and other consequences, creating financial stress on the family.	Younger teens may be affected by financial pressure in family or protected from financial consequences of use due to financial support of family. Older youth may be delayed in ability to individuate financially due to use.
High-risk behaviours	Some risk taking is a normative part of adolescence. Use may lead to high-risk behaviour and exposure to potential trauma. Self-harming behaviour, disordered eating or other mental health risks may be present.	Younger teens may need education in potential risks. Older youth may benefit from exploring potential impact and interaction of various behaviours they engage in, in the context of a harm reduction approach to mitigate effects of risk.
Legal history	Use may put youth at risk for involvement in illegal activities related to illicit substance use or associated illegal behaviour.	Younger teens may benefit from education on underage drinking or consequences of illegal drug use. Older youth may seek treatment related to charges or probation orders.
Housing	Use may be exacerbated by homelessness, marginal housing or an unsafe living environment. Neighbourhood and community context may affect substance use (i.e., in terms of crime levels).	Younger teens who live with family may need intervention to create a supportive, safe environment. Older youth may need help obtaining housing in an environment that is safe and supports reduced use.

ASSESSMENT AREA	ISSUES TO CONSIDER	DEVELOPMENTAL PERSPECTIVE
Physical health	Substances may be used to cope with physical discomfort or underlying medical conditions. Some medical conditions may be masked by use or mistaken for substance use (e.g., seizures, diabetic coma). Use may create or exacerbate medical problems.	Younger teens who are not finished with development may be at risk for permanent consequences from use. Older youth may be more likely to experience withdrawal.
Ethnic and cultural identification	Cultural values, beliefs, assumptions or traditions may be associated with substance use and mental health difficulties. Culture may be looked at in terms of ethnicity, race, age, gender, sexual orientation and ability. Strong cultural and/or spiritual connections may be a protective factor.	Younger teens may struggle with a clash between family values and those of the mainstream or peers. Older youth may struggle with their own cultural identity and how it defines their values and beliefs related to substance use or other issues.

Source: Adapted from Centre for Addiction and Mental Health (2004), pp. 71–73.

Treatment

Because youth usually present for service with multiple complex issues, an integrated, "ecologically grounded," systems-oriented treatment approach has been found to be most helpful (Bender et al., 2006). Treatment may be required to address various concerns at the same time, possibly using many resources and engaging the client, along with significant people in his or her life, such as family members, peers and school personnel. Ideally, treatment includes individual and/or group interventions for the young person, parent or family education and support, and joint sessions for the young person and family together.

Current evidence supports a number of integrated treatment models, largely based in cognitive-behavioural therapy (CBT) and trauma-informed care (see Chapters 1 and 17 for further discussion of these approaches).

The Continuum of Care

Meeting youth "where they're at" is the hallmark of youth-centred work. Approaches that use various levels of coercion have their proponents, but they are not considered to be best practice (Health Canada, 2001). Youth-specific programs need to provide a youth-friendly, safe environment. Features that help to retain youth in treatment include a harm reduction philosophy; a flexible, open-ended approach; a holistic perspective; and cultural appropriateness (Health Canada, 2001; National Treatment Strategy Working Group, 2008; Ontario Youth Strategy Project, 2008).

A key principle of treatment matching is to consider and recommend the least intensive, least intrusive treatments that the service provider can expect to be effective. This is particularly important with youth because, during this formative stage of life, it is important to emphasize strengths and help young people regain balance so they can move on with their life tasks. Since many young people require assistance at various points along their developmental journey, their early experiences of the treatment system must be helpful and appropriate, so they are more likely to re-engage later if necessary.

The National Treatment Strategy (National Treatment Strategy Working Group, 2008) provides a framework for considering pathways to care and the continuum of care for individuals, including youth.

FIGURE 22-1: Potential Pathways of Youth within a Tiered Continuum of Care

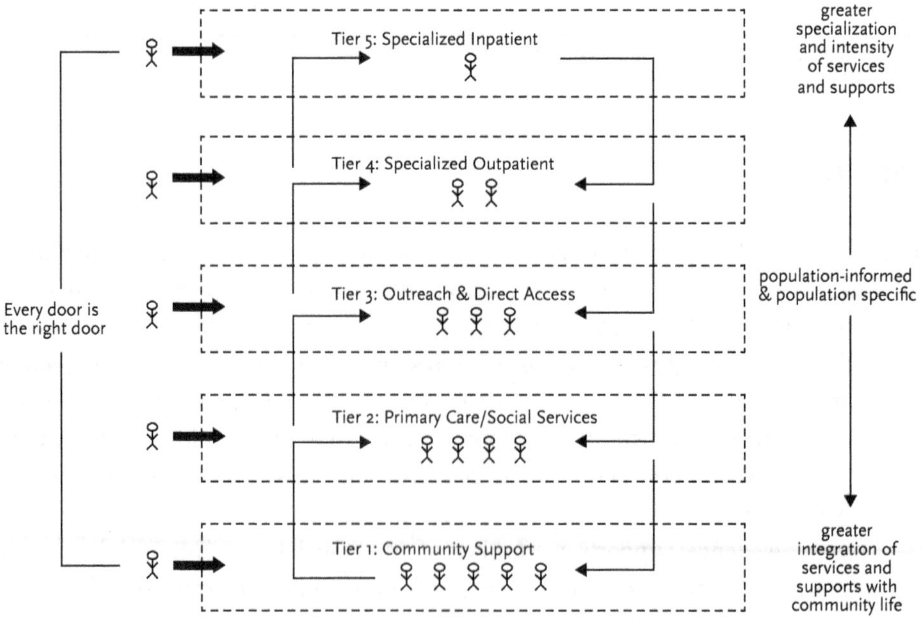

Source: National Treatment Strategy Working Group. (2008). National Treatment Strategy report [PowerPoint slides].

The continuum of treatment offers a range of options, varying in intensity and modality. As illustrated in Figure 22-1, note that some services and supports are offered in more than one tier and some are exclusively available in certain tiers. Comprehensive care, which involves addressing the complexity of issues with which youth may present, often requires a collaborative model, where a service plan includes service from more than one provider, simultaneously or sequentially. Planning must consider agency mandate, service provider expertise and youth need, particularly with respect to acuity and severity of the issues. The following section describes the major options across the continuum of care.

Outreach and early intervention (Tiers 1–3)

Reaching out to youth in the community who might not access services in a traditional or institutional setting can be an important way to intervene early with substance use and mental health issues. Best practices support the use of motivational enhancement approaches, considering the stages of change that are strength-based and respectful of youth and families and that consider the community and cultural context. Outreach activities can take place in natural settings for youth, such as schools, community centres, treatment agencies, drop-in centres and shelters. Preliminary outreach activities may focus on building trust, fostering positive interactions and screening for substance use and mental health and related concerns, and can help link youth to further assessment, treatment and ongoing services. Group-based approaches that incorporate culturally based activities, discussion and incentives (such as meals or snacks) appear most promising, although the risk for reinforcing negative peer associations in group settings should be considered (Health Canada, 2008).

Outpatient treatment (Tiers 3 & 4)

Outpatient treatment is usually a more formal arrangement, consisting of regular appointments with a therapist in a youth mental health or substance use treatment setting. Outpatient treatment can be offered in a group or individual format. Group treatment is a good choice for many young people, as it offers a sense of belonging and encourages them to find a balance between conformity and individual expression, and to experiment with roles and skills. However, for youth with particularly sensitive issues, or with cognitive challenges or oppositional and disruptive behaviour, group treatment may not be optimal. Flexibility and a range of options are crucial (Health Canada, 2001). The ideal treatment plan for youth, whether outpatient or residential, would include family work along with any individual work. (Family involvement and intervention are discussed later in this chapter.)

Because of the high rate of concurrent disorders among youth, some treatment approaches target particular co-occurring issues. The Cannabis Youth Treatment Study evaluated various approaches and found them all to be effective with youth. These included multidimensional family therapy (Liddle, 2002), combined motivational enhancement therapy and CBT (Dennis et al., 2004) and an adolescent community reinforcement approach (Harrington et al., 2006).[1] Some treatments were designed initially for adults but have been successfully adapted for youth. Examples include Seeking Safety for concurrent substance use and trauma (Najavits, 2002; Najavits et al., 2006), dialectical behaviour therapy for concurrent substance use and self-harming behaviour (Miller et al., 2007) and multi-systemic therapy for young offenders with concurrent substance use and mental health issues (Henggeler et al., 1999). In addition, the American Academy of Child and Adolescent Psychiatry ([AACAP], 2005) practice parameter states that 12-step approaches such as developmentally appropriate Alcoholics Anonymous or Narcotics Anonymous groups may be helpful as an adjunct to professional treatment for youth who have chosen an abstinence goal.

Day treatment (Tier 4)

Day treatment allows youth to benefit from the more intensive aspects of a residential program while remaining at home or in a community residence. Day programs can provide long-term support and allow young people to transition to less intense involvement more gradually. These programs may incorporate academic programming, vocational training and leisure and recreation, in addition to substance use treatment.

Residential programs (Tier 5)

Residential programs allow youth to "take a break" from their using environment, and can be particularly helpful when the situation is extreme. Programs that are youth-specific are the most appropriate, and can incorporate leisure activities, as well as alternative therapies such as art and music therapy as a holistic approach. Longer-term programs may include academic programming.

Withdrawal management and brief inpatient stabilization (Tier 5)

Withdrawal management and hospital-based concurrent disorder services are rarely available for youth, and when they are, they are rarely youth specific. These approaches can be useful in extreme situations, such as when the young person is homeless or when other severe psychosocial factors are present. If only adult facilities are available, emotional and physical safety must be considered, particularly for younger adolescents. Withdrawal and stabilization in a supervised setting are particularly useful for young people with suspected or confirmed concurrent mental health disorders because a period of abstinence is often necessary to make an accurate diagnosis and determine appropriate medication management. Young people with concurrent disorders often find it especially difficult to withdraw or stabilize on their own, as their symptoms may be more distressing and difficult to cope with when they are abstinent.

---

[1] Free manuals for these specific treatment approaches are available at http://store.samhsa.gov.

Alternative and complementary therapies (Tiers 1–5)

Alternative and complementary therapies can be an important part of individualized treatment, particularly with diverse populations. What may be alternative or complementary in one setting or with one population may be the accepted, expected or primary approach in others. This is particularly true of culture- or religion-based approaches, such as the healing circles and sweats often used by traditional Aboriginal healers.

Stress management, art therapy, nutrition, massage and recreation therapies are often integrated into comprehensive treatment programs as adjuncts to more traditional "talk" therapies.

As we have discussed, the diagnosis and treatment of adolescents is extremely complex. There is a high rate of concurrent emotional, physical and learning problems. Each person processes information and makes changes in a unique way. Alternative and complementary therapies and approaches provide options for tapping into the young person's unique strengths, thereby optimizing the possibility of matching approaches to his or her needs and learning and personal styles. Integrating some of these components in the community component of some of the systemic approaches mentioned above is a good fit. For example, a multi-systemic therapist may work with youth to involve them in a meaningful way in recreational activities in their community.

Continuing Care (Tiers 2 & 3)

Continuing care has generally been a less prominent part of youth treatment programs, likely due to the high dropout rate and preference for briefer treatment (Breslin et al., 1999). Given the high prevalence of return to pre-treatment patterns of substance use among youth, the Cannabis Youth Treatment Study developed the Assertive Continuing Care as part of the multidimensional approach described earlier in order to minimize the time between discharge and the first continuing care appointment. It involves home visits and telephone support. These "assertive" methods of reaching clients require that the service provider assume responsibility for arranging continuing care appointments, in contrast to the traditional office-based appointment model. This manualized intervention involves procedures and techniques for initiating and providing community-based services to adolescents with substance use disorders. Assertive continuing care is provided as part of the adolescent community reinforcement approach also developed for the Cannabis Youth Treatment Study (Godley et al., 2009; Liddle, 2002). These kinds of outreach and reinforcement strategies (i.e., engaging family and community supports) have been shown to increase maintenance of changes youth make in treatment.

Family intervention (Tiers 1–5)

Family involvement and intervention are supported by strong evidence that "the engagement of even one family member . . . is considered critical," and can improve treatment retention and outcome (Health Canada, 2001, p. 31). Each young person may define and experience "family" differently. It may include caregivers in the immediate or extended family and/or supportive others (i.e., peers, partners). In the absence of any available family, or in the event that meeting with family may create an unsafe situation for the young person, the AACAP practice parameter (2005) supports addressing family issues with the young person alone.

Although, historically, dealing with substance use issues was considered an "individual problem," it is logical—particularly with youth—to involve and work with families. Young people, especially adolescents, are often involved and living with their families of origin, and parental authority and care are expected. The family milieu and relationship dynamics can have a significant effect on youth substance use (i.e., a strong bond with a caring adult and healthy role models are protective factors, and family stress and parental substance use and mental health issues are risk factors). The AACAP practice parameter (2005) and the Alberta Alcohol and Drug Abuse Commission (2006) recommend family involvement at every stage of assessment and treatment, particularly with adolescents, because including family work has been shown to be most effective in treating substance use disorders in adolescents.

A number of specific approaches have empirical support for addressing youth substance use and concurrent disorders. These approaches include multi-systemic therapy (Henggeler et al., 1999), family behavioural therapy (Donohue et al., 2009), ecologically based family therapy (Slesnick & Prestopnik, 2005), multidimensional family therapy (Liddle, 2002) and the adolescent community reinforcement approach (Godley et al., 2009). All of these approaches are ecologically based and systems oriented. They include individual and/or group sessions, generally using a cognitive-behavioural approach; individual and/or group psychoeducational and support sessions for caregivers; and joint sessions with the young person and caregivers. Interventions that involve other significant people in the young person's life (e.g., peers, teachers and school personnel, probation officers) are also backed by empirical support.

Family approaches work best if the family can be involved at the start of service involvement, as part of the assessment. For youth who are reluctant to have their families involved, it may be helpful to discuss the purpose of including families so the young person can appreciate how family involvement can benefit them. Explaining that their privacy and confidentiality will be protected even if their families are involved can be reassuring. Young people need to understand that they will be able to decide what information can be shared with their family, and that the therapist will not share information about their substance use or anything else without their consent. Families, too, need to understand this, in order to feel comfortable themselves and be clear about the treatment process.

It is not uncommon for families to be reluctant to participate in treatment, particularly with older youth, where there is a history of treatment attempts that the family has perceived to be unsuccessful and where there is a history of significant conflict, anger and resentment. In these situations, it can be helpful for the service provider to offer outreach to these families by explaining the purpose and process of the intervention, using motivational enhancement strategies that create a sense of hope and possibility.

However, it is not always feasible, given resource and mandate constraints, to provide these types of comprehensive intervention packages. They are not appropriate for all families, and some families may not be able to commit to such involvement. Table 22-3 outlines the different levels of family involvement that benefit families.

TABLE 22-3

Categories of Family Involvement

LEVEL OF INTERVENTION	ACTIVITY	OBJECTIVES
Family orientation	Orient the family to the philosophy and approaches of the service	Provide information and education Enlist family support
Psychoeducation sessions	Provide education and information on substance use and mental illness	Understand interaction between substance use and mental illness Reduce anxiety Assist in anticipating high-risk situations Develop coping strategies Educate parents
Support groups	Provide support and counselling	Reduce isolation Assist in coping Help family members consider their own goals and needs
Conjoint family or couples counselling	Contract with each member of the family/ couple for interventions aimed at resolving relationship problems related to substance use and mental illness	Improve family functioning Provide support for client treatment through resolution of related family problems

Source: Adapted from Boudreau et al. (1998).

It is important to match families to the most appropriate level of intervention available, considering the needs of the family and its readiness to engage. Agencies must also be sensitive to the barriers families may face. Health equity and access issues significantly affect the ability of youth and their families to participate in and benefit from any level of service, and may need to be addressed to enable involvement. Barriers include child or elder care obligations; requirements for translation and interpretation services so the young person and/or family members are not required to provide the service; proximity to treatment and transportation (i.e., in rural and remote settings and in urban settings where travel time and/or costs may be prohibitive); and workplaces that make it difficult for parents or other caregivers to miss work to attend appointments.

Educating families about the stages of change can help them understand how to match their interactions with their child to the stage of change their child may be in. For example, in the "precontemplation" phase, education and discussion can help the young person perceive his or her parents as responsive and understanding, and may facilitate communication and decrease conflict. Table 22-4 lists tasks for youth and family members, considering the young person's stage of change.

TABLE 22-4
Stages of Change: Tasks for Youth and Family Members

STAGE	YOUTH TASKS	FAMILY MEMBER TASKS
Precontemplation	Acknowledge that a problem exists.	Learn about substance use. Allow the young person to experience the consequences of his or her use.
Contemplation	Resolve ambivalence about behaviour. Weigh the pros and cons of behaviour. Recognize the need to change.	Support family member when leaning toward change. Support engagement with the treatment system. Practise self-care throughout the stages.
Preparation/ determination	Learn about alternatives and steps toward change. Develop an action plan for change.	Support realistic expectations and goals. Support positive behaviour change.

STAGE	YOUTH TASKS	FAMILY MEMBER TASKS
Action	Take steps toward goals.	Reinforce positive steps.
	Prevent repeating problematic behaviours and deal with lapses.	
	Learn about triggers.	
	Develop new ways of behaving and coping.	
	View lapses as opportunities for learning.	
	Get back on track quickly after lapses.	
Maintenance	Continue to do what works.	Reinforce positive, healthy behaviour.
	Prevent relapses and deal with lapses.	
	Get back on track quickly after lapses.	

Source: Bubbra, S., Himes, A., Kelly, C., Shenfeld, J. Sloss, C. & Tait, L. (2008). *Families Care: Helping Families Cope and Relate Effectively: Facilitator's Manual* (p. 267). Toronto: Centre for Addiction and Mental Health.

Harm Reduction

Once family members understand the concept of stages of change, the idea of harm reduction also makes more sense. Families can begin to accept the notion of change as a process and let go of unrealistic expectations, for example that a young person in the precontemplation stage will commit to abstinence. Understanding the stages of change helps families support changes the young person is ready to make, which facilitates improved outcomes.

If conjoint work does not seem appropriate, or parents and/or the young person are not willing, there are still ways to maintain a family-oriented approach. Individual or group treatment for the young person, with education or support groups for parents, as described earlier, can be very helpful. The family models referred to earlier have components or modules for parents alone.

A note about prevention: given the relationship between family-related risk and protective factors and youth substance use and mental health, it is important to provide families with the skills and resources they need to create nurturing, resilience-building environments. Programs such as Strengthening Families (Kumpfer et al., 2003) offer skill-building groups for parents and children, followed by a joint group where parents and children practise their skills together. Strengthening Families includes a family dinner before the group session to build family and group cohesion and provide a forum for supported skill practice. There are groups tailored for parents with children of various ages. In Ontario, Strengthening Families programs are available in some jurisdictions for families with children age 7 to 11. A pilot adaptation is currently underway in Toronto for families with youth age 12 to 16. Strengthening Families has been shown to be effective in building resilience among youth, demonstrated by delayed and decreased involvement with substance use.

Revisiting the Case Study

Anja, whose story began this chapter, was struggling with escalating substance use, deteriorating school performance and family conflict and stress. Her parents saw her use and behaviour as the cause of all their problems, and hoped that treatment could remove Anja from the environment and fix everything.

> A comprehensive assessment revealed that Anja has underlying learning issues and some symptoms of depression. She was offered psycho-educational testing, psychiatric treatment and a structured group focused on engagement, motivation and substance use reduction. Once the testing was complete, Anja was given the option of attending a day treatment academic program. Her parents were provided with education around substance use and mental health issues so they could have more empathy for Anja and understand how to support and respond to her better. Family sessions created a more neutral environment for discussing conflict. Anja's father was offered treatment for his own substance use, which helped him understand how his alcohol use affected Anja and the family.

Conclusion

As Anja's situation illustrates, flexibility, a broad perspective and a holistic approach are among the most important aspects of treatment for youth. A harm reduction framework helps to reach young people "where they are" and facilitates the change process by offering goal choices, including non-abstinence, in all areas of young people's lives. By being accepting and non-judgmental, and recognizing developmental challenges characteristic of adolescence and emerging adulthood, therapists were able to engage Anja in treatment. They addressed both her difficulties and obvious strengths, while also reaching out to her family, and including them in the treatment and recovery process.

Early screening and comprehensive assessment are important for treatment planning, and can provide opportunities to engage youth in setting goals and increase their motivation for change. Service providers in systems that encounter youth must be trained to identify substance use and mental health issues and related problems, and must ensure that young people receive comprehensive care. This includes reaching out to family, peers and community supports, and working collaboratively across services and sectors to ensure that young people have access to the broad range of services, resources and supports they require.

As with most youth, Anja's situation was multi-faceted and complex. While the young person's response and the treatment provider's service may not be as ideal as in Anja's case, her example illustrates the importance of comprehensive assessment and treatment. By starting to address several areas of difficulty and taking a flexible approach, the change process can begin.

Practice Tips

1. Use a two-stage screening approach at the point of entry into the service system to facilitate early identification of substance use and mental health issues and related concerns.
2. Provide a thorough assessment that identifies and highlights strengths and protective factors and considers the impact of the determinants of health (e.g., gender, income security, ethnicity) to understand the unique needs of each young person.
3. Engage youth in a process that allows them to identify things they would like to change, and work with them at their pace.
4. Use motivational enhancement strategies, which are effective in facilitating youth engagement in a process of change.
5. Determine what is developmentally appropriate given the age and stage of the young person you are working with. For example, consider the degree of supervision required and the degree of responsibility that can be expected.
6. Working with families is integral to working with youth and may include parenting education and support, joint sessions with youth and family members and working with youth on family issues without the family present. Families may need help identifying and addressing barriers to participating in treatment, such as the need for child or elder care, translation and interpretation services and work schedule accommodation.
7. Collaborative, cross-sectoral service plans are most effective in addressing the breadth of youth needs.

Resources

Publications

Adair, C.E. (2009). *Concurrent Substance Use and Mental Disorders in Adolescents: A Review of the Literature on Current Science and Practice.* Edmonton, AB: Alberta Centre for Child Family and Community Research.

Bender, K., Springer, D.W. & Kim, J. (2006). Treatment effectiveness with dually diagnosed adolescents: A systematic review. *Brief Treatment and Crisis Intervention, 6,* 177–205.

Centre for Addiction and Mental Health. (2004). *Youth & Drugs and Mental Health: A Resource for Professionals.* Toronto: Author.

Internet

Canadian Centre on Substance Abuse
 www.ccsa.ca

Centre for Addiction and Mental Health Knowledge Exchange portal for professionals
 http://knowledgex.camh.net

Chestnut Health Systems
 www.chestnut.org

Toronto Harm Reduction Task Force
 http://canadianharmreduction.com

References

Alberta Alcohol and Drug Abuse Commission. (2006). *Youth Detoxification and Residential Treatment Literature Review: Best and Promising Practices in Adolescent Substance Use Treatment.* Edmonton, AB: Author.

American Academy of Child and Adolescent Psychiatry (AACAP). (2005). Practice parameter for the assessment and treatment of children and adolescents with substance use disorders. *Journal of the American Academy of Child and Adolescent Psychiatry, 44,* 609–621.

Arrington, E.G. & Wilson, M.N. (2000). A re-examination of risk and resilience during adolescence incorporating culture and diversity. *Journal of Child and Family Studies, 9,* 221–230.

Barbara, A., Chaim, G. & Doctor, F. (2002). *Asking the Right Questions: Talking about Sexual Orientation and Gender Identity during Assessment for Drug and Alcohol Concerns.* Toronto: Centre for Addiction and Mental Health.

Bava, S. & Tapert, F. (2010). Adolescent brain development and the risk for alcohol and other drug problems. *Neuropsychological Review, 20,* 398–413.

Bender, K., Springer, D.W. & Kim, J. (2006). Treatment effectiveness with dually diagnosed adolescents: A systematic review. *Brief Treatment and Crisis Intervention, 6,* 177–205.

Boudreau, R., Chaim, G., Pearlman, S., Shenfeld, J. & Skinner, W. (1998). *Working with Couples and Families: Skills for Addiction Workers. Trainer's Guide.* Toronto: Addiction Research Foundation.

Breslin, F.C., Kathy, S.J., Tupker, E. & Pearlman, S. (1999). *First Contact: A Brief Treatment for Young Substance Users.* Toronto: Centre for Addiction and Mental Health.

Canadian Centre on Substance Abuse (CCSA). (n.d.). Youth overview. Retrieved from www.ccsa.ca/Eng/Topics/Populations/Youth/Pages/YouthOverview.aspx

Center for Substance Abuse Treatment (CSAT). (2005). *Substance Abuse Treatment for Persons with Co-occurring Disorders.* Treatment Improvement Protocol (TIP) series 42. Rockville, MD: Substance Abuse and Mental Health Services Administration. Retrieved from www.ncbi.nlm.nih.gov/books/NBK64197/pdf/TOC.pdf

Centre for Addiction and Mental Health. (2004). *Youth & Drugs and Mental Health: A Resource for Professionals.* Toronto: Author.

Chaim, G. & Henderson, J. (2009). *Innovations in Collaboration: Findings from the GAIN Collaborating Network Project, A Screening Initiative Examining Youth Substance Use and Mental Health Concerns.* Toronto: GAIN Collaborating Network.

Connor, D.F. (2002). *Aggression and Antisocial Behaviour in Children and Adolescents: Research and Treatment.* New York: Guilford Press.

Dennis, M., Godley, S.H., Diamond, G., Tims, F.M., Babor, T., Donaldson, J. et al. (2004). The Cannabis Youth Treatment (CYT) study: Main findings from two randomized trials. *Journal of Substance Abuse Treatment, 27,* 197–213.

Donohue, B., Azrin, N., Allen, D.N., Romero, V., Hill, H.H., Tracy, K. et al. (2009). Family behavior therapy for substance abuse: A review of its intervention components and applicability. *Behavior Modification, 33,* 495–519.

Godley, S.H., Smith, J.E., Meyers, R.J. & Godley, M.D. (2009). Adolescent community reinforcement approach. In D.W. Springer & A. Rubin (Eds.), *Substance Abuse Treatment for Youth and Adults: Clinician's Guide to Evidence-Based Practice* (pp. 109–201). Bloomington, IL: Lighthouse Institute Publications.

Harrington, S., Godley, M.D., Godley, S.H., Karvinen, T., Slown, L.L. & Wright, K.L.S. (2006). *The Assertive Continuing Care Protocol: A Clinicians's Manual for Working with Adolescents after Residential Treatment for Alcohol and Other Substance Use Disorders* (2nd ed.). Bloomington, IL: Lighthouse Institute Publications.

Health Canada. (2001). *Best Practices: Treatment and Rehabilitation for Youth with Substance Use Problems.* Ottawa: Author. Retrieved from www.hc-sc.gc.ca/hc-ps/alt_formats/hecs-sesc/pdf/pubs/adp-apd/youth-jeunes/youth-jeunes-eng.pdf

Health Canada. (2008). *Best Practices: Early Intervention, Outreach and Community Linkages for Youth with Substance Use Problems.* Ottawa: Author. Retrieved from www.hc-sc.gc.ca/hc-ps/pubs/adp-apd/bp-mp-intervention/index-eng.php

Henggeler, S.W., Pickrel, S.G. & Brondino M.J. (1999). Multisystemic treatment of substance-abusing and dependent delinquents: Outcomes, treatment, fidelity, and transportability. *Mental Health Services Research. 1*, 171–184.

Hershberger, S.L. & d'Augelli, R. (2000). Issues in counseling lesbian, gay, and bisexual adolescents. In R.M. Perez, K.A. DeBord & K.J. Bieschke (Eds.), *Handbook of Counseling and Psychotherapy with Lesbian, Gay and Bisexual Clients* (pp. 225–247). Washington, DC: American Psychological Association.

Kumpfer, K.L., Alvarado, R. & Whiteside, H.O. (2003). Family-based interventions for substance abuse prevention. *Substance Use and Misuse, 38,* 1759–1789.

Liddle, H.A. (2002). *Multidimensional Family Therapy for Adolescent Cannabis Users.* Cannabis Youth Treatment series, vol. 5. Rockville, MD: Substance Abuse and Mental Health Services Administration. Retrieved from www.chestnut.org/li/cyt/products/MDFT_CYT_v5.pdf

Miller, A.L., Rathus, J.H. & Linehan, M.M. (2007). *Dialectical Behavior Therapy with Suicidal Adolescents.* New York: Guilford Press.

Najavits, L.M. (2002). *Seeking Safety: A Treatment Manual for PTSD and Substance Abuse.* New York: Guilford Press.

Najavits, L.M., Gallop, R.J. & Weiss, R.D. (2006). Seeking Safety therapy for adolescent girls with PTSD and substance abuse: A randomized controlled trial. *Journal of Behavioral Health Services & Research, 33,* 453–463.

National Treatment Strategy Working Group. (2008). *A Systems Approach to Substance Use in Canada: Recommendations for a National Treatment Strategy.* Ottawa: National Framework for Action to Reduce the Harms Associated with Alcohol and Other Drugs and Substances in Canada. Retrieved from www.nationalframework-cadrenational.ca/uploads/files/TWS_Treatment/nts-report-eng.pdf

Ontario Youth Strategy Project. (2008). *Best Practices in Treating Youth with Substance Use Problems: A Workbook for Organizations That Serve Youth.* Retrieved from www.addictionsontario.ca

Paglia-Boak, A., Mann, R.E., Adlaf, E.M., Beitchman, J.H., Wolfe, D. & Rehm, J. (2010). *The Mental Health and Well-Being of Ontario Students, 1991–2009: Detailed OSDUHS Findings.* CAMH Research Document series no. 29. Toronto: Centre for Addiction and Mental Health.

Public Health Agency of Canada. (2006). *Street Youth in Canada: Findings from Enhanced Surveillance of Canadian Street Youth, 1999–2003.* Ottawa: Author. Retrieved from www.phac-aspc.gc.ca/std-mts/reports_06/youth_e.html

Rush, B., Castel, S., Somers, J., Duncan, D. & Brown, D. (2009). *Systematic Review and Research Synthesis of Screening Tools for Mental and Substance Use Disorders Appropriate for Children and Adolescents: Technical Report.* Toronto: Centre for Addiction and Mental Health & Vancouver: Centre for Applied Research in Mental Health and Addiction.

Schulenberg, J., Maggs, J.L., Steinman, K.J. & Zucker, R.A. (2001). Development matters: Taking the long view on substance abuse etiology and intervention during adolescence. In P.M. Monti, S.M. Colby & T.A. O'Leary (Eds.), *Adolescents, Alcohol, and Substance Abuse: Reaching Teens through Brief Interventions* (pp. 19–57). New York: Guilford Press.

Slesnick, N. & Prestopnik, J.L. (2005). Ecologically based family therapy outcome with substance abusing runaway adolescents. *Journal of Adolescence, 28,* 277–298.

Smith, P. & Chaim, G. (2000). Adolescent substance use and the family. In B. Brands (Ed.), *Management of Alcohol, Tobacco and Other Drug Problems: A Physician's Manual* (pp. 371–386). Toronto: Centre for Addiction and Mental Health.

Statistics Canada. (2008). Motor vehicle accident deaths, 1979 to 2004. Ottawa: Author. Retrieved from www.statcan.gc.ca/pub/82-003-x/2008003/article/10648-eng.htm#3

Statistics Canada. (2012). Victims and persons accused of homicide, by age and sex. Ottawa: Author. Retrieved from www.statcan.gc.ca/tables-tableaux/sum-som/l01/cst01/legal10a-eng.htm

Toronto Harm Reduction Task Force. (n.d.). Mission. Retrieved from http://canadianharmreduction.com/about

Trupin, E. & Boesky, L.M. (2001). *Working Together for Change: Co-occurring Mental Health and Substance Abuse Disorders among Youth/Adults in Contact with the Justice System.* Rockville: MD: GAINS Center for People with Co-occurring Disorders in the Justice System.

White, H.R., Labouvie, E.W. & Papadaratsakis, V. (2005). Changes in substance use during the transition to adulthood: A comparison of college students and their non-college age peers. *Journal of Drug Issues, 35,* 281–306.

Appendix

Best Practices Recommendations

The Ontario Youth Strategy Project (2008) developed the following best practices recommendations for organizations that serve youth with substance use problems.

Orientation to youth

- Be individualized, client centred and client directed.
- Trust and respect the young person's inherent motivation for treatment.
- Involve the family, as defined by the young person.
- Consider youth within their system of relationships, including peers, family, community and others.

Approach to practice

- Have an explicit framework that directs practice and leads to demonstrable outcomes.
- Use a holistic, biopsychosocial approach.
- Use a harm reduction approach.
- Be strength based and experiential, and focus on skill building.

Appreciating the context

- Provide safe, respectful service.
- Involve youth in meaningful ways in developing, delivering and evaluating services.
- Recognize that youth are not a homogeneous group.
- Manage tension between the young person's needs, choices and program resources.

References

Ontario Youth Strategy Project. (2008). *Best Practices in Treating Youth with Substance Use Problems: A Workbook for Organizations That Serve Youth*. Retrieved from www. addictionsontario.ca

Chapter 23

Older Adults and Substance Use

Jennifer Barr and Virginia Carver[*]

Mrs. Ray is a recently widowed 79-year-old woman who lives in a retirement home. She has a long history of social alcohol use with occasional episodes of overdrinking. Her doctor has advised her to seek help to reduce her alcohol use due to medical complications arising from a combination of drinking and having diabetes, blood pressure problems and bouts of confusion and depression. Not long ago, Mrs. Ray had a fall, which the attending physician in the emergency department attributed to frailty. Mrs. Ray does not consider her alcohol use to be a problem and is unwilling to meet with the substance use professional that her physician recommends.

Mr. Bo is a 65-year-old man living alone in a boarding house, who has a long history of excessive drinking. His children have little to do with him, but are occasionally in contact. They are concerned that, although he has been abstinent for several years, he has begun drinking again, is not eating well and seems increasingly depressed. Mr. Bo says he feels unwell at times and is very lonely, but he is not keen on accepting help.

A Clinical and Demographic Imperative

With a growing proportion of Canadians living well into their 80s and 90s and beyond, due to increased life expectancy and lower fertility rates, the proportion of people over age 65 is projected to increase from 13.2 per cent currently to 24.5 per cent over the next three decades (Turcotte & Schellenberg, 2007). This will reverse the demographic curve of past generations and pose interesting challenges in housing, pensions, health care, consumer goods and other aspects of life more traditionally geared to a younger society. Most Canadians enjoy increased mental well-being and contentment with age. However, a small but substantial number of older Canadians experience problems with substance use, including alcohol, tobacco, medications and, although previously rare in

[*] Special thanks to Jane Baron, the original author of this chapter, and Margaret Flower, who contributed to the revised chapter in the third edition of this book. Thanks also to the clinical experts who generously shared their knowledge and experience: Dallas Smith, Carolyn Thomas, Ida King and Marilyn White-Campbell.

this age group, illicit drugs. Some people will experience chronic substance use problems that continue as they age, whereas others will develop substance use problems as a consequence of age-related stresses. Mrs. Ray and Mr. Bo, presented in the opening vignettes, represent these two situations—the losses of aging precipitating relapse or new substance use problems.

Addiction services are beginning to notice the "greying" of their clientele. Data from the Ontario Drug and Alcohol Treatment Information System (personal communication, 2012) shows a steady increase in the number of older adults being admitted for treatment over the last several years.[1] Most of this increase has occurred among people age 55 to 64. In fact, experts are raising concerns about the potential increase in the number of older adults needing help with substance use problems. One U.S. study estimates that the number of adults age 50 and older who require substance abuse treatment will more than double by 2020, driven not simply by the proportionate increase in the number of older adults, but also by an increase in the non-medical use of prescription drugs and illicit drug use associated with the aging baby boomer generation (Gfroerer et al., 2003).

The purpose of this chapter is to provide clinicians with an understanding of older people's special issues, their exciting and proven potential for change and best practices for improving access to care and supporting that change. We discuss the prevalence of substance use problems in this population, in particular highlighting the fact that today's older adults are more likely to be current drinkers who, like Mrs. Ray, often take prescription drugs that can interact with one another, and that lower tolerance and physiological changes that come with age can exacerbate these effects. We also discuss considerations for screening and assessing substance use problems in older adults, and implications for treatment, which vary depending on whether the person's substance use began early in adulthood and is more chronic, or developed later.

We hope this introductory chapter will inspire clinicians to respond to what is considered a clinical and demographic imperative by developing comfort, proficiency and enthusiasm for working with older adults.

An Underserved Group

Historically older adults have been "underestimated, underidentified, underdiagnosed, and undertreated" (Center for Substance Abuse Treatment [CSAT], 1998, p. 1) as a clinical population. This is due to several factors, such as the erroneous perception that older adults simply do not have alcohol or other drug problems. (They in fact do use at much lower rates than other age groups, but this does not mean the absence of serious problems.) While many people mature out of alcohol or other drug problems as they age, for some, signs and symptoms of substance use problems, such as confusion, falls or fractures, forgetfulness and self-neglect, can be mistaken for conditions thought to

---

1 For women, the number of individual admissions rose from 1,444 in 2003–2004 to 2,354 in 2009–2010. The number for men increased from 2,801 to 4,077 over the same period.

be typical signs of aging. Some presentations are atypical, most are complex, and many physical and mental health conditions mimic one another, making it difficult to screen, assess and accurately diagnose substance use problems (Menninger, 2002; O'Connell et al., 2003).

Failing to recognize problems in this age group is exacerbated by the fact that older adults themselves may be unaware that they have problems or may be reluctant to ask for help. Substance use problems carried even more shame and stigma for previous generations, particularly women. Older adults may minimize problems and have poor information about the harmful effects of alcohol or other drugs (Menninger 2002; O'Connell et al., 2003).

Last Pleasures

Professional attitudes toward aging have also been linked to overlooking problems in older adults. These attitudes are reflected in the stereotype that older adults cannot change or improve, and the belief that they are entitled to their alcohol as a "last pleasure" or an "earned privilege." Clients report feeling there is a prevailing belief that older adults should be able to have a few drinks if they want (Ruth, 2008). This reveals ageism, or negative and discriminatory attitudes about older people and their abilities, which directly affects the individual, as well as the availability and design of programs and services. These attitudes suggest that the older person's quality of life is not as important as that of a younger person (Ontario Human Rights Commission, 2001).

Other professionals have described not wanting to pry, perceiving alcohol use as a private matter or considering substance use an understandable coping mechanism given the losses of aging (O'Connell, et al., 2003). These attitudes lead to what O'Connell calls "therapeutic nihilism," which results in a tendency not to refer older adults to addiction treatment, creating an under-representation in the treatment service system (Menninger, 2002; O'Connell et al., 2003) and the self-fulfilling prophecy that older adults do not seek help.

Family members may share the attitudes of professionals. They may also seek help institutionalizing their loved one, because they are concerned about the person's safety, rather than seeking addiction treatment for their loved one, as they might for a younger person.

These factors can combine to create serious barriers for older people in finding and accessing appropriate treatment and care. Without encouragement to seek help on the part of the family doctor and family members, and without accessible addiction services well-attuned to the nuances of working with older adults, it is unlikely that Mr. Bo or Mrs. Ray would receive the help they require.

Improved Outcomes

Research has demonstrated that older adults do as well as, if not better than, their younger counterparts in addiction treatment, and that reducing substance use can improve their health-related quality of life. Recovery for those with serious problems has led to overall improvements in activities of daily living, and in a reversal of alcohol-related and alcohol-exacerbated cognitive impairment (Oslin, 2004). The improvement in health and quality of life from reducing or stopping alcohol use, and the knowledge that older adults are able to succeed with the help of addiction treatment, form a supremely sound argument for encouraging older adults to enter treatment.

Prevalence of Problems

Alcohol

Compared to younger adults, older adults are generally less likely to drink, and they consume smaller amounts if they do drink, although even one or two drinks a day can be problematic for some. A recent Ontario survey found a significant upward trend in older adults' reported alcohol use in the past 12 months, from 58.8 percent in 1997 to 73.5 percent in 2007 (Ialomiteanu et al., 2009). Similar results have been found nationally (Health Canada, 2008).

Older adults who are current drinkers are more likely than younger adults to drink daily or several times a week, although in smaller amounts. In Ontario, the percentage of people who drink daily increases with age and is highest among those age 65 years and older (Ialomiteanu et al., 2009). Nationally, compared to other age groups, more than 80 per cent of past-year drinkers age 65 and older report drinking one to two drinks on a typical drinking day, while having the lowest reported rate of drinking five or more drinks on a typical drinking day (Adlaf et al., 2005).

Older adults generally have low rates of exceeding low-risk drinking guidelines or drinking hazardously compared to younger people (Ialomiteanu et al., 2009). For example, across Canada, 10.9 per cent and 13.6 per cent of people age 65 to 74 years, and 75+ years, respectively, report exceeding low-risk drinking guidelines compared to 38 per cent for people in their early 20s (Adlaf et al., 2005). However, between 2006 and 2007, Ontarians age 50 to 64 years had a significant increase in hazardous or high-risk drinking (8.3 per cent to 13.5 per cent), as measured by the Alcohol Use Disorders Identification Test (AUDIT)[2] (Ialomiteanu et al., 2009).

Compared to men, women in general are less likely to be current or daily drinkers, and more likely to be lifetime abstainers. Women consume less on average per

---

2 The AUDIT was developed by the World Health Organization to screen for hazardous or harmful alcohol use in primary care settings and includes items that identify hazardous drinking (quantity/frequency), dependence symptoms and harm from alcohol use. The pattern of responses to the AUDIT items as well as the overall score will determine whether a brief intervention or referral for more in-depth assessment and treatment is required (Babor et al., 2001).

week, and are also less likely to exceed low-risk drinking guidelines and drink hazardously. However, among Ontario women across all age groups, a number of measures indicate that more women are drinking, and they are drinking more. Survey results indicate a significant increase in the prevalence of women drinking between 2006 and 2007 (Ialomiteanu et al., 2009). Other measures of women's drinking show increases in daily drinking between 1996 and 2007, estimated number of drinks consumed over the past year and hazardous drinking as measured by the AUDIT, where rates almost doubled between 1998 and 2007 (Ialomiteanu et al., 2009). These findings suggest that as younger cohorts age, there will be more similarity in drinking patterns between men and women.

Prescription Drugs

Older adults report high rates of medication use. Data from the 2003 Canadian Community Health Survey found that 92 per cent of adults age 65 years and over reported taking at least one type of medication in the previous month (Statistics Canada, 2006). The survey also found that 27 per cent of older women and 16 per cent of older men reported taking at least five types of medication, most commonly non-narcotic pain relievers, blood pressure medication, heart medication, diuretics and stomach remedies (Statistics Canada, 2006).

The variety of prescribed and over-the-counter medications used by older adults may have additive effects when used together and with other substances. For example, an older adult may be simultaneously using several drugs that depress the central nervous system (CNS), such as alcohol, a prescribed sleeping medication and an over-the-counter painkiller containing codeine, such as 222s. Taking many substances together that have similar effects on the CNS may produce a stronger effect and increase the risk of becoming dizzy and confused, falling or experiencing other negative consequences (Simoni-Wastila & Yang, 2006).

Overmedication, particularly in the case of CNS depressants, can lead to problems with motor function, falls and injuries, co-ordination problems, confusion and forgetfulness (CAMH, 2008). Older adults may also unknowingly develop a dependence on certain types of prescription medication. A recent study of community-dwelling French-speaking older adults in Quebec found that 25 per cent were using benzodiazepines, and 9.5 per cent met the *Diagnostic and Statistical Manual of Mental Disorders* (American Psychiatric Association, 2000) criteria for dependence (Voyer et al., 2010).

Illicit Drugs

To date, few older adults report lifetime or past-year use of illicit drugs. However the most recent survey of Ontario adults (Ialomiteanu et al., 2009) found a significant increase in past-year use of cannabis by people age 50 and older, from 1.4 per cent in

1998 to 4.6 per cent in 2007. A similar trend of greater reported use by the boomer cohort compared to people now age 65 years and over was found nationally, with 0.3 per cent, 1.1 per cent and 4.4 per cent of older adults age 75+, 65–74 and 55–64 years, respectively, reporting past-year cannabis use (Adlaf et al., 2005). Geriatric addiction services in Ontario also report an increase in rates of illicit drug use among clients.

Tobacco and Gambling

Although older adults in Ontario have lower rates of smoking compared to other age groups (only 8.9 per cent report smoking) those older adults who do smoke smoke on average more cigarettes per day than other age groups (Ialomiteanu, 2009). Regular smoking is also associated with heavy drinking (Selby & Els, 2004; Sullivan & Covey, 2002), and smoking exacerbates the health consequences of heavy drinking (Hurt et al., 1996; Selby & Els, 2004).

The expansion of legal gambling is not confined to casinos, but can take many widely accessible forms, including buying inexpensive lottery tickets. As well as the vulnerability of older adults to gambling, there are concerns about combining drinking and gambling: a recent study found that among older adults, higher levels of alcohol use are associated with at-risk problem gambling (Wiebe et al., 2004). Similarly, McCready and colleagues (2008) found that dependence on alcohol or other drugs increased the risk of developing a gambling problem.

Diversity Issues

Older adults are a spectacularly diverse group, spanning more than 40 years (age 55–100+). Older adults are much more unique than any stereotype might portray.

Ethnocultural Diversity

In 2001, 28 per cent of older adults in Canada were immigrants (41 per cent in Ontario). While in the past most immigrants came from western or northern Europe or the United States, new immigrants are increasingly from Asian countries (Turcotte & Schellenberg, 2007) and are progressively representing a greater proportion of the older adult population. While most immigrants can speak one of Canada's two official languages, about five per cent of those age 75 and older speak neither, and this proportion is increasing— as is the proportion of those speaking a language other than French or English at home (Turcotte & Schellenberg, 2007). Older immigrant women are somewhat less likely than older immigrant men to speak an official language. Rates of substance use problems, as well as awareness, acceptance and approaches to problems, vary greatly within cultural groups; therefore, providing culturally competent care is essential.

Aboriginal People

Although Canada's Aboriginal population is much younger than the non-Aboriginal population, Ontario has the highest number of Aboriginal older adults in Canada. They are far less urbanized than their non-Aboriginal counterparts. Many experience poorer health than non-Aboriginal Canadians, have less access to health care and are vulnerable to mental health and substance use problems. Aboriginal older adults may also have endured the residential school system and other negative circumstances.

Sexual Orientation

Lesbian, gay, bisexual and transgendered (LGBT) older adults may have struggled to hide their sexuality their entire lives, having grown up as part of a generation where homosexuality was socially unacceptable, considered a criminal offence and classified as a mental health disorder. Alcohol or other substances may have played a role in helping LGBT people cope with shame and the fear of being discovered. Many suppressed their true identities and lived the accepted heterosexual norm. Many who decide to "come out" to their families and friends may face challenges that include losing significant relationships.

Few services exist for older LGBT people, and even those services and retirement and long-term care resources that people can access may leave them vulnerable to further discrimination. Providing a sensitive, accepting therapeutic environment is essential, as is advocacy for older LGBT adults: open dialogue and collaborative problem solving are encouraged, respecting the autonomy of the older adult.

Issues of Aging

Physiological Changes

Older adults who continue the same pattern of drinking from their younger years may not be aware that they have less tolerance as they age. Physical changes associated with aging include less alcohol dehydrogenase available to break down alcohol before it reaches the bloodstream, reduced body water and lean body mass, and increased body fat. Thus, water-soluble drugs, such as alcohol, can be more concentrated in the body, and drugs such as benzodiazepines that are stored in the fat stay in the body longer (Centre for Addiction and Mental Health [CAMH], 2008). Older people may also experience a decline in kidney and liver function, resulting in higher concentrations and slower elimination of some drugs from the body. Some medical conditions that are common among older adults, such as diabetes, hypertension or dementia, can increase sensitivity to alcohol.

As a result, older adults can have a higher blood alcohol concentration than younger people after consuming the same amount of alcohol (Barnes et al., 2010; National Institute on Alcohol Abuse and Alcoholism, 1998; Simoni-Wastila & Yang, 2006). Because women are generally smaller and have less body water and more fat than men, they are even more vulnerable to the effects of substances.

This greater sensitivity among older adults can result in problems, such as adverse reactions when a medication is used with alcohol or overmedication even within therapeutic doses. Because of the daily or almost daily drinking pattern of many older adults, there is a high potential for combining alcohol with medications: more than 150 prescribed and over-the-counter drugs interact with alcohol (CAMH, 2008). When older people are prescribed medication by a physician, they generally assume the drug is safe, without necessarily realizing its potential interactions with other medication or the hazards of long-term use, particularly with benzodiazepines and opioids.

It is important for older adults to understand the increased risks associated with using medication and other substances. Older adults should avoid driving or using machinery and must be particularly careful negotiating unfamiliar tasks or situations when they are using alcohol, CNS depressant medications or illicit drugs. Older adults who use illicit drugs such as cannabis, heroin and cocaine are also at risk for physical health problems, particularly if these substances are mixed with prescribed medications (Boddiger, 2008).

Concurrent Problems

Substance use problems are associated with an increased risk of mental health problems, particularly depression and dementia, in older adults (Bartels et al., 2005; Dar, 2006; Oslin, 2004; Tjepkema, 2004). Rates of substance use problems are reported to be higher among people in psychiatric and general medical settings, with U.S. studies reporting prevalence rates from 18 to 44 per cent (Center for Substance Abuse Treatment, 1998). Depression is both a precursor and a consequence of heavy drinking (Tjepkema, 2004). It can increase the risk of suicide and in general complicate recovery from substance use problems, with poorer health outcomes and more service use (Bartels et al., 2005; Dar, 2006; Oslin, 2004). Alcohol can directly and indirectly increase the risk for dementia. Longstanding use may lead to cognitive impairment and head injuries. Furthermore, people with Alzheimer's and other dementias may inadvertently over-consume alcohol or double dose on medications simply because they cannot remember how much they have already taken.

Early and Late Onset, and Intermittent Problems

Three typologies of substance use problems appear in older persons, based on patterns of use and age of onset: "early onset," "late onset" and "intermittent" problems are useful typologies in helping to increase identification and understanding, and facilitate the development of appropriate treatment plans. Early onset refers to alcohol or other drug problems that develop early in life and continue into old age. For people with long histories of chronic substance use problems, alcohol and other drug use habits may be manifested in significant health problems, cognitive impairment, few material or social resources and risk of homelessness.

Late onset refers to problems that develop later in life, often in reaction to stresses associated with aging, which are usually losses or illnesses. Many older adults begin to have problems with substance use in times of transition or loss (e.g., forced retirement, bereavement, new or escalating health concerns, loss of independence). Their relationship to the substance can be based on an emotional need to feel better or deal with loss. Usually late onset means there are more resources and supports in place. The third typology, intermittent problems, refers to substance use issues that occur periodically throughout adult life but that become more serious or consistent as a person ages. Previous problem use is a risk factor for problems occurring later in life.

Treatment Approaches

Geriatric Addiction Best Practice

Older adults with alcohol and other drug problems will enter treatment when it is tailored to meet their needs. Generalist treatment services can inadvertently pose barriers or provide treatment that is ill suited to the special needs of older adults. Clients have reported that they felt unsafe in generalist programs, that younger group participants were dismissive of them, and that they did not feel welcome. They had the impression that staff found older people difficult and tiring to work with (Ruth, 2008).

If you are an addiction service provider or are referring a client to an addiction program, it is important to ensure that the program's content, pace and delivery are compatible with the client's abilities, needs and life circumstances, and that the service is accessible. Identifying clients' achievements and strengths, and reminiscing about the past are appropriate therapeutic tasks, as is future life planning. Planning for the future could involve determining new ways of spending time, rather than setting out employment or other goals.

The following best practices help to remove barriers to treatment, address age-specific issues and ensure the best outcomes. These core principles have emerged from clinical experience, formal evaluations and qualitative research of client feedback (Health Canada, 2002).

1. A harm reduction philosophy

Many older people do not consider their use of alcohol or other drugs to be a problem, which may exclude them from treatment programs that require clients to be motivated to stop using substances immediately upon entry or that require them to be abstinent prior to entry. Also, some programs may not allow clients to use certain medications, particularly if they are mood altering, even if they are medically required. According to the harm reduction philosophy, there is no requirement that the client admit to having an alcohol or other drug problem. In the initial stages of treatment, the client may only be willing or able to change the use of one substance, or none at all while addressing other more immediate concerns. Treatment needs to focus not necessarily on the substance use, but on what the client identifies will make life better and more comfortable, and make him or her more content.

2. A holistic problem-solving approach and intensive case management

Problems among older adults are usually complex, as older adults often have a wide range of needs; for instance, they may have chronic or acute physical health problems; financial concerns; mental health problems; and social and emotional issues, including feelings of loneliness and isolation. Treatment requires longer episodes of care and needs to be slower, gentler and more flexible, and provided over six months to three years.

3. Home visiting or outreach

Substance use treatment for older adults ideally involves outreach: working with the client in his or her own home or neighbourhood, or in a location where the person is most comfortable. Outreach is a cornerstone of appropriate care for older people and overcomes barriers that require clients to travel to or be in residence to participate in programs. Some older people are not ready or able to leave their homes because of a lack of transportation, mobility problems, hearing or vision loss, emotional problems such as anxiety or depression, financial constraints and other psychological or physical issues.

Outreach can also involve psychologically reaching out to offer help in a way that accommodates the older person's needs. This means addressing the problems that are of most concern to the client and not having unrealistic expectations. It may be necessary to adjust the program or efforts to help the client's situation, rather than expecting the client to adjust his or her needs to suit the program or the form of help being offered.

4. Age- and gender-specific groups

The kinds of issues discussed in many programs may not be relevant to older people. Older adults may also be uncomfortable in a group that requires them to talk about themselves. They may have difficulty following group interaction because of hearing or vision problems, cognitive decline or limited stamina. Regardless of age, women who have experienced trauma, such as family violence, may feel more comfortable in an all-women's group.

5. Social and recreational programs to improve social inclusion

Specialized geriatric addiction programs offer meals, outings and other recreational programming, not only for the intrinsic value of the social event, but also to allow clients to practise social skills and develop non–substance-using relationships. These kinds of activities, as well as individual counselling and group treatment, should be offered and adequately resourced.

6. Involvement and support of families and significant others

It is ideal to involve family and friends when possible. The social and family supports that older adults have or that can be nurtured as part of therapy are an important resource. Social and family relationships can ease loneliness and the sense of loss that older people often experience and provide assistance with practical tasks, such as getting to appointments. Including family or a close friend in aspects of treatment allows for others to understand and support the person's treatment goals.

Screening and Brief Intervention

The purpose of screening is to explore potential problem substance use and determine whether a more in-depth assessment or referral is required. Screening also provides an opportunity to educate the client about safe drinking levels, medication management and alternative ways of coping with stress, anxiety or sleep problems, for example, through relaxation techniques, exercise, non-chemical sleep aids and diet.

Screening may involve an interview, a paper-and-pencil questionnaire or a computerized standardized screening instrument. It can be helpful to include questions about substance use as part of a general lifestyle assessment. This helps normalize the process, since many people, including older adults, are sensitive to being asked about substance use. Oslin (2004) recommends that this check-in be done annually in a health care setting.

Identifying Substance Use Problems

Identifying a substance use problem can be challenging. While some older adults do not connect their drinking or other substance use to their current problems, families and even health care professionals often interpret this as "denial." It is important to reframe "denial" and understand that reluctance to recognize a problem can be related to fears that revealing substance use will result in a loss of independence, or to feelings of shame or stigma, which are especially strong in older generations. Identifying a problem may be hampered by the attitudes of those around the older person; for example, family, friends and even health and social service professionals may feel that substance use is a private matter. As well, cognitive changes can affect insight, and some people may not be used to thinking about or analyzing themselves. Ageism can be a factor when family or care providers do not see the benefit harm reduction can play in enhancing an older person's life, and when they make comments like "What is it going to hurt at this stage?"

When possible, screening for at-risk alcohol use is best done by using the concept of a standard drink and including questions about frequency of drinking; how much is consumed on a typical drinking day; the circumstances of use (e.g., to help with sleep or anxiety); whether there are days of the week when the person consumes more than usual; whether the person may be driving, operating machinery or engaging in other risky behaviour after drinking; and whether the person has experienced any negative consequences that might be associated with alcohol use.

Several alcohol screening instruments may be used with older adults—most commonly the Short Michigan Alcoholism Screening Test—Geriatric version (SMAST-G), and the Alcohol Use Disorders Identification Test (AUDIT) (Oslin, 2004). However, these screening tests can have some limitations when used with older adults, even if they have been validated with this age group (CAMH, 2008; Dar, 2006). Limitations include difficulty responding to items because of memory problems or cognitive impairment; not detecting binge drinking (Blazer & Wu, 2009); and not having high validity with older adults, particularly older women (Adams et al., 1996). Several other alcohol screening tests for older adults exist, including the Alcohol-Related Problems Survey (ARPS) and a shorter version, the Short ARPS (SHARPS) (see CAMH, 2008).

The Senior Alcohol Misuse Indicator ([SAMI], Busto et at., 2003) has been found to work well as a more subtle health-focused approach.[3] It asks the following questions:

1a. Have you recently (in the last few months) experienced problems with any of the following:
☐ changes in sleep?
☐ drowsiness?
☐ falls?
☐ changes in appetite or weight?
☐ dizziness?
☐ difficulty remembering things?
☐ poor balance?

1b. Have you recently (in the last few months) experienced problems with any of the following:
☐ feelings of sadness?
☐ loneliness?
☐ lack of interest in daily activities?
☐ feelings of anxiety?
☐ feelings of worthlessness?

2.   Do you enjoy wine/beer/spirits? Which do you prefer?

3.   As your life has changed, how has your use of (selected) wine/beer/spirits changed?

4.   Do you find you enjoy (selected) wine/beer/spirits as much as you used to? Yes/No

---

3 Information about using and scoring the SAMI and other screening tools can be found in *Improving Our Response to Older Adults with Substance Use, Mental Health and Gambling Problems* (CAMH, 2008).

5.   You mentioned that you have difficulties with_____ (from answers to questions
     1a and 1b). I am wondering if you think that (selected) wine/beer/spirits might be
     connected? Yes/No.

Identifying Medication Problems

There are few standardized instruments for screening problems related to using psychoactive medications (Health Canada, 2002). However, the following questions may be
helpful in determining whether a medication problem exists. Let the client know that
these questions refer to prescription, over-the-counter and health food supplements and
herbal remedies.

- Can you tell me the names of medications you are taking?
- What was [name or indicate the medication] prescribed for?
- How long have you been taking these medications?
- Do you take them regularly (at the recommended time)?
- Do you skip days or forget days?
- Do you ever have difficulty remembering when to take your medication?
- Does the pharmacy provide you with your medications in a dosette or bubble pack?
- Do you have difficulty opening medication containers?
- Do you ever use medications from another person?
- Do you have any difficulty reading the written directions on how to take the medication?
- Can you tell me the names of the medications (or pills) you are taking that were not
  prescribed by a doctor?

Assessment

The purpose of an assessment is to help the client and the practitioner determine next
steps for treatment and assess risk. When an assessment is appropriate, the context will
help guide the process, such as the reason for the assessment, who has requested it,
where it is taking place, whether the client is a willing participant and whether he or she
is aware that the concern is substance use.

  An in-depth assessment provides a critical opportunity to establish a trusting and
therapeutic relationship. The desired outcome may be simply that the older person will
continue with the service offered, enabling change to evolve based on his or her needs.

  The initial presenting problem, or in some cases a crisis, may have to be dealt with
first. Often, this is not related to substance use, but to another health problem, a crisis
in the family or a change in living situation (e.g., loss of a spouse, impending eviction).
The counsellor should attend to the most immediate concern in order to engage the client in a process of change. The substance use issue is best introduced when the client
is most receptive—preferably after the initial concern is attended to and a therapeutic,
caring relationship has developed.

While it is critical to be up front with the client and explain the treatment model, sometimes clients are reluctant to engage with an addiction treatment agency. If this is the case, request that the client meet with you once so you can explain the approach and that you will focus on the issues most pressing to the client to start with, and will discuss substance use later if he or she is comfortable doing so.

Older adults may find the assessment process intrusive or tiring, although they may comply because they perceive the health care professional as being in a position of authority. Some older adults may not be willing or able to complete forms or other structured tests and will need time to "tell their stories." Here are some suggestions for simplifying and enhancing the process:

- Allow time to conduct an assessment over a number of contacts, rather than in one structured, time-limited interview.
- Access information (with required consent) from other involved health professionals to avoid repeating a questioning process that may feel invasive or tiring
- Listen closely to the client's story, as you can gain much information that can be applied to the formal assessment, including information that indicates a client's self-perception and coping abilities, and identifies areas that may require further investigation.
- Be aware of language: some older adults may not have a high level of education; some terms that may be common for a practitioner may be unfamiliar to an older generation; cognitive changes or impairment may affect the person's ability to understand complex sentences or longer words; and clients may lose the ability to understand English if they learned it as a second language.
- Avoid common pitfalls such as "talking down" to clients, speaking to them as if they are children, or ignoring them and conducting the interview through other caregivers who may be present.

Explore areas such as sensory functioning, mobility, living environment, lifestyle, losses, diet, mental condition, physical health, social support, literacy and speech (each area is discussed in detail below). The level of functioning in these areas determines the person's ability to make changes in his or her life. Someone who is in poor health, cannot get around, is living in unhealthy circumstances or is confused will not be able to deal with issues related to substance use until these immediate problems are addressed.

The following areas are important to assess with older clients:

Sensory function: How well does the person see (e.g., read labels on medication containers, books, newspapers)? This knowledge reflects the person's communication and comprehension. How long since the last prescription for glasses? Has sense of taste been lost? This could result in a loss of interest in diet. Assume some age-related hearing loss: have hearing aids been prescribed?

Mobility: Can the person move about inside and outside, walk without aids, bathe and dress independently, shop for himself or herself? Lack of self-care may be a physical problem, not a self-esteem indicator. Living environment and lifestyle: Is the person happy in his or her living situation? Have there been housing problems because of substance use? Can the person maintain his or her living environment? Are there fire hazards or sanitation problems? Does the person live close enough to stores, buses, etc.? Does the person go out? How often does he or she see other people?

Diet and nutrition: What are the person's eating habits (e.g., does he or she eat alone)? Does the person have a good appetite and enjoy food? How is food prepared and stored? Does the person know the importance of good nutrition and its effect on daily living?

Losses: Has the person lost family, friends, physical health (hearing, sight), a job, role in life or home?

Mental health: Is the person confused or experiencing memory problems? Does he or she appear depressed? Mental health symptoms can present differently in older adults; for example, depression may present as complaints about physical discomfort or boredom, or with words such as "low" or "sad." Anxiety may be expressed as "worries." Irritability can accompany depression. It can be difficult to distinguish a substance use problem from depression, dementia or many other issues because of similar indicators or because of the atypical presentations common in older people. If the person seems to avoid the issue of mental health, the avoidance may not be due to alcohol or medication use—it could be a genuine indicator of an age-related mental illness. It is critical to ask the person if he or she has had thoughts about dying, both passive or active suicide ideation.

Useful screening and assessment tools include the Beck Depression Inventory (Beck et al., 1961) and Folstein's Mini Mental Status exam (Folstein et al., 1975). The Geriatric Depression Scale (GDS) is a commonly used tool for assessing depression in older adults and is available in English, French and other languages (Yesavage et al., 1983). Substance use counsellors can add these and other tools to their assessment protocols to help identify the early stages of an underlying depression or dementia.

Capacity: Distinguishing between normal forgetfulness, dementia, depression and delirium is extremely important, but can be challenging. A referral to a psychogeriatric specialist may be helpful or necessary. Where possible, caregiver input is essential. Executive functioning (i.e., carrying out plans), abstract thinking and other crucial functions can be affected and need to be considered before treatment plans are developed. The person may seem to be in denial or may be acting difficult, but these may be signs of neurological problems. In addition, older people with chronic substance misuse may have alcohol-induced persistent dementia with acute and/or chronic effects on cognitive functioning. They may also have had multiple head injuries, resulting in symptoms of acquired brain injury, which may affect reasoning and decision-making capabilities.

Physical health: Ask about sleeping patterns, weight change, disabilities and illnesses, dizziness, foot care, digestion/elimination and dental problems, or difficulty with eating because of dentures. Has there been a recent hospital admission? Has the person had recent surgery? Is there a physical problem that has not been addressed? Is the person in regular contact with a doctor?

Social support: Does the person have contact with family and friends? How much contact does he or she have with other people? Does the person have close support or only acquaintances? Knowing how the person's support has changed will help identify strategies to replace missing supports.

Alcohol and other drug use: How often and how much does the person drink alcohol? Has the pattern of drinking changed (increased, decreased, periods of abstinence)? Has drinking affected other areas of functioning? What medications (prescribed, over-the-counter or herbal remedies) are being used? Has the person ever experienced withdrawal? How did he or she cope with withdrawal? Is the person afraid to stop using alcohol or other drugs? Does he or she smoke?

Abuse: Physical, emotional, financial or other forms of abuse may need to be assessed. Is neglect a factor? Drinking problems can affect self-determination, and the ability to assess personal risk can be a problem for both the victim and the perpetrator of the abuse.

Finances: Is the person managing his or her finances? Is there concern about the person's ability to manage finances (competence to manage finances where there is evidence of cognitive decline)?

Risk: Assess the level of immediate risk. Does the person drive? Is he or she at risk of fire due to careless smoking habits? Is there a risk of suicide? Risk of falls? Is the person extremely frail? Does he or she wander or get lost?

Literacy and speech: Does the person have reading or writing problems? Are the problems a result of limited education or loss of ability? Is the person comfortable communicating in English or French? As memory problems develop, people tend to revert to their original language. Are there other issues that might limit the person's literacy or speech pattern, such as a stroke?

Culture: Being sensitive to cultural diversity helps build trust. Be especially attentive to cultural values around age, gender, education, social time and position in the family. Communication may be a challenge depending on language and literacy levels. Stigma and shame of addiction may have a greater impact in some cultures and can affect self-esteem and the ability to make changes. Cultural differences may make it very difficult to meet with a person individually, or may mean that there is close familial support to be drawn on. Culture should be understood in the broadest sense: all of us are influenced by factors such as our beliefs, ethnicity, age, sexual orientation and religion.

Treatment

Older people may represent a wide range of ages and stages of problem use in treatment. In spite of this remarkable diversity, people whose substance use problems are classified as early onset or late onset form two fairly distinct groups. They share some similarities in terms of the developmental tasks of aging, but also have different needs and require different treatment approaches.

For people whose substance use problems are intermittent, or who have relapsed, treatment must be tailored to the person and will depend on his or her symptoms. It is encouraging to note that there is no difference in treatment outcomes between chronic and late-onset drinkers (Graham et al., 1995).

When working with older adults with concurrent disorders, the approach will also depend on their symptoms, and will mean addressing the substance use and mental health issues at the same time or over time, once the most pressing issue is stabilized.

Withdrawal

Some older people may be abstinent for one reason or another when they enter treatment, often in response to an acute injury or illness associated with their substance use. Signs and symptoms that may indicate a drug withdrawal in a younger person do not necessarily apply to an older person. For example, among older adults, falls, tremors, memory problems and hallucinations may not be symptoms of withdrawal. Acute confusion, behavioural changes, fluctuating levels of consciousness and changes in cognition indicating delirium may be in response to withdrawal from alcohol or other substances such as benzodiazepines. Withdrawal is better tolerated with gradual tapering unless the person is experiencing a health crisis.

Withdrawal in older people, particularly with early onset, is more severe and protracted and can last up to 10 days rather than the more usual three days. Seizures may be more likely. Psychoactive substances can harm the physical system, so it is important to be aware of the client's physical condition while also focusing on withdrawal from the drug. The older person may have to withdraw from alcohol and other substances under the supervision of a physician with appropriate medication available, rather than in a non-medical detoxification setting. For older people, very slow tapering off mood-altering medications is recommended, as it causes less distress and allows the person to plan for coping without the substance. It is invaluable to have the support of the doctor who has prescribed the medication and who can provide consultation and oversee other medical needs. If the doctor does not recognize the substance use as a problem, it may be necessary to seek other medical advice and support for the process of withdrawal.

Due to post-acute withdrawal effects, it can take weeks or even months for confusion to clear, which will affect the pace of treatment and make it necessary to repeat information and provide it in different formats. Many of the physical, psychological and social problems associated with long-term substance use will still be active. These problems range from physical illnesses such as diabetes, arthritis, digestive disorders, heart disease, cancer and respiratory diseases (many who drink also smoke) to the social and psychological problems of depression, isolation, loneliness and low self-esteem.

Early Onset

People with early onset substance use problems may enter treatment in their 50s, but have problems more often associated with older people (e.g., chronic illnesses, isolation, multiple losses). For this reason, most addiction programs for older adults accept clients as young as age 55.

The early onset client usually presents for treatment in the chronic stage and often presents with major problems, such as poor health, chronic illness, mobility issues, loneliness, low self-esteem, poor coping mechanisms, isolation, depression and loss of meaning in life. These problems often create a sense of helplessness and hopelessness and require a specialized holistic intervention that responds to the person's physical, psychological, emotional and spiritual needs, as well as to the alcohol or other drug use issues.

Older adults who still use addictive substances often use less than they did when they were younger. But this can mislead the client and others to believe that the severity of the problem has decreased, when in fact the person is still using at hazardous levels for his or her age and physical condition.

Clinicians may find that the client's income is spent on alcohol, that he or she is not eating properly, is neglecting self-care or is not paying the rent, therefore risking eviction. It is helpful to know whether the client with early onset problems has tried treatment before, what was and was not helpful, and whether the person has concerns and fears about trying treatment again.

Physical needs

Alcohol affects every system of the body. It adversely affects appetite and digestion, sleep patterns, and nerve, muscle and joint functioning. Poor nutrition, inadequate sleep and lack of exercise over many years weaken the person's physical condition and predispose him or her to chronic illnesses. Long-term alcohol use can cause or exacerbate diseases such as hypertension, diabetes and disorders of the digestive system, as well as cognitive changes.

Psychological needs

If the client has had drinking problems most of his or her adult life, the drinking may have interfered with or prevented the person from completing earlier developmental tasks, such as pursuing his or her life's work, becoming productive in a job, developing intimacy with a partner and learning to be interdependent, becoming responsible to others in a family or similar situation and finding a place in society.

Failing to fully develop one's potential and losing employment as a result of substance use lead to psychological problems associated with failure, insecurity and condemnation by family, friends and society. Poorly developed work habits and skills are accompanied by feelings of low self-esteem and inadequacy. In most cases, the older client will not return to the workforce, so treatment should focus more on addressing the person's use of time because days without structure tend to be filled with drinking. A common treatment goal is to help the client rediscover earlier skills and interests or develop new ones.

Providing a safe environment to explore the older person's life story is crucial. Many older adults have experienced trauma (incest, physical hardships, rape, loss of children in infancy, war) that may have been suppressed: "family secrets" may never have been uttered, and the wounds connected to these secrets have never healed.

Clients may have used substances to deal with difficulty developing relational skills. The result is poor social skills, the inability to relate to others at a deep-feeling level and the loss of family and friends due to behaviour associated with alcohol and other drug use. Service providers may need to help clients move away from dwelling on past failures and toward recognizing strengths, and helping them focus on planning for future activities and successes, while responding to their immediate problems.

Treatment that includes an opportunity to socialize and helps the client become comfortable expressing feelings helps to alleviate loneliness. Although many older people initially prefer individual counselling, one goal of counselling could be to help the client feel comfortable joining a group. A group can often be a key to developing new friendships and finding alternatives to drinking, and can provide a stepping stone to moving out into the wider community. At the same time, it is important to respect that group work is not for everyone.

People with long-term substance use problems have usually not developed the ability to be interdependent—to be responsible to and for others, and to allow others to be responsible to and for them. This may present in various ways: not showing up for appointments, or displaying demanding behaviour or overdependence on the counsellor. The client may fluctuate between angry feelings—"I don't need anyone, leave me alone"—to clinging to the counsellor. At this juncture, approaches should work toward strengthening the client–counsellor relationship, without resulting in overdependence. The goal is to gradually broaden the client's base of support and help him or her learn to interact with others in a give-and-take relationship.

Social needs

Social isolation is a major problem for clients with early onset problems. The physical and psychological limitations mentioned above affect the person's ability to form and maintain friendships. Compounding this is the loss of family and friends because of past behaviour.

Social isolation can be a problem for many older people as they lose the company of work colleagues, children who have left home and partners or other close friends who have died. For the person with early onset substance use problems, these changes often occur earlier in life and are more extensive than for others of a similar age. Friends and family have been replaced with "drinking friends" and places, and drinking friends may have died. The long-term effects of substance use may have decreased the ability to actively participate in relationships, and communication skills may be underdeveloped. The person may have limited energy for social activities, and underlying depression can affect the ability to be an active participant.

Relationships may be limited to those who also drink or use other drugs. Find out how the person obtains the substances if he or she is not able to get out, as this reliance on others may increase susceptibility to financial and other forms of abuse.

Social isolation promotes feelings of loneliness and fear, as well as anxiety when with people. The person must be helped in treatment to gradually rebuild those social skills—skills that are easily lost when they are not actively used. A relationship with one caring person is often a good place to start, followed by encouraging the client to gradually extend his or her circle of contacts. Encourage the client to join a group for older adults. Access to the community offers important opportunities for socializing.

Financial needs

Older adults may be affected by low income and poverty and the additional challenges that face low socio-economic groups. Pensions and disability insurance are not always sufficient to cover the increasing costs of rent, food or medication. Help with budgeting, connecting with community resources such as food and transportation programs, and ensuring the client receives all applicable financial supplements is an important aspect of a holistic approach to treatment.

Spiritual needs

The spiritual issues associated with long-term use of alcohol and other drugs usually concern the meaning of life and feelings of guilt and remorse. Older clients may feel they have wasted their lives, that life was particularly hard on them, or that they deserve their hardship because of things that have happened related to their substance use.

Freedom to talk about these issues is a necessary part of treatment. Understanding and accepting their substance use problem can help older clients feel less guilty and accept the personal strengths that have allowed them to survive the negative consequences of substance use. This might also be the opportunity the person needs to forgive others who brought them pain and sadness.

Finally, it is important to consider the effect of other people's attitudes toward the person with a substance use problem. Frequently this attitude is extremely pessimistic. Family and caregivers have observed many years of substance use, promises made and broken, efforts to stop using followed by even greater use. Attempts to control the substance use are often brief, and then the cycle begins again. The family reaches the end of its coping ability and moves away in an effort to reclaim its own health. Eventually, friends and colleagues look on from a distance, and it is left to the professional caregiver to offer support and try once again to inspire hope.

Without understanding and accepting the chronic relapsing nature of the problem, even the health care professional may give up. If this happens, the client's feelings of hopelessness and helplessness are reflected by others. Using creative interventions to engage the person in a process of change will break this impasse. It is essential to find areas of change that are important to the client and in which he or she feels some confidence for success. As previously discussed, the focus of change initially is often not substance use. However, as people become stronger, both physically and emotionally, and with support, they can change their use of alcohol and other drugs.

Summary of best approaches

The best approaches to helping a person with an early onset substance use problem include:

- an individual approach focusing on areas for change that the client sees as important and achievable; for example, a relationship with a counsellor can be the first step toward alleviating loneliness, to be followed later by other social activities; addressing basic needs such as food and shelter
- developing trust by helping the client address the problem that he or she identifies by giving the clear message that help will be provided, and that it is not based on clients having to first "prove" themselves by addressing the substance use
- a supportive one-on-one relationship, which is non-confrontational and nurturing, recognizing that the client might initially need frequent contact regarding a variety of concerns
- outreach—working with the client in his or her own home, allowing for physical and emotional comfort; reaching out to offer help instead of waiting for the person to seek help
- group activities that offer support and social interaction with peers (these may take the form of a supportive counselling group, as well as recreational activities undertaken by the group)
- a thorough knowledge and use of available health and social services in the community.

Late Onset

People with late onset problems usually enter treatment at a later age than early onset clients, commonly 65 to 75 years or older, with fewer years of substance use problems and fewer associated losses. Thus, these clients present quite a different picture than people with early onset problems. Often, they have lived a full life, having successfully managed a career and family. The person has developed skills and interests during the adult years, and family ties are more likely to be intact.

A late onset substance use problem can develop through two routes. Some people may have been social drinkers all their lives. After retirement, with more leisure time and drinking-related social activities, and fewer work-related constraints, their drinking may escalate. Increased use, combined with greater physical sensitivity to the effects of alcohol and other drugs as people age, is sufficient to initiate major health and possibly other problems related to substance use.

The other route to late onset problems is when an older person self-medicates with alcohol or other psychoactive drugs, or is prescribed psychoactive drugs to alleviate stress caused by a crisis, physical ill health, the loss of someone close or other age-related stresses. Benzodiazepines are frequently prescribed to help people, particularly older women, cope with these losses or stressors, putting them at risk of psychological and physical dependence over time.

Like early onset problems, late onset problems may affect many dimensions of people's lives—physical, psychological, social and spiritual. However, late onset problems may present somewhat differently.

The person finds it hard to recognize and accept that he or she has crossed the line from social to harmful use, as is the case with younger people. In addition, symptoms or problems associated with heavy alcohol or other drug use (e.g., confusion, disorientation, recent memory loss, tremors, inflammation of joints, gastritis, hypertension, depression, heart disease, sleep disturbances) are often erroneously accepted as "normal" signs of aging. Thus, the client, family and professional caregivers may fail to identify the problem in its early stages.

Important treatment approaches for older adults include providing education about substance use, attending to the presenting crisis, fostering healthy ways of dealing with distress and providing support.

If the client is dealing with a crisis, it is important to identify the stressor and attend to it along with the substance use problem. Crises in later years most often pertain to loss (e.g., of a life partner, friends, pets, health, independence, autonomy, status). As one client aptly described it after reading about the stages of grief, "I am perpetually in several stages of grief at the same time. I never get out of it." Feelings of acute fear, anger, sadness and anxiety often accompany the experience of loss. Cognitively, the person may fluctuate between preoccupation with the object of loss and denial of it. Multiple losses and consequent grief are best responded to by providing support and social contact, and by offering opportunities to reflect, reminisce and openly grieve without the use of medication. Careful listening with empathetic responses allows the person to feel and express grief safely.

Other Aspects of Care

Case management

Agencies that provide services to older adults benefit their clients by connecting and collaborating with one another because the complexity of the issues older adults face usually requires links with a variety of resources. Building partnerships between service providers, and consulting on behalf of individual clients greatly improves services and limits the possibility of misdiagnosis. Helping with the practical aspects of a client's situation and supporting the person's understanding of the different services available builds trust and enhances engagement with the client.

A program that focuses on substance use problems may not meet all of the client's needs, in which case referrals to other agencies may be appropriate. For example, you may need to refer someone for grief counselling.

Concurrent disorders

Clients can be helped to achieve stability using a collaborative approach between mental health and addiction services and, where possible, involving the client's physician. Addressing the most urgent issues first will allow for stabilizing one area, then moving on to address other areas, for example stabilizing alcohol use before addressing underlying depression. Applying a holistic approach that addresses many aspects of lifestyle change means that change in one area will affect other areas of the client's life.

Integrated services

A push toward integrating services allows a much greater opportunity for clients of any age to access services and for service providers to benefit from one another's expertise. Innovative partnerships can be created. In one local example,[4] a full-time geriatric addiction specialist (a social worker who has clinical training and expertise working with older adults) has been embedded into a specialty community-based geriatric mental health outreach team consisting of geriatric psychiatrists and other transdisciplinary workers. Clients receive a full geriatric mental health assessment, including addiction screening, followed by treatment and case management in a harm reduction model. Services are provided to clients in their own environment (e.g., house, retirement home, long-term care home) and at a pace that meets their needs. Working in close partnership, the mental health outreach program and the addiction program collaborate to enhance the local continuum of services and supports available to older adults and their families affected by concurrent disorders. They also facilitate geriatric addiction and mental health cross-training within and beyond the program.

---

4 This partnership involves the Halton Geriatric Mental Health Outreach Program (St. Joseph's Healthcare Hamilton) and Halton ADAPT (Alcohol, Drug and Gambling, Assessment, Prevention and Treatment Services). For information about each program, visit www.hgmhop.ca and www.haltonadapt.org.

Social inclusion and recreation

There are many reasons for providing planned programs for socializing and recreation, which can take the form of organized outings, social gatherings, communal meals and peer support.

Older adults may have difficulty finding social groups in the community that have alcohol-free events. Even retirement homes have "happy hours." Older adults may have a different concept of leisure and recreation. Depending on the generation, some believe that work is the only meaningful activity, and reading and playfulness are a waste of time. Counsellors may need to help clients see the benefits of recreation, exploring with them the value of play, past experiences of play and how they can now view play as purposeful. Socializing can be a challenge for late onset clients who may feel they are the "only one" to have developed problems like these. Embarrassment about others finding out is acute— social and recreational programming is very important to reduce the sense of shame.

Finally, it can be difficult for clients to appreciate and accept the positive rewards of being around other people. Clients often will have accepted that they are "loner types"— stemming from a long history of discomfort or feelings of being judged in groups. The person may be so socially isolated that being with strangers is overwhelming.

Counsellors may need to follow up individually with clients about any challenges they have in social groups, checking in to help them feel comfortable and reviewing communication and other interpersonal skills. There are benefits to mixing clients at different stages of treatment; peer involvement from clients who have made changes can help inspire others that change is possible later in life.

Family and caregiver involvement and support

While confidentiality is the same as for any other client, it is ideal if family or friends can be included in the treatment plan. The client may not want others involved—the person may feel too ashamed to have family know the full extent of the substance use—or may simply not be ready. Gaining family involvement will need to be approached at the same pace as other therapeutic interventions. It may take a while before the person is prepared to involve the family; the counsellor may need to act as mediator with family members who have been estranged.

Family and loved ones who are involved may have very different goals for treatment (e.g., they want the person to stop using substances right away). Education is needed to help the family understand the treatment model and rationale, and the benefits of harm reduction and the change process, so they can be supportive of the client's treatment. Families or other caregivers may need access to their own counsellor who is not involved with their loved one. They may need group or individual sessions to understand the best ways to care for themselves and to be able to provide optimal support.

Revisiting the Case Studies

At the beginning of this chapter, we introduced two case examples. In one, Mrs. Ray's heavy alcohol use became chronic in older age, and is particularly problematic because of its interaction with medications for which concurrent use of alcohol is contraindicated. In the second case, Mr. Bo has been a chronic drinker from an early age, and faces a number of challenges with few social supports or material resources. Both are examples of the types of substance use problems that older adults often confront—Mr. Bo's pattern reflects early onset problems, while Mrs. Ray experienced late onset problems. Both have experienced crises in response to the significant losses so common to older people.

> Mrs. Ray's children—after several gentle conversations—convince her to see a counsellor by reassuring her that the referral is to help her with her grief, which is normal with loss. The counsellor, over several meetings, establishes a rapport with Mrs. Ray, provides education about the effects of her medications and offers supportive feedback regarding her physician's concerns. In telling her personal story to the counsellor over time, Mrs. Ray is able to express her worries in her own way. Involving her children in a supportive role helps Mrs. Ray stay motivated and reminded of her goals.

> A treatment professional meets with Mr. Bo at his home, develops a rapport with him and arranges for a friendly visitor from a seniors' agency to visit him weekly. This visitor is interested in hearing about Mr. Bo's life, and listens as Mr. Bo expresses his grief about losing so many friends, while beginning to introduce Mr. Bo to other opportunities for outings and activities in the community. Mr. Bo's substance use is introduced gradually as a topic for discussion, while the treatment service continues to provide intensive case management over the period of a year. Mr. Bo's family notices that he is eating better with the help of a nutrition program, and he has begun to cut down on his drinking as he looks forward to contact with others in the program.

Conclusion

With a burgeoning older adult population, the new face of substance use problems in aging baby boomers, and the fact that older adults with substance use problems have long been underserved, addressing substance use problems with this population has become a clinical imperative. Addiction counsellors need to prepare to serve older adults. In addition to understanding the unique treatment needs of older adults and applying long-honed best practice approaches, this also means consulting and collaborating with the many community-based organizations that serve older adults in order to address the needs of individual clients.

We hope this introductory chapter has sparked an interest and passion in serving older adults and will inspire you to develop comfort, proficiency and enthusiasm for working with this population.

Practice Tips

- Older adults' physiology can mean heightened vulnerability to problems with much lower amounts of alcohol or other drugs. Practitioners must be vigilant and prepared to screen for substance use problems to improve identification and referral for treatment for people age 55 and older.
- Older adults will enter treatment when it is tailored to meet their needs. Overcoming barriers to treatment requires that practitioners recognize and support older adults' right to treatment and their capacity for change through outreach and improved accessibility.
- Older adults do well in treatment and can make significant life changes. Helping older clients requires developing a therapeutic alliance; the initial contact is crucial to successfully engaging the client. The essence of working with older adults is to identify the problem from the client's perspective—the process of change does not necessarily begin with changing substance use.
- Diversity among older adults necessitates individual treatment plans, but recognizing early and late onset typologies can help to improve identification and develop suitable treatment.
- Case management is an integral aspect of treating older adults and requires a thorough knowledge of the range of services available. Consulting, connecting and sharing with mental health and other professionals ensures optimum treatment.

Resources

Publications

Center for Substance Abuse Treatment. (2012). *Substance Abuse among Older Adults.* Treatment Improvement Protocol (TIP) series 26. Rockville, MD: Author. Retrieved from www.ncbi.nlm.nih.gov/books/NBK64419/pdf/TOC.pdf

Centre for Addiction and Mental Health. (2008). *Improving Our Response to Older Adults with Substance Use, Mental Health and Gambling Problems.* Toronto: Author.

Health Canada. (2002). *Best Practices: Treatment and Rehabilitation for Seniors with Substance Use Problems.* Ottawa: Author. Retrieved from www.hc-sc.gc.ca/hc-ps/pubs/adp-apd/treat_senior-trait_ainee/index-eng.php

Registered Nurses' Association of Ontario. (2003). *Nursing Best Practice Guideline: Screening for Delirium, Dementia and Depression in Older Adults.* Toronto: Author. Retrieved from http://rnao.ca/sites/rnao-ca/files/Screening_for_Delirium_Dementia_and_Depression_in_the_Older_Adult.pdf

Internet

Alzheimer Knowledge Exchange Resource Centre—Mental Health, Addictions and Behavioural Issues
www.akeresourcecentre.org/MentalHealth

Canadian Coalition for Seniors Mental Health
www.ccsmh.ca

References

Adams, W.L., Barry, K.L. & Fleming, M.F. (1996.). Screening for problem drinkers in older primary care patients. *JAMA, 276,* 1964–1967.

Adlaf, E.M., Begin, P. & Sawka, E. (Eds.). (2005). *Canadian Addiction Survey (CAS): A National Survey of Canadians' Use of Alcohol and Other Drugs: Prevalence of Use and Related Harms.* Ottawa: Canadian Centre on Substance Abuse. Retrieved from www.ccsa.ca/2005%20CCSA%20Documents/ccsa-004028-2005.pdf

American Psychiatric Association. (2000).*Diagnostic and Statistical Manual of Mental Disorders* (text rev.). Washington, DC: Author.

Babor, T.F., Higgins-Biddle, J.C., Saunders, J.B. & Monteiro, M. (2001). AUDIT, The Alcohol Use Disorders Identification Test: Guidelines for Use in Primary Care (2nd ed.). Geneva, Switzerland: World Health Organization. Retrieved from http://whqlibdoc.who.int/hq/2001/who_msd_msb_01.6a.pdf

Barnes, A.J., Moore, A.A., Ang, A., Tallen, L., Mirkin, M. & Ettner, S. (2010). Prevalence and correlates of at-risk drinking among older adults: The project SHARE study. *Journal of General Internal Medicine, 25,* 840–846.

Bartels, S.J., Blow, F.C., Brockmann, L.M. & Van Citters, A.D. (2005). *Substance Abuse and Mental Health among Older Americans: The State of the Knowledge and Future Directions.* Rockville, MD: Substance Abuse and Mental Health Services Administration.

Beck, A.T., Ward, C.H., Mendelson, M., Mock, J. & Erbaugh, J. (1961). An inventory for measuring depression. *Archives of General Psychiatry, 4,* 561–571.

Blazer, D.G. & Wu, L. (2009). The epidemiology of at-risk and binge drinking among middle-aged and elderly community adults: National Survey on Drug Use and Health. *American Journal of Psychiatry, 166,* 1162–1169.

Boddiger, D. (2008). Drug abuse in older US adults worries experts. *The Lancet, 372,* 1622.

Busto, U., Flower, M.C. & Purcell, B. (2003). Senior Alcohol Misuse Indicator. Toronto: Centre for Addiction and Mental Health.

Center for Substance Abuse Treatment. (1998). *Substance Abuse among Older Adults.* Treatment Improvement Protocol (TIP) series 26. Rockville, MD: Substance Abuse and Mental Health Services Administration. Retrieved from http://www.ncbi.nlm. nih.gov/books/NBK64422/

Centre for Addiction and Mental Health (CAMH). (2008). *Improving Our Response to Older Adults with Substance Use, Mental Health and Gambling Problems.* Toronto: Author.

Dar, K. (2006). Alcohol use disorders in elderly people: Fact or fiction? *Advances in Psychiatric Treatment, 12,* 173–181.

Folstein, M.F., Folstein, S.E. & McHugh, P.R. (1975). "Mini-mental state": A practical method for grading the cognitive state of patients for the clinician. *Journal of Psychiatric Research, 12,* 189–198.

Gfroerer, J., Penne, M., Pembnerton, M. & Folsom, R. (2003). Substance abuse treatment need among older adults in 2020: The impact of the aging baby-boom cohort. *Drug and Alcohol Dependence, 69,* 127–135.

Graham, K., Saunders, S.J., Flower, M.C., Birchmore, T.C., White-Campbell, M. & Pietropaolo, A.Z. (1995). *Addictions Treatment for Older Adults: Evaluation of an Innovative Client-Centred Approach.* New York: Haworth Press.

Health Canada. (2002). *Best Practices: Treatment and Rehabilitation for Seniors with Substance Use Problems.* Ottawa: Author. Retrieved from www.hc-sc.gc.ca/hc-ps/ pubs/adp-apd/treat_senior-trait_ainee/index-eng.php

Health Canada. (2008). *Canadian Addiction Survey (CAS): A National Survey of Canadians' Use of Alcohol and Other Drugs. Focus on Gender.* Ottawa: Author. Retrieved from www.hc-sc.gc.ca/hc-ps/pubs/adp-apd/cas_gender-etc_sexe/index-eng.php

Hurt, R.D., Offord, K.P., Croghan, I.T., Gomez-Dahl, L., Kottke, T.E., Morse, R.M. & Melton, L.J., III. (1996). Mortality following inpatient addictions treatment. Role of tobacco use in a community-based cohort. *JAMA, 276,* 783–784.

Ialomiteanu, A.R., Adlaf, E.M., Mann, R.E. & Rehm, J. (2009). *CAMH Monitor eReport: Addiction and Mental Health Indicators among Ontario Adults, 1977–2007.* CAMH Research Document series 25. Toronto: Centre for Addiction and Mental Health.

McCready, J., Mann, R.E., Zhao, J. & Evans R. (2008). Correlates of gambling-related problems among older adults in Ontario. *Journal of Gambling Issues, 22,* 174–194.

Menninger, J. (2002). Assessment and treatment of alcoholism and substance-related disorders in the elderly. *Bulletin of the Menninger Clinic, 66,* 166–183.

National Institute on Alcohol Abuse and Alcoholism. (1998). *Alcohol and Aging.* Alcohol Alert series 40. Bethesda, MD: Author. Retrieved from http://pubs.niaaa.nih.gov/publications/aa40.htm

O'Connell, H., Chin, A.V., Cunningham, C. & Lawlor, B. (2003). Alcohol use disorders in elderly people—redefining an age old problem in old age. *British Medical Journal, 327,* 664–667.

Ontario Human Rights Commission. (2001). *Time for Action: Advancing Human Rights for Older Ontarians.* Toronto: Author. Retrieved from www.ohrc.on.ca/en/time-action-advancing-human-rights-older-ontarians

Oslin, D.W. (2004). Late-life alcoholism: Issues relevant to the geriatric psychiatrist. *American Journal of Geriatric Psychiatry, 12,* 571–583.

Ruth, S. (2008). Developing a model of community based alcohol and drug treatment for an ageing population. Unpublished manuscript.

Selby, P. & Els, C. (2004). Tobacco interventions for people with alcohol and other drug problems. In S. Harrison & V. Carver (Eds.), *Alcohol and Drug Problems: A Practical Guide for Counsellors* (3rd ed., pp. 709–731). Toronto: Centre for Addiction and Mental Health.

Simoni-Wastila, L. & Yang, H.K. (2006). Psychoactive drug abuse in older adults. *American Journal of Geriatric Pharmacotherapy, 4,* 380–394.

Statistics Canada. (2006, February 7). Health Reports: Seniors' health care use. *The Daily.* Catalogue no. 11-001-XIE. Retrieved from www.statcan.gc.ca/daily-quotidien/060207/dq060207a-eng.htm

Sullivan, M.A. & Covey, L.S. (2002). Current perspectives on smoking cessation among substance abusers. *Current Psychiatry Reports, 4,* 388–396.

Tjepkema, M. (2004). Alcohol and illicit drug dependence. Supplement to *Health Reports* Vol. 15. Statistics Canada Catalogue no. 82-003. Ottawa. Retrieved from www.statcan.gc.ca/pub/82-003-s/2004000/pdf/7447-eng.pdf

Turcotte, M. & Schellenberg, G. (2007). *A Portrait of Seniors in Canada, 2006.* Statistics Canada Catalogue no. 89-519-XIE. Retrieved from www.statcan.gc.ca/pub/89-519-x/89-519-x2006001-eng.pdf

Voyer, P., Préville, M., Cohen, D., Berbiche, D. & Béland, S-G. (2010). The prevalence of benzodiazepine dependence among community-dwelling older adult users in Quebec according to typical and atypical criteria. *Canadian Journal on Aging, 29,* 205–213.

Wiebe, J., Single, E., Falkowski-Ham, A. & Mun, P. (2004). *Gambling and Problem Gambling among Older Adults in Ontario.* Toronto: Responsible Gambling Council. Retrieved from www.responsiblegambling.org/docs/research-reports/gambling-and-problem-gambling-among-older-adults-in-ontario.pdf?sfvrsn=10

Yesavage, J.A., Brink, T.L., Rose, T.L., Lum, O., Huang, V., Adey, M.B. & Leirer, V.O. (1983). Development and validation of a geriatric depression screening scale: A preliminary report. *Journal of Psychiatric Research, 17,* 37–49.

Chapter 24

Colonization, Addiction and Aboriginal Healing

Peter Menzies

When Anthony was three years old, an Indian Agent (an official representative of the federal government to First Nations communities) removed him from his birth home in a First Nations community in northern Ontario. He later attended a residential school for 10 years, where he was physically and sexually abused by his caretakers. He was regularly reminded of the primitive nature of his culture, customs and language. When the school closed, Anthony was placed into the care of the Children's Aid Society because his family was deemed incapable of providing for his needs. Until he was 18, he remained in care and lived in numerous group homes and foster homes. He did not complete high school and was regularly in conflict with the law due to his substance use issues. At age 47, after several periods of incarceration, Anthony has decided he no longer wants substances to control his behaviour and has begun addiction treatment.

There is growing evidence that problem substance use among Aboriginal people is symptomatic of broader systemic issues. As this case scenario suggests, the colonization of Aboriginal people has resulted in personal, familial and community trauma, and substance use may be one manifestation of this trauma. Substances are often used as "self-medication" to mask such mental health problems as depression and anxiety arising from experiences of colonization.

Both Aboriginal and mainstream service providers are recognizing that these issues can be addressed by implementing holistic treatment strategies. An Aboriginal holistic approach can also be considered in combination with western intervention strategies. Such efforts build on indigenous healing methods and help both the person and the community to sustain long-term health. Culturally congruent service delivery requires the counsellor's commitment to learning about a client's cultural history, values, beliefs and norms, and to joining him or her in a change process. This process may involve engaging other community members, including Elders, in the healing process. Healing thus becomes not just an individual process, but a community development effort.

Prevalence of Substance Use and Mental Health Issues among Aboriginal People

Not all First Nations communities have higher rates of mental health or addiction problems compared to the general population (Ponting & Voyageur, 2005; Wuttunee, 2004). However, when health data are aggregated across Aboriginal populations, Aboriginal people are disproportionately represented among those experiencing mental health and addictions issues, as detailed below:

- The rate of suicide among First Nations people is 2.1 times that of the general Canadian population (Health Canada, 2003).
- National rates of suicide among Aboriginal youth are estimated to be five to six times higher than among non-Aboriginal youth (Health Canada, 2003).
- The smoking rate among First Nations adults is twice as high as that among members of the general population (58.8 per cent vs. 24.2 per cent) (Health Canada, 2009).
- Alcohol-related deaths among First Nations people are six times higher than among the general population (Tremblay, 2009).
- Aboriginal youth are two to six times more at risk for alcohol-related problems than non-Aboriginal youth (Health Canada, 1999).
- About 16 per cent of Aboriginal people have faced major depression, which is twice the Canadian average (Statistics Canada, 2008).
- Of the estimated 1 million Aboriginal people living in Canada, more than one third has been affected either directly by residential school experiences or indirectly as family or community members linked to residential school survivors (Standing Senate Committee on Social Affairs, Science and Technology, 2006).

Given the disproportionate number of Aboriginal communities dealing with these issues, we must have a common historical, social and cultural understanding of what is meant by "Aboriginal."

History of Aboriginal People in Canada

Identity

The term *Aboriginal* generally refers to the original inhabitants of North America and their descendants. However, while most people or communities define themselves as belonging to a particular ethnic group based on place of birth or residence, language, cultural practices and beliefs, the definition of Aboriginal has largely been imposed by government statute.

Statutory designations

Status and non-status Indians

The *Indian Act* of 1876 codified biological and cultural factors, designating as "status" Indians those who were recognized by the federal government as having treaty rights, and as "non-status" Indians those who did not. These designations ignored members of "mixed race" and disenfranchised women who married non-Aboriginal men (Mawhiney, 1994).[1] The Act continues to apply these status and non-status designations, consequently limiting which members of the community can "enjoy" benefits provided under the Act. Restoule (2000) observes that "this definition has had a profound impact not only in how we are understood by non-Aboriginal people, but also in how we have come to understand ourselves" (p. 106).

Métis

Métis was another designation under the *Indian Act*. It refers to people of mixed Aboriginal and European descent. In order to reduce the number of people labelled "Indian," by 1880, people of mixed blood no longer met the criteria to be registered as Indians (Frideres, 1998). The federal government relinquished responsibility to the provinces for all Métis people. As a result, many Métis formed their own distinct communities and developed political and economic institutions reflecting their distinct heritage (Frideres, 1998).

However, on January 8, 2013, the Federal Court of Canada ruled that Métis and non-status Aboriginal people are considered to be "Indian" under the *Constitution Act, 1867*, and fall under federal jurisdiction. The decision did not address whether the federal government has a fiduciary responsibility to the two groups, but the assumption is that such responsibilities would flow through the ruling (*Daniels v. The Queen*, 2013).

Inuit

Inuit people (historically referred to as "Eskimo") form the fourth group of Canada's Aboriginal people. Although they are referred to collectively as *Inuit*, language, cultural practices and belief systems are distinct within many Inuit communities. Although after 1867 the Inuit were placed under federal jurisdiction, they continue to be distinct from those defined as "Indian" under the *Indian Act*.

Increasingly, Canada's Aboriginal people are asserting their right to identify membership from within their own communities, rather than allowing membership to be imposed. As this new millennium unfolds, Aboriginal people are increasingly renewing ties with their families of origin and developing links to their historical roots.

---

1 In 1985, Bill C31 amended the *Indian Act* to allow women with non-Aboriginal husbands and their children access to benefits, with the consent of the band. It also restored the rights of those who had been considered "enfranchised" through post-secondary education, employment or participation in a federal election.

Identity and current population data

Evidence that an increasing number of Aboriginal people are identifying with their heritage is found in Canadian population data. According to the 2006 census (Statistics Canada, 2008), 1,172,790 people identified their ancestry as linked to the Aboriginal Peoples of Canada, which accounted for 3.8 per cent of Canada's total population (31,241,030 people). This is an increase from 3.3 per cent in 2001 and 2.8 per cent in 1996 (See Table 24-1).

TABLE 24-1

Size and Growth of the Population by Aboriginal Identity, Canada, 1996 and 2006

ABORIGINAL IDENTITY	2006	% CHANGE FROM 1996 TO 2006[3]
Total population	31,241,030	9
Aboriginal identity population	1,172,790	45
First Nations people[1]	698,025	29
Métis[1]	389,785	91
Inuit[1]	50,485	26
Multiple and other Aboriginal responses[2]	34,500	34
Non-Aboriginal population	30,068,240	8

[1] Includes people who reported a North American Indian, Métis or Inuit identity only.

[2] Includes people who reported more than one Aboriginal identity group (North American Indian, Métis or Inuit) and those who reported being a registered Indian and/or band member without reporting an Aboriginal identity.

[3] Data have been adjusted to account for incompletely enumerated reserves in 1996 and 2006.

Source: Statistics Canada (2008).

As Canada's fastest-growing group, the Aboriginal population's median age is 27 years, compared with 40 years for non-Aboriginal people (Statistics Canada, 2008). This is due to a higher birth rate and lower life expectancy for Aboriginal adults. As noted in the census, the senior population represented only five per cent of the Aboriginal population, compared with 13 per cent of the non-Aboriginal population.

According to the 2006 census (Statistics Canada, 2008), in 2006, 54 per cent of the Aboriginal population reported living in urban areas (up from 47 per cent in 2001). In 2006, Winnipeg was home to the largest urban Aboriginal population (68,380). Edmonton had the second largest number of Aboriginal people (52,100). Vancouver ranked third (40,310). Toronto (26,575), Calgary (26,575), Saskatoon (21,535) and Regina (17,105) were also home to relatively large numbers of urban Aboriginal people.

It is estimated that by 2016, Canada's urban Aboriginal population will total almost half a million people (Statistics Canada, 1998).

The Aboriginal profile within urban centres is distinct from that on reserves. Consider the following:

- Aboriginal people are much younger than the general population: one out of three Aboriginal people are under 15 years of age (Statistics Canada, 1998).
- Single-parent families constitute nearly half of all migrants from First Nations reserves to Canada's urban centres (Royal Commission on Aboriginal Peoples [RCAP], 1996a).
- Young teenagers represent 35 per cent of the total number of people leaving reserves to settle in urban centres (RCAP, 1996a).

Social conditions on reserves (i.e., limited housing, limited employment and educational opportunities, limited access to health care and social services) are generally cited as the main stimulus for people leaving the reserves (RCAP, 1996b).

Historical Relationships in Aboriginal Communities

The social conditions described above exist as a result of the historical relationship between Aboriginal people and the federal government. The *Indian Act* established the federal government as the "guardian" of regulated status Indians; Inuit were not included because they were not considered "Indian" at the time the Act was created. The Act established a power relationship between the government and Indians; for example, the Act:

- established where Indians could live
- determined what traditional ceremonies they could practise
- prevented them from leaving or travelling off the reservations without written approval
- determined what support they would receive from government agencies
- prescribed how they could interact with others outside of the community (Mawhiney, 1994).

The Act created a hierarchy of decision-making authorities within these artificial settlements (reserves) that did not reflect traditional values and practices. Indian Agents were hired to administer the Act, and served as justices of the peace when it came to infractions, with penalties ranging from being forbidden to leave the reserve to imprisonment. The Act essentially became a "legislative straightjacket" (RCAP, 1996b) controlling the daily lives of Aboriginal people.

Residential schools

The Act also allowed for the institutionalization of Aboriginal people in a manner unrivalled in Canadian history. Recognizing the importance of education in the transmission of social values, the government used various religious institutions, including the Roman Catholic, United, Presbyterian, Salvation Army and Anglican churches, to force widespread social change on Aboriginal communities. From 1870 until the last residential school closed in 1996, an estimated 150,000 Aboriginal people were placed in residential schools across Canada (Commission to Promote Sustainable Child Welfare, 2011).

An estimated 80,000 residential school survivors are still living (Truth and Reconciliation Commission of Canada, 2012). The Assembly of First Nations (1994) chronicled the role of residential schools in relation to changing government policy concerning Aboriginal people. It found that the government used the schools, over time, for three different purposes: assimilation, segregation and integration. The 1996 Royal Commission on Aboriginal Peoples (RCAP, 1996a, 1996b, 1996c) and the more recent Truth and Reconciliation Commission (2012) chronicled the abuses experienced by students and the resulting impact on individuals, families and communities.

In 1969, the federal government withdrew from its partnership with the churches in residential schools. The last residential school in Canada—the Gordon Residential School in Saskatchewan—closed in 1996 (Claes & Clifton, 1998). With the integration of Aboriginal children into the public school system, child welfare became the new instrument of government assimilation policies.

Child welfare

Many studies indicate that a disproportionate number of Aboriginal children were taken into care by provincial child welfare authorities (Canadian Council on Children and Youth, 1978; Hepworth, 1980). Other studies identify how the child welfare system decimated Aboriginal communities across Canada (Johnston, 1983).

From 1951 until the late 1960s, the federal government negotiated with the provinces over the cost of providing child welfare services to First Nations communities. The interim agreement struck between the two levels of government provided that the needs of Aboriginal children would be met only if the government staff involved reported a life-or-death situation (Timpson, 1990).

No preventative measures were implemented to minimize the impact of this funding vacuum, and families faced a plethora of social issues without resources. In response, the provincial governments adopted a crisis intervention approach to child welfare. Johnston (1983) introduced the term "the '60s scoop" to describe the period when an overwhelming number of Aboriginal children were permanently removed from their homes and communities and placed in foster care or made Crown wards (Andres, 1981; Johnston, 1983; Richard, 1989; Timpson, 1990).

The 1996 Royal Commission on Aboriginal Peoples concluded that First Nations children are six times more likely to be placed in care than children from the general population. To compound this situation, the Commission found that placement of children in non-Aboriginal foster care homes has been as high as 90 per cent in some provinces (RCAP, 1996a). Children sent for adoption to the United States and Europe felt even more intense isolation from their families and their Aboriginal identity (Bagley et al., 1993). Lederman (1999) observes:

Children's Aid Societies perpetuated the same belief as residential schools: that a well-meaning white, cultural institution was better than a Native child's family and community. Many, perhaps even most, of the child welfare workers were compassionate and well-intentioned. But, however well-meaning Children's Aid Society intrusions may have been, they further continued the traumatization of Native people and likely compounded it. (p. 64)

By 1969, widespread demonstrations and co-ordinated efforts by Aboriginal groups prevented further federal devolution of responsibilities for Aboriginal programs and services to the provinces and territories, as proposed in the federal government's white paper on Indian policy (Timpson, 1990). However, by that time, the child welfare system was well established as a new instrument of colonization (Armitage, 1993; Hudson & McKenzie, 1981). In fact, about three times more Aboriginal children are in care today than when residential schools were at capacity (Blackstock, 2003).

The Legacy of Colonialism

As instruments of colonization, the *Indian Act* and the residential school and child welfare systems left many Aboriginal people without the resources required to build healthy communities (Deiter, 1999).

Child welfare studies describe the long-term effects of removing Aboriginal children from their birth families and placing them in non-Aboriginal homes (Couchi & Nabigon, 1994; Frideres, 1998; Locust, 1999). Warry (1991) reported that as these children matured, they became "apples": racially "red," or Aboriginal, on the outside, but culturally "white" on the inside. Locust (1999) coined the term "split feather syndrome" to describe the long-term psychological problems of these children, whose cultural isolation and loss of familial connections left them feeling isolated from both mainstream and Aboriginal culture. Without belonging to either culture, many described their socialization as being split between two worlds. Gagne (1998) proposes that colonialism has been the "seed of trauma" for many First Nations communities and has left a legacy of dependence for many individuals and communities.

Former residential school students and child welfare system survivors have rates of substance use problems, anxiety disorders, depression, suicide and low self-esteem as adults that are significantly higher than those of the general population (Beisner & Attneave, 1982; Gagne, 1998; Hodgson, 1990; Mussell et al., 1991).

It is important to understand how the loss of connection to culture and the erosion of communities have contributed to the higher rates of substance use problems among Aboriginal people. According to McCormick (2000), "for many Aboriginal people, consumption of alcohol has been their attempt to deal with the state of powerlessness and hopelessness that has arisen due to the devastation of traditional cultural values" (p. 27).

Intergenerational Trauma

While approaches to understanding and treating posttraumatic stress and associated disorders usually focus on the direct or individual impact, recent studies of Aboriginal communities note that trauma has affected more than one generation within families and communities (Braveheart-Jordan & De Bruyn, 1995; Lederman, 1999; Phillips, 1999; Waldram, 1997). In a review of morbidity factors in Aboriginal communities, Waldram (1997) acknowledges this legacy: "The current state of affairs can be clearly linked to the traumatic effects of colonialism, including geographic and economic marginalization, and attempts at forced assimilation" (p. 184).

Napier (2000) described this intergenerational trauma, in which "the bonds between many hundreds of Aboriginal children and their families and nations were bent and broken, with disastrous results" (p. 3). Hodgson (1990) summarized the cumulative impact across generations:

> If you subject one generation to that kind of parenting and they become adults and have children, those children become subjected to that treatment and then you subject a third generation to a residential school system the same as the first two generations. You have a whole society affected by isolation, loneliness, sadness, anger, hopelessness and pain. (p. 17)

Gagne (1998) identified the residential school experience as a key component within the cycle of trauma. In a discussion of the sociological causes of intergenerational trauma among First Nations people, he concluded that the effect of the residential school experience has been felt beyond the generation that attended the school: "At least two subsequent generations were also 'lost.' The children of these students became victims of abuse as their parents became abusers because of the residential school experience" (Gagne, p. 363).

Both mainstream and Aboriginal health practitioners have challenged the *Diagnostic and Statistical Manual of Mental Disorders* (American Psychiatric Association, 2000) diagnosis of posttraumatic stress disorder (Waldram, 1997), which ignores the role of culture and intergenerational or community trauma and does not connect a person's experience to broader, systemic conditions that perpetuate and exacerbate the problem. According to Waldram (2004), "Approaching trauma through DSM by and large precludes a meaningful discussion of culture, and virtually excludes notions of history and collective, community or cultural trauma" (p. 235). Similarly, Root (1992) suggests that racism and discrimination compound the impact of direct or personal trauma by allowing for the oppression of a community. This insidious trauma becomes "normalized" to the point that the group does not realize that social conditions continue to be oppressive. Rather than focusing on a single event that makes the person feel unsafe, this insidious trauma leads to a view that the world is an unsafe place for a whole group of people (Root, 1992). Kirmayer and colleagues (2000) concur that the focus on individual trauma does not adequately reflect the Aboriginal experience:

> The emphasis on narrating personal trauma in contemporary psychotherapy is problematic because many forms of violence against Aboriginal people are structural or implicit and so may remain hidden in individual accounts. . . . Individual events are part of larger historical formations that have profound effects for both individuals and communities. (Kirmayer et al., 2000, p. 613)

Toward an Aboriginal Model for Health Care Service Delivery

Historical social policies have affected many generations of Aboriginal people. The severing of family ties has left a legacy of trauma, with many Aboriginal people unable to function in mainstream society, and alienated from their indigenous roots. Left dependent on social institutions, many are unable to meet their individual needs. Increasingly, Aboriginal researchers and front-line workers are advocating culturally congruent service delivery based on local values and culture. They suggest that to strengthen communities in distress, western methods of mental health practice must recognize and validate traditional methods of healing. Duran and colleagues (1998) explain the necessity for this approach: "Until traditional Indigenous therapies are implemented and considered legitimate, there will be a struggle, and sadly, the suffering of historical legacy and ongoing trauma will continue" (p. 349).

Cultural differences between Aboriginal people and the majority culture in North America have been well documented (Cross, 1986; Horejsi & Pablo, 1993; Johnston, 1983; Morrissette et al., 1993; Red Horse, 1980). (See Appendix A for a summary of these differences.) Aboriginal values necessitate a holistic approach to health care service delivery. Because the physical, mental, emotional and spiritual elements of health of individuals, families and communities are interwoven and interdependent, "wellness" can be achieved only when all four elements—body, mind, emotions, spirit—of personal health are balanced.

Cultural Competence

Braveheart-Jordan & De Bruyn (1995) discuss the need for cultural competence in working with women in Aboriginal communities across North America. Their work has demonstrated that effective therapeutic relationships require knowledge of the history and values of a community. The counsellor must not only understand the nuances of a person's cultural background, but must also actively explore the client's cultural community—both with the client, and by approaching members of the community.

To work effectively in Aboriginal communities, it is important to find out how closely individuals, families or communities identify with Aboriginal values. Morrissette and colleagues (1993) have developed a practical framework for working with Aboriginal people; they suggest asking clients to identify themselves on a cultural continuum that describes their cultural awareness, ranging from "traditional" to "neo-traditional" to "non-traditional."

On this continuum, traditional Aboriginal people closely regard the teachings of Elders and acknowledge a strong interdependence between people and the earth or nature. For a client who identifies as traditional, referral to an Elder or other traditional expert may facilitate that client's personal development. Counsellors can also help by facilitating access to traditional healing methods such as the pipe ceremony, storytelling, traditional medicines, sweat lodge ceremonies, vision quests, shaking tent ceremonies and teaching circles.

Neo-traditional Aboriginal people identify with a blend of traditional spirituality and practices that reflect the dominant society and Christian beliefs. Counsellors can support clients who identify as neo-traditional through a blend of traditional teachings and conventional approaches to substance use treatment. The role of the counsellor is to facilitate the person's healing and recognize his or her need to become a more "balanced" community member.

Non-traditional Aboriginal people have adopted most of the norms and practices of the dominant society. They may experience ambivalence as a result of internal conflict between dominant values and exposure to Aboriginal values, and may feel culturally alienated because they do not fit into either the dominant or Aboriginal society. The client may need the counsellor's help to discover his or her culture and heritage, which could involve working with an Elder. However, some Aboriginal people may not identify a role for their traditional culture in the treatment process. The treatment choice always rests with the client. Following what the client wants from treatment reflects a strong traditional value, as well as a mainstream one.

Traditional Healing Strategies

Traditional healing strategies are gaining recognition in mainstream health care and social service settings. Waldram (1997) notes that Aboriginal people are regaining control of the healing process in mainstream treatment through the use of traditional approaches that include the medicine wheel (to guide the process), sweat lodge ceremonies, healing circles and sweet grass ceremonies. Healing centres, such as Poundmaker's Lodge in Alberta, affirm the value of Aboriginal people controlling their own healing processes.

Role of Elders

Increasingly, Elders and traditional healers are being recognized for their critical role as part of a client's treatment team; their respected place in their communities means that their participation sanctions the healing process (Cross, 1986). The traditional role of

Elders is reemerging as communities recognize that Elders' knowledge and experience support and enhance community activities.

Community empowerment

In their work addressing abuse in Aboriginal communities in northern Manitoba, Duck and colleagues (1997) recognized the need for a community-based approach to healing in Aboriginal communities. They entrenched their work in community empowerment: "A key aspect of healing communities is the recapturing of community values: rebuilding the family, respecting the wisdom of the Elders in sharing essential teachings, allowing women and children to voice their opinions, and recreating a strong nation" (p. 2).

The medicine wheel

The medicine wheel represents traditional theology, philosophy and psychology for some Aboriginal people (Morrisseau, 1998). It is based on a world view in which the spiritual, mental, physical and social aspects of life are inseparably connected and continuously interacting (Swinomish Tribal Mental Health Project, 1991). By learning the four directions of the medicine wheel (east, south, west and north), the counsellor is better able to understand Aboriginal culture and develop an effective way of working with these communities. (See Appendix B for a description of one way to use the medicine wheel.)

Stories

It is also important to be able to take other teachings, such as those of Nanabush, a character in an Ojibway tale, and explore the client's problems through these teachings. In Ojibway teaching, Nanabush was sent to the people to teach about the mystery of life through his adventures. It is through such stories that Ojibway people learn about our values and place within creation.

When these teachings are incorporated into therapy, the client not only receives the therapeutic interpretation; he or she also learns about the cultural teachings. But in order to use these teachings, the clinician must know how particular ones might apply to the client's situation. The clinician gives the client the teaching as a "gift" and encourages the person to meditate over the teaching and how it might apply to his or her life. The client can then choose whether or not to share his or her interpretation or understanding of the teaching.

This approach may seem at odds with the therapeutic intervention, but by forcing the client to give an interpretation, the clinician would be interfering, and potentially putting his or her own values or reflections on the teaching, rather than deferring to what it means for the client. (See the table in Appendix A under the section called "non-interference.") The client most likely has thought about the teaching and may not be ready to discuss it. In my practice, I have found it best to assess the client in terms of culture readiness before using Nanabush teachings.

Integrating Aboriginal and Non-Aboriginal Practices

The blending of traditional healing and western assessment and treatment processes is gaining recognition in mainstream institutions, such as the Centre for Addiction and Mental Health (CAMH) in Toronto. CAMH's urban Aboriginal Services links western approaches to assessing and treating substance use and mental health concerns with traditional healing strategies. The services are provided under the guidance of a community advisory committee, which consists of Aboriginal agencies and non-Aboriginal services that have many Aboriginal clients. A team of therapists and an Elder visit both mainstream and Aboriginal agencies to provide intensive therapy and help link Aboriginal people to services in the community. CAMH offers healing circles, talking circles, one-on-one support from an Elder, individual therapy sessions (pre-treatment and aftercare), a 21-day inpatient treatment cycle for men and women and sweat lodge ceremonies. The team also shares information about traditional healing strategies and cultural norms and values with other CAMH staff, as well as developing culturally congruent assessment and treatment skills.

In partnership with First Nations communities, the northern Aboriginal team provides clinical mentorship and capacity building, facilitates access and transitions to CAMH programs and supports training and research strategies and applications.

Depending on where the client identifies on the cultural continuum, the therapist needs to consider with the client other programs, including non-indigenous ones, that may support the client's healing journey. Broadening the client's choices allows both cultural reintegration and rediscovery of the positive aspects of the client's identity as an indigenous person, linked to centuries of tradition and wellness based on balance and wholeness. It also facilitates access to the full diversity of conventional and complementary healing and health approaches, while respecting and encouraging the client's potential for continuing change and growth. Rooted in these foundations, recovery becomes an ongoing and constructive process.

This range of treatment approaches is important not just for Aboriginal people, but also for families and communities, and for the systems of care and support that are designed to support them. System building has been recently manifested in important work led by a partnership of Aboriginal, government, community and academic agencies across the country. Together, they produced *Honouring Our Strengths* (Health Canada et al., 2011), which offers a holistic model of integrative care, starting with health promotion and including early identification, secondary-risk reduction, active treatment and specialized interventions, all joined by care facilitation. (The model is presented graphically in Appendix C.) Such a model provides a template against which current systems resources and gaps can be identified, and a map on which systems growth and development can be planned and evaluated.

All too often, clinicians must help change happen one case at a time, usually without a broader system of support to draw from. Even if change can only happen for one person, one family or one community at a time, the ability to do change work successfully is radically enhanced if the system supports are there to empower and facilitate that action.

Revisiting the Case Study

Anthony is determined not to end up incarcerated for the rest of his life. His healing journey will require exploring how his substance use is intrinsically linked to systemic issues that have affected him, his family and his community. Anthony's therapist helps him examine his social location within this story. The therapist recognizes that Anthony has never considered how attending a residential school and being in the child welfare system have affected him, and that he has not made the connection between his addictions and these early life experiences. With the therapist, Anthony examines his deep-seated anger and frustration about his life course. Together they also explore Anthony's birth culture and how his feelings about being an Aboriginal person are affecting his behaviours. Therapy creates opportunities for Anthony to reconfigure his beliefs about himself, his family, his community and his cultural identity that lead to self-destructive behaviours.

Conclusion

A growing number of Aboriginal people are moving into urban centres, seeking both health care and new life opportunities. Given the high rates of mental health and addiction issues within Aboriginal communities, health care providers must be prepared to support Aboriginal people in a way that recognizes their unique history within the Canadian experience. In order to effectively meet the needs of Aboriginal people with substance use and/or mental health issues, counsellors and health care agencies must understand the Aboriginal world view. History has played a critical role in the experiences of Aboriginal people: intergenerational trauma is rooted in public policies related to the *Indian Act*, and experiences with the residential school system and child welfare authorities. These experiences have left a legacy of individual, family and community distress. Assessment and treatment strategies must be based on this knowledge and provide choices to Aboriginal people around their own healing processes. These indigenous processes must form the root of any healing strategy, and cannot be employed simply as an adjunct to western healing methods.

Practice Tips

- Understand both the historical and ongoing impact of colonization on Aboriginal people.
- Be aware of the continuing intergenerational impact of residential schools and the child welfare system on the mind, body, spirit and emotions of Aboriginal people across Canada. Healing may be a lifelong process, given the many traumas Aboriginal people have experienced over the last 500 years.
- Explore the role of trauma in the lives of your Aboriginal clients, including intergenerational trauma.
- Do not become the expert: let the client tell his or her story. Your role is to help guide the client in exploring the colonization process and how it has affected him or her.
- Allow the client to choose and walk his or her own healing path.
- Do not assume that all Aboriginal people are aware of the practices and beliefs of their traditional culture, or that they want these interventions.
- Be patient: working with people experiencing oppression can be a long-term process, lasting months, even years.
- Be hopeful. Despite daunting challenges created by systemic disadvantages over many generations, a growing number of stories of change and healing exist, offering pathways to health and healing for Aboriginal individuals, families and communities.
- Participate in Aboriginal ceremonies in order to understand cultural practices.

Resources

Internet
Aboriginal Canada Portal
    www.aboriginalcanada.gc.ca
Aboriginal Healing Foundation
    www.ahf.ca
Aboriginal Nurse's Association of Canada
    www.anac.on.ca
Commission on First Nations & Métis Peoples and Justice Reform
    www.justice.gov.sk.ca/justicereform/
First Nations Child and Family Caring Society
    www.fncaringsociety.com

Health Canada, First Nations and Inuit Health
   www.hc-sc.gc.ca/fniah-spnia/index-eng.php
National Native Addictions Partnership Foundation
   http://nnapf.com
National Native Alcohol and Drug Abuse Program renewal
   http://nnadaprenewal.ca

References

American Psychiatric Association (APA). (2000). *Diagnostic and Statistical Manual of Mental Disorders* (text rev.). Washington, DC: Author.

Andres, R. (1981). The apprehension of Native children. *Ontario Indian, 46,* 32–37.

Armitage, A. (1993). Family and child welfare in First Nation communities. In B. Wharf (Ed.), *Rethinking Child Welfare in Canada* (pp. 131–171). Toronto: McClelland & Stewart.

Assembly of First Nations. (1994). *Breaking the Silence: An Interpretive Study of Residential School Impact and Healing as Illustrated by the Stories of First Nations Individuals.* Ottawa: Author.

Bagley, C., Young, Y. & Scully, A. (1993). *International and Transracial Adoptions: A Mental Health Perspective.* Aldershot, United Kingdom: Avebury Press.

Beisner, M. & Attneave, C. (1982). Mental disorders among Native American children: Rates and risk periods for entering treatment. *American Journal of Psychiatry, 139,* 193–198.

Blackstock, C. (2003). First Nations child and family services: Restoring peace and harmony in First Nations communities. In K. Kufedlt & B. McKenzie (Eds.), *Child Welfare: Connecting Research Policy and Practice* (pp. 331–342). Waterloo, ON: Wilfrid Laurier University Press.

Braveheart-Jordan, M. & De Bruyn, L. (1995). So she may walk in balance: Integrating the impact of historical trauma in the treatment of Native American Indian women. In J. Adelman & G. Enguidanos (Eds.), *Racism in the Lives of Women: Testimony, Theory and Guides to Ethnoracist Practice* (pp. 345–368). New York: Haworth Press.

Canadian Council on Children and Youth. (1978). *Admittance Restricted: The Child as Citizen in Canada.* Ottawa: Author.

Claes, R. & Clifton, D. (1998). *Needs and Expectations for Redress of Victims of Abuse at Residential Schools.* Retrieved from http://dalspace.library.dal.ca/bitstream/handle/10222/10440/Sage%20Research%20Redress%20EN.pdf?sequence=1

Commission to Promote Sustainable Child Welfare. (2011). *Aboriginal Child Welfare in Ontario: A Discussion Paper.* Ottawa: Minister of Children and Youth Services.

Couchi, C. & Nabigon, H. (1994). A path towards reclaiming birth culture. In F. Shroff (Ed.), *The New Midwifery* (pp. 41–50). Toronto: LPC Inbook.

Cross, T. (1986). Drawing on cultural tradition in Indian child welfare practice. *Social Casework, 67*, 283–289.

Daniels v. The Queen, 2013. FC 6. Retrieved from http://cas-ncr-nter03.cas-satj.gc.ca/rss/T-2172-99%20reasons%20jan-8-2013%20ENG.pdf

Deiter, C. (1999). *From Our Mothers' Arms: The Intergenerational Impact of Residential Schools in Saskatchewan.* Toronto: Plenum Press.

Duck, J., Ironstar, V. & Ricks, F. (1997). Healing and the community. *Journal of Child and Youth Care, 11* (3), 1–13.

Duran, E., Duran, B., Yellow Horse Brave Heart, M. & Yellow Horse-Davis, S. (1998). Healing the American Indian soul wound. In Y. Danieli (Ed.), *International Handbook of Multigenerational Legacies of Trauma* (pp. 341–354). New York: Plenum Press.

Frideres, J. (1998). *Aboriginal Peoples in Canada: Contemporary Conflicts* (5th ed.). Toronto: Prentice Hall Allyn & Bacon Canada.

Gagne, M. (1998). The role of dependency and colonialism in generating trauma in First Nations citizens. In Y. Danieli (Ed.), *International Handbook of Multigenerational Legacies of Trauma* (pp. 355–372). New York: Plenum Press.

Health Canada. (1999). *A Second Diagnostic on the Health of First Nations and Inuit People in Canada.* Ottawa: Author.

Health Canada. (2003). *Acting on What We Know: Preventing Suicide in First Nations Youth. The Report of the Suicide Prevention Advisory Group.* Ottawa: Author.

Health Canada. (2009). *A Statistical Profile on the Health of First Nations in Canada: Determinants of Health, 1999 to 2003.* Ottawa: Author.

Health Canada, Assembly of First Nations & National Native Addictions Partnership Foundation. (2011). *Honouring Our Strengths: A Renewed Framework to Address Substance Use Issues among First Nations People in Canada.* Ottawa: Author. Retrieved from http://nnadaprenewal.ca/wp-content/uploads/2012/01/Honouring-Our-Strengths-2011_Eng1.pdf

Hepworth, P. (1980). *Foster Care and Adoption in Canada.* Ottawa: Canadian Council on Social Development.

Hodgson, M. (1990). *Impact of Residential Schools and Other Root Causes of Poor Mental Health.* Edmonton, AB: Nechi Institute on Alcohol and Drug Education.

Horejsi, C. & Pablo, J. (1993). Traditional Native American cultures and contemporary U.S. society: A comparison. *Human Services in the Rural Environment, 16* (3), 24–27.

Hudson, P. & McKenzie, B. (1981). Child welfare and Native people: The extension of colonialism. *The Social Worker, 49* (2), 63–88.

Johnston, P. (1983). *Native Children and the Child Welfare System.* Ottawa: Canadian Council on Social Development.

Kirmayer, L., Brass, G. & Tait, C. (2000). The mental health of Aboriginal peoples: Transformations of identity and community. *Canadian Journal of Psychiatry, 45*, 607–616.

Lederman, J. (1999). Trauma and healing in Aboriginal families and communities. *Native Social Work Journal, 2* (1), 59–90.

Locust, C. (1999). Split feathers: Adult American Indians who were placed in non-Indian families as children. *Pathways, 14* (1), 1–5.

Mawhiney, A. (1994). *Towards Aboriginal Self-Government: Relations between Status Indian Peoples and the Government of Canada 1969–1984.* New York: Garland Publishing.

McCormick, R. (2000). Aboriginal traditions in the treatment of substance abuse. *Canadian Journal of Counselling, 34* (1), 25–32.

Morrisseau, C. (1998). *Into the Daylight: A Wholistic Approach to Healing.* Toronto: University of Toronto Press.

Morrissette, V., McKenzie, B. & Morrissette, L. (1993). Towards an Aboriginal model of social work practice. *Canadian Social Work Review, 10* (1), 91–108.

Mussell, W., Nicholls, W. & Adler, M. (1991). *Making Meaning of Mental Health Challenge in First Nations.* Chilliwack, BC: Sal'i'shan Institute Society.

Napier, D. (2000, May 2). Sins of the fathers. *Anglican Journal.* Retrieved from www.anglicanjournal.com/articles/sins-of-the-fathers-6853

Phillips, G. (1999, November). *How we heal.* Paper presented at Link-Up Queensland's 1999 meeting of the National Stolen Generations Conference, Gold Coast, Australia.

Ponting, R. & Voyageur, C. (2005). Multiple points of light: Grounds for optimism among First Nations in Canada. In D. Newhouse, C. Voyageur & D. Beavon (Eds.). *Hidden in Plain Sight: Contributions of Aboriginal Peoples to Canadian Identity and Culture* (pp. 425–454). Toronto: University of Toronto Press.

Red Horse, J.G. (1980). American Indian elders: Unifiers of families. *Social Casework, 61,* 490–493.

Restoule, J.P. (2000). Aboriginal identity: The need for historical and contextual perspectives. *Canadian Journal of Native Education, 24* (2), 102–113.

Richard, K. (1989). Kenn Richard fights racism within child welfare. *Metropolis, 2* (11), 3–4.

Root, M. (1992). Reconstructing the impact of trauma on personality. In L. Brown & M. Ballou (Eds.), *Personality and Psychopathology: Feminist Reprisals* (pp. 229–265). New York: Guilford Press.

Royal Commission on Aboriginal Peoples. (1996a). *Volume 1: Looking Forward, Looking Back.* Ottawa: Minister of Supply and Services.

Royal Commission on Aboriginal Peoples. (1996b). *Volume 4: Perspectives and Realities.* Ottawa: Minister of Supply and Services.

Royal Commission on Aboriginal Peoples. (1996c). *Volume 3: Gathering Strength.* Ottawa: Minister of Supply and Services.

Standing Senate Committee on Social Affairs, Science and Technology. (2006). *Out of the Shadows At Last: Transforming Mental Health, Mental Illness and Addiction Services in Canada.* Ottawa. Retrieved from www.parl.gc.ca/Content/SEN/Committee/391/soci/rep/pdf/rep02may06part1-e.pdf

Statistics Canada. (1998, January 13). 1996 census: Aboriginal data. The Daily. Ottawa: Author. Retrieved from www.statcan.gc.ca/daily-quotidien/980113/dq980113-eng.htm

Statistics Canada. (2008). *Aboriginal Peoples in Canada in 2006: Inuit, Métis and First Nations, 2006 Census.* Ottawa: Author.

Swinomish Tribal Mental Health Project. (1991). *A Gathering of Wisdoms: Tribal Mental Health; A Cultural Perspective.* LaConner, WA: Swinomish Tribal Community.

Timpson, J.B. (1990). Indian and Native special status in Ontario's child welfare legislation. *Canadian Social Work Review, 7,* 49–68.

Tremblay, P. (2009, February 26). *Getting it right: Using population specific, community-based research to advance the health and well-being of First Nations, Inuit and Métis in Canada.* Paper presented at the 4th Annual Aboriginal Health Forum, Calgary, Alberta. Retrieved from www.naho.ca/documents/naho/english/pdf/AboriginalHealthforum_insight_2009_01_23.pdf

Truth and Reconciliation Commission of Canada. (2012). *Truth and Reconciliation Commission of Canada: Interim Report.* Winnipeg, MB: Author. Retrieved from www.attendancemarketing.com/~attmk/TRC_jd/Interim_report_English_electronic_copy.pdf

Waldram, J. (1997). The Aboriginal Peoples of Canada. In I. Al-Issa & M. Tousignant (Eds.), *Ethnicity, Immigration and Psychopathology.* New York: Plenum Press.

Waldram, J.B. (2004). *Revenge of the Windigo: The Construction of the Mind and Mental Health of North American Aboriginal Peoples.* Toronto: University of Toronto Press.

Warry, W. (1991). Ontario's first people: Native children. In L. Johnson & D. Barnhorst (Eds.), *Children, Families and Public Policy in the '90s* (pp. 207–230). Toronto: Thompson Educational Publishing.

Wuttunee, W. (2004). *Living Rhythms: Lessons in Aboriginal Economic Resilience and Vision.* Montreal: McGill-Queen's University Press.

Appendix A

TABLE 24-2

Cultural Value Conflict Areas

MAINSTREAM	ABORIGINAL
Family	
The person is perceived as a separate entity.	The person is perceived in the context of his or her family.
Individual responsibility is considered important.	Involvement and dependence on family is encouraged.
Decision making must involve the person affected as much as possible.	Decision making must involve the older, respected members of the family.
Family is usually defined as biological parents and their offspring (nuclear family).	Family consists of biological parents, their children, grandparents, aunts and uncles (extended family). A child's cousins may be viewed as sisters and brothers.
Acceptance of others	
People relate to others in terms of their roles (e.g., their job).	Native people usually relate to other people in terms of the whole person.
People do not need to like or agree with someone to use his or her services (e.g., student and teacher).	People tend to accept or reject others completely and have difficulty working with those they have rejected.
Assertiveness, directness, eye contact and a firm handshake are signs of a confident, trustworthy person.	Directness and assertiveness are offensive. In interpersonal relations, a person must be patient, humble, quiet and respectful, especially toward older people.
Social relations	
Differences in status and rank are noted and stressed.	Differences in status are minimized to make others feel comfortable.
Communication follows predictable, formal steps to make others feel comfortable.	An informal style of communicating is used to make others feel comfortable.

MAINSTREAM	ABORIGINAL
Relationship to nature Humankind is rational and can construct machines and develop techniques to solve problems.	Nature guides and rules humanity. Humans must be accepting of such things as disease and suffering. Nature is the Creator. Nature is us. Nature is everything.
Time Time is perceived in terms of the clock (e.g., supper is at 5:00 p.m.). Time moves quickly from past to present to future; one must keep up with time and use it to change and master one's environment.	Time is perceived in terms of the right time to do something (e.g., supper is when you eat.) Time moves slowly; people must integrate themselves with the environment and adapt to it rather than change it.
Children Some children are "planned," while others may be viewed as an "accident" or unwanted. Children belong to the biological parents, who take primary responsibility for their care. Young adults are expected to leave home and become independent. Corporal punishment is often used in an attempt to control a child's behaviour. Shaming and teasing are commonly used to control a child.	All children are gifts from the Creator and are valued, regardless of the circumstances of their birth. Children are members of the community, and all members are responsible for them. Adult children feel little pressure to leave home and establish an independent household. Children learn through direction and instruction. Children learn through modelling and observation.
Older adults Because older people are no longer economically productive, they are not highly valued.	Elders are held in high esteem and are often asked for advice and guidance. They are expected to be wise and understanding.
Non-interference Giving advice, exerting influence and providing direction are important roles for people as they mature. A person receiving advice is expected to accept it in good grace.	People are allowed to explore their environment and make decisions without direction and interference. Any interference is perceived as rude, bad behaviour. Power or dominance over another is not acceptable.

MAINSTREAM	ABORIGINAL
Competition Competition between people or groups is seen as healthy and good for the person's development, as well as for society.	Non-competition is valued, as it avoids intra-group rivalry, prevents "showing off" and promotes the family, clan or tribe over the individual.
Sharing Acquiring material goods is a sign of success and power. The status of a person or family is enhanced in the community by the accumulation of goods and wealth.	Sharing with others is a sign of honour and respect for the person and the group. Survival of the family, clan and tribe is promoted. No person is better off or more powerful than others in the group.
Language patterns Speech is loud and fast with frequent interruptions. Responses to others are quick, using direct eye contact. Verbal skills are highly valued.	Speech is slow and soft with few interjections. Responses to others are delayed, with very little eye contact. Non-verbal communication is highly regarded.
Self A person learns to control himself or herself through trial and error. Aggressive use of self and competition with others are strengths. Value is placed on controlling the environment and other people, as well as one's own behaviour.	A person participates only when certain of his or her ability. People allow others to go first to learn from them. Individual privacy and non-interference are highly regarded.

Adapted from Brant, C. (1990), Horejsi & Pablo (1993) & Sanders, P. (1987).

References

Brant, C. (1990). Native ethics and rules of behaviour. *Canadian Journal of Psychiatry, 35*, 534–539.

Horejsi, C. & Pablo, J. (1993). Traditional Native American cultures and contemporary U.S. society: A comparison. *Human Services in the Rural Environment, 16* (3), 24–27.

Sanders, P. (1987). Cultural conflicts: An important factor in the academic failures of American Indian students. *Journal of Multicultural Counseling and Development, 15*, 81–90.

Appendix B

The Medicine Wheel as a Counselling Tool[1]

The medicine wheel represents traditional spirituality, philosophy and psychology for Aboriginal people, and presents a way of understanding and assessing the progress of the therapeutic relationship from a cultural perspective. The path suggested by the four directions of the medicine wheel can help identify tasks or strategies the counsellor can use with the client. The wheel must be used in conjunction with the core values as a guide to action and in relating to other people.

The East door

The East door is the beginning of change or an opportunity for individual or community renewal. According to traditional teachings, the East door brings illumination and provides an opportunity to see more clearly. It is in the east that a person develops self-reliance and a sense of what needs to be done. There is an emphasis on meeting physical needs in order to build strength. Additional traditional healing methods and teachings, such as sweat lodges and fasting, may be required. These spiritual activities help the person and the community work through issues, and identify a path along which to move toward the next door.

The South door

The South door is important, as it provides an opportunity for unlearning as well as learning. For Aboriginal people, or those who do not share the world view of the dominant culture, it is an opportunity to develop an understanding of how they have been oppressed or limited. People learn from one another, share ideas and feelings and reflect on their understanding of a shared vision; it is an opportunity to develop and nurture relationships. This door symbolizes time, patience and relationships. Personal realities and attitudes may shift as people become part of a collective; they may gain new insight and knowledge by reviewing previously held beliefs and ideals. For Aboriginal people, it is an opportunity to understand the impact of history, colonization and oppression; the South door encourages growth, change and understanding identity.

The West door

The West door presents a time for meditation, reflection and development of inner strength before the process turns external. Before moving forward, the person (or family or community) must confront the issues that prevent him or her from meeting his or

---

1 Based on Coggins, K. (1990), Cross, T. (1986), Morrisseau, C. (1998), Morrissette et al. (1993) & Native Council of Canada (1990).

her goals. It is a time of healing and an opportunity to regain balance and harmony. This opportunity for introspection requires that the counsellor support the person, family or community as they attempt to regain balance in their lives and respect for themselves.

The North door

This is the door of wisdom, where a person analyzes, imagines, understands, organizes, synthesizes, predicts, calculates and interprets hidden meanings. At the North door, action plans are devised and caring behaviours are emphasized; social action, economic development, devising appropriate political structures and spiritual support can be explored. The existing network of Aboriginal social agencies and community members can be brought together to develop strategies for problem solving, with Elders facilitating the individual and group process of healing.

References

Coggins, K. (1990). *Alternative Pathways to Healing: The Recovery Medicine Wheel.* Deerfield Beach, FL: Health Communications.

Cross, T. (1986). Drawing on cultural tradition in Indian child welfare practice. *Social Casework, 67,* 283–289.

Morrisseau, C. (1998). *Into the Daylight: A Wholistic Approach to Healing.* Toronto: University of Toronto Press.

Morrissette, V., McKenzie, B. & Morrissette, L. (1993). Towards an Aboriginal model of social work practice. *Canadian Social Work Review, 10* (1), 91–108.

Native Council of Canada. (1990). *Native Child Care: The Circle of Care.* Ottawa: Author.

Appendix C

FIGURE 24-1: Systems Model

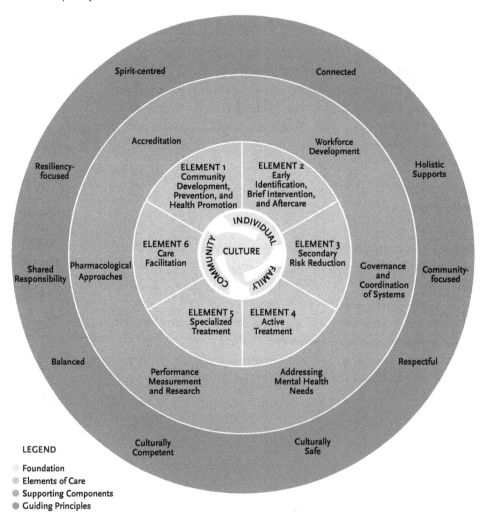

Source: Health Canada. (2011). *Honouring Our Strengths: A Renewed Framework to Address Substance Use among First Nations People in Canada* (p. 16). http://publications.gc.ca/collections/collection_2011/sc-hc/H14-63-2011-eng.pdf. Reproduced with permission of the Minister of Public Works and Government Services Canada, 2013.

Chapter 25

People with Diverse Sexual Orientations and Gender Identities Who Have Substance Use Concerns

Jim Cullen, Dale Kuehl and Nick Boyce*

> Abhay is a 31-year-old Indo-Canadian from a medium-sized city. He self-identifies as a female-to-male (FtM) transman seeking support to reduce his use of crystal meth (methamphetamine), which he has been using daily for the last year. Abhay lost his job six months ago due to his use, and his housing and relationship are at risk. He reports having used illicit drugs since he was 12, with the only period of "non-use" being the two years during which he transitioned into his male gender. Abhay discloses that he transitioned more than eight years ago and has struggled with depression and interpersonal relationship problems since childhood. Abhay (whose birth name was Harjeet) was kicked out of his home at 16 for being a lesbian, but since transitioning, he identifies his sexual orientation as that of a straight male. Recent interpersonal relationships have been emotionally painful for him. When he confides to a new partner that he is trans, he often gets rejected.

In this case scenario, what strengths does Abhay bring to the counselling relationship? What are some of the key issues he is struggling with, and how would you respond if he were your client? What are the issues you imagine having to triage first in a care plan? What overarching struggles do you think will need to be addressed in the support you provide? Finally, do you feel competent to provide addiction treatment to Abhay? If not, how and where would you get the support you need to better understand and provide service?

This case scenario highlights the complexity of working with individuals and communities with diverse sexual orientations and gender identities. As the transsexual/transgender community becomes more visible and attempts to access service, clinicians—even those who are comfortable providing care and treatment to gay, lesbian or bisexual clients—may need additional training to work effectively with both transgendered or transsexual clients, and clients who cannot or will not be "compartmentalized" into

---

* With special thanks to Farzana Doctor, the original author of this chapter.

categories or boundaries of specific gender identities. The ability to integrate macro (i.e., social-structural-political) perspectives with micro (i.e., individual clinical) perspectives in providing care can also present challenges to clinicians and treatment services alike.

The clinician may grapple with such questions as:

- What is the difference between gender identity and sexual orientation?
- How can I construct a treatment plan for clients with multiple, co-occurring issues?
- Do I need to be a member of the (lesbian, gay, bisexual, transgendered, transsexual, two-spirit, intersex, queer (LGBTTTIQ) community to work effectively with clients?
- Are certain treatment approaches more relevant for people of varying genders and sexualities?

People working in the addiction treatment field who want to develop and expand their clinical skills may face challenges in understanding specific clients or populations of clients. This can be particularly true for clients who have diverse and wide-ranging gender and sexual identities. Challenges can also arise when trying to translate research findings into clinical practice, as well as in using practice to inform research studies. This chapter shares that knowledge with people working with diverse communities.

Clinicians who work in the substance use field still receive little education and training around working with people from LGBTTTIQ communities. As a result, clinicians may not understand the unique issues, concerns and needs of clients from these communities, and may even stereotype, stigmatize or discriminate against certain clients. Perhaps for this reason, LGBTTTIQ people have historically been underserved by substance use treatment agencies (Craft & Mulvey, 2001; Finlon, 2002; Senreich, 2010).

With higher rates of substance use among LGBTTTIQ people, developing appropriate and relevant services is important. This chapter discusses the unique needs and concerns of LGBTTTIQ people with substance use problems to increase clinicians' understanding, skill and competence in working with these clients. (For definitions of relevant terms, see the glossary at the end of the chapter.)

Prevalence of Substance Use in LGBTTTIQ Communities

Hughes & Eliason (2002), leaders in prevalence research about this population, state that "writing a state of the science paper on substance use among lesbians, gay men, bisexual and transgender (LGBT) persons is a daunting task" (p. 263). They cite many reasons, including:

- lack of research on LGBT communities
- methodological problems in previous research, such as small and non-random samples
- inconsistent definitions of sexual orientation and substance use.

Furthermore, bisexual, transgendered and transsexual people are largely missing from research about substance use. Bisexuals are often either grouped with gays and lesbians, or excluded from analyses due to low numbers. One exception is a large U.S. study that compared drinking habits among bisexual, homosexual and heterosexual groups: 25 per cent of bisexual women reported heavy drinking, the highest rate of any other group in the study, including homosexuals (McCabe et al., 2009). However, overall, more research is needed. Sell and Becker (2001) describe this lack of quality research as "one of the greatest threats to health" for LGBTTTIQ communities (p. 876).

Various studies have found that, overall, LGBTTTIQ communities have disproportionately higher rates of substance use problems. McKirnan and Peterson (1989) compared a large sample of Chicago gays and lesbians with an earlier study of men and women from a general rural and urban population. Among their findings:

- Lesbians were less likely than heterosexual women (15 per cent vs. 35 per cent) to abstain from alcohol, but were more likely to be moderate drinkers (76 per cent vs. 59 per cent). Lesbians and heterosexual women had similar rates of heavy drinking (9 per cent vs. 7 per cent).
- Despite similar rates of heavy drinking, lesbians reported higher rates of alcohol-related problems than heterosexual women (23 per cent vs. 8 per cent).
- Lesbians and gay men had similar rates of marijuana and cocaine use.
- Gays and lesbians showed less age-related decline in alcohol and other drug use than is typical in the general population.
- Gay men were less likely than heterosexual men to abstain from alcohol (13 per cent vs. 23 per cent) and less likely to report heavy drinking (17 per cent vs. 21 per cent), but were more likely to report alcohol-related problems (23 per cent vs. 16 per cent).
- Gay men were more likely than heterosexual men to report lifetime use of marijuana and cocaine, but the two groups did not differ in how frequently they used these substances.
- Gay men and their heterosexual counterparts in the same age group reported different use of substances. For example, gay men over age 35 were more likely to use cocaine frequently.
- 14 per cent of gay men reported using amyl nitrate (poppers) regularly, and 7 per cent reported daily use.

Hughes and Wilsnack (1997), whose study involved lesbian and heterosexual women in Chicago, New York and Minneapolis-St. Paul, reported these findings:

- Lesbians were more likely than heterosexual women to abstain from alcohol (24 per cent vs. 17 per cent), a finding that contrasts with that of McKirnan and Peterson (1989).
- Most lesbians (73 per cent) and heterosexual women (82 per cent) reported light to moderate drinking (fewer than two drinks per day on average).
- Only 3 per cent of lesbians and 1 per cent of heterosexual women reported heavy drinking (more than two drinks per day on average).
- More lesbians than heterosexual women reported participation in 12-step programs (14 per cent vs. 6 per cent).
- The incidence of an age-related decline in drinking, commonly found with heterosexual women, was lower among lesbians.

Hughes and Wilsnack (1997) also found that alcohol use among lesbians may be declining. They suggest that this may be due to increased awareness of health and substance use issues, decreased stigma of gays and lesbians, and changing norms in the gay and lesbian communities.

Aaron and colleagues (2001) compared the prevalence of smoking and alcohol use among lesbians and women in the general population and found that:

- More lesbians than general population women currently smoked (35.5 per cent vs. 20.5 per cent).
- Fewer lesbians than general population women abstained from alcohol (42.5 per cent vs. 55.4 per cent).
- More lesbians than general population women indicated that they drank heavily (4.7 per cent vs. 1.1 per cent).

In a study of circuit parties (dance parties that can attract up to 20,000 mostly gay men) in the San Francisco / Bay Area, Mansergh and colleagues (2001) found that 25 per cent of attendees reported having "overused" drugs, along with engaging in unprotected sex. Clements-Nolle and colleagues (2001) studied male-to-female (MtF) and female-to-male (FtM) transgendered people in San Francisco and found that lifetime use of intravenous drugs was prevalent among both MtF people (34 per cent) and FtM people (18 per cent).

Reback and Lombardi (1999) studied MtF people in West Hollywood, 35 per cent of whom were sex-trade workers, and found that:

- In the past month, 37 per cent reported drinking alcohol, 13 per cent reported marijuana use, 11 per cent reported crack use, 11 per cent reported methamphetamine use, 7 per cent reported cocaine use and 2 per cent reported heroin use.
- More of the sex-trade workers than the general MtF group reported methamphetamine use (21 per cent vs. 5 per cent) and crack use (25 per cent vs. 3 per cent).

Kelly and Parsons (2010) found that prescription drug use was prevalent among men who have sex with men (MSM). They also found that white MSM, HIV-positive MSM, gay-identified MSM and MSM over age 40 are more likely to have recently used a range of prescription drugs than straight men in general.

Various explanations have been suggested for these high prevalence rates. Some people working in the field theorize that while the bar, rave and circuit party cultures in LGBTTTIQ communities are important because they provide safe places to socialize without fear of discrimination, these cultures also normalize substance use (Collins & Howard, 1997; Kauth et al., 2000).

Most, however, explain the higher rates of substance use in LGBTTTIQ communities in relation to the experiences of marginalization and oppression (Doctor, 2003; Ghindia & Kola, 1996; Hughes & Eliason, 2002). It is not being LGBTTTIQ, but rather, coping with oppression that may increase the risk of substance use. These experiences may also cause higher rates of mood and anxiety disorders, and thoughts and plans of suicide (Gilman et al., 2001). New international evidence links high prevalence rates of mental health problems among LGBTTTIQ populations to social stressors (Chakraborty et al., 2011), which make these communities highly vulnerable to substance use problems. With a greater awareness of the concurrence of substance use and mental health problems among the LGBTTTIQ population, interventions should be comprehensive (Swendsen et al., 2010).

Anti-oppression Framework and Cultural Competence

An anti-oppression framework and cultural competence (understanding concepts of gender and sexual orientation and the unique issues that concern LGBTTTIQ communities, specifically societal oppression) are requirements for working well with LGBTTTIQ clients. For example, a recent survey of transgendered people found that the expertise of a gender specialist is important to those who seek help for gender-related issues. Clinicians without updated information about transgender issues and communities were not as helpful (Rachlin, 2002), and in fact, may do harm. Many LGBTTTIQ people may not access care due to fear of stigma and discrimination (Clark et al., 2001).

It is not uncommon for LGBTTTIQ clients to experience oppression in a social service environment (Barbara, 2002; Coalition for Lesbian and Gay Rights in Ontario, 1997). In 1976, after lobbying by gay organizations, psychologists and psychiatrists, the American Psychiatric Association (APA) removed the designation of homosexuality as a sexual deviation from the *Diagnostic and Statistical Manual of Mental Disorders* (DSM). However, gender identity disorder was included in the DSM-IV-TR (APA, 2000), and some LGBTTTIQ organizations argued that the label pathologizes transgendered, transsexual, gender-diverse and gender-variant people (Van Wormer et al., 2000), and lobbied to have it removed. Gender identity disorder has been replaced in the newly released DSM-5 (APA, 2013) by the term "gender dysphoria," which is considered to be a more neutral diagnosis of emotional distress over one's gender. Clients of substance use treatment agencies have reported the following examples of oppression:

- A gay male client at a mainstream residential treatment centre is told not to speak about his sexual orientation because it is not relevant to his substance use, while other clients are encouraged to talk about their relationships and families.
- A preoperative transsexual woman (someone who cannot afford the very costly gender reassignment surgery not covered by her health plan) is asked to wear "masculine" clothing while she is in treatment.
- A lesbian is asked at intake if she is married. When she tells the intake worker that she has a partner, the intake worker asks, "What's his name?"
- A transgendered woman is asked not to sit in the women's lounge of a treatment agency.

LGBTTTIQ people and communities also face societal oppression. "Homophobia," "biphobia" and "transphobia" are terms for overt and covert fear and hatred of gays and lesbians, bisexuals and transgendered and transsexual people, respectively. Examples include derogatory jokes, name calling, bashing and pathologizing. Feinberg (2001) provides an example of transphobia:

Five years ago, while battling an undiagnosed case of bacterial endocarditis, I was refused care at a Jersey City emergency room. After the physician who examined me discovered that I am female bodied, he ordered me out of the emergency room despite the fact that my temperature was above 104 °F (40 °C). He said I had a fever "because you are a very troubled person." . . . Had I died from this illness, the real pathogen would have been bigotry. (pp. 897–898)

Key concepts in understanding oppression

Heterosexism refers to the systemic, or societal, discrimination encountered by gay, lesbian and bisexual people (it is assumed that heterosexuality is the normal and preferred sexual orientation).

Genderism refers to the systemic discrimination encountered by transgendered, transsexual and gender–non-conforming people (it is assumed that the binary construct of gender is preferred and normal). Some examples of heterosexism and genderism include the exclusion of LGBTTTIQ people from marriage and adoption rights, intake and application forms that do not include options other than "M" and "F" or "married" and "single," and lack of resources and services available to these communities.

Heterosexual privilege refers to the unearned and often invisible privileges afforded to those who do not challenge dominant sexual orientation norms. Examples include the privilege to hold hands in public with one's partner without fear of harassment, discrimination or physical violence. Or, when a non-heterosexual moves to a new town or starts a new job, always having to gauge when or whether to come out and to whom. Recent legal victories such as same-sex marriage in Canada have occurred in the last decade; yet stigma and harassment are still very real for many people in the LGBTTTIQ community.

Gender privilege refers to the unearned and often invisible privileges afforded to those who do not challenge dominant gender norms. Examples include being able to use a public bathroom without being challenged by other patrons, and seeking medical care without facing scrutiny about one's gender identity. These privileges, while often invisible to those who receive them, are usually strikingly obvious to those who are not afforded them.

When you think of Abhay, the client whose case scenario begins this chapter, how do you imagine that genderism and heterosexism may have affected his life, and how would you provide care? Recall the multiple forms of oppression Abhay experienced from the trauma of growing up in a heterosexist and transphobic environment; for example,

Abhay was rejected by his family and friends when he came out first as a lesbian. He was also stigmatized as a drug user living with depression. Of equal importance was his experience transitioning from female to male in a world with rigid gender roles. The clinician needs to be empathic and willing to explore whether there is a correlation between Abhay's sexual orientation and/or gender identity and his depression and crystal meth use. The clinician can begin by validating Abhay's experience, challenging the dominant discourse of male/female constructs, and allowing him to reflect on the impact heterosexism and transphobia have had on him and how they are influencing his current substance use and mental health concerns. This kind of exploration can provide a solid foundation to building the therapeutic relationship.

In a society that supports genderism and heterosexism, it can be difficult for us as clinicians to identify and change our own biases. However, we must recognize and challenge our homophobia, biphobia and transphobia to become more competent in this area. Clinicians must also learn more about their local LGBTTTIQ community, and its specific needs, challenges, resources and strengths. To do this, they can:

- access print, electronic and visual media to expand awareness
- attend workshops and conferences on LGBTTTIQ issues
- encourage discussion with colleagues and members of local LGBTTTIQ communities
- reflect on their own pre-existing areas of bias, privilege and marginalization, life experience and history, and assumptions.

LGBTTTIQ communities include people of different ages, races, classes, abilities, rural or urban locations, religions and politics. Although glossy gay magazines tend to depict the LGBTTTIQ community as homogeneous, white, male and affluent (Plumb, 2001), research suggests that gay men may earn less on average than their straight counterparts, and that transgendered and transsexual people, as well as people of colour, tend to face the most employment-related discrimination. The myth of affluence ignores the diversity of LGBTTTIQ communities (Anastas, 2001). LGBTTTIQ clients who are poor, older, of colour or who have disabilities may face double or triple marginalization, and their experiences of being LGBTTTIQ cannot be separated from their other identities.

Appropriate Use of Language

The use of appropriate language and terminology is important when working with members of LGBTTTIQ communities. Because words are often used to oppress marginalized groups, it is key that these groups name themselves rather than be labelled by others. For example, a word such as "homosexual," used to refer to people with same-gender desire, is rarely used by people to refer to themselves (most prefer the terms "gay" or "lesbian") (Broido, 2000). Language issues can be confusing because sometimes terminology changes as a particular group gains strength and voice. For example, some LGBTTTIQ people have reclaimed words such as "queer," "fag" and "dyke" to proudly describe themselves. "Queer" is often used as an umbrella term for all LGBTTTIQ people. A person's decision about how or whether to label himself or herself may be connected to factors such as geographical location, degree of "outness" (openness about sexual orientation), political beliefs and the relative safety of the person's situation, age or culture (Hughes & Eliason, 2002; Liu & Chan, 1996; Savin-Williams, 1996; Stone & Women's Survey Group, 1990). Furthermore, each LGBTTTIQ community uses terminology differently, depending on its size and culture. Given the variety of labels and ways in which people may identify their gender and sexual orientation, it is wise to ask LGBTTTIQ clients how they prefer to be described and identified. This may include asking transgendered, intersex, transsexual and two-spirit clients which gender pronoun(s) they want you to use to refer to them (Pazos, 1999). The glossary at the end of this chapter may be a helpful guide to understanding and using appropriate language.

Gender Identity and Sexual Orientation

To better understand LGBTTTIQ clients, one must first understand key concepts and the meanings of "gender identity" and "sexual orientation."

"Gender identity" refers to how individuals identify and understand their core or innate sense of maleness or femaleness (Mallon, 1999). Society generally views gender as a binary construct, in which people are either male/masculine or female/feminine, with little tolerance for those who conform to neither. Manifestations of this binary construct are found in many cultural norms (e.g., our custom of asking whether a newborn is a boy or a girl). As a result, transgendered, transsexual and intersex people are often pathologized for their gender variance or diversity (Cooper, 1999; Raj, 2002), although some clients may accept a binary construct and reject a more fluid notion of gender. Some transsexuals, for example, who hope to live as the opposite gender, may view gender identity in a more traditional way (Raj, 2002).

An alternative to the binary construct of gender is to view identity as a continuum (Feinberg, 2001) that contemplates genders along a spectrum of gender expression, where particular expressions are not favoured or seen to be normal or abnormal.

This is a challenge for many of us. We are trained from a very young age to understand gender in a rigid, "either/or" way. In the English language, there are no gender pronouns for people who do not see themselves as "he" or "she." But what if we were not to assume that a newborn's genitals would necessarily predict its gender identity? What if a parent said, "I can't wait to see what gender my child becomes"?

Feinberg (1998) has coined the gender neutral pronouns *hir* (pronounced "here") and *sie* (pronounced "see") to replace "him"/"her" and "he"/"she."

"Sexual orientation" is a term for the emotional, physical, sexual and sometimes spiritual attractions a person has for others. This attraction may be experienced through fantasy, desire or behaviour, and may or may not be acted upon. Sexual orientation is distinct from sexual behaviour; the former is a way of identifying attraction and the latter is a way of identifying what we do. For example, a person may be gay, but celibate. A woman may be in a long-term, monogamous relationship with another woman, but consider herself bisexual. Some people may not label their sexual orientation at all. As with gender identity, it can be useful to consider sexual orientation as a continuum, where sexuality is fluid and changeable over time (Broido, 2000).

Sexual orientation is distinct from gender identity, although the two are often confused. A transgendered, transsexual, two-spirit person may identify as heterosexual, gay, lesbian, bisexual, transensual (sexually attracted to a transgendered person) or polysexual. These two dimensions of identity overlap in crucial ways for many LGBTTTIQ people. It is often gender non-conformity that schoolyard bullies identify when they tease a child they perceive to be gay. Identifying where sexual orientation and gender identity intersect is important for many clients. For example, some lesbians identify as "butch," a gender expression that does not conform to gender norms of how women are supposed to look and act. These women, as they "come out" and begin to understand themselves, affirm both same-gender desire and non-conforming gender expression. A transsexual man who, pre-transition, identified as a lesbian, may need, post-transition, to re-evaluate his sexual orientation. Partners of transitioning transsexual people may also face this re-evaluation process themselves in relation to their partner's gender transition.

Figure 25-1 shows the relationships among biological sex, gender identity, gender expression and sexual orientation in the predominant ways most people and cultures have constructed and thought about them (e.g., born female, identify as a woman, dress in "female" clothes, take on gender-specific roles or jobs, attracted to men). This normative construct leaves out many variations. Figure 25-2 illustrates the complexities and interrelations of biological sex, gender identity, gender expression and sexual orientation.

FIGURE 25-1: "Normative" Diagram of Sex, Gender and Attraction

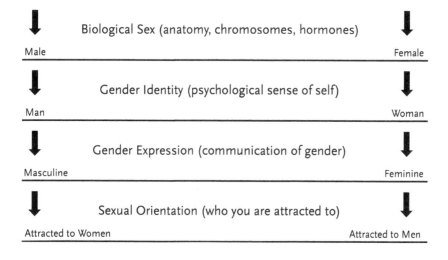

Source: Reprinted with permission from Rebecca Hammond and Jordan Zaitzow.

FIGURE 25-2: Inclusive Diagram of Sex, Gender and Attraction

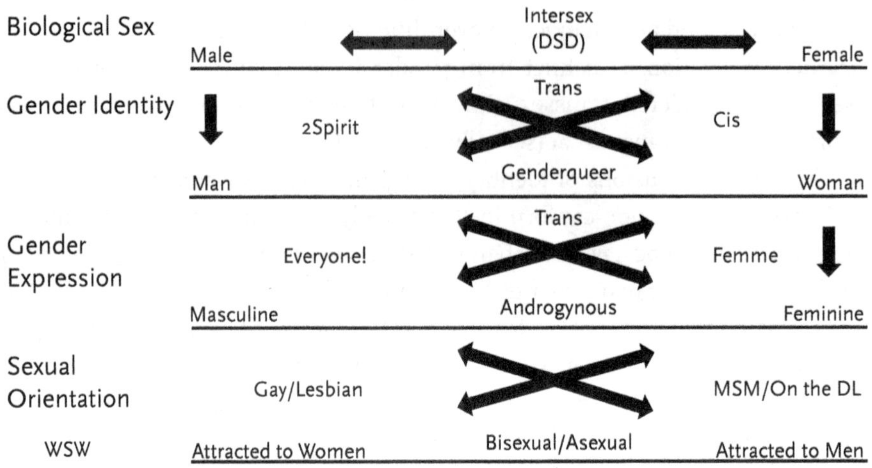

Source: Reprinted with permission from Rebecca Hammond and Jordan Zaitzow.

Unique Issues in Assessment and Treatment

LGBTTTIQ people with substance use issues may share many of the same concerns as the general population. What makes LGBTTTIQ communities distinct is the effect of oppression and the different cultural norms in some of the communities. This section discusses both considerations.

Coming Out

Coming out—or realizing, identifying and disclosing one's "non-normative" gender, sexuality or sexual orientation to oneself or others—is a process, not a destination. Various stage models exist for this process, and have been both embraced for facilitating understanding of a complex process, and criticized for being too simplistic. According to the Cass (1979) model, the beginning of the coming-out process is usually marked by uncertainty or confusion around identity. The process traverses acceptance and pride until, finally, the person integrates their sexual orientation into their overall identity. A person may move back and forth through this process at different times, depending on the situation. Moving to a new neighbourhood, city, job or school may prompt a person to become more out or closeted, depending on the circumstances.

Nearly all LGBTTTIQ people go through this process of coming out; it is unique to each person and is ongoing. "Transitioning" is a term to describe the process transgendered or transsexual people may go through as they begin to express a different gender identity. A transition process may involve a name change, or hormonal, aesthetic or surgical treatments. However, not all transgendered or transsexual people wish to transition:

> While some transgendered individuals desire to "transition" from one sexed body to another by means of hormones, electrolysis and surgery, not all do and fewer still have the economic ability to do so. An increasing number of transgendered individuals are choosing to identify as neither male nor female and are claiming unique contours of sex and gender that offer new and unlimited possibilities. Understanding the nature of these possibilities requires a language that challenges cultural assumptions of sex and gender. The language and literature of transgendered existence is only now emerging as the transgendered community develops and we begin to think beyond the binary of male and female, man and woman, masculine and feminine. (Cooper, 1999, p. 112)

Coming out and community

An important part of coming out is finding a community of other LGBTTTIQ people. Reynolds and Hanjorgiris (2000) write that for gay people, "identification with the gay community has been found to promote understanding of, coping with, and ultimately accepting of a gay identity and behaviour" (p. 42).

Racialized minority LGBTTTIQ people face racism from both mainstream society and LGBTTTIQ communities, and homo/transphobia from their ethnoracial communities (Walters et al., 2001). For those who are negotiating identity development and are from more than one marginalized group, it is important to find communities that recognize and support the intersection of both identities (Duruz, 1999). For example, a Chinese lesbian may find she experiences affirmation for both "parts" of herself in an organization for Chinese lesbians, and a deaf gay man facing ablism from LGBTTTIQ communities and homophobia from a deaf community may find support from a group for LGBTTTIQ people with hearing impairments. If such resources are not available, as is likely in rural areas and smaller centres, web resources such as chat groups and e-mail distribution lists may be good alternatives.

Delaying or choosing not to come out

It is uncertain whether healthy identity development for LGBTTTIQ people depends on being "out" to everyone they know, including family (Van Wormer et al., 2000). There are good reasons to avoid or delay coming out. For some adolescents, coming out while living with their families may mean abuse or a loss of support, as illustrated in this description of the experience of transgendered youth:

> If the child continues to express her/himself outside of the gender expectations into adolescence . . . the interventions become more swift and severe. . . . Parents or guardians take out their own discomfort with gender non-conformity on their child, resulting in strained relations and further isolation of the adolescent. . . . In the event of extreme and/or persistent gender non-conformity, or if youths disclose to their parents that they are transgender, the family may react with extreme behaviours in turn. Physical, emotional and verbal abuse may occur, or the youth might be thrown out of the home. (Burgess, 1999, p. 42)

A young person in this situation might benefit from waiting until he or she is more independent before coming out to parents, and might first seek allies in the family and community to provide a support network.

Some people of colour may choose not to come out to their families for fear of losing an important support that affirms their ethnoracial identity (Fukuyama & Ferguson, 2000). Liu and Chan (1996), referring to the specific cultural context of Asian Americans, state:

> Because Asian Americans' individual identities are so tied to family identity, even if sexuality is not disclosed or openly discussed, the adult daughter or son may still feel very secure and cared for and may not be willing to risk jeopardizing this relationship by coming out. (p. 94)

Racism within the larger society and within LGBTTTIQ communities (Ridge et al., 1999) can make a connection with their family and their ethnoracial community even more important to LGBTTTIQ people of colour (Diaz et al., 2001; Kanuha, 1990).

Interestingly, recent studies suggest there is greater acceptance from families of gay and lesbian people of colour than from families of white gay men and lesbians. Washington (2001) suggests that although the former do not necessarily celebrate their LGBTTTIQ children, fewer families of colour tend to disown their children in these circumstances.

Families and other loved ones of LGBTTTIQ people appear to go through a process themselves during which their attitudes and beliefs change as they become more aware of, and comfortable with, their loved one's coming out. One family response to coming out model includes the following eight stages: repulsion, pity, denial, tolerance, acceptance, support, celebration and activism (Charania & Surani, 2002). Family members may need to come to terms with their loved one's changes and grieve for perceived losses. For example, some parents may initially worry that they won't have grandchildren (even though LGBTTTIQ people can and often do have children). Families of transgendered and transsexual people may also need time to adjust to new pronouns, names and expectations associated with their loved one's transition (Cooper, 1999).

The clinician's role in supporting the coming out process

Clinicians should encourage discussing sexual orientation and gender identity to help clients with the coming out process (Van Wormer et al., 2000). Without such discussion, many clients may not disclose or question their identity (Reynolds & Hanjorgiris, 2000), which may result in care that is not as relevant to them as it could be. To encourage disclosure, clinicians should be "intentionally inclusive," a term used to describe the explicit communication needed to help marginalized clients discuss taboo subjects. One way to be intentionally inclusive is to ask direct questions, in a non-judgmental way, about gender identity and sexual orientation issues.

Asking the Right Questions 2: Talking with Clients about Sexual Orientation and Gender Identity in Mental Health, Counselling and Addiction Settings (Barbara et al., 2007) provides a guide for asking relevant questions. (See "Asking intentionally inclusive questions" sidebar.) The Gay and Lesbian Medical Association ([GLMA], 2002a) has produced a similar guide. Another way to be welcoming to LGBTTTIQ clients is to change agency forms. For example, on an intake form, replace the terms "husband / wife" with "partner." When asking about gender, in addition to "female/male," include "transgendered" or "intersexed." Modify the decor in waiting areas to include a rainbow flag, which has become a symbol of LGBTTTIQ diversity, as well as pamphlets, signs or a poster depicting issues relevant to LGBTTTIQ clients. Unless a clinician is intentionally inclusive, clients may not come out or may feel that the clinician is judgmental or rejecting, or will pathologize their LGBTTTIQ identity.

Asking intentionally inclusive questions

These questions are to be administered by a therapist or counsellor during an assessment interview or early in counselling.

1. Can you tell me about any particular problems you have faced because of discrimination based on your sexual orientation/gender identity?
2. Can you tell me about your coming out and/or transitioning process?*
3. How open are you about your sexual orientation/gender identity? At work? At school? At home? With new acquaintances?
4. Tell me about your family. How has your sexual orientation / gender identity affected your relationship with your family? Do you have support from your family?
5. How are you involved in the LGBTTTIQ communities?
6. Do you have concerns about body image? Do you have concerns about aging? Do body image pressures and ageism in the LGBTTTIQ communities affect you?

---

7. HIV is a big concern for a lot of people. Can you tell me in what ways this may be true for you?

8. Do you use alcohol and/or other drugs to cope with any of these issues we mentioned? Are your mental health concerns related to any of these issues we mentioned? If yes . . . in what ways?

not at all ☐   a little ☐   somewhat ☐   a lot ☐

*Authors' note: You may also choose to ask: At what age did you first realize you were ___? What has it been like for you after coming out or transitioning to yourself and to others?

Source: Barbara et al. (2007). Reprinted with permission.

The clinician can help the client understand the process of coming out by emphasizing its ongoing, developmental nature, and that it is unique for each person. Clients may not understand that it is normal to experience many different feelings during this time, including joy, fear, loss of heterosexual or gender privilege, awkwardness around other LGBTTTIQ people, freedom and anger at societal oppression. On this last point, clinicians should help clients understand that the coming out process is not only a personal issue, but also one that is affected by community and societal oppression. A clinician can play an important role by advocating for a client within the social service agency, or when the client's family, school or community is involved (Burgess, 1999; Reynolds & Hanjorgiris, 2000). Clients may also need help with what Reynolds and Hanjorgiris (2000) call "the process of identity management," in which the clinician helps clients understand how their "identity intersects with and affects other aspects of their life such as career, relationships with family of origin, religion or faith, and coming out to others" (p. 50).

Coming out and substance use

There are many links between coming out and substance use. Most clients we have spoken with about identity development and substance use identify a connection between coming out, internalized oppression and substance use. For example, clients may increase their substance use to cope with feeling different, being closeted or fitting in with other LGBTTTIQ people, or to deal with internalized oppression, fear of rejection or discomfort in sexual situations. Some clients notice that stopping or reducing substance use makes them more conscious of identity issues. Other clients find that their substance use decreases as their identity becomes more integrated. Some clients notice no link between coming out and substance use and may instead connect their substance use to other stressors, such as childhood trauma.

Discrimination and Bashing

LGBTTTIQ people often encounter verbal assaults, violence and other forms of discrimination because they challenge dominant sexual orientation and gender norms (Swigonski, 2001). The harm caused by such encounters can manifest in hypervigilance, fear, lack of trust and decreased self-worth (Walters et al., 2001). However, despite the harm caused by discrimination, LGBTTTIQ people can also develop resilience and strength by living with adversity (Shernoff, 2002). Social activism can be an important strategy for a client who, by creating change, may cope better with oppression (Diaz et al., 2001; Jones, 2002). Counselling that acknowledges the existence of oppression and allows clients to explore its impact is also helpful.

A study of experiences of homophobia, racism and poverty among gay and bisexual Latino men in the United States found links among all three forms of oppression and suicidal thoughts (Diaz et al., 2001). Most striking was the presence of suicidal ideation among those who "as a child heard that gays are not normal" (Diaz et al., 2001, p. 930). Some LGBTTTIQ people may use alcohol and other drugs to feel more empowered when enduring discrimination. For example, a lesbian client who at work encountered daily teasing, put-downs and threats about her lesbian identity would often cope by drinking before and after her shift. Another client with gender identity issues felt more confident in public in masculine clothing, and used amphetamines to make himself less aware of people's reactions to him.

Internalized Oppression

Internalized oppression refers to how people internalize negative messages, beliefs and myths about their identities (Chen-Hayes, 2003; Mascher, 2003). Internalized oppression can affect a person's self-esteem and health, which can result in increased substance use (Cabaj, 2000; Diaz et al., 2001; Hughes & Eliason, 2002). Addressing internalized oppression and teaching clients how to affirm their identity (or identities) may lead to more successful treatment (Craft & Mulvey, 2001). Here are some points to consider when working with LGBTTTIQ clients:

- Internalization of oppression is a normal reaction to societal discrimination. Internalized homophobia, biphobia and transphobia may become apparent through a person's negative statements about, discomfort with or isolation from LGBTTTIQ communities.
- Clinicians, whether they belong to the LGBTTTIQ communities or not, need to be aware of their own heterosexism and genderism when working with clients. Given that oppression is prevalent in society, if a clinician does not have this self-awareness, negative beliefs about LGBTTTIQ people can be easily transferred to the client. This is particularly the case for LGBTTTIQ clinicians who may be seen as role models to clients who are coming out or transitioning.
- Many tools are available for clinicians to help clients understand how these pressures can affect identity. Allan Downs' *The Velvet Rage* (2006) uses a staged model to

capture the pain of growing up gay in a straight world. The first stage, "Overwhelmed by shame," most often occurs in childhood; the child feels, or knows, that he is different from his friends who are perceived as straight and learns to hide his true self to gain acceptance and validation. This leads to internalized anger and rage because he is hiding his authentic self. This is followed by the second stage, "Compensation of shame"; in his quest not to feel inferior, he seeks acceptance and validation by becoming an overachiever or by becoming successful in his personal and professional life. In the final stage, "Discovering authenticity," he has accepted his true self and is able to cultivate relationships and activities that are genuine and fulfilling.

Resolving internalized oppression issues

The clinician can help clients resolve internalized oppression by gently challenging expressions of homophobia, biphobia and transphobia. For example, some effective responses to the statement "Lesbian relationships don't last" might be, "What do you mean when you say that?" "How does that fit with your own experience?" "Where did you learn that?" "Do you think that's true for all lesbians?" A clinician can also disagree, or give examples of LGBTTTIQ people who contradict the client's expressed myth. Boyd and Whitman (2003) provide a list of questions to help clinicians explore the causes of a client's internalized oppression. Bowers (2003) suggests using a technique known as semi-hypnotic visualization to explore internalized negative beliefs. The clinician asks the client to reflect on early memories of hearing homophobic, biphobic or transphobic comments, jokes or descriptions about LGBTTTIQ people and how those experiences shaped his or her sense of self-worth growing up and in the present.

Internalized oppression and multiple marginalization

A client who experiences multiple marginalization may have to integrate several aspects of his or her identity to resolve internalized oppression (Walters et al., 2001). Chen-Hayes (2003) suggests identifying and rating with the client the importance of multiple forms of identity (i.e., social class, citizenship status, disability status, gender) and present and past levels of internalized oppression connected to each. These dimensions are explored in greater detail below.

Body Image

Body image and eating disorders are concerns for LGBTTTIQ people. Negative body image relates to substance use in different ways. Some substances, such as cocaine and crystal methamphetamine, can be used to reduce appetite. Other substances help a person cope with negative perceptions about his or her appearance. It is useful to ask LGBTTTIQ clients to assess how, for them, community and societal pressures, substance use and body image intersect with one another (Barbara et al., 2002).

Some studies suggest that lesbian and bisexual women are less affected by negative body image than heterosexual women and gay men. Explanations for this include:

- an appreciation for larger body sizes
- less concern with appearance
- more satisfaction with their bodies (Kauth et al., 2000; Lakkis et al., 1999).

Yet lesbians, as women, remain affected by societal messages that emphasize the "relentless pursuit of thinness" (Szekely, 1988) and are likely to internalize them to some degree.

Gay and bisexual men face greater body image challenges (Barbara, 2002; Kauth et al., 2000; Lakkis et al., 1999) because of both pressure to conform to the "ideal body" image prevalent in gay culture—that of a young, white, muscular, masculine male (Ayres, 1999)—and internalized homophobia (Pytluk, 2003). LGBTTTIQ people with disabilities may have additional trouble developing a positive self-image because of the stereotype that people with disabilities are asexual (Schneider, 2003).

Ayres (1999) describes his experience as a gay Chinese man in Australia, and how body image pressures have race and age dimensions:

> [The gay bar] is an environment where being physically desirable is closely related to being socially desirable . . . as I became a participant in the gay world, I found myself increasingly influenced by the imagery which determined what was desirable. . . . There is no single Ideal Body. Advertisements are variously filled with blondes, brunettes, Latinos, chunky men, lean men. But the closer you look at what is considered "sexy," "hunky," "desirable," the more you realize that there is a limited range of parts which make up Ideal Bodies. The recurring themes are youth, masculinity and race . . . how can we as Asian men see ourselves as desirable? This is true not only for Asian men, but for all excluded categories: old men, fat men, short men, Aboriginal men. (p. 91)

Research on transgendered and transsexual people and body image is scarce. For some transpeople, eating problems and poor body image may intersect with gender issues (Marone et al., 1998). For example, a large-framed transsexual woman may diet in an attempt to become smaller and conform to the dominant standards of feminine beauty: young, thin, with long hair and a flawless complexion. But transpeople are not that different from non-transpeople when it comes to conforming to societal gender norms. Many women remove facial and body hair, and wear makeup (to appear more "feminine"), and men often work out to achieve a more "masculine" physique (Cooper, 1999).

Despite an overall lack of research, there is some published literature demonstrating that it is possible to build culturally sensitive substance use prevention and treatment for transgendered populations (Lombardi, 2001).

Aging

Older LGBTTTIQ people are largely invisible to mainstream and LGBTTTIQ communities because of society's obsession with youth, and because it is often wrongly assumed that older people are non-sexual (Van Wormer et al., 2000). Penny Coleman's (2000) photodocumentary of older LGBTTTIQ people is an example of this group's efforts to become more visible. It includes an interview with "Gerry," an older lesbian, who describes the ageism in the lesbian community:

> These days, Gerry spends much of her time alone. It's a little quieter than she would like. The last time she walked into a gay bar by herself was to meet some friends on her seventieth birthday. "The whole wall was lined with leather jacketed kids, and I heard somebody say, 'Geez, did you see what just walked in?'" Gerry got off a well-aimed rejoinder, but it stuck and it stopped her. . . . "But really, the only difference between me now and me thirty years ago is I ain't getting laid. Go find me another ninety-year-old lesbian who wants to go to bed with me! That's my problem now." (pp. 4–5)

According to a report from the 519 Church Street Community Centre in Toronto, which serves LGBTTTIQ communities, services for older adults, including LGBTTTIQ-positive housing, geriatric care and social activities need great improvement (Harmer, 2000). The report also suggested that LGBTTTIQ organizations include older LGBTTTIQ people in leadership roles and advocate efforts to change how the community views, recognizes and celebrates its elders. When working with LGBTTTIQ older adults who have substance use concerns, it is important to be aware of the issues of ageism and invisibility. Do they affect the ability of older adults to access appropriate services and supports? Do they identify any impact on self-esteem? In what ways does substance use help them cope with ageism and invisibility?

HIV/AIDS

Research into HIV/AIDS and its risk factors has focused mostly on men who have sex with men (MSM), a term that includes:
- gay or bisexual men
- men who may not identify as gay or bisexual but who engage in same-gender sex
- transgendered and transsexual people who identify as male and who have sex with other men (Hughes & Eliason, 2002).

HIV/AIDS affects both those infected and their loved ones (Kauth et al., 2000; Van Wormer et al., 2000). Highly active antiretroviral therapy (HAART) has decreased HIV/AIDS–related mortality, but it is costly and the side-effects make it difficult to maintain (Wolitski et al., 2001). The availability of these medications may also lead some MSM to believe they can be less vigilant about safer-sex behaviour.

In recent years, an increasing number of people have been charged and convicted for not telling a sexual partner that they are HIV positive. While this is not an issue unique to LGBTTTIQ people, it is something to consider when having conversations about sex with clients—either individually or in group sessions (confidentiality within LGBTTTIQ groups is discussed below). The clinician's place of employment should implement policies and procedures to address situations where clients who are HIV positive disclose risky behaviours (e.g., unprotected sex with other clients). Some situations may warrant a "duty to warn" (e.g., reporting a client to public health), but this needs to be weighed against breaking a client's confidentiality. More often, the clinician can talk directly to clients, reminding them of legal precedents (which indicate the need for HIV-positive people to disclose their status before engaging in high-risk behaviours), or facilitate conversations between clients and their partners, thus maintaining client confidentiality.

Safer Sex and Substance Use

Studies with MSM have shown that substance use often precedes unsafe sex (Calzavara et al., 2003; Halkitis & Parsons, 2002). In a Washington, DC–based survey of MSM, 66 per cent of men reported having had sex while under the influence of alcohol or other drugs during the previous year, and 58 per cent stated they were more likely to engage in unprotected sex when drinking (District of Columbia Department of Health & Whitman-Walker Clinic, 2002). The respondents also reported using the following substances:

- alcohol (79 per cent)
- poppers (amyl nitrate) (39 per cent)
- marijuana (30 per cent)
- ecstasy (28 per cent).

Substance use also helps gay and bisexual men and transpeople cope with the loss, due to HIV/AIDS, of others in their social and support networks; it can also help people cope with an uncertain HIV status or a new diagnosis (Halkitis & Parsons, 2002).

Substance use plays a role in HIV infection in transgendered and transsexual people as well. Because HIV risk increases with sex work, the transgendered and transsexual people who do this work (due to limited job options and employment discrimination) are at greater risk (Clements-Nolle et al., 2001; Hughes & Eliason, 2002; Reback & Lombardi, 1999). Namaste (1999), in her study of female-to-male people in Quebec, found that many did not believe they were at risk for HIV/AIDS. However, she did find that in areas of Quebec where new needles were not readily available (for the injection of hormones), there was a higher HIV rate in the female-to-male population.

In our clinical experience, lesbian and bisexual women report not being affected by HIV/AIDS, but they do discuss the impact of caring for or losing gay and bisexual male friends with the disease. There is a perception that lesbians are at a low risk for HIV/AIDS because woman-to-woman contact has not shown conclusive risks of transmission.

However, sexual orientation does not necessarily match with sexual behaviour; some lesbians and bisexual women have had or do have sex with men. Some may use injection drugs, which can also increase their risk (Kauth et al., 2000).

More recent studies have begun to address the gap in research about the transgender community and the intersection of risky sexual behaviour and substance use. Operario and colleagues (2005) highlight that within these communities, cultural minorities such as Asian Pacific Islanders are at even greater risk.

See Chapters 4 and 7 for more discussion about HIV/AIDS and other blood-borne diseases.

Family Issues

The role of the family is often different for LGBTTTIQ people than for heterosexual or gender-conforming people, and presents different issues.

Coping with estrangement, alienation and rejection from one's family of origin after coming out or transitioning can cause distress. Fear of rejection may cause some LGBTTTIQ people to avoid disclosure (Barbara, 2002). This may also be true when already "out" LGBTTTIQ people raised in adoptive families are reunited with their biological families.

Substance use may help one cope with this distress. From our clinical experience, some clients find that a visit (or even anticipation of a visit) with a homophobic, transphobic or biphobic family member who seems not to accept them can trigger substance use. Relapse prevention planning and education about boundaries can help a client resist turning to substance use in these circumstances. Family therapy may also be appropriate (Anderson, 1996). If this is not possible, a "chosen family" (a close network of, for example, friends, ex-partners, lovers and some biological family members) may provide much-needed support (Siegel & Walker, 1996). Parents and Families of Lesbians and Gays (PFLAG) offers support to families coming to terms with loved ones' gender identity or sexual orientation, and has chapters all over North America. Although couples therapy is often not considered in traditional substance use treatment due to heterosexist bias (Anderson, 1996), it can be appropriate because it addresses issues of trust, intimacy and support; it may also be useful for a couple where one or both partners are reducing or stopping substance use, or to investigate whether the substance use of one partner has influenced the other to use (Hughes & Eliason, 2002).

While the role of family is increasingly being recognized as an important component in recovery, incorporating the "family" or "chosen family" into treatment is often overlooked in addiction settings. This oversight is occurring despite significant evidence that family involvement plays an important role in recovery. CRAFT (community reinforcement and family training approach) is one model in which including family or "chosen family" in treatment improves outcomes (Meyers et al., 2005).

For Abhay, who was presented in this chapter's opening case scenario, offering sessions to him and his family of origin may not be realistic or desirable, given the family's unwillingness to accept Abhay's sexual orientation and subsequent gender transition. However, collaborating with Abhay's chosen family creates the potential to build care teams that reinforce behavioural changes Abhay can make when he leaves clinical care and returns to the community.

LGBTTTIQ people are also affected by issues involving children, including:

- having children and/or coming out to them (Van Wormer et al., 2000)
- beginning a relationship with someone with a child or children (Hollingsworth & Didelot, 2003)
- coping with societal discrimination toward LGBTTTIQ parents and their children (McLean, 2003).[1]

Sexuality

Substance use may help men and women feel less inhibited about same-gender sexual activity. Lesbians and bisexual women are more likely to use alcohol for this purpose, whereas gay and bisexual men are more likely to use drugs such as:

- methamphetamine (to increase sexual potency)
- amyl nitrate (poppers) (to prolong orgasm and relax the anal sphincter)
- Viagra (to enhance sexual performance) (Hughes & Eliason, 2002).

Gay social venues such as community events, dances, bathhouses, circuit parties, sex clubs and dance clubs, while providing havens from homophobia, normalize substance use. The link between sexuality and substance use in these venues is problematic because, as discussed earlier, there is a higher risk of unprotected sex. These are often also sexualized environments, where LGBTTTIQ people flirt, cruise or have sex (Barbara, 2002; Halkitis & Parsons, 2002).

LGBTTTIQ people in urban centres might have a range of other social venues available to them (e.g., sports, social, support, spiritual and hobby groups), and it is important to encourage clients to explore these alternatives (Cooper, 1999). But many clients choose to socialize at venues where substance use occurs; these venues are central to LGBTTTIQ communities, and their historical importance as the "first gay community centres" lives on. The clinician can help the client develop a plan to avoid high-risk behaviours at these venues. This plan might include:

- learning and exercising refusal skills
- going with a "buddy"
- going late and leaving early to reduce exposure to triggers
- taking very little money to avoid impulsive substance use.

Some clients also use substances to relieve shyness or discomfort with their bodies (physical pain or poor body image) or to block intrusive traumatic imagery (related to past sexual abuse) during sex. A number of lesbian clients we have worked with who

---

1 The LGBT Parenting Network, created in 2002, provides a newsletter, activities and a website dedicated to these issues. Visit http://familypride.uwo.ca.

had had heterosexual relationships reported that they first used substances while having non-pleasurable heterosexual sex, hoping this would improve the experience. These women were later unable to break the habit when having pleasurable sex with women.

Intersex children, who often have scarred, insensitive or painful genitals as a result of intrusive surgeries, can have difficulty exploring their sexuality. Support groups, where intersex people can meet others with similar experience, can help (Cooper, 1999).

Like their gender-conforming queer counterparts, transgendered and transsexual people (and their sexualities) have been portrayed as exotic, repulsive or immoral through pornography and popular media (Cooper, 1999). For them, forging a healthy sex life requires examining and challenging internalized transphobia. With more and more transgendered and transsexual clients presenting for service, it is vitally important that we understand the distinction between sexual orientation and gender identity.

Clinicians, too, should consider the messages they have internalized about sexuality in general and LGBTTTIQ sexualities in particular. Most of us have personal beliefs about what types of sexual behaviour are "normal." These beliefs are socially constructed, and challenging them is necessary when working with the diversity of human sexuality. Ask yourself how you feel about non-monogamy or S/M (sado-masochism), or how you would react to seeing two men kissing on the street? Where did you learn these beliefs, and how do you think they might affect your work with clients? Our beliefs about sexuality are likely a creation of our social norms, which in many cases (and not just in relation to sexuality) tend to marginalize those who do not fit within them.

A careful psychosocial assessment should be provided to support the client around interpersonal relationships if this is a concern for him or her; the assessment could include determining both the client's strengths and areas that may require further discussion and support. In Abhay's case, the therapist could support him around issues of disclosing or not disclosing his trangendered identity, as this is clearly triggering and anxiety-provoking when Abhay is seeking sexual partners.

Creating LGBTTTIQ-Positive Spaces and Services

In order to make a social service organization more welcoming to LGBTTTIQ clients, it is helpful to assess its overall sensitivity to LGBTTTIQ people. The organization should have:
- LGBTTTIQ-positive policies and procedures
- an environment that communicates LGBTTTIQ related policies
- forms that are LGBTTTIQ positive
- services (both generic and LGBTTTIQ specific) that acknowledge the needs of LGBTTTIQ communities
- staff who are LGBTTTIQ positive and trained in LGBTTTIQ issues, or who are out themselves

- community outreach activities and support local celebrations and Pride
- LGBTTTIQ representation on program advisory committees and boards.

Policies and Procedures

The organization's policies and procedures should:
- be sufficiently specific to and inclusive of LGBTTTIQ people
- stipulate how to address discrimination from staff and clients
- communicate to staff the expected code of conduct.

Physical Space

The office, group rooms, agency hallways and waiting areas can communicate to marginalized people that they are in a safe and sensitive environment. You can do this by:
- putting up posters that communicate anti-oppression and appreciation of diversity
- displaying pamphlets, magazines and newspapers from diverse communities in waiting areas
- installing unisex bathrooms in your organization (GLMA, 2002a).

LGBTTTIQ-Positive Forms

Heterosexist and genderist questions on intake forms (e.g., "Are you married?" or those that limit gender to "M" and "F") communicate very quickly to LGBTTTIQ clients that they are not welcome. Ensure that your forms encourage clients to disclose their sexual orientation and gender identity.[2]

Services

LGBTTTIQ-specific services

For some clients, LGBTTTIQ-specific services are more appropriate than generic services (Hicks, 2000; Senreich, 2010). Group counselling can help LGBTTTIQ clients address life issues and transitions, behaviour change and the intersection of substance use with coming out, internalized oppression and other issues mentioned in this chapter (Gillespie & Blackwell, 2009). LGBTTTIQ-specific groups create an environment in which people feel safe addressing these issues (Debord & Perez, 2000; Barbara, 2002). Without these specific services, clients attending generic programs might "closet" themselves; they might avoid discussing personal issues or lie about a same-gender partner (Cullen, 2004). In smaller communities, there may not be enough people to offer an

2 See *Asking the Right Questions 2* (Barbara et al., 2007) and *MSM: Clinician Guide to Incorporating Sexual Risk Assessment in Routine Visits* (GLMA, 2002b) for more information about creating LBGTTTIQ-positive intake forms.

LGBTTTIQ group. Depending on the comfort level of the client, individual counselling may be the best alternative, or group facilitators must provide a "safe space" for clients to participate in a generic group.

Confidentiality issues, particularly with LGBTTTIQ-specific groups, need to be considered further. The nature and realities of smaller, more tight-knit, LGBTTTIQ communities and sexual networks may factor into discussions, group dynamics, boundaries and confidentiality issues among participants and between participants and professionals. For example, if Abhay is in an LGBTTTIQ-specific group, he may have had sex with someone else in the group, "chatted" to another group member on an Internet site or used drugs with another member. Seeing that person in the group may be triggering or may prevent the person from fully disclosing. Confidentiality outside the group could also be compromised regardless of group guidelines around this.

Safer Generic Groups

Clinicians can make their generic or mixed groups safer for all marginalized groups, including LGBTTTIQ clients, by being intentionally inclusive. For example, during a first session, when guidelines and group norms are discussed, the clinician can review some common differences among people (the group can generate a list through brainstorming or a pairs exercise) and remind clients that discriminatory remarks will not be tolerated. The facilitator might begin a session on a specific topic by reminding clients that the discussion will include diverse experiences and opinions. A discussion about relationship issues, for example, could start with a reference to the variety of relationships that exist, including opposite-gender and same-gender relationships; this reference invites clients to raise issues and sets a group norm of openness to, and affirmation of, difference.

Clinicians should address and challenge discriminatory remarks as they arise during groups (Bush & Sainz, 2001). They can do this by:
- asking clients to clarify the meaning of statements
- reminding them of group guidelines
- asking group members to share their feelings about the statements being made.

A clinician who does not address discriminatory statements lowers the safety level of the group. However, a therapy group with a particular purpose such as addiction treatment is not the place to process one member's long-held prejudicial attitudes. Turning the group's focus away from its purpose in order to devote multiple sessions to homophobia may only further alienate the LGBTTTIQ member from the rest of the group. You can often control behaviour in a group, but attitudes and prejudice require much longer interventions. Therefore, it is essential that anti-discrimination policies be backed with consequences for a person who makes the group unsafe. Depending on the circumstance, removing that person is often the best clinical intervention if the situation presents an ongoing issue.

In the example of Abhay, part of the treatment plan may involve referring him to a generic skills group. Let's say that in the course of group, Abhay outs as a transgendered man while disclosing his triggers for substance use, and one male group member reacts by calling him a freak. The clinician then intervenes, reminding the group of the discrimination policy. Discussion then ensues, as Abhay tries to explain his identity, family and community rejection. After some time, the clinician gently brings the group back to the triggers discussion. However, the offending client continues to mumble under his breath, staring angrily at Abhay for the rest of the session. The clinician faces this conundrum:

If you remove the offending client, do you lose an opportunity because that client, through the group, may be in contact with an LGBTTTIQ person for the first time in his life? This contact could help reduce the client's ignorance and prejudicial feelings as he gets to know Abhay as a human being struggling with issues of addiction similar to his.

If you allow the offending client to stay (depending on the behaviour), do you run the risk of Abhay dropping out of service because he feels unsafe? You can see the complexity of this scenario. There is no easy answer. A culturally competent clinician may ask to speak separately with Abhay and the client after the group has ended or during a requested group break. Always meet first with the person who has experienced the discrimination to ensure he or she is okay. Tell the person that you will not tolerate any forms of homophobia, biphobia or transphobia, and that the purpose of the group is to provide peer support, not reinforce past traumatic events. You may also wish to check in with Abhay mid-week. Then meet with the offending client, outline the anti-discrimination rules of the group or agency, and emphasize that those comments and behaviours will not be tolerated. Perhaps the client has never met an LGBTTTIQ person before, or is unwilling to challenge his own prejudices, and a referral to another group or agency may be the only alternative. The overriding principle, however, must always be emotional and physical safety for all members in the group.

LGBTTTIQ-Positive, -Trained and Out Staff

We are often asked if non-LGBTTTIQ clinicians should work with the community. The answer is an absolute *yes*! Being an ally to communities that are oppressed and face discrimination is a significant way to change how society functions. It does require more effort than simply being well meaning. Clinicians who wish to work with the community (including clinicians who are LGBTTTIQ) need anti-heterosexism and anti-genderism training, as well as information about LGBTTTIQ communities. Such training can be facilitated in various ways:

- Ask (and pay) local LGBTTTIQ groups to help train your staff.
- Subscribe to journals and listservs that keep your staff up to date (see the Resources section for ideas).
- Recruit LGBTTTIQ staff to work at your organization, listening carefully to them and seeking their advice, and encourage all staff to be LGBTTTIQ positive.

- Become allies to LGBTTTIQ staff, making it safe for them to come out to other staff and clients; don't expect them to do all the work to make your organization LGBTTTIQ-positive.
- Ensure that human resources forms and practices are not genderist and heterosexist (Clark et al., 2001).
- Ensure that staff, whether LGBTTTIQ or not, are comfortable talking about sex, sexuality and drugs. Self-reflection exercises may be a helpful way for staff to examine their own attitudes and values.

Outreach

Outreach is crucial to ensure the involvement of LGBTTTIQ people from the wider community. Consider in your outreach plan:
- where and how you advertise your services
- whether your flyers indicate that LGBTTTIQ people are welcome and that your services reflect their needs
- contacting LGBTTTIQ services and groups in your area by accessing a local paper, listserv or community bulletin board, or leaving flyers in bars or coffee shops
- participating and, if possible, hosting LGBTTTIQ community events in a way that is visible and meaningful
- involving past clients who are LGBTTTIQ (either as volunteers or as paid peer models) to do outreach to the community
- reaching out or even providing basic counselling through LGBTTTIQ-specific websites and forums. LGBTTTIQ people are often quite familiar with using technology to connect with others. For example, some gay men rely on phone apps to find romantic or sexual partners, rather than meeting in bars or other traditional social venues. Some HIV/AIDS organizations have had staff provide outreach and education in Internet chat rooms.

LGBTTTIQ Representation

Without the participation of LGBTTTIQ communities, your other efforts, such as policy development, service provision and outreach, may not be successful (Feinberg, 2001). Make sure you have LGBTTTIQ staff and community members involved in:
- hiring committees
- strategic planning
- other decision making.

Conclusion

Throughout this chapter, we have explored the unique experiences of LGBTTTIQ communities: discrimination, societal and internalized oppression; the decision about whether to come out or transition, and the stress of this process for the person and sometimes the family. We have also addressed the preoccupation with body image and "passing" (a transgendered or transsexual person's ability to be accepted as his or her preferred gender) and how aging is perceived within these communities, the impact of HIV/AIDS and the effect of substance use on safer sex practices. We have also discussed the specialized clinical skills required to provide culturally competent addiction assessment and counselling to this population, using the case example of Abhay.

As LGBTTTIQ communities continue to mobilize and be empowered, people will expect services that are culturally sensitive and inclusive. A clinician does not need to be an expert in the field to work with this population, build a therapeutic alliance and commit to ongoing training and education in this area.

Practice Tips

- Educate yourself about the unique experiences of LGBTTTIQ clients, and appreciate that each client has a unique lived experience based on his or her social location (e.g., age, gender, race).
- Provide a welcoming and inclusive setting for LGBTTTIQ clients.
- Ask clients about discrimination, oppression, family, community involvement, HIV and intimate relationships; do not wait for them to tell you.
- Learn about the unique issues that LGBTTTIQ clients bring to the counselling relationship, whether or not you are a member of this community yourself, and approach clients without judgment: this openness is essential to fostering trust and building a therapeutic alliance.
- Use individual and/or group counselling sessions as an opportunity to examine the implications of these new identities. The process and decision about whether to come out or transition is often stressful for both the person and the family, so counselling can be helpful.

Glossary

The discourse around LGBTTTIQ issues and the definitions in this glossary will change over time. Changes in thinking and attitudes toward sexual orientation and gender identity are continually taking place in society as a whole and within LGBTTTIQ communities. These terms and definitions are not standardized and may be used differently by different people and in different regions.

Asexual: a person who is not sexually and/or romantically active, or not sexually and/or romantically attracted to other persons.

Autosexual: a person whose significant sexual involvement is with oneself, or a person who prefers masturbation to sex with a partner.

Biphobia: irrational fear or dislike of bisexuals. Bisexuals may be stigmatized by heterosexuals, lesbians and gay men.

Bisexual: a person whose sexual orientation is directed toward men and women, though not necessarily at the same time.

Coming out: the process by which LGBTTTIQ people acknowledge and disclose their sexual orientation or gender identity, or in which transsexual or transgendered people acknowledge and disclose their gender identity to themselves and others (see also "Transition"). Coming out is thought to be an ongoing process. People who are "closeted" or "in the closet" hide the fact that they are LGBTTTIQ. Some people "come out of the closet" in some situations (e.g., with other gay friends) and not in others (e.g., at work).

Crossdresser: a person who dresses in the clothing of the other sex for recreation, expression or art, or for erotic gratification. Formerly known as "transvestites," crossdressers may be male or female, and can be straight, gay, lesbian or bisexual. Gay/bisexual male crossdressers may be "drag queens" or female impersonators; lesbian/bisexual female crossdressers may be "drag kings" or male impersonators.

Dyke: traditionally used as a derogatory term for lesbians. Other terms include lezzie, lesbo, butch, bull dyke and diesel dyke. Many women have reclaimed these words and use them proudly to describe their identity.

Fag: traditionally used as a derogatory term for gay men. Other terms include fruit, faggot, queen, fairy, pansy, sissy and homo. Many men have reclaimed these words and use them proudly to describe their identity.

Family of choice: the circle of friends, partners, companions and perhaps ex-partners with which many LGBTTTIQ people surround themselves. This group gives the support, validation and sense of belonging that is often unavailable from the person's family of origin.

Gay: a person whose primary sexual orientation is to members of the same gender or who identifies as a member of the gay community. This word can refer to men and women, although many women prefer the term "lesbian."

Gender conforming: abiding by society's gender rules, e.g., a woman dressing, acting, relating to others and thinking of herself as feminine or as a woman.

Gender identity: a person's own identification of being male, female or intersex; masculine, feminine, transgendered or transsexual. Gender identity most often corresponds with one's anatomical gender, but sometimes people's gender identity doesn't directly correspond to their anatomy. Transgendered people use many terms to describe their gender identities, including pre-op transsexual, post-op transsexual, non-op transsexual, transgenderist, crossdresser, transvestite, transgendered, two-spirit, intersex, hermaphrodite, fem male, gender blender, butch, manly woman, diesel dyke, sex radical, androgynist, female impersonator, male impersonator, drag king, drag queen, etc.

Genderqueer: this very recent term was coined by young people who experience a very fluid sense of both their gender identity and their sexual orientation, and who do not want to be constrained by absolute or static concepts. Instead, they prefer to be open to relocate themselves on the gender and sexual orientation continuums.

Gender role: the public expression of gender identity. Gender role includes everything people do to show the world they are male, female, androgynous or ambivalent. It includes sexual signals, dress, hairstyle and manner of walking. In society, gender roles are usually considered to be masculine for men and feminine for women.

Gender transition: the period during which transsexual people begin changing their appearance and bodies to match their internal identity.

Genderism: the belief that the binary construct of gender, in which there are only two genders (male and female), is the most normal, natural and preferred gender identity. This binary construct does not include or allow for people to be intersex, transgendered, transsexual or genderqueer.

Hate crimes: offences that are motivated by hatred against people based on their actual or perceived race, colour, religion, national origin, ethnicity, gender, disability or sexual orientation.

Heterosexism: the assumption, expressed overtly or covertly, that all people are or should be heterosexual. Heterosexism excludes the needs, concerns and life experiences of lesbian, gay and bisexual people, while it gives advantages to heterosexual people. It is often a subtle form of oppression that reinforces silence and invisibility for lesbian, gay and bisexual people.

Heterosexual: a person whose primary sexual orientation is to members of the opposite gender. Heterosexual people are often referred to as "straight."

Heterosexual privilege: the unrecognized and assumed privileges that people have if they are heterosexual. Examples of heterosexual privilege include holding hands or kissing in public without fearing threat, not questioning the normalcy of your sexual orientation, raising children without fears of state intervention or worries that your children will experience discrimination because of your heterosexuality.

Homophobia: irrational fear, hatred, prejudice or negative attitudes toward homosexuality and people who are gay or lesbian. Homophobia can take overt and covert, as well as subtle and extreme, forms. Homophobia includes behaviours such as jokes, name-calling, exclusion and gay bashing.

Homosexual: a person whose primary sexual orientation is to members of the same gender. Most people prefer to not use this label, preferring to use other terms, such as gay or lesbian.

Internalized homophobia: fear and self-hatred of one's own sexual orientation that occurs for many lesbians and gay men as a result of heterosexism and homophobia. Once lesbians and gay men realize they belong to a group of people that is often despised and rejected in our society, many internalize and incorporate this stigmatization, and fear or hate themselves.

Intersex: a person who has some mixture of male and female genetic and/or physical sex characteristics. Formerly called "hermaphrodites," many intersex people consider themselves to be part of the trans community.

Lesbian: a female whose primary sexual orientation is to other women or who identifies as a member of the lesbian community.

LGBTTTIQ: a common acronym for lesbian, gay, bisexual, transsexual, transgendered, two-spirit, intersex and queer individuals and communities. This acronym may or may not be used in a particular community. For example, in some places, the acronym LGBT (lesbian, gay, bisexual and transgendered/transsexual) is more common. Sometimes a second "Q" is added to represent "questioning" (people who are unsure of their identity). Also, "two-spirit" is often represented as "2-S."

MSM: any man who has sex with a man, whether he identifies as gay, bisexual or heterosexual. This term highlights the distinction between sexual behaviour and sexual identity (i.e., sexual orientation). A person's sexual behaviour may manifest itself into a sexual identity, but the reverse is not always true; sexual orientation does not always reflect sexual behaviour. For example, a man may call himself heterosexual, but may engage in sex with men in certain situations (e.g., prison, sex work).

Out, or Out of the closet: varying degrees of being open about one's sexual orientation or gender identity.

Passing: transgendered or transsexual people's ability to be accepted as their preferred gender. The term refers primarily to acceptance by people the person does not know, or who do not know the person is transgendered or transsexual. Typically, passing involves a mix of physical gender cues (e.g., clothing, hairstyle, voice), behaviour, manner and conduct when interacting with others. Passing can also refer to hiding one's sexual orientation, as in "passing for straight."

Polysexual: an orientation that does not limit affection, romance or sexual attraction to any one gender or sex, and that further recognizes there are more than two sexes.

Queer: traditionally, a derogatory and offensive term for LGBTTTIQ people. Many LGBTTTIQ people have reclaimed this word and use it proudly to describe their identity. Some transsexual and transgendered people identify as queers; others do not.

Questioning: people who are questioning their gender identity or sexual orientation and who often choose to explore options.

Sexual behaviour: what people do sexually. Sexual behaviour is not necessarily congruent with sexual orientation or sexual identity.

Sexual identity: one's identification to self (and others) of one's sexual orientation. Sexual identity is not necessarily congruent with sexual orientation or sexual behaviour.

Sexual minorities: people who identify as LGBTTTIQ.

Sexual orientation: emotional, physical, romantic, sexual and spiritual attraction, desire or affection for another person. Examples include heterosexuality, bisexuality and homosexuality.

Straight: often used to describe people who are heterosexual.

Transgendered: a person whose gender identity is different from his or her biological sex, regardless of the status of surgical and hormonal gender reassignment processes. Often used as an umbrella term to include transsexuals, transgenderists, transvestites (crossdressers), and two-spirit, intersex and transgendered people.

Transgenderist: someone who is in between being a transsexual and a transgendered person on the gender continuum, and who often takes sex hormones, but does not want genital surgery. Transgenderists can be born male (formerly known as "she-males") or born females (once called "he/shes"). The former sometimes obtain breast implants and/or have electrolysis.

Transition: the process (which for some people may also be referred to as the "gender reassignment process") whereby transsexual people change their appearance and bodies to match their internal (gender) identity, while living their lives full time in their preferred gender role.

Transphobia: irrational fear or dislike of transsexual and transgendered people.

Transsensual: a person who is primarily attracted to transgendered or transsexual people.

Transsexual: a person who has an intense long-term experience of being the sex opposite to his or her birth-assigned sex and who typically pursues a medical and legal transformation to become the other sex. There are transmen (female-to-male transsexuals) and transwomen (male-to-female transsexuals). Transsexual people may undergo a number of procedures to bring their body and public identity in line with their self-image, including sex hormone therapy, electrolysis treatments, sex reassignment surgeries and legal changes of name and sex status.

Transvestite: see "Crossdresser."

Two-spirit: an English term coined to reflect specific cultural words used by First Nations and other indigenous peoples for those in their cultures who are gay, lesbian, transgendered or transsexual, or who have multiple gender identities. The term reflects an effort by First Nations and other indigenous communities to distinguish their concepts of gender and sexuality from those of western LGBTTTIQ communities. Two-spirit may also be represented as "2-S" in acronyms (e.g., LGBTT2-SIQ).

WSW: a term that refers to any woman who has sex with a woman, whether she identifies as lesbian, bisexual or heterosexual. This term highlights the distinction between sexual behaviour and sexual identity (i.e., sexual orientation). For example, women who identify as lesbian can also have sex with men, and not all WSW identify as lesbian or bisexual.

Resources

Publications

Barbara, A.M., Chaim, G. & Doctor, F. (2007). *Asking the Right Questions 2: Talking with Clients about Sexual Orientation and Gender Identity in Mental Health, Counselling and Addiction Settings.* Toronto: Centre for Addiction and Mental Health. Retrieved from http://knowledgex.camh.net/amhspecialists/screening_assessment/assessment/arq2/Pages/default.aspx

Guss, J.R. & Drescher, J. (2000). *Addictions in the Gay and Lesbian Community.* Binghamton, NY: Haworth Medical Press.

Lev, A.I. (2004). *Transgender Emergence: Therapeutic Guidelines for Working with Gender-Variant People and Their Families.* New York: Routledge.

Mallon, G. (1998). *Foundations of Social Work Practice with Lesbian and Gay Persons.* Binghamton, NY: Haworth Press.

Internet

AIDS Committee of Toronto
  www.torontovibe.com
International Advisory Council for Homosexual Men and Women in Alcoholics Anonymous
  www.iac-aa.org
Substance Abuse and Mental Health Services Administration—lesbian, gay, bisexual and transgender section
  www.samhsa.gov/obhe/lgbt.aspx
U.S. National Association of Gay and Lesbian Addiction Professionals
  www.nalgap.org

References

Aaron, D.J., Markovic, N., Danielson, M.E., Honnold, J.A., Janoky, J.E. & Schmist, N.J. (2001). Behavioural risk factors for disease and preventative health practices among lesbians. *American Journal of Public Health, 91,* 972–975.

American Psychiatric Association (APA). (2000). *Diagnostic and Statistical Manual of Mental Disorders* (4th ed., text rev.). Washington, DC: Author.

American Psychiatric Association (APA). (2013). *Diagnostic and Statistical Manual of Mental Disorders* (5th ed.). Washington, DC: Author.

Anastas, J.W. (2001). Economic rights, economic myths, and economic realities. *Journal of Gay and Lesbian Social Services, 13* (1/2), 99–116.

Anderson, S.C. (1996). Addressing heterosexist bias in the treatment of lesbian couples with chemical dependency. In J. Laird & R. Green (Eds.), *Lesbians and Gays in Couples and Families* (pp. 316–340). San Francisco: Jossey-Bass.

Ayres, T. (1999). China doll—the experience of being a gay Chinese Australian. *Journal of Homosexuality, 36* (3/4), 87–97.

Barbara, A.M. (2002). Substance abuse treatment with lesbian, gay and bisexual people: A qualitative study of service providers. *Journal of Gay and Lesbian Social Services, 14* (4), 11–17. Retrieved from http://knowledgex.camh.net/amhspecialists/screening_assessment/assessment/arq2/Pages/default.aspx

Barbara, A.M., Chaim, G. & Doctor, F. (2007). *Asking the Right Questions 2: Talking with Clients about Sexual Orientation and Gender Identity in Mental Health, Counselling and Addiction Settings.* Toronto: Centre for Addiction and Mental Health.

Bowers, R. (2003). Semihypnotic visualization: Treating internalized homophobia in sexual and gender minorities. In J. Whitman & C. Boyd (Eds.), *The Therapist's Notebook for Lesbian, Gay and Bisexual Clients* (pp. 20–24). New York: Haworth Clinical Practice Press.

Boyd. C. & Whitman, J. (2003). Who told me that? Challenging internalized homophobic messages. In J. Whitman & C. Boyd (Eds.), *The Therapist's Notebook for Lesbian, Gay and Bisexual Clients* (pp. 56–59). New York: Haworth Clinical Practice Press.

Broido, E.M. (2000). Constructing identity: The nature and meaning of lesbian, gay and bisexual identities. In R.M. Perez, K.A. Debord & K.J. Bieschke (Eds.), *Handbook of Counseling and Psychotherapy with Lesbian, Gay and Bisexual Clients* (pp. 13–34). Washington, DC: American Psychological Association.

Burgess, C. (1999). Internal and external stress factors associated with the identity development of transgendered youth. *Journal of Gay and Lesbian Social Services. 10* (3/4), 35–47.

Bush, I.R. & Sainz, A. (2001). Competencies at the intersection of difference, tolerance, and prevention of hate crimes. *Journal of Gay and Lesbian Social Services, 13* (1/2), 205–224.

Cabaj, R. (2000). Substance abuse, internalized homophobia, and gay men and lesbians: Psychodynamic issues and clinical implications. *Journal of Gay and Lesbian Psychotherapy, 3,* 5–24.

Calzavara, L., Burchell, A.N., Remis, R.S., Major, C., Corey, P., Myers, T. et al. (2003). Delayed application of condoms is a risk factor for Human Immuno-deficiency Virus infection among homosexual and bisexual men. *American Journal of Epidemiology, 157,* 210–217.

Cass, V.C. (1979). Homosexual identity development: A theoretical model. *Journal of Homosexuality, 4,* 219–235.

Chakraborty, A., McManus, S., Brugha, T.S., Bebbington, P. & King, M. (2011). Mental health of the non-heterosexual population of England. *British Journal of Psychiatry, 198,* 143–148.

Charania, G. & Surani, T. (2002). *Rewriting the Script Discussion Guide.* Toronto: Equity Logistics.

Chen-Hayes, S. (2003). Challenging multiple oppressions with GLBT clients. In J. Whitman & C. Boyd (Eds.), *The Therapist's Notebook for Lesbian, Gay and Bisexual Clients* (pp. 20–24). New York: Haworth Clinical Practice Press.

Clark, M.E., Landers, S., Linde, R. & Sperber, J. (2001). The GLBT Health Access Project: A state-funded effort to improve access to health care. *American Journal of Public Health, 91,* 895–896.

Clements-Nolle, K., Marx, R., Guzman, R. & Katz, M. (2001). HIV prevalence, risk behaviors, health care use, and mental health status of transgender persons: Implications for public health intervention. *American Journal of Public Health, 91,* 915–921.

Coalition for Lesbian and Gay Rights in Ontario. (1997). *Systems Failure: A Report on the Experiences of Sexual Minorities in Ontario's Health-Care and Social-Services System.* Toronto: Author. Retrieved from www.rainbowhealthontario.ca/home.cfm

Coleman, P. (2000). *Village Elders.* Chicago: University of Illinois Press.

Collins, B. & Howard, B. (1997). Working with lesbians and gay men. In S. Harrison & V. Carver (Eds.), *Alcohol & Drug Problems: A Practical Guide for Counsellors* (2nd ed., pp. 293–318). Toronto: Addiction Research Foundation.

Cooper, K. (1999). Practice with transgendered youth and their families. *Journal of Gay and Lesbian Social Services, 10* (3/4), 111–129.

Craft, E.M. & Mulvey, K.P. (2001). Addressing lesbian, gay, bisexual and transgender issues from the inside: One federal agency's approach. *American Journal of Public Health, 91,* 889–891.

Cullen, J. (2004). *Understanding the experiences of gay men in addiction treatment: A phenomenological study.* Unpublished doctoral dissertation, University of Toronto, Toronto, Ontario.

Debord, K.A. & Perez, R.M. (2000). Group counseling theory and practice with lesbian, gay, and bisexual clients. In R.M. Perez, K.A. Debord & K.J. Bieschke (Eds.), *Handbook of Counseling and Psychotherapy with Lesbian, Gay and Bisexual Clients* (pp. 183–206). Washington, DC: American Psychological Association.

Diaz, R.M., Ayala, G., Bein, E., Henne, J. & Marin, B. (2001). The impact of homophobia, poverty, and racism on the mental health of gay and bisexual Latino men: Findings from 3 US cities. *American Journal of Public Health, 91,* 927–932.

District of Columbia Department of Health & Whitman-Walker Clinic. (2002). *Men Who Have Sex with Men (MSM), Survey Results 2001.* Washington, DC: Author.

Doctor, F. (2003). Examining links between drug and alcohol use and experiences of homophobia/biphobia and coming out. In J. Whitman & C. Boyd (Eds.), *The Therapist's Notebook for Lesbian, Gay and Bisexual Clients* (pp. 262–267). New York: Haworth Clinical Practice Press.

Downs, A. (2006). *The Velvet Rage: Overcoming the Pain of Growing Up Gay in a Straight Man's World.* Cambridge, MA: Da Capo Press.

Duruz, A. (1999). Sister outsider, or "just another thing I am": Intersections of cultural and sexual identities in Australia. *Journal of Homosexuality, 36* (3/4), 87–97.

Feinberg, L. (1998). *Trans Liberation: Beyond Pink or Blue.* Boston: Beacon Press.

Feinberg. L. (2001). Trans health crisis: For us it's life or death. *American Journal of Public Health, 91,* 897–900.

Finlon, C. (2002). Health care for all lesbian, gay, bisexual and transgender populations. *Journal of Gay and Lesbian Social Services, 14* (3), 109–116.

Fukuyama, M.A. & Ferguson, A.D. (2000). Lesbian, gay and bisexual people of colour: Understanding cultural complexity and managing multiple oppressions. In R.M. Perez, K.A. Debord & K.J. Bieschke (Eds.), *Handbook of Counseling and Psychotherapy with Lesbian, Gay and Bisexual Clients* (pp. 81–106). Washington, DC: American Psychological Association.

Gay and Lesbian Medical Association (GLMA). (2002a). *Creating a Safe Clinical Environment for Lesbian, Gay, Bisexual, Transgender and Intersex (LGBTI) Patients.* Retrieved from www.glma.org

Gay and Lesbian Medical Association (GLMA). (2002b). *MSM: Clinician Guide to Incorporating Sexual Risk Assessment in Routine Visits.* Retrieved from www.glma.org

Ghindia, D.J. & Kola, L.A. (1996). Co-factors affecting substance abuse among homosexual men: An investigation within a midwestern gay community. *Drug and Alcohol Dependence, 41,* 167–177.

Gillespie, W. & Blackwell, R.L. (2009) Substance use patterns and consequences among lesbians, gays, and bisexuals. *Journal of Gay and Lesbian Social Services, 21* (1), 90–108.

Gilman, G.E., Cochran, S.D., Mays, V.M., Hughes, M., Ostow, D. & Kessler, R.C. (2001). Risk of psychiatric disorders among individuals reporting same-sex sexual partners in the National Comorbidity Survey. *American Journal of Public Health, 91,* 933–939.

Halkitis, P.N. & Parsons, J.T. (2002). Recreational drug use and HIV risk sexual behaviour among men frequenting gay social venues. *Journal of Gay and Lesbian Social Services, 14* (4), 19–38.

Harmer, J. (2000). *Older Gay, Bisexual, Transgender, Transsexual Persons; Community Services Challenges and Opportunities for the 519 Community Centre and the GLBT Community. A Review.* Toronto: The 519 Community Centre.

Hicks, D. (2000). The importance of specialized treatment programs for lesbian and gay patients. *Journal of Gay and Lesbian Psychotherapy, 3,* 81–94.

Hollingsworth, L.A. & Didelot, M.J. (2003). Coming out of marriage: Developing an emerging gay, lesbian, or bisexual identity. In J. Whitman & C. Boyd (Eds.), *The Therapist's Notebook for Lesbian, Gay and Bisexual Clients* (pp. 50–55). New York: Haworth Clinical Practice Press.

Hughes, T.L. & Eliason, M. (2002). Substance use and abuse in lesbian, gay, bisexual and transgender populations. *Journal of Primary Prevention, 22,* 263–298.

Hughes, T.L. & Wilsnack, S.C. (1997). Use of alcohol among lesbians: Research and clinical implications. *American Journal of Orthopsychiatry, 67,* 20–36.

Jones, T. (2002). Characteristics of a group of lesbian and gay radical street activists. *Journal of Gay and Lesbian Social Services, 14* (4), 39–54.

Kanuha, V. (1990). Compounding the triple jeopardy: Battering in lesbian of color relationships. In L.S. Brown & M.P. Root (Eds.), *Diversity and Complexity in Feminist Therapy* (pp. 169–184). New York: Harrington Park Press.

Kauth, M., Hartwig, M. & Kalichman, S. (2000). Health behavior relevant to psychotherapy with lesbian, gay and bisexual clients. In R.M. Perez, K.A. Debord & K.J. Bieschke (Eds.), *Handbook of Counseling and Psychotherapy with Lesbian, Gay and Bisexual Clients* (pp. 435–456). Washington, DC: American Psychological Association.

Kelly, B.C. & Parsons, J.T. (2010). Prevalence and predictors of non-medical prescription drug use among men who have sex with men. *Addictive Behaviors, 35,* 312–317.

Lakkis, J., Ricciardelli, L.A. & Williams, R.J. (1999). Role of sexual orientation and gender-related traits in disordered eating. *Sex Roles, 41* (1/2), 1–16.

Liu, P. & Chan, C.S. (1996). Lesbian, gay and bisexual Asian Americans and their families. In J. Laird & R. Green (Eds.), *Lesbians and Gays in Couples and Families* (pp. 137–152). San Francisco: Jossey-Bass.

Lombardi, E. (2001). Enhancing transgender health care. *American Journal of Public Health. 91,* 869–872.

Mallon, G.P. (1999). Knowledge for practice with transgendered persons. *Journal of Gay and Lesbian Social Services, 10* (3/4), 1–17.

Mansergh, G., Colfa, G.N., Marks, G., Rader, M., Guzman, R. & Buchbinder, S. (2001). The Circuit Party Men's Health Survey: Findings and implications for gay and bisexual men. *American Journal of Public Health, 91,* 953–958.

Marone, P., Iacoella, S., Cecchini, M.G. & Ravenna, A.R. (1998). An experimental study of body image and perception in gender identity disorders. *International Journal of Transgenderism, 2* (3). Retrieved from www.wpath.org/journal/www.iiav.nl/ezines/web/IJT/97-03/numbers/symposion/ijtco501.htm

Mascher, J. (2003). Overcoming biphobia. In J. Whitman & C. Boyd (Eds.), *The Therapist's Notebook for Lesbian, Gay and Bisexual Clients* (pp. 78–83). New York: Haworth Clinical Practice Press.

McCabe, E.S, Hughes, T.L., Bostwick, W.B., West, B.T. & Boyd, C.J. (2009). Sexual orientation, substance use behaviors and substance dependence in the United States. *Addiction, 104,* 1333–1345.

McKirnan, D.J. & Peterson, P.L. (1989). Alcohol and drug use among homosexual men and women: Epidemiology and population characteristics. *Addictive Behaviours, 14,* 545–553.

McLean, Ron. (2003). Family care planning for gay, lesbian, bisexual and transgendered parents: Creating healthy living environments for adults and children. In J. Whitman & C. Boyd (Eds.), *The Therapist's Notebook for Lesbian, Gay and Bisexual Clients* (pp. 249–255). New York: Haworth Clinical Practice Press.

Meyers, R.J., Smith, J.E. & Lash, D.N. (2005). A program for engaging treatment-refusing substance abusers into treatment: CRAFT. *International Journal of Behavioral Consultation and Therapy, 1,* 90–100.

Namaste, V. (1999). HIV/AIDS and female to male transsexuals and transvestites: Results from a needs assessment in Quebec. *International Journal of Transgenderism, 3* (1/2), 1030–1033.

Operario, D., Nemoto, T., Ng, T., Syed, J. & Mazrai, M. (2005). Conducting HIV interventions for Asian Pacific Islander men who have sex with men: Challenges and compromises in community collaborative research. *AIDS Education and Prevention, 17,* 334–346.

Pazos, S. (1999). Practice with female-to male transgendered youth. *Journal of Gay and Lesbian Social Services, 10* (3/4), 65–82.

Plumb, M. (2001). Undercounts and overstatements: Will the IOM Report on lesbian health improve research? *American Journal of Public Health, 91,* 873–875.

Pytluk, S.D. (2003). Body as self: Resolving body image disturbances in gay men. In J. Whitman. & C. Boyd (Eds.), *The Therapist's Notebook for Lesbian, Gay and Bisexual Clients* (pp. 215–219). New York: Haworth Clinical Practice Press.

Rachlin, K. (2002). Transgender individuals' experiences of psychotherapy. *International Journal of Transgenderism, 6* (1). Retrieved from www.wpath.org/journal/www.iiav.nl/ezines/web/IJT/97-03/numbers/symposion/ijtvoo6noo1_03.htm

Raj, R. (2002). Towards a transpositive therapeutic model: Developing clinical sensitivity and cultural competence in the effective support of transsexual and transgendered clients. *International Journal of Transgenderism, 6* (2). Retrieved from www.wpath.org/journal/www.iiav.nl/ezines/web/IJT/97-03/numbers/symposion/ijtvoo6noo2_04.htm

Reback, C.J. & Lombardi, E.L. (1999). HIV risk behaviors of male-to-female transgenders in a community-based harm reduction program. *International Journal of Transgenderism, 3* (1/2).

Reynolds, A.L. & Hanjorgiris, W.F. (2000). Coming out: Lesbian, gay and bisexual identity development. In R.M. Perez, K.A. Debord & K.J. Bieschke (Eds.), *Handbook of Counseling and Psychotherapy with Lesbian, Gay and Bisexual Clients* (pp. 35–55). Washington, DC: American Psychological Association.

Ridge, D., Hee, A. & Minichiello, V. (1999). "Asian" men on the scene: Challenges to the "gay communities." *Journal of Homosexuality, 36* (3/4), 43–68.

Savin-Williams, R.C. (1996). Self-labeling and disclosure among gay, lesbian and bisexual youths. In J. Laird & R. Green (Eds.), *Lesbians and Gays in Couples and Families* (pp. 153–183). San Francisco: Jossey-Bass.

Schneider, K. (2003). An alphabet of GLBT and disability issues. In J. Whitman & C. Boyd (Eds.), *The Therapist's Notebook for Lesbian, Gay and Bisexual Clients* (pp. 262–267). New York: Haworth Clinical Practice Press.

Sell, R.L. & Becker, J.B. (2001). Sexual orientation data collection and progress toward healthy people 2010. *American Journal of Public Health, 91,* 876–882.

Senreich, E. (2010). Are specialized LGBT program components helpful for gay and bisexual men in substance abuse treatment? *Substance Use & Misuse, 45,* 1077–1096.

Shernoff, M. (2002). Terrorist attacks in America: Impact on queer clients and clinicians. *Journal of Gay and Lesbian Social Services, 14* (3), 95–102.

Siegel, S. & Walker, G. (1996). Connections: Conversations between a gay and straight therapist. In J. Laird & R. Green (Eds.), *Lesbians and Gays in Couples and Families* (pp. 316–340). San Francisco: Jossey-Bass.

Stone, S.D. & the Women's Survey Group. (1990). Lesbian life in a small centre: The case of St. John's. In S.D. Stone (Ed.), *Lesbians in Canada* (pp. 94–105). Toronto: Between the Lines.

Swendsen, J., Conway, K.P., Degenhardt, L., Glantz, M., Jin, R., Merikangas, K.R. et al. (2010). Mental disorders as risk factors for substance use, abuse and dependence: Results from the 10-year follow-up of the National Comorbidity Survey. *Addiction, 105,* 1117–1128.

Swigonski, M.E. (2001). Human rights, hate crimes and Hebrew-Christian Scripture. *Journal of Gay and Lesbian Social Services, 13* (1/2), 33–46.

Szekely, E. (1988). *Never Too Thin.* Toronto: Women's Press.

Van Wormer, K., Wells, J. & Boes, M. (2000). *Social Work with Lesbians, Gays and Bisexuals.* Toronto: Allyn and Bacon.

Walters, K.L., Simoni, J.N. & Horwath, P.F. (2001). Sexual orientation bias experiences and service needs of gay, lesbian, bisexual, transgendered, and two-spirited American Indians. *Journal of Gay and Lesbian Social Services, 13* (1/2), 133–149.

Washington, P. (2001). Who gets to drink from the fountain of freedom? Homophobia in communities of colour. *Journal of Gay and Lesbian Social Services, 13* (1/2), 1117–1131.

Wolitski, R.J., Valdiserri, R.O., Denning, P.H. & Levine, W.C. (2001). Are we headed for a resurgence of an HIV epidemic among men who have sex with men? *American Journal of Public Health, 91,* 883–888.

SECTION 5

PROFESSIONAL PRACTICE AND SYSTEM ISSUES

Chapter 26

Legal Issues

Robert M. Solomon and Sydney J. Usprich

Without question, the legal environment has become more challenging for all professionals in the last 35 years. Thus, it is not surprising that health care professionals are increasingly being sued, and called upon in disciplinary hearings and other legal contexts to explain and justify their conduct. There has been a parallel trend toward recognizing and protecting the legal rights of clients, especially those who are young. Legal issues will continue to play a greater role in the working lives of all health care professionals, including those in the substance use field. This chapter aims to help substance use workers understand the basic legal principles governing assessment and treatment.

In addition to the legal issues inherent in any treatment relationship, several complicating factors can arise in the substance use field. First, some clients only reluctantly enter treatment, in response to a probation order or at the insistence of an employer, spouse, parent or registrar of motor vehicles. What impact do such pressures have on your legal obligations to the client?

Second, some clients may be under the provincial age of majority, yet still have the legal capacity to give a valid consent to treatment. It may sometimes be difficult to determine whether an underage client is competent to consent to the proposed treatment. Assuming that a client is competent to consent, how should you respond to inquiries about the case from parents, school officials, welfare workers or the police?

Third, the use of alcohol and other drugs frequently involves conduct that is not only illegal, but which also may endanger the client and others. Do you have any legal obligation to inform the police of a client's criminal activities? Moreover, can you be held civilly liable for failing to warn third parties of the dangers posed by a client?

Such issues arise because substance use treatment often cuts across the criminal justice, health care, child welfare, education and employment systems. Rather than provide an exhaustive legal analysis of these systems and their possible effects on treatment, this chapter focuses on basic legal principles governing treatment relationships and explains their special application to substance use workers.

Equally, we do not have the space to review the relevant statutes and cases in every jurisdiction in Canada. Consequently, the body of this chapter outlines the major principles, while the References section points to more specific principles. The exact legal rules vary from jurisdiction to jurisdiction, reflecting differences in provincial case law and statutes.

The first section of this chapter examines the law governing consent to treatment, counselling and care. A brief discussion of liability in negligence is provided in the second section. The third section examines confidentiality, disclosure, reporting obligations and the duty to warn.

Consent to Treatment, Counselling and Care

Introduction to Consent Issues

One hallmark of our legal system is the importance it attaches to the protection of a person's physical integrity. Whether couched in terms of physical inviolability, autonomy, self-determination or privacy, the principle is the same—namely, a person's right to control his or her own body. However, this concept is a double-edged sword, in that the law protects the individual's right to decide, whether the person's decision is wise or foolish.

Virtually any physical interference with another person may result in both criminal liability (*Criminal Code*, s. 265(1)) and civil liability.[1] In the absence of consent, the defendant will be held liable unless he or she can legally justify the interference on some other ground. In these situations, however, treatment professionals are rarely charged with a criminal offence. Rather, the issue of consent typically arises in determining whether the health care professional has a valid defence to a civil action for the tort (wrongful act) of battery.

Battery is defined as intentionally bringing about a harmful or socially offensive physical contact with another person (see, for example, *Bettel v Yim*, 1978). Merely touching a client may give rise to liability; he or she need not suffer any physical injury. Any surgical procedure, administration of drugs or treatment involving physical contact may constitute battery. Once the client establishes that physical contact occurred, the burden of proof shifts to the professional to establish a valid defence (*Non-marine Underwriters, Lloyd's of London v Scalera*, 2000). If the defendant cannot prove that the client consented or that there is another defence, the defendant will be held liable for all the consequences of the battery. In most cases, the key issue is not whether physical contact occurred, but whether the clinician can establish the defence of consent.

The legal principles governing the defence of consent have developed almost exclusively from cases involving surgery and other physical interventions. However, the tort of battery is also relevant to substance use treatment programs that include physical examinations, taking blood samples, administering drugs or other physical contact. Treatment that involves only the taking of a history, questionnaires, counselling or similar non-physical interactions cannot give rise to a battery claim. Nonetheless, the issue of consent and the principles governing it are still relevant in these situations.

---

1 Depending on the facts, a physical interference can give rise to one or more civil actions in tort: battery (physical contact), assault (threat of immediate physical contact) and false imprisonment (imposition of a total restraint of movement).

General Principles of Consent

Several provinces and territories have enacted statutes governing specific aspects of consent to treatment, counselling and care (see, for example, Ontario's *Health Care Consent Act, 1996*, ss. 10–11; and British Columbia's *Health Care (Consent) and Care Facility (Admission) Act*, ss. 4–6). However, in the absence of applicable statutory provisions to the contrary, the relationship between health care professionals and their clients is governed by the common law principles of consent, which are summarized below.

As a general rule, a treatment professional must obtain consent for any test, procedure, surgery, counselling or physical examination. Consent should be obtained in advance, and should cover the intervention, as well as any related issues regarding record keeping, confidentiality, reporting obligations and other disclosures of information. The consent must relate to the specific treatment or counselling undertaken (*Parmley v Parmley and Yule*, 1945; *Schweizer v Central Hospital*, 1974). If the client is competent to give a valid consent, then his or her consent alone is required (*C. v Wren*, 1986; *Starson v Swayze*, 2003; *Hughes Estate v Hughes*, 2007). The consent of the next-of-kin is relevant only if the client is not competent to give consent. Even then, the validity of a substitute consent is limited (*Re Superintendent of Family & Child Services and Dawson*, 1983; *"Eve" v "Mrs. E.,"* 1986).

To be valid, consent must be given voluntarily. However, the concept of volition is defined broadly, and rests on whether the client's decision was the product of his or her conscious mind (*Smith v Stone*, 1647; *Gilbert v Stone*, 1648). For example, clients who reluctantly consent to drug treatment because it is a term of probation, or because they have been threatened with being fired from a job or expelled from school, will still be held to have consented "voluntarily" (*Deacon v Canada (Attorney General)*, 2006).

A client may consent implicitly or explicitly (*Strachan v Simpson*, 1979; *O'Bonsawin v Paradis*, 1993; *Battrum v British Columbia*, 2009). The fact that a client comes for treatment provides a broad measure of implicit consent. Clients may seek treatment for alcohol or other drug problems, and yet expressly limit the scope of their consent. A substance use worker may refuse to treat the client if these limitations are unreasonable. However, the worker cannot ignore or override the client's stated prohibitions (*Mulloy v Hop Sang*, 1935; *Malette v Shulman*, 1990).

Informed Consent: Battery or Negligence?

Traditionally, a health practitioner's failure to obtain a valid consent was viewed as a basis for a battery action, whether the lack of consent was due to a failure to disclose the risks or to misrepresentation. Consistent with American practice, the Canadian courts began to analyze some medical consent cases in terms of negligence: Has the doctor failed to exercise a reasonable standard of care in advising the patient of the nature of the procedure and its risks? As in the United States, this development created uncertainty as to the boundary between medical battery and medical negligence.

The Supreme Court of Canada resolved this issue in two 1980 cases (*Reibl v Hughes* and *Hopp v Lepp*), holding that once patients are aware of the general nature of the treatment, they cannot bring a battery action alleging that they were not informed of the risks. Rather, battery actions are limited to cases in which the patient did not consent at all, the consent was exceeded or the consent was obtained fraudulently. In all other cases, the plaintiff must bring a negligence action for failure to obtain an informed consent. By requiring a plaintiff to frame these actions in negligence, the Supreme Court significantly limited the scope of health professionals' potential liability.

Exceptions to General Principles of Consent

The courts have relaxed the strict requirements of consent in three situations. First, in an unforeseen medical emergency where it is impossible to obtain the patient's consent, a health professional is allowed to operate without consent to preserve the patient's health or life (*Marshall v Curry*, 1933; *Murray v McMurchy*, 1949). This right is granted to health care professionals in order to save lives. This is the basis upon which emergency room staff are permitted to operate on unconscious accident victims.

The second exception involves clients who have given a general consent to a course of therapy, treatment program or operation. In such situations, a client will be viewed as implicitly consenting to any subordinate tests, procedures or interventions that are necessarily incidental to the broader course of treatment (*Male v Hopmans*, 1967; *Villeneuve v Sisters of St. Joseph*, 1971). However, this implied consent will be negated if the client objects. While it may not be legally necessary, it is prudent to obtain a specific consent for any subordinate procedures that pose significant risks or involve sensitive sexual, legal or emotional issues.

Third, the courts at one time permitted health care professionals to withhold information from a client if the disclosure would undermine the client's morale or discourage him or her from having needed treatment (*Kenny v Lockwood*, 1932; *Male v Hopmans*, 1967). However, consistent with the increased emphasis on patients' rights, the courts have rejected or narrowed this "therapeutic privilege" doctrine. For example, the judge in *Meyer Estate v Rogers* (1991) stated that the doctrine is no longer part of Ontario law. In *Pittman Estate v Bain* (1994), the court acknowledged that the therapeutic privilege to withhold information continues to exist, but defined it very narrowly. Health care professionals do have some discretion, but it is best viewed as being limited to how they inform clients, the technical matters they discuss and the emphasis they place on the relative risks of undergoing versus forgoing treatment.

Consent Forms and the Burden of Proof

Unless a statute states otherwise, a client may give consent orally or in writing. Since the client's presence provides some measure of implied consent, it is not legally necessary to obtain written consent for routine treatment sessions. However, it is wise to obtain written consent for treatment that involves significant risks, is complex or innovative, or entails potentially sensitive legal, sexual or emotional issues. Similarly, written consent is recommended if the client is immature, unstable or lacks good judgment. Based on these criteria, it would be prudent for substance use workers to obtain written consent at the outset of the treatment relationship. Moreover, many agencies require staff to obtain a signed consent to initiate any counselling or treatment.

A signed consent form provides only some evidence of consent, not conclusive proof. The key legal issue is not whether a client signed a consent form, but rather whether he or she understood the nature of the proposed treatment and its risks, benefits and alternatives. In other words, was the client given sufficient information to make an informed decision, and did he or she consent to the treatment? A signed consent form is only as good as the information it contains and the circumstances in which it is presented to the client. A signed consent form is of little value if:

- it is written in technical language that the client cannot understand
- it is presented as a mere technicality
- there is no opportunity to read it
- it is written in general language that did not identify the specific treatment and its risks
- the client's questions were not adequately answered
- the client was in severe pain, intoxicated or drugged when signing it.

Competency or Capacity to Consent

The terms "competency" and "capacity" are often used synonymously, but practice in this regard varies. To be valid, a consent must be given by a client who is legally competent. The general test of competency is whether the client can understand the information relevant to making an informed decision and appreciate the reasonably foreseeable consequences of that decision. The test of competency relates to the ability to comprehend information, not to the ability to make a prudent decision.

A client may be competent to make some decisions, but not others. Similarly, a client may be competent to make a certain decision one day, but not the next. Finally, the law presumes that all individuals are competent, unless there is clear evidence to the contrary (*Re C (Adult: refusal of medical treatment)*, 1994). This very low threshold test is applied on a case-by-case basis.

As stated earlier, if the client is competent to consent, then his or her consent alone is relevant. Indeed, it would be inappropriate even to discuss a client's treatment with the next-of-kin without the client's consent, because this would involve a breach of confidence. Consequently, the assessment of a client's competency to consent is a critically important preliminary issue.

Minors
General principles
The age of majority varies across Canada. Moreover, this legislation typically does not govern the age of consent to treatment. In the absence of a statute to the contrary, the test of competency is the same whether the client is a minor or an adult. Generally, the court will assess whether the client understands the proposed treatment and its risks, benefits and alternatives, and appreciates the consequences of having or forgoing it. If a minor meets this test, then his or her consent is valid and parental consent is unnecessary (*Walker (Litigation Guardian of) v Region 2 Hospital Corp.*, 1994). In some jurisdictions, the issue is framed in terms of whether the person is a "mature minor" and the courts rely on indications of independence as a guide to this determination (*Re Dueck*, 1999). As the following case illustrates, Canadian courts increasingly recognize the right of young people to make their own treatment decisions.

In *C. v Wren* (1986), the plaintiffs sought an injunction to prevent a doctor from performing an abortion on their 16-year-old daughter. As was then required by the *Criminal Code*, the daughter had obtained approval from a therapeutic abortion committee. The court sympathized with both the parents and their daughter in this "painful dispute" over the ethics of the proposed abortion. However, the legal issue was clear: Could this 16-year-old girl give a valid consent to a therapeutic abortion? The court concluded that the daughter understood the nature of the procedure and its risks, and therefore was competent to give a valid consent. Consequently, the parents' application for an injunction was dismissed.

Statutory age-of-consent provisions
The general test of competency applies unless a statute states otherwise. In any one jurisdiction, several statutes may impose age-of-consent requirements for specific types of treatment. For Ontario examples, see the *Trillium Gift of Life Network Act*, s. 3 and the *Child and Family Services Act* (CFSA), ss. 27, 28 & 132. Since this chapter cannot review all the relevant legislation in each province, the Ontario *CFSA* is used to illustrate the operation of the statutory provisions.

The *CFSA* applies only to specified service providers, which include the Minister of Community and Social Services, approved agencies, children's aid societies and licensees (s. 3(1)). The Act is also limited to stipulated services, including child development, child treatment, child welfare, community support and young offender services (ss. 3(1), 88 & 89). Thus, the *CFSA*'s age-of-consent provisions do not apply to treatment provided under the *Health Care Consent Act, 1999*, such as substance use counselling from a psychologist in the outpatient clinic of a public hospital. In contrast, a social worker providing identical counselling in an approved agency would be subject to the *CFSA*'s provisions.

The *CFSA* establishes different age requirements for consent, depending on the type of service or counselling in question:

- A person 16 years or older may consent, without parental knowledge or approval, to any services or care (s. 27(1)).
- A person under age 16 needs parental consent for residential care services (s. 27(2)) or the administration of psychotropic drugs (s. 132).
- A child 12 years or older may consent to counselling services without parental knowledge or consent. However, if the person is younger than 16, the counsellor must advise the person that it is desirable to involve his or her parents (s. 28).

In *A.C. v Manitoba (Director of Child and Family Services)* (2009), the Supreme Court of Canada held that statutory age provisions must comply with the requirements of the *Canadian Charter of Rights and Freedoms*. The provision must take increasing account of a young person's views in accordance with his or her maturity. Moreover, a child's maturity must be assessed individually, having regard to the nature of the treatment and the severity of the potential consequences.

Summary

Unless a statute states otherwise, minors can give a valid consent to alcohol and other drug treatment. The key issue is whether the minor is capable of understanding the proposed treatment and its risks. If the minor meets this test of competency, the consent of the parent or guardian is not required. As in Ontario, several provincial statutes may impose age-of-consent requirements for certain limited types of treatment. The end result is that the age of consent to substance use treatment is governed by a complex tangle of common law and statutory provisions that vary from province to province. However, the trend is to recognize that young people can make their own treatment, counselling and care decisions if they have the ability to understand the relevant information and appreciate the consequences of their decisions.

Adults

The general test of competency is the same whether the client is a minor or an adult. The principles apply equally to those in custody or under other legal restraints, unless there is express statutory authority to the contrary (*Attorney General of British Columbia v Astaforoff*, 1984; *Attorney General of Canada v Notre Dame Hospital*, 1984). If the person is competent, his or her consent to treatment must be obtained. Although a client's refusal to consent to treatment may constitute a breach of probation or a violation of parole, that does not alter the treatment worker's obligation to abide by the client's decision.

The issue of an adult's competency may also arise in cases involving mental illness or dementia. However, the mere fact that a client is, for example, mentally ill does not mean he or she is incapable of giving a valid consent. Rather, clinicians must assess each client's ability to understand the proposed treatment and its risks. Although this principle is easy to state, it may be difficult to apply in many situations, such as that of an occasionally disoriented person with a severe alcohol problem (*Starson v Swayze*, 2003; *Neto v Klukach*, 2004; *Isber v Zebrowski*, 2009).

One area that has caused confusion is the role of health care professionals in treating people suspected of impaired driving. Although this issue is more relevant to hospital emergency staff than to substance use workers, a brief summary of the current law follows. Health care professionals must refuse police requests to take blood samples or conduct other tests on unwilling or unconscious suspects for enforcement purposes. These situations must be distinguished from medical emergencies in which it is impossible to obtain the suspect's consent. In such cases, the staff may perform any medical procedures needed to save the life or preserve the health of the suspect. Even in these situations, the blood samples or test results should not simply be given to the police. Rather, the police must obtain a search warrant authorizing them to seize the evidence (*Pohoretsky v The Queen*, 1987; *R. v Dyment*, 1988; *R. v Greffe*, 1990).

In 1985, Parliament introduced a special warrant that authorizes blood samples to be taken from unconscious impaired driving suspects in limited circumstances. A health care professional acting under this warrant is protected from both civil and criminal liability. Nonetheless, the legislation permits health care professionals to refuse to participate in the procedure (*Criminal Code*, ss. 256(1) & 257).

Substitute Consent

The issue of substitute or next-of-kin consent arises only if the client is not competent to give or withhold consent, or a statute requires a parental or other third-party consent. In such circumstances, the law permits the client's substitute decision maker to give or refuse consent on the incompetent client's behalf. In Ontario, the *Health Care Consent Act, 1996*, sets out a ranked list of those who may give substitute consent for treatment (s. 20). However, it can be hard to find a substitute decision maker in some cases, such as those involving people living on the street. The Act states that if no one else higher on the list is competent, readily available and willing to serve as a substitute decision maker, then the Public Guardian and Trustee (PGT) has authority to make the decision (s. 20(5)). Similarly, the PGT will exercise substitute consent if two substitute decision makers at the same rank disagree on whether to give or refuse consent (s. 20(6)).

The power to exercise substitute consent is not absolute. The decision to give or withhold consent must accord with any prior known wish of the individual that was expressed when he or she was competent (*Malette v Shulman*, 1990; *Fleming v Reid*, 1991). If there is no such wish, the substitute decision maker must make the decision in the best interest of the patient deemed incompetent (*T.(I.) v L.(L.)*, 1999). Thus, a court can invalidate a parental decision to refuse drug treatment for their incompetent child if the parents' refusal is not in the child's best interest (*"Eve" v "Mrs E."*, 1986). The court can order that the child be given treatment or be made a ward of the provincial child welfare agency. The agency would then give the necessary consent for the child to receive the needed treatment.

Factors That Invalidate Consent

Once it is established that a client has consented, it must be determined whether any factors negate consent. If the consent is negated, the practitioner's legal position would be the same as if there had been no consent. There are four factors that the courts may consider in negating consent: mistake, duress (coercion), deceit (fraud) and public policy.

If a client consented to treatment under a mistaken belief created by the treatment professional, the client's consent would be negated (*Parmley v Parmley and Yule*, 1945; *Guimond v Laberge*, 1956). This issue would arise if a clinician inadvertently overstated the benefits of the treatment or failed to adequately answer the client's concerns about the risks, and the client consented based on these misconceptions. While it is important to encourage clients to have beneficial treatment, care must be taken not to overstate the benefits or understate the risks.

Consent is invalid if it was obtained under duress, which the courts have defined narrowly as an immediate threat of physical force (*Latter v Braddell*, 1880; *Re Riverdale Hospital and C.U.P.E.*, 1985). As long as the courts continue to use this restrictive definition, the issue is unlikely to arise in a typical drug treatment situation. The fact that a client consented only reluctantly (e.g., to avoid being thrown out of the house, expelled from school or charged with breach of probation) does not constitute duress. However, the issue of duress would arise if a client consented because of an unlawful threat of being physically restrained or drugged.

A client's consent is also invalid if it was obtained through deceit, which the courts have limited to a person's lying or acting in total disregard for the truth. Deceit will negate consent only if it relates to the nature of the proposed treatment or its potentially harmful consequences, as opposed to any other matter (*R. v Cuerrier*, 1998 and *R. v Williams*, 2003). The issue of deceit would arise if, for example, a counsellor knowingly misled research participants into believing they were receiving an active drug, when they were being given a placebo.

The courts have increasingly recognized public policy factors in negating the defence of consent. For example, in *Lane v Holloway* (1968), the court refused to accept the defence of consent, because it was obvious from the outset of the fight that the elderly plaintiff was no match for the young defendant. Consent may also be negated if it would be "unconscionable" to allow the defendant to raise the defence, as in the case of a foster father who had consensual sexual relations with his 15-year-old stepdaughter (*M.(M.) v K.(K.)*, 1989). Similarly, consent may be negated if it was obtained by exploiting a relationship of trust. Thus, the fact that the patient consented to sexual contact in exchange for drugs did not provide her doctor with a defence in a battery action (*Norberg v Wynrib*, 1992).

Conclusion

With limited exceptions, treatment relationships in our legal system are based on consent. Although consent issues usually relate to medical procedures, they apply equally to psychological assessment, treatment and counselling. Therefore, before beginning counselling or treatment, substance use workers should ensure they have obtained a valid consent. The following checklist will help with this task.

Consent checklist

- Is the client capable of giving or refusing consent? (Can the client understand the procedure and its risks, and appreciate the likely consequences of having or failing to have the proposed treatment?)
- If the client is capable of giving consent, has he or she explicitly consented to the proposed treatment?
- If not, has the client implicitly consented and how was that implicit consent demonstrated?
- Is the consent valid in that the client consented voluntarily?
- Is the consent valid in that it is an informed consent? (Have the risks and benefits of the proposed treatment and its alternatives been explained? Have the material risks been disclosed? Have the client's questions been fully and frankly answered?)
- Is there adequate proof of consent? Is this a situation in which the consent should be in writing?
- If the client is not capable, is this an emergency in which the health practitioner is authorized to intervene without consent?
- If this is not an emergency, has a valid substitute consent been given?
- Do any factors—mistake, duress, deceit or public policy—invalidate the consent or substitute consent?

Liability in Negligence

The term "negligence" is used in two distinct ways. In its broader sense, it refers to a major branch of tort or civil liability law. In its narrower sense, the term refers to one element of this cause of action, namely whether the defendant's conduct breached the standard of care. It is generally easy to determine from the context when the term is being used to describe the branch of law or the breach of the standard of care.

Health practitioners can be held accountable in negligence for acts arising from any aspect of their professional responsibilities. For example, the liability of a psychologist or social worker is not limited to counselling, but can stem from interviewing and assessing a client; designing a treatment plan; record keeping; making a referral or placement; failing to control or protect a client; and hiring, training, assigning or supervising staff.

Our courts recognize that health, counselling and care professionals cannot be expected to guarantee the outcome of the services that they provide. Rather, negligence is reflected in the standard of care that these and other professionals are required to meet. The fact that an operation fails; a patient dies; or a client reoffends, resumes drinking or remains depressed does not constitute negligence. Nor are individuals held to have breached the standard of care simply because their decision in hindsight proved to be wrong.

Rather, negligence refers to a breach of the standard of care that would be expected of a reasonable person in the circumstances. The standard is geared to the specific education, experience and professional qualifications of the defendant (*Crits v Sylvester*, 1956; *T.(S.) v Gaskell*, 1997; *B.(K.L.) v British Columbia*, 2003). Thus, a social worker providing addiction counselling to a teenager would be held to the standard of care of a reasonable social worker with the same training and experience. It may be helpful to view negligence in this context as conduct that is substandard in terms of one's profession. In essence, a counsellor's or therapist's liability in negligence turns on meeting the standards of his or her peers and profession, and not on some external legal principle.

It is important to distinguish between negligence and errors in judgment. There is no liability in negligence for errors in judgment. Assume that a social worker, after conducting a thorough assessment, places a child in a foster home and the child is subsequently abused by one of the foster parents. Although the social worker's decision had tragic consequences for the child, placing the child in that home would be viewed as an error in judgment and not negligence. In other words, the issue is not whether a decision was right, but rather whether it was reasonable (*Wilson v Swanson*, 1956; *D.(B.) v British Columbia*, 1997).

It is also crucial to distinguish between the concepts of negligence and incompetence. An allegation of negligence is generally made in terms of a specific act, placement, referral or decision. The fact that a practitioner's conduct on one occasion or in one regard was negligent does not mean that he or she is incompetent. The term "incompetence" generally refers to situations in which an individual is viewed as being unable to meet the standards or discharge the responsibilities of his or her profession. Depending on the context, a finding of incompetence can result in the person being disciplined by his or her governing college, sued by the client in negligence or fired by the employer for cause without notice.

The Standard of Care and Its Breach

Compliance with and breach of customary practice

A customary practice is generally defined as a well-established approach, technique, process or procedure that has been widely accepted within a profession, trade or industry. The party relying on customary practice has the burden of proving that such a custom exists. If the practitioner can prove that he or she complied with the relevant customary practice, this will provide some evidence that he or she met the standard of care. Conversely, if the client can prove that the practitioner breached the relevant customary practice, this will provide some evidence that the practitioner was negligent (*Chasney v Anderson*, 1950; *Emmonds v Makarewicz*, 1995). The Canadian courts have held that a judge may reject a customary practice if that practice is patently unsafe or fraught with risk (*ter Neuzon v Korn*, 1995; *Comeau v Saint John Regional Hospital*, 2001).

Negligence liability of students, trainees and volunteers

Organizations can be held vicariously or indirectly liable for the conduct of those providing gratuitous services if their duties are carried out under the organization's direction or control. Students, trainees and volunteers are not held to the same standard of care as fully qualified staff, but rather that of a reasonable student, trainee or volunteer in the circumstances. Nevertheless, they should have the training, skills and knowledge necessary to competently perform their assigned duties. They should also be trained to know their own limits and when it is necessary to refer a case to, or seek assistance from, more qualified staff (*S.(C.) (Next Friend of) v Miller*, 2002).

Supervisors, managers and professional staff may be held personally liable in negligence if their inadequate screening, placing or supervising of a trainee or volunteer results in injury to a client or third party. They must also exercise reasonable care to safeguard trainees and volunteers. Thus, for example, a supervisor could be held liable in negligence for assigning a naïve trainee to work with an aggressive client who subsequently injures the volunteer.

The standard of care expected of supervisors

An increasing number of suits are being brought against supervisory staff for negligence in the screening, hiring, placing, training, monitoring and disciplining of subordinate staff. Supervisory staff are expected to know the capabilities of their workers and ensure that the workers can competently complete the tasks they are assigned (*Granger (Litigation Guardian of) v Ottawa General Hospital*, 1996; *Till v Walker*, 2000).

The standard of care expected in counselling

Psychologists, therapists and social workers will face relatively few suits for their approach to counselling, given the broad range of accepted approaches. As the following case illustrates, any claims that are made will likely fail unless the practitioner's approach constitutes a marked departure from that of his or her peers. In *T. (S.) v Gaskell* (1997), the plaintiff sued her social worker in negligence, claiming that the counselling evoked memories of childhood sexual abuse that caused her to descend into self-destructive behaviour that included criminal acts, alcoholism, substance use problems and suicidal depressions. The court dismissed the claim. The social worker met the standard of care expected in providing such counselling. She had not forced or pressured the plaintiff to recall these memories; the plaintiff did not exhibit any outward signs of distress; and both external and internal support mechanisms appeared to be in place for the plaintiff. The social worker thought that the therapeutic alliance with the plaintiff was very strong.

The courts have held that counsellors owe professional duties to their clients, and not to the client's partner or family. In *N.(M.) v Froberg* (2009), a psychologist who had assessed two children at the request of their mother was sued by the children's father. In dismissing the suit, the court stated that the psychologist owed a common law duty and a fiduciary duty to her clients, the children, and not to the plaintiff. The counsellor's paramount concern must always be the best interests of her clients (*D.(B.) v Halton Region Children's Aid Society*, 2007).

Those who represent themselves as providing counselling services are expected to meet minimum standards of competency in counselling, even if they do not have any professional qualifications or training. Thus, a private addiction withdrawal program was held liable in negligence for the conduct of a live-in patient who served as a supervisor on the premises. The patient/supervisor ignored a resident's suicide attempt earlier in the day on which the resident killed himself on the premises (*Roy c. Taxi-Go-Gîtes inc.*, 2004).

Liability for Failing to Obtain Informed Consent

In keeping with the rise of patients' and clients' rights, the courts require that clients be given enough information to make an informed decision about the proposed treatment and its alternatives. This does not mean that clients must be told of all the possible risks (*Reibl v Hughes*, 1980; *Hopp v Lepp*, 1980; *Haughian v Paine*, 1987). The key legal principles governing informed consent are summarized below. A practitioner's failure to adequately inform a client of the risks of a procedure or treatment may result in the practitioner being held liable in negligence.

- Practitioners have a legal duty to disclose to their patients or clients all the material risks associated with a proposed procedure. The term "material risk" includes a small risk of a serious consequence. In the foundation case, a four per cent chance of death and a 10 per cent chance of paralysis were held to constitute material risks (*Reibl v Hughes*, 1980). The courts have increasingly held that very small and even remote risks of death or serious injury are material. Examples include:
  - a very small risk of stroke during a neck manipulation by a chiropractor (*Leung v Campbell*, 1995)
  - an extremely small chance of stroke from taking oral contraceptives (*Buchan v Ortho*, 1986)
  - a 1/40,000 to 1/100,000 chance of death as a result of a severe reaction to a diagnostic dye (*Meyer Estate v Rogers*, 1991)
  - a 1/220 chance of having a baby with Down's syndrome (*Zhang v Kan*, 2003).
- The term "material risk" also includes a substantial probability of a relatively minor consequence, such as a 35 per cent risk of a minor infection.

- In addition to informing the patient of the physical nature of the risk (e.g., cutting a nerve), the practitioner must explain the impact of such an eventuality on the patient's life (*Tremblay v McLauchlan*, 2001).
- Practitioners must also disclose non-material risks that they know, or ought to know, would be of particular concern to the client or patient.
- Practitioners should discuss with the client or patient the consequences of leaving the problem untreated.
- The courts have increasingly required full disclosure of the alternatives to the proposed treatment, particularly if the proposed treatment involves significant risks (*Haughian v Paine*, 1987; *Thibault v Fewer*, 2002; *Remtulla v Zeldin*, 2005).
- Practitioners must answer all questions openly and honestly, even if the answers would discourage the patient or client from consenting (*Hartjes v Carmen*, 2004).
- Responsibility for obtaining an informed consent rests with the person performing the service. While practitioners may delegate this task to a subordinate, they are ultimately accountable for ensuring that an informed consent was obtained (*Semeniuk v Cox*, 1999).
- Practitioners may use videos, pamphlets and other similar means of informing patients and clients, but they must ensure that the person understands the information and its significance (*Byciuk v Hollingworth*, 2004).
- Practitioners do not have any clear therapeutic privilege to withhold information because they feel that a patient or client is unable to cope with the information. They do, however, have the freedom to decide how they will present the information and what they will emphasize.
- Practitioners do not have to disclose information to patients or clients who have expressly stated that they do not want to be informed of the risks, benefits and alternatives.
- Practitioners who do not meet these standards of disclosure are in breach of their duty of care. However, the patient or client must also establish that the failure to be informed caused or contributed to his or her injuries. In effect, the failure to inform must have induced the plaintiff to consent to treatment to which he or she would not otherwise have agreed, and that treatment must have caused the plaintiff's loss (*Arndt v Smith*, 1997; *Turkington v Lai*, 2007; *Sterritt v Shogilev*, 2009).

Liability for Omissions

Traditionally, the common law did not impose liability in negligence on a person for failing to act for the benefit of another. While the courts continue to pay lip service to this general principle, they have recognized a growing number of "special relationships" in which one person may be held civilly liable for negligently failing to control or protect another. It is well established that a "special relationship" giving rise to a duty to control and protect exists between:

- children and their parents and teachers (*Myers v Peel County Board of Education*, 1981; *Eichmanis (Litigation Guardian of) v Prystay*, 2003; *Hussack v Chilliwack School District No. 33*, 2009)
- police and corrections staff and prisoners (*Williams v New Brunswick*, 1985; *S.(J.) v Clement*, 1995; *Rhora (Litigation Guardian of) v Ontario*, 2006)
- probation/parole officers and probationers/parolees (*Hendrick v De Marsh*, 1984; *H.(D.) v British Columbia*, 2008)
- employers and employees (*Jacobsen v Nike Canada Ltd.*, 1996; *Sulz v Canada*, 2006).

The courts have consistently held that a special relationship exists between health care professionals and their patients and clients. As the following cases illustrate, practitioners are not held liable simply because their decision turns out to have been wrong. Rather, the plaintiff must establish that the practitioner's conduct fell below the standard of care expected of a reasonable professional in the circumstances.

In *Villemure v L'Hôpital Notre-Dame* (1973), a patient was admitted to the psychiatric ward of a hospital after attempting suicide. On his physician's recommendation, the patient was moved from the psychiatric ward that had barred windows to a semi-private room that did not. The patient's requests to be returned to the psychiatric ward were ignored and he was left in the room unsupervised. Shortly thereafter, he died by suicide by jumping from the window. The patient's attending physician and the hospital's nursing staff were held liable in negligence for failing to properly supervise and safeguard the patient.

In *Holan Estate v Stanton Regional Health Board* (2001), a voluntary patient suffering from severe depression died by suicide while on a pass issued by his treating physician. Before she allowed the patient to leave, a psychiatric nurse with 15 years experience conducted her own assessment and determined that the patient did not pose an undue risk to himself or others. The doctor and nurses were not held liable in negligence because they had undertaken an appropriate assessment and exercised their clinical judgment accordingly. Although in hindsight their decision was incorrect and had tragic consequences, they exercised reasonable care in making that decision.

In *Yelle v Children's Aid Society of Ottawa-Carleton* (2002), the plaintiffs sued Children's Aid and the foster parent of a youth who set their homes on fire. The youth had a long history of serious psychological and behavioural problems that started when he was three years old. Numerous assessments had indicated that he needed ongoing counselling and a very structured environment. His conduct improved substantially in the Roberts/Smart Centre where he received counselling. However, his conduct deteriorated rapidly after he was discharged. In the year prior to the fires, he was involved in a series of break and enters, thefts and other property offences, fights and threats. An experienced foster parent, who had temporary care of the youth and knew of his previous arsons, warned Children's Aid that the youth was going to set fires, given his history. During this year, Children's Aid repeatedly transferred the youth from one short-term or emergency foster placement to another. The last placement was in an untried foster home with an inexperienced and untrained foster parent. Children's Aid took no steps to obtain counselling for the youth, despite his escalating pattern of serious criminal offences. Nor did Children's Aid pursue the possibility of obtaining the youth's consent to return to the centre where he had done well, or obtaining a court order for secure custody if he refused to consent. The court held that Children's Aid owed the plaintiffs a duty of care, given the youth's clear pattern of escalating criminality in the community. Children's Aid was held to be negligent in failing to provide counselling, support and a structured environment, which the youth "so desperately needed." The claim against the foster parent was dismissed because she had acted in good faith to discharge her responsibilities.

Several challenging issues may arise around an addiction worker's duty to control and protect. Consider a situation in which a client who is intoxicated attends a counselling session and causes a car crash while driving home. The counsellor may be sued for negligently allowing the client to leave in a condition that posed a foreseeable risk of injury to the client or others. Such a case might succeed if the counsellor had been negligent in failing to recognize the client's intoxication, or had realized that the client was impaired but did not make a reasonable effort to stop him or her (see *Monteith v Hunter*, 2001).

Confidentiality and Disclosure of Client Information

Confidentiality

The term "confidentiality" has several meanings in common usage. However, when used in a legal context, confidentiality refers to the legal obligation not to *willingly* disclose information that has been received in confidence, without the client's consent (*Halls v Mitchell*, 1928; *Cronkwright v Cronkwright*, 1971; *R. v Dersch*, 1993). Consequently, a substance use worker who disclosed information without a client's consent would not be in breach of confidentiality if he or she was *required* to do so by a search warrant, subpoena or other court order. Nor would a counsellor breach confidentiality if he or she complied with the province's mandatory child abuse reporting provisions or disclosed information as required by other statutes.

The public tends to view confidentiality as an absolute guarantee of silence. Many people believe that information given in confidence to health care professionals will never be disclosed without explicit consent. As a result, counsellors may find themselves caught between their legal obligation to comply with court orders or mandatory reporting provisions and their clients' reasonable, but mistaken, understanding of confidentiality. To avoid being seen as betraying a client's trust, counsellors should explain the meaning and limits of confidentiality at the outset of the relationship.

An obligation of confidentiality will not usually arise until a health care professional has entered a counselling or other treatment relationship with a client. The courts will likely hold that a confidentiality obligation begins when it would be reasonable for the client to expect privacy. Although not all telephone requests for appointments or information would give rise to such an obligation, some might. For example, a reminder for an eye appointment left with a client's secretary is likely to be treated differently from a reminder for an appointment with a substance use counsellor. Obviously, the more serious the matter, and the more emotionally, sexually or legally sensitive the issue, the greater the expectation of privacy.

An obligation of confidentiality applies to all information that a client gives in confidence, whether it relates to the client or to other people. However, the confidentiality requirement is generally limited to statements and observations made within the professional relationship. Thus, no confidentiality obligation would apply to a substance use counsellor who happens to see an intoxicated client stagger to his car at a shopping mall. Like any other member of the public, the counsellor could choose to call the police. However, the counsellor would have to limit his or her statements to what was seen at the mall, and would breach confidentiality if he or she disclosed any information arising from the treatment relationship, including that the person was a client.

Depending on the circumstances, a health care practitioner may be subject to several overlapping confidentiality obligations at any one time. First, a number of provincial statutes impose confidentiality obligations on health care professionals in specific situations. Second, counsellors may be subject to ethical and professional codes of confidentiality. Third, a clinician who promises, either implicitly or explicitly, to maintain confidentiality will have a common law duty to honour that obligation. Fourth, the courts are likely to assume that confidentiality is an inherent element of all therapeutic relationships. Thus, even in the absence of a statute, professional code or promise of confidentiality, those who present themselves to the public as counsellors may be expected to treat client information as confidential.

Depending on the source of the obligation, a breach of confidentiality can lead to penal, professional and civil liability. A person who breaches a statutory confidentiality obligation may be prosecuted. For example, a substance use worker in Ontario who wrongfully discloses information from the clinical record of a psychiatric patient may be prosecuted under the *Mental Health Act* and fined up to $25,000 (ss. 35 & 80). If a clinician is a member of a regulated profession, such as social work or psychology, breaching confidentiality may be grounds for a finding of professional misconduct and may lead to a fine, reprimand or licence suspension. A breach of confidentiality may also result in civil liability in negligence or in the emerging tort action for intentional breach of confidence.

Privilege

The legal term "privilege" refers to the right to refuse to disclose confidential information when testifying, when faced with a subpoena for client records or when subject to a mandatory reporting obligation (*R. v O'Connor*, 1995; *R. v McLure*, 2001; *R. v National Post*, 2010). As a general rule, people called as witnesses in court or before other legal tribunals must answer all relevant questions put to them (see, for example, *Canada*

Evidence Act, s. 46). Similarly, those served with subpoenas or other court orders must provide the records or files that are sought. Privilege is an exception to these general rules. In the absence of privilege, a person who defies a court order or refuses to answer questions when testifying may be found in contempt of court (*Cornwall Public Inquiry (Commissioner of) v Dunlop*, 2008).

Traditionally, the only professional relationship to which privilege applied was that between solicitors and their clients. Solicitor-client privilege is based on the view that our legal system requires clients to speak freely with their lawyers. This will only occur if such communications remain confidential. However, even solicitor-client privilege is limited. It applies only to statements about past criminal offences, and not to statements about ongoing or future crimes. Nor does it apply to physical evidence. Although other professionals, such as priests, police, psychologists, journalists and social workers, have claimed a comparable need for privilege, common law has not granted such automatic protection to these relationships.

Courts have discretion to grant privilege on a case-by-case basis to confidential communications other than solicitor-client relationships (*Slavutych v Baker*, 1976). The party seeking privilege must establish four requirements: the communication must have originated in confidence; confidentiality must be essential to maintaining the relationship; the relationship must be one that society values and wishes to foster; and the injury to the relationship from disclosure of the information must outweigh the benefit of having the relevant evidence available to resolve the case.

Communications made in the course of most care relationships would likely satisfy the first three requirements. First, clients expect that the information they give to counsellors or other health care professionals will be kept confidential. Indeed, most professionals explicitly state that all information their clients provide will be kept confidential. Second, successful treatment relationships are largely built on trust. Most clients would not disclose intimate details about their lives unless they were assured of confidentiality. Without such information, a substance use worker would be unable to accurately assess the client's problems and provide proper care. Third, society has an interest in promoting successful treatment relationships.

The fourth requirement has been the most difficult to satisfy. If the confidential information is relevant to the case, the courts have tended to deny privilege and order disclosure. Not surprisingly, some judges may rule that the interests of justice in resolving cases outweigh the importance of granting privilege and maintaining confidentiality. As the following case illustrates, this is particularly true in criminal, child abuse and child custody cases. The courts also appear more reluctant to grant privilege when it is sought by an accused, as opposed to a victim (*R. v R.S.*, 1985; *R. v Gruenke*, 1991).

In *Gibbs v Gibbs* (1985), an estranged husband and wife were involved in custody proceedings. The wife had a long history of mental illness that required hospitalization on several occasions, and was reportedly displaying those symptoms again. The husband argued that his wife could not be relied upon to care for their two children and that he should be granted custody. In order to support his claim, the husband requested that his wife's psychiatric records be disclosed. The court ordered disclosure of the records despite the doctor's conclusion that this would likely have an adverse effect on the wife's treatment. The judge stated that the potential harm to the children far outweighed any risks to the wife.

Despite frequent recommendations that privilege be extended, legislatures have been reluctant to grant immunity from disclosure. Even where legislation purports to provide privilege, the courts have tended to interpret privilege narrowly, on the basis that the interests of justice require disclosure of all relevant information. Furthermore, a provincial statute that privileges specific communication may be challenged if it conflicts with federal legislation that authorizes disclosure of that same communication (see, for example, *R. v B.*, 1979). However, note that Parliament has enacted special statutory privileging provisions to provide greater protection from disclosure to the records of sexual assault victims (*Criminal Code*, ss. 278.1–278.91).

In summary, while almost all information that treatment workers obtain in providing treatment is confidential, little, if any, is privileged. Perhaps more importantly, privilege is granted on a case-by-case basis and a treatment worker can never know at the time of making a record whether it will be privileged. Consequently, treatment workers should assume that some day they will have to testify and that their records may be examined in court. This realization should encourage treatment workers to take their record-keeping obligations seriously and to adopt a professional and objective tone in preparing client records.

Disclosure of Client Information

Clients' access to their records

Treatment and care records do not belong to clients. Rather, they are the property of the agency and the people providing the service. Nonetheless, in the absence of a statute to the contrary, the client has a right of reasonable access to this information (*McInerney v MacDonald*, 1992). The professional does not have to produce the records immediately or turn over original documents. He or she may offer to provide a summary of the records or to review the file with the client. However, if the client demands access to, or a copy of, the complete treatment record, the court will uphold the client's right. Agencies can charge clients for the administrative and duplicating costs of copying the record for the client.

If the treatment professional believes that allowing the client access would harm or endanger the client or a third party, the professional can refuse the request and apply to the court. However, the burden of proof is on the treatment professional to justify denying a client access. This has two important implications. First, substance use workers should assume that their clients may read the entire file some day. Second, professionals should not promise colleagues or other third parties that their comments about the client will remain confidential because they may not be able to keep such a promise.

Disclosure with clients' consent

In the absence of a statute to the contrary, a substance use worker ordinarily cannot disclose client information without that client's consent—not even to the client's employer, family members, probation officer or the police. Even simple inquiries, such as whether a person is a client, are best left unanswered, with an explanation that all client information is confidential. Even if the client was referred by an employer, probation officer or other third party, the treatment worker must generally obtain the client's consent before disclosing information to that other party.

Although the client's express consent is usually required, implied consent may be assumed in several situations. First, treatment professionals may share confidential client information without express consent for the purposes of providing proper care.[2] For example, a counsellor who is concerned about a client who is potentially suicidal may consult a colleague to determine how best to proceed, whether or not the colleague works in the same agency. The counsellor should only disclose identifying client information if it would be helpful to the colleague in formulating his or her advice. The colleague would be subject to the same confidentiality obligations as the counsellor. Second, professionals may be permitted to disclose client information without consent in compassionate circumstances. For example, hospitals treating unconscious accident victims routinely notify the next-of-kin. Third, there is also a right to share confidential information for internal administrative purposes, such as audits and quality assurance reviews.

Depending on the circumstances, there may also be an implicit right to share confidential information with a client's parents, spouse, employer or other referring agency. For example, if the client's parents attended the initial session, the substance use worker may discuss with them, at a later date, information from that session. Clients often approach treatment professionals to document their claim for an employment, insurance or government benefit. In many such cases, it is obvious that there is implied consent to disclose client information to the party providing the benefit. It has been suggested that client information may also be used without consent for research or teaching purposes, provided the client cannot be identified. Although some statutes authorize such disclosures in limited circumstances, there does not appear to be any common law authority for this proposition. Given the increasing concern about privacy, clinicians are advised to obtain express consent in all of these situations.

Reporting Obligations

Reporting criminal offences

In addition to disclosing information when faced with a court order or search warrant, treatment professionals may be required by various statutes to report certain information to designated authorities. However, contrary to what many people believe, there is

---

2 However, some discretion must be exercised in disclosing confidential information even to colleagues (see *Re: Lavasseur and College of Nurses of Ontario* (1983), 18 A.C.W.S. (2d) 126 (Ont. H.C.)).

no general obligation to report federal or provincial offences, to assist the police or to answer police questions (see, for example, *Koechlin v Waugh*, 1957; *R. v Carroll*, 1959; *Rice v Connolly*, 1966; *Kenlin v Gardiner*, 1967; *Colet v The Queen*, 1981). With the exception of treason and high treason (*Criminal Code*, s. 50(1)(b)), it is not a federal criminal offence to fail to report to police crimes that have been, or may be, committed.

Consequently, substance use workers are not required by federal law to report a client's illicit drug use to the police, nor even to acknowledge that a client is in treatment. Professionals can refuse to respond to a police or probation officer's request for client information, but they cannot lie or deliberately mislead officers. Staff who do so may be charged with obstructing justice or similar offences (*Criminal Code*, ss. 129, 139 & 140).

Provincial reporting obligations

In contrast to the *Criminal Code*, various provincial statutes impose mandatory reporting obligations on health care professionals and others. These obligations vary from province to province. Moreover, they tend to be defined precisely, applying to named categories of professionals in very specific circumstances. The common reporting obligations relate to communicable diseases, unfit drivers, sexual impropriety with a client and child abuse. In these situations, the perceived threat to the public is viewed as outweighing the client's right to confidentiality, thus justifying the reporting obligation.

Most provinces have legislation that requires medical professionals to report to public health officials patients who have specified communicable diseases. Physicians providing services to patients who are not hospitalized may be required to report any patient who they believe has a communicable disease. Hospital administrators have a similar reporting obligation with respect to hospital patients (see, for example, the Ontario *Health Protection and Promotion Act*, ss. 25–26).

Educators may also be required to report any student who they suspect has a communicable disease (see, for example, the Ontario *Education Act*, s. 265(k) & (l)). The list of diseases is extensive and typically includes HIV/AIDS, hepatitis, tuberculosis, venereal diseases and various types of influenza. Failure to report is an offence in some provinces and can result in fines. Generally, no action or other proceeding may be brought against a person who makes the required report in good faith.

Most provinces require physicians to report the name, address and clinical condition of any patient of driving age who has or may have a medical condition that may make driving hazardous. Although these provisions were probably intended to deal with medical conditions, such as failing eyesight, heart disease and epilepsy, they are broad enough to encompass substance use problems. However, the legislation is usually limited to medical practitioners and optometrists.[3] Consequently, addiction counsellors would have no statutory obligation to report a client who admits to alcohol- or drug-induced blackouts while driving. Indeed, if they were to report such clients, they might be in breach of their confidentiality obligations. Such dilemmas can occur in various circumstances, and approaches to handling these problems are covered later in this chapter.

---

3 See, for examples, Manitoba, *The Highway Traffic Act*, C.C.S.M. c. H.60, s. 157(1) & (2); British Columbia, *Motor Vehicle Act*, R.S.B.C. 1996, c. 318, s. 230; and Ontario, *Highway Traffic Act*, R.S.O. 1990, c. H.8, ss. 203 and 204.

Several jurisdictions require health care professionals to report to the relevant governing body any reasonable suspicion that any other health care professional has engaged in sexually inappropriate conduct with a patient (see, for example, Ontario's *Regulated Health Professions Act, 1991 (RHPA)*, s. 4, and the *RHPA*'s *Schedule 2, Health Professions Procedural Code*, ss. 85.1–85.7). Thus, for example, a nurse or occupational therapist who was informed by a female patient that the patient's family doctor had made sexual advances would be required to report this information to the College of Physicians. Similar legislation has been enacted for social workers, but it requires them to report sexual improprieties committed by other social workers and social service workers (see, for example, the Ontario *Social Work and Social Service Work Act*, ss. 43–45).

The most comprehensive reporting obligations are contained in the provincial child protection legislation. Two sets of reporting obligations may apply—one that applies to everyone and a broader set that applies to those who have contact with children in a professional capacity, such as educators, child care workers and the police. The obligation to report is defined broadly, usually in terms of having a reasonable suspicion that a child has been, or may be, abused. Child abuse is also defined broadly to include physical and sexual mistreatment, as well as the failure to provide proper medical and psychological treatment. This broad definition would include children who are not receiving treatment for alcohol or other drug problems, and children who are endangered by their parents' substance use problems. Thus, a substance use worker may be required to report to provincial child welfare officials a parent who drives with his or her children while high or intoxicated.

The failure to report child abuse may be a provincial offence that is subject to a substantial fine. The legislation usually states that no civil action can be brought against a person who has reported as required, even if it turns out that there was no abuse. Child protection legislation takes precedence over any conflicting provisions of other provincial statutes, and over professional confidentiality obligations, except for solicitor-client privilege (see, for example, Manitoba's *The Child and Family Services Act*, C.C.S.M. c. C.80, ss. 18–18.4).

The following summary of Ontario's legislation illustrates several common features of various child abuse reporting provisions.

Reporting obligations: Ontario's Child and Family Services Act

Despite the provisions of any other Act, anyone who has reasonable grounds to suspect any of the following circumstances must immediately report the suspicion and the grounds upon which it is based to a Children's Aid Society (s. 72(1)):

- A child has suffered or is at risk of suffering physical harm that is inflicted by the parent or person in charge of the child; resulted from that person's failure to adequately care or provide for, supervise or protect the child; or resulted from that person's pattern of neglect.
- A child has suffered or is at risk of suffering emotional harm, as demonstrated by serious anxiety, depression, withdrawal, self-destructive or aggressive behaviour, or

delayed development, which is caused or contributed to, as described above, by the parent or person in charge of the child.

- A child has suffered or is at risk of suffering sexual molestation or exploitation inflicted by the parent or person in charge of the child, or caused by that person's failure to protect the child when that person knows or ought to know of the possibility.
- A child requires medical treatment, treatment for emotional harm, or treatment for a mental, emotional or developmental condition that could seriously impair the child's development, and the parent or person in charge of the child fails or refuses to provide the treatment, or is unavailable or unable to consent.
- A child has been abandoned; the child's parent has died or is unavailable to exercise custodial rights and has not made adequate arrangements for the child's care; or the parent is unable or unwilling to resume responsibility for his or her child in residential care.
- A child under age 12 has killed or seriously injured another person or caused serious property damage and needs treatment to prevent a recurrence, but the parent or person in charge of the child fails or refuses to provide it, or is unavailable or unable to consent.
- A child under age 12 has, on more than one occasion, injured another person or damaged another's property with the encouragement of the person in charge of the child or because of that person's failure or inability to adequately supervise the child.

Under section 72(1), the duty to report applies to those who perform professional or official duties with regard to children, including health care professionals, teachers, counsellors, clergy, youth and recreation workers, service providers, peace officers, coroners and solicitors. It is an offence for these people to fail to report as required and, upon conviction, they may be fined up to $1,000 (s. 72(4) and (6.2)). The reporting obligation is ongoing. Any person who has additional grounds to suspect one of the above circumstances must promptly report these grounds to a Children's Aid Society, even if he or she has made previous reports regarding the child (s. 72(2)). Reports must be made directly to a Children's Aid Society. A person must not rely on a third person to report on his or her behalf (s. 72(3)). The term "child" is defined, for the purposes of reporting, as a person under 16 years of age. These duties to report apply even if the information is confidential or privileged (s. 72(7)). However, nothing in this section overrides the privilege that may exist between a solicitor and his or her client (s. 72(8)).

No action can be brought against a person for complying with these reporting obligations, unless he or she acted unreasonably or in bad faith (s. 72(7)).

Failing to Warn

Duty to warn cases involve a conflict between a practitioner's confidentiality obligation and his or her duty to protect patients or clients and those whom the patient or client may foreseeably endanger. Assume that a client with a history of violence makes an unequivocal threat during counselling to kill a third party and that there is no relevant mandatory reporting obligation. If the counsellor breaches confidentiality, he or she may be subject to penal, professional and civil liability. If the counsellor remains silent and the threat is carried out, then the counsellor may be sued for failing to protect the victim.

The leading case in this area is *Tarasoff v Regents of the University of California* (1976), which held that counsellors could be held liable for failing to warn intended victims, even if doing so required breaching client confidentiality. In this case, a client told his psychologist at the University Hospital that he intended to kill his former girlfriend when she returned from vacation. The psychologist concluded that the client was dangerous and contacted the campus police. The client was picked up, briefly detained and then released. Neither the woman nor her family were warned of the potential danger. When the woman returned, the client killed her. The family sued the psychologist for failing to warn. The court acknowledged the psychologist's arguments about the difficulty of predicting dangerousness, but indicated that this was not the issue. The psychologist was not being sued because he had negligently assessed his client. Rather, he was being sued because he had concluded that the client was dangerous and failed to warn the intended victim. The psychologist also argued that there should be no duty to warn because it would necessitate breaching his ethical obligation to maintain confidentiality. In rejecting this argument, the court emphasized that the confidentiality obligation to the client ends when the public peril begins. Consequently, the judge rejected the psychologist's request to dismiss the family's claim and sent the case to trial. The psychologist and the university settled out of court for close to $2 million dollars before the trial.

Although Canadian courts have not addressed the civil liability issue that arose in *Tarasoff*, it appears that they would also give priority to public safety. In *Smith v Jones* (1999), a psychiatrist interviewed the accused at the request of his lawyer. The accused, who was charged with the aggravated sexual assault of a prostitute, told the psychiatrist that he planned to kill prostitutes. The psychiatrist told the lawyer that the accused was dangerous and would likely commit future crimes. The accused pleaded guilty, but the psychiatrist's concerns were not addressed at the sentencing hearing. The psychiatrist sought a declaration allowing him to disclose the privileged information in the interest of public safety. The Supreme Court of Canada upheld the psychiatrist's request for a declaration authorizing disclosure of the privileged information. The Court stated that danger to public safety may, in appropriate circumstances, justify setting aside solicitor-client privilege. The Court stated that there must be a clear risk of imminent serious bodily harm or death to an identifiable person or group.

Although *Smith* is not a duty to warn case, it strongly suggests that the Canadian courts will go at least as far as *Tarasoff* in requiring professionals to warn and take other steps to protect the public. However, both *Tarasoff* and *Smith* involve unequivocal death threats made against an identified victim or class of victims by a person who the professional concluded was capable of murder. What remains to be resolved is whether this duty will be imposed in other high-risk situations. For example, would a duty arise if the client was only threatening suicide, or was incapable of operating a crane, driving a train or otherwise continuing to work in a safety-sensitive position? Would a HIV-positive client's admitted failure to practise safe sex require or justify breaching confidentiality? It may be some time before the Canadian courts address these issues and clarify the scope of the duty to warn.

Conclusion

Treatment professionals should assume that all client information is confidential, but that nothing will be privileged. As a working guideline, information should not be disclosed without the client's consent, unless the professional is compelled by law to do so.

The statutory requirements governing disclosure and reporting are complex and varied. They may be supplemented by the rules that agencies or institutions adopt. Moreover, additional requirements may be imposed by the governing bodies of particular professions. This chapter covered the general principles and specific examples of common situations, but it is up to each substance use worker to determine the requirements that pertain to his or her specific situation.

References

Statutes
Child and Family Services Act, R.S.O. 1990, c. C.11.
The Child and Family Services Act, C.C.S.M. c. C.80.
Criminal Code, R.S.C. 1985, c. C-46.
Education Act, R.S.O. 1990, c. E.2.
Health Care Consent Act, 1996, S.O. 1996, c. 2.
Health Care (Consent) and Care Facility (Admission) Act, R.S.B.C. 1996, c. 181.
Health Protection and Promotion Act, R.S.O. 1990, c. H.7.
Mental Health Act, R.S.O. 1990, c. M.7.
Regulated Health Professions Act, 1991, S.O. 1991, c. 18.
Regulated Health Professions Act, 1991, S.O. 1991, c. 18, *Schedule 2: Health Professions Procedural Code.*
Social Work and Social Service Work Act, 1998, S.O. 1998, c. 31.
Trillium Gift of Life Network Act, R.S.O. 1990, c. H.20.

Cases
A.C. v Manitoba (Director of Child and Family Services), [2009] 2 S.C.R. 181.
Arndt v Smith (1997), 35 C.C.L.T. (2d) 233 (S.C.C.).
Attorney General of British Columbia v Astaforoff, [1984] 4 W.W.R. 385 (B.C.C.A.).
Attorney General of Canada v Notre Dame Hospital (1984), 8 C.R.R. 382 (Que. S.C.).
B.(K.L.) v British Columbia (2003), 19 C.C.L.T. (3d) 66 (S.C.C.).

Battrum v British Columbia (2009), 70 C.C.L.T. (3d) 164 (B.C.S.C.).

Bettel v Yim (1978), 20 O.R. (2d) 617 (Co. Ct.).

Bolduc v R. (1967), 63 D.L.R. (2d) 82 (S.C.C.).

Buchan v Ortho Pharmaceutical (Can.) Ltd. (1986), 25 D.L.R. (4th) 658 (Ont. C.A.).

Byciuk v Hollingworth (2004), 27 C.C.L.T. (3d) 116 (Alta. Q.B.).

C. v Wren (1986), 35 D.L.R. (4th) 419 (Alta. C.A.).

Chasney v Anderson, [1950] 4 D.L.R. 223 (S.C.C.).

Colet v The Queen, [1981] 1 S.C.R. 2.

Comeau v Saint John Regional Hospital (2001), 9 C.C.L.T. (3d) 233 (N.B.C.A.).

Cornwall Public Inquiry (Commissioner of) v Dunlop (2008), 90 O.R. (3d) 524 (S.C.J.).

Crits v Sylvester, [1956] O.R. 132 (C.A.), aff'd. [1956] S.C.R. 991.

Cronkwright v Cronkwright (1971), 14 D.L.R. (3d) 168 (Ont. H.C.).

D.(B.) v British Columbia, [1997] 4 W.W.R. 484 (B.C.C.A.).

D.(B.) v Halton Region Children's Aid Society (2007), 284 D.L.R. (4th) 682 (S.C.C.).

D.(M.) (Guardian ad litem of) v British Columbia, [2000] B.C.T.C. 287 (S.C.).

Deacon v Canada (Attorney General), [2006] F.C.J. No. 1153 (Fed. C.A.).

Eichmanis (Litigation Guardian of) v Prystay (Jan. 29, 2003), File No. 99-0708 (Ont. S.C.J.).

Emmonds v Makarewicz (2000), 2 C.C.L.T. (3d) 255 (B.C.C.A.).

"Eve" v "Mrs. E.", [1986] 2 S.C.R. 388.

Fleming v Reid (1991), 4 O.R. (3d) 74 (C.A.).

Gibbs v Gibbs (1985), 1 W.D.C.P. 6 (Ont. S.C.).

Gilbert v Stone (1648), 82 E.R. 539 (K.B.).

Granger (Litigation Guardian of) v Ottawa General Hospital (1996), 7 O.T.C. 81 (Ont. S.C.J.).

Guimond v Laberge (1956), 4 D.L.R. (2d) 559 (Ont. C.A.).

H.(D.) v British Columbia (2008), 57 C.C.L.T. (3d) 36 (B.C.C.A.).

Halls v Mitchell, [1928] 2 D.L.R. 97 (S.C.C.).

Hartjes v Carmen (2004), 53 C.C.L.T. (3d) 195 (Ont. Div. Ct.).

Haughian v Paine (1987), 40 C.C.L.T. 13 (Sask. C.A.).

Hendrick v De Marsh (1984), 6 D.L.R. (4th) 713 (Ont. H.C.).

Holan Estate v Stanton Regional Health Board (2001), 11 C.C.L.T. (3d) 34 (N.W.T.S.C.).

Hopp v Lepp (1980), 112 D.L.R. (3d) 67 (S.C.C.).

Hughes Estate v Hughes (2007), 51 C.C.L.T. (3d) 16 (Alta. C.A.).

Hussack v Chilliwack School District No. 33 (2009), 70 C.C.L.T. (3d) 98 (B.C.S.C.).

Isber v Zebrowski, [2009] O.J. No. 4514 (Ont. S.C.J.).

Jacobsen v Nike Canada Ltd. (1996), 133 D.L.R. (4th) 377 (B.C.S.C.).

Kenlin v Gardiner, [1967] 2 Q.B. 510 (Q.B.).

Kenny v Lockwood, [1932] 1 D.L.R. 507 (Ont. C.A.).

Koechlin v Waugh (1957), 11 D.L.R. (2d) 447 (Ont. C.A.).

Lane v Holloway, [1968] 1Q.B. 379 (C.A.).

Latter v Braddell (1880), 50 L.J.Q.B. 166 (C.P.).

Leung v Campbell (1995), 24 C.C.L.T. (2d) 63 (Ont. Gen. Div.).

M.(M.) v K.(K.) (1989), 38 B.C.L.R. (2d) 273 (C.A.).

Male v Hopmans (1967), 64 D.L.R. (2d) 105 (Ont. C.A.).

Malette v Shulman (1990), 67 D.L.R. (4th) 321 (Ont. C.A.).

Marshall v Curry, [1933] 3 D.L.R. 260 (N.S.S.C.).

McInerney v MacDonald (1992), 93 D.L.R. (4th) 415 (S.C.C.).

Meyer Estate v Rogers (1991), 6 C.C.L.T. (2d) 102 (Ont. Gen. Div.)

Monteith v Hunter (2001), 8 C.C.L.T. (3d) 268 (Ont. S.C.J.).

Mulloy v Hop Sang, [1935] 1 W.W.R. 714 (Alta. S.C.).

Murray v McMurchy, [1949] 2 D.L.R. 442 (B.C.S.C.).

Myers v Peel County Board of Education (1981), 123 D.L.R. (3d) 1 (S.C.C.).

Neto v Klukach (2004), 12 Admin. L.R. (4th) 101 (Ont. S.C.J.).

Non-marine Underwriters, Lloyd's of London v Scalera (2000), 185 D.L.R. (4th) 1 (S.C.C.).

Norberg v Wynrib, [1992] 2 S.C.R. 226.

O'Bonsawin v Paradis (1993), 15 C.C.L.T. (2d) 188 (Ont. Gen. Div.).

Parmley v Parmley and Yule, [1945] 4 D.L.R. 81 (S.C.C.).

Pittman Estate v Bain (1994), 112 D.L.R. (4th) 257 (Ont. Gen. Div.)

Pohoretsky v The Queen (1987), 33 C.C.C. (3d) 398 (S.C.C.).

R. v B. (1979), 2 Fam. L. Rev. 213 (Ont. Prov. Ct.).

R. v Carroll (1959), 23 D.L.R. (2d) 271 (Ont. C.A.).

R. v Cuerrier (1998), 162 D.L.R. (4th) 513 (S.C.C.).

R. v Dersch, [1993] 3 S.C.R. 768.

R. v Dyment (1988), 45 C.C.C. (3d) 244 (S.C.C.).

R. v Greffe, [1990] 1 S.C.R. 755.

R. v Gruenke, [1991] 3 S.C.R. 263.

R. v McLure (2001), 195 D.L.R. (4th) 513 (S.C.C.).

R. v National Post, 2010 S.C.C. 16.

R. v O'Connor, [1995] 4 S.C.R. 411.

R. v R.S. (1985), 19 C.C.C. (3d) 115 (Ont. C.A.).

R. v Williams, [2003] 2 S.C.R. 134.

Re C (Adult: refusal of medical treatment), [1994] 1 All E.R. 819 (Fam. Div.).

Re Dueck (1999), 171 D.L.R. (4th) 761 (Sask. Q.B.).

Re Lavasseur and College of Nurses of Ontario (1983), 18 A.C.W.S. (2d) 126 (Ont. H.C.).

Re Riverdale Hospital and C.U.P.E. (1985), 19 L.A.C. (3d) 396.

Re Superintendent of Family & Child Services and Dawson (1983), 145 D.L.R. (3d) 610 (B.C.S.C.).

Reibl v Hughes (1980), 114 D.L.R. (3d) 1 (S.C.C.).

Remtulla v Zeldin, [2005] O.J. No. 3424 (S.C.J.)(Q.L.).

Rhora (Litigation Guardian of) v Ontario (2006), 43 C.C.L.T. (3d) 78 (Ont. C.A.).

Rice v Connolly, [1966] 2 Q.B. 414 (Q.B.).

Roy c. Taxi-Go-Gîtes inc. (2004), 33 C.C.L.T. (3d) 87 (C.S. Que.).

S.(C.)(Next Friend of) v Miller (2002), 11 C.C.L.T. (3d) 136 (Alta. Q.B.).

S.(J.) v Clement (1995), 22 O.R. (3d) 495 (Gen. Div.).

Schweizer v Central Hospital (1974), 6 O.R. (2d) 606 (H.C.).

Semeniuk v Cox (1999), 48 C.C.L.T. (2d) 286 (Alta. Q.B.).

Slavutych v Baker, [1976] 1 S.C.R. 254.

Smith v Jones, [1999] 1 S.C.R. 455.

Smith v Stone (1647), 82 E.R. 533 (K.B.).

Starson v Swayze (2003), 225 D.L.R. (4th) 385 (S.C.C.).

Sterritt v Shogilev, [2009] O.J. No. 2063 (S.C.J.).

Strachan v Simpson, [1979] 5 W.W.R. 315 (B.C.S.C.).

Sulz v Canada (Attorney General) (2006), 54 B.C.L.R. (4th) 328 (S.C.), aff'd. (2006), 60 B.C.L.R. (4th) 43 (C.A.).

T.(I.) v L.(L.) (1999), 46 O.R. (3d) 284 (C.A.).

T.(S.) v Gaskell (1997), 147 D.L.R. (4th) 730 (Ont. Gen. Div.).

Tarasoff v Regents of the University of California, 17 Cal. Rptr. 3d 425 (U.S. 1976).

ter Neuzen v Korn, [1995] 10 W.W.R. 1 (S.C.C.).

Thibault v Fewer, [2002] 1 W.W.R. 204 (Man. Q.B.).

Till v Walker, [2000] O.J. No. 84 (S.C.J.) (Q.L.).

Tremblay v McLauchlan (2001), 6 C.C.L.T. (3d) 238 (B.C.C.A.).

Turkington v Lai (2007), 52 C.C.L.T. (3d) 254 (Ont. S.C.J.).

Villemure v L'Hôpital Notre-Dame, [1973] S.C.R. 716.

Villeneuve v Sisters of St. Joseph of Diocese of Sault Ste. Marie (1971), 18 D.L.R. (3d) 537 (Ont. H.C.).

Walker (Litigation Guardian of) v Region 2 Hospital Corp. (1994), 116 D.L.R. (4th) 477 (N.B.C.A.).

Williams v New Brunswick (1985), 34 C.C.L.T. 299 (N.B.C.A.).

Wilson v Swanson (1956), 5 D.L.R. (2d) 113 (S.C.C.).

Yelle v Children's Aid Society of Ottawa-Carleton (2002), 13 C.C.L.T. (3d) 53 (Ont. S.C.J.).

Zhang v Kan (2003), 15 C.C.L.T. (3d) 1 (B.C.S.C.).

Chapter 27

Tips for Testifying in Court

Sydney J. Usprich, Robert M. Solomon and Cate Sutherland

Why Me?

Addiction workers who deal with clients involved in the criminal justice system may, at some point, be required to appear in criminal court. The most common reasons for an addiction worker being called to testify are (1) to provide evidence about a client's attendance (or non-attendance) or participation in a treatment program; and (2) to explain addiction assessment findings or treatment recommendations relating to a client.

Addiction workers may also be required to appear in family court to testify in child welfare matters. Some children in our society are, unfortunately, affected by the substance use problems of adults. When such a situation comes to the attention of an authority, the matter is often referred to court for resolution. Specific situations that may require a counsellor's testimony include court cases in which the Children's Aid Society (CAS) is following a complaint that a child needs protection; and disagreements between parents or others regarding custody of, or access to, children. Family court also handles criminal matters involving young offenders (age 12 to 17).

Testifying in court does not rank high on anyone's list of enjoyable activities, but if you are subpoenaed as a witness in a trial or other hearing, you are obligated to attend and give evidence. Remember that you are not on trial. You are simply doing your duty by telling the court what you know in order to help the court arrive at a fair decision.

For the layperson, the courtroom can be an intimidating place and appearing there can be stressful. But the experience need not be as unpleasant as some people fear. The more you understand about the process of testifying, and the better prepared you are, the less uncomfortable the experience will be.

Providing testimony in an efficient, professional manner is an easily learned skill. This chapter outlines a number of steps you can take to reduce your stress and ensure that the image you present in court reflects the credibility and quality of your program. It offers advice on preparing for court appearances and testifying, and provides tips on courtroom deportment.

Preparation

Learn about Courts

Preparation should start long before you are required to appear in court. If you have never been to criminal court before, sit through some criminal proceedings to familiarize yourself with the procedures. Pay close attention to how things are done so you will know what to expect. This will help eliminate the fear of the unknown.

If you want to observe the proceedings in family court, prior arrangements may be required. Since matters handled by family court involve children, the proceedings are closed to the public for the obvious reason of preserving the child's privacy. However, you can usually arrange to observe in family court by calling the court office to explain your purpose.

After you have observed some court proceedings, envision yourself on the stand, calmly responding to questions. Before your first court appearance, it may help to have someone rehearse, or role play, with you.

Talk to the Lawyers

Once you learn that you may be called as a witness, determine whether you will appear for the Crown or the defence counsel (the client's lawyer). You will probably have been contacted by a lawyer for the side planning to call you as a witness. It is wise to advise the lawyer as early as possible about any dates on which it would be difficult to attend court. For example, you may have vacation travel plans that would make it extremely disruptive and expensive to attend court on certain dates. The earlier the lawyer knows this, the easier it will be to arrange a more convenient date.

As part of their preparation, most lawyers try to meet their prospective witnesses to review the witnesses' evidence. Accordingly, you may be contacted long before the trial by the lawyer or someone else from his or her law firm to discuss your testimony.

There is no legal requirement for you to participate in this sort of discussion. In a strict legal sense, a subpoena obligates you only to appear in court and give evidence. However, although you are not required to co-operate, you might benefit from doing so. In addition to being helpful to the lawyer, the pre-trial discussion can help you as a witness. You will learn in advance the type of questions you will be asked when you testify.

The lawyer for the other side may also contact you to discuss the case and the evidence you will be giving. You are not required to participate in any such discussion, but there is nothing improper about doing so. The side calling a witness does not "own" that witness; any witness is free to talk to the other side to the extent that he or she wishes. You may wish to seek guidance from your employer or from the lawyer for whom you will be testifying as to whether, and to what extent, you should co-operate with the lawyer for the other side.

After reviewing your records and speaking to the lawyer(s), you will have some idea of what you plan to say in court. But remember, sometimes questioning takes unexpected turns. For example, the Crown attorney may tell you that you will be asked to testify on the client's poor attendance in the program, but on cross-examination the defence lawyer may focus on the subject matter of the client's sessions.

Review Your Client's Records

Preparation for testifying also involves reviewing your client's records. Thorough and accurate records are indispensable to witnesses. Records help reconstruct the facts of a case. A trial often takes place several years and hundreds of clients after an event occurred, and the records may be the only way the addiction worker can recall sufficient details about the case.

In addition, the records themselves can be invaluable during the trial or hearing. A record that the witness made or approved close to the time of the event can be used by the witness while testifying (see Sopinka et al., 1999, ss. 16.77–16.98). Furthermore, the actual record may be admissible as documentary evidence, even if the witness does not testify (see *Ares v. Venner*, 1970; for an example of a statutory provision, see the Ontario *Evidence Act*, 1990, ss. 35 & 52). At times this use of the record is vital. For example, if the potential witness has died or is otherwise unavailable, the record may become the sole source of information and evidence.

The state of the records can influence a witness's credibility in court. A witness who faces the court armed with a complete record of facts and observations is in a strong position. If the record is accurate, objective and complete, the witness will be perceived as organized, methodical and conscientious.

But be forewarned that if you use a file on the witness stand, it can be taken from you to be entered as an exhibit. When you take a file to court, always photocopy the contents beforehand and leave the copies in your office.

Make Notes

Apart from reviewing official records, it is often useful to make additional notes as soon as you are informed that you will be a witness. Litigation is a slow process, and considerable time may elapse before the trial takes place. As soon as you know that you may be a witness, make notes of everything you can remember about relevant matters to help preserve your memory of those events. Since these notes are made some time after the events in question, the witness cannot use them when testifying. Nonetheless, the notes can be useful later, to refresh your memory prior to testifying and to help you recall the events about which you will be giving evidence.

Day of the Trial

When the day comes, arrive at the courthouse a few minutes early. Let the lawyer for whom you are appearing know that you are there. Ask if there are any last-minute changes, and briefly review your testimony.

If the trial is in progress, you should check with the court usher to see whether there has been an order excluding witnesses. At some trials, the presiding judge may make such an order at a lawyer's request. With this order, witnesses are not allowed to be in court to hear other witnesses prior to giving their own testimony. In that event, it would be improper for you as a witness to enter the courtroom, so you could simply wait, or ask the usher to take a note to the lawyer.

Bring any relevant records or documents, as instructed by the lawyer who requested your testimony. In addition, bring any personal notes that you have made, which you can review to refresh your memory prior to testifying.

When you are called to the witness stand, you will be "sworn in" before providing evidence. The usual procedure is to be sworn in by taking an oath on the Bible. Since the Christian Bible contains the Old Testament, many members of the Jewish faith are content to swear on the standard Bible. If your religious beliefs require that the oath be taken in a different way, this is permissible, but you should inform the lawyer in advance so that arrangements can be made. For example, a Muslim may wish to take the oath on the Koran, which may not be routinely available. As well as informing the lawyer in advance of any special requirements, it may be simplest for the witness to bring along the appropriate holy book or other objects needed.

Witnesses who object to swearing a religious oath have the option of "affirming" the truth. (e.g., see *Canada Evidence Act*, 1985, s. 14). This is simply a solemn promise, without any religious connotations, to tell the truth. It is best if you advise the lawyer in advance that you intend to affirm, rather than take an oath.

Giving Evidence

After the oath or affirmation formalities are done, you are ready to give your evidence. The lawyer calling a witness begins with what is known as "examination-in-chief" or "direct examination." Once the lawyer who called you as a witness finishes asking questions, it then becomes the turn of the lawyer for the other side. This latter questioning is called "cross-examination." At the conclusion of the cross-examination, the witness's testimony has usually ended, but sometimes the original lawyer may ask further questions in "re-examination."

The judge, who may ask questions at any stage, usually tells you when you are finished as a witness and may leave the witness stand. Unless you have been told that you are subject to recall as a witness, which rarely occurs, you may either leave the court or take a seat in the courtroom audience. Even if there has been an order excluding witnesses, the exclusion no longer applies to you after you have finished giving evidence.

Be Clear and Concise

When giving evidence, as a rule, give brief, direct answers to direct questions. Do not elaborate unless specifically requested to do so and, even then, be concise.

Answer only what is asked of you. Do not offer information that is not requested, even if you think it is important. Remember, you are not in court to tell a story, but merely to provide evidence. In addition, do not allow yourself to get caught up in explaining the rationales of your field. Speak only about the particular client in his or her particular situation.

Provide your testimony in a clear, well-modulated voice, loud enough to be heard by all. Speaking inaudibly implies that you do not have confidence in the information you are providing and makes it difficult for others to understand you.

Take your time. Hurried answers are sometimes incorrect answers. Give your answers in words so that a proper record can be made. For example, answer "yes," rather than nodding your head. If you happen to respond with physical motions or gestures, the lawyer questioning you may describe your response by "talking it onto the record." For example:

Lawyer: *How big was the knife?*

Witness: *About this long.*

Lawyer: *The witness is indicating with her hands a length of about six inches.*

In assessing a witness's evidence, the court often considers not only what you say, but also how you say it. Your credibility can be affected by both your verbal and non-verbal presentation on the stand. You should answer in a clear, straightforward manner and avoid being either hesitant or arrogant. Nevertheless, if you are unsure about something, it is not fair to anybody to answer with a confidence you do not feel.

Court Decorum

Stand (or sit, if invited to do so) in the witness box as calmly as you can, without giving the impression that you are a mannequin. There is a fine line here. You do not want to appear so relaxed that you seem indifferent to the proceedings. On the other hand, you do not want a ramrod posture to project an air of nervousness and rigidity. Also, if you are standing, keep your hands out of your pockets.

Wear your "poker face" to court. Do not visibly react to what you hear by rolling your eyes or shaking your head, or through other body-language editorializing. (This applies whether you are in the witness box or sitting elsewhere in the court.) You should appear totally objective—and thus, professional—at all times.

Courts generally have rather specific, though unwritten, rules on what is considered proper attire—conservatism is the name of the game. This usually means suits, or at least a shirt and tie for men, and suits or dresses for women. Generally, hats are not permitted in court.

When sitting in court before or after giving evidence, do not talk during the proceedings. If you find it necessary to communicate with someone, speak in the most discreet whisper. Better yet, pass a note.

Addressing Members of the Court

When giving evidence, speak directly to the person asking the question, and make eye contact. Never address the defendant directly while you are on the stand. Do not refer to an adult client by his or her first name; use "Mr." or "Ms."

Lawyers are also addressed as "Mr." or "Ms.," or simply "sir" or "ma'am" (madam). Although it will rarely arise, you may wish to refer to a trial lawyer other than the one who is currently questioning you. Aside from referring to the lawyer by name ("Mr./Ms. Smith"), you may—especially if you don't know the lawyer's name—refer to him or her as "counsel" (e.g., counsel for the plaintiff, counsel for Mr. Jones, counsel for the hospital).

In most jurisdictions, you should address the judge as "Your Honour." The correct terminology will depend on the level of court and the province in which the trial takes place. You can ask the lawyer beforehand, or simply listen to how the lawyers address the judge and copy their terminology. As an easy alternative, simply address the judge as "sir" or "ma'am" (madam). If you need to refer to the judge in the third person, the correct form is "His/Her Honour."

Do not address the judge directly unless he or she has spoken to you first. The only exception to this rule is when you need to refer to the file or your notes. Generally, you are expected to provide your testimony without looking in the file while you are on the stand. If you need to do so, turn to the judge and ask, "May I refer to my notes, Your Honour?" The judge will probably give permission. But if the witness must rely on notes rather than his or her recollection, lawyers have the right to determine whether the notes are reliable. This typically consists of questions about when the notes were made.

Direct Examination

Direct examination typically begins with mundane matters such as the witness's name and relevant qualifications. Rather than the witness being asked questions to elicit this routine introductory material, the lawyer will often recite the information and simply expect the witness to agree.

> Lawyer: *You are Mary Smith and are employed as a counsellor at the Central Addictions Centre?*

Witness: *Yes, sir.*

Lawyer: *The Central Addictions Centre is located at 123 Main Street in downtown Blankville?*

Witness: *That's right.*

Lawyer: *I understand that in your professional capacity you were providing counselling to John Doe in May 2010?*

Witness: *Yes, he had been seeing me professionally from March through June of that year.*

Particularly if you are being called as an "expert" witness, the lawyer may wish to bring out extensive details of your professional qualifications such as education, experience and membership in professional bodies. Such issues should be discussed well before the trial, so the witness can be properly prepared with the appropriate information. Indeed, the lawyer may have requested a curriculum vitae or resumé for this purpose.

Cross-Examination

The opposing lawyer (i.e., a lawyer who did not call the witness to testify) may try to achieve several goals through cross-examination. The lawyer may try to get additional information from the witness that will help the other side, or additional facts that may weaken evidence already given. The lawyer may try to get the witness to qualify an earlier answer, concede that there is some doubt on a particular point or admit that an alternative explanation is possible.

Sometimes, the lawyer may attempt to weaken evidence by discrediting a witness. There may be an effort to suggest that the witness is mistaken, biased, forgetful or not credible for a variety of other reasons.

Some lawyers will ask convoluted or awkward questions, and it can be difficult to understand just what they want to know. Listen carefully to the question and make sure you understand before you reply. Do not hesitate to admit your confusion. Simply say, "I'm sorry, I do not understand the question. Could you please repeat it?" This forces the lawyer to rephrase the question in a clearer form, and has the added advantage of giving you a few extra seconds to form an answer.

Although lawyers should not do so, sometimes they ask "double-barrelled" questions. This is especially likely in cross-examination where the lawyer is permitted to ask leading questions that require only a "yes" or "no" answer. If you simply answer yes or no, it may be unclear whether your single answer is in response to both halves of the question or only the last part. It is best to respond to such double questions by explicitly answering both halves. For example, a witness might be asked, "Was the client intoxicated and attempting to attack you?" Rather than answering "yes," it is clearer if the witness were to say, "Yes, he appeared drunk and attempted to attack me."

Another awkward type of question is one framed in the negative. For example: "You didn't see him do it, did you?" A simple reply of "no" could mean either "No, I didn't see" or "No, I disagree with you. I did see." Make sure that your answer is properly understood by responding fully: "No, I did not see."

A device that lawyers commonly use in cross-examination is to cut a witness off before he or she can give a full answer or a qualification to an answer. The result may be that a particular answer may be misleading because it is incomplete. If that should happen, ask the lawyer, firmly and courteously, to let you complete your answer. Often, however, the judge or the other lawyer will intercede on your behalf, asking that you be allowed to finish.

Sometimes, cross-examination gets rough. While it may feel like a personal attack, it is not. Remember, a lawyer's first obligation is to his or her client, and it is the lawyer's duty to test all evidence vigorously. While the lawyer may be aggressive toward you on the stand, you will probably find that this ends at the courtroom door.

Must I Answer?

Generally, witnesses must answer all relevant questions put to them. Privilege is one of the few exceptions to that general rule. The legal term "privilege" means the right to refuse to disclose confidential information when giving testimony. (For a more detailed discussion of privilege, refer to Chapter 26 on legal issues.) Traditionally, the only professional relationship to which privilege applied was that between solicitors and their clients. In the absence of privilege, a person who refuses to answer a question when required to do so may be jailed for contempt of court.

Canadian law has no equivalent to the American device of "taking the Fifth." Under the Fifth Amendment to the U.S. Bill of Rights, a witness may refuse to answer a question that tends to incriminate him or her. In Canada, a witness would have to answer such a question. However, section 13 of the *Canadian Charter of Rights and Freedoms* (1982) protects a witness from having any incriminating answer used against him or her in any other proceedings (except a prosecution for testifying falsely). This protection automatically applies to all the witness's answers without the witness having to ask for it.

Limits on Testimony

Generally, a witness's testimony is confined to information within his or her personal knowledge—that is, evidence based on his or her own observations rather than on what other people may have told the witness. As a result, a witness is not usually allowed to give what lawyers call "hearsay" evidence.

The rule against hearsay means you will often not be allowed to repeat what other people have told you. The hearsay rule is complex and not always easy to apply. First, the rule has many exceptions that permit hearsay evidence to be given. Second, hearsay evidence will not always be in the obvious form ("Charlie told me . . ."). For example, information that the witness obtained from someone else's notes may be considered hearsay.

As a witness, you are not expected to be a lawyer with expert knowledge of the hearsay rule. In discussing your evidence with the lawyer before the trial, he or she can advise you as to what conversations you may or may not be allowed to repeat because of the hearsay rule. If the issue arises while you are giving evidence and you are unsure, for example, whether you can repeat a given conversation, it is always appropriate to ask the trial judge whether you may say what someone has told you.

In situations where you are allowed to repeat statements that other people have made, these statements may sometimes involve obscene or offensive language. There is no need to be embarrassed. The judge and the lawyers have undoubtedly heard such language before. Bear in mind that it is not you who used that language; you are merely quoting what someone else has said. The importance of the evidence might depend on the fact that the speaker used that sort of language. While it is best to quote the speaker's words as accurately as possible, you could paraphrase the words if you are truly uncomfortable repeating them. In that case, you should make it clear that you are doing so.

Another area with restrictions on testimony involves the giving of opinions or conclusions by a witness. Only an "expert" witness testifying specifically on a matter within his or her area of expertise may give an opinion. An ordinary witness must give only his or her observations, not the opinions or conclusions that the witness may have drawn from those observations. However, a witness may give opinions about common matters on which, in a sense, everybody is an "expert." For example, a witness could testify that someone appeared drunk, was happy or sad, and so forth. Again, you are not expected to be a lawyer and to know all the fine distinctions. The lawyers and the judge will provide guidance on what you may or may not say.

The lawyers and the judge have a shared responsibility to keep inadmissible evidence out of the trial. If some evidence that you are about to give is inadmissible because of the hearsay rule, the opinion rule or some other reason, you may be interrupted and instructed not to give that evidence. Sometimes this interruption will take the form of an objection by the lawyer who is not currently questioning you. He or she will interrupt by saying "Objection" or "I object." If that happens, you should stop what you are saying. The trial judge, after listening to both lawyers' arguments, will decide whether the evidence is admissible and will advise you whether you can continue.

Family Court

Many of the procedures and principles related to testifying in criminal court also apply to family court. However, a few differences between these courts are noted in this section. For example, as a witness in family court, you are—because of the privacy concerns mentioned earlier—less likely to be permitted in the courtroom during other testimony in the case. In this situation, you will be instructed to wait in the outer area until called to provide your testimony.

Another minor difference involves the number of lawyers who participate in the proceedings. In criminal matters, there are typically two lawyers—the Crown and the defence. Child welfare cases, however, often have more than two lawyers, as anyone who is a party in the case could be represented. A child could have a separate lawyer, as could the Children's Aid Society, if involved, and other parties, such as the parents (separately or together) or a third party seeking custody or access. This does not necessarily mean that each lawyer will have many questions or that you will be on the stand longer, although both are possible. Typically, one or two lawyers will elicit the main parts of your testimony. The others may ask a few more questions to clarify or obtain slightly different types of information.

This leads to the most important differences between family and criminal court—the nature of the testimony and the scope allowed to the witness. In child welfare matters, there can be a wider interpretation of the relevance of evidence, giving lawyers more latitude in the questions asked or the avenues that may be explored with witnesses. The court has to make decisions, based on the testimony before it, that may profoundly affect the lives of children. Thus, it is understandable that the court would wish to hear any information that could be pertinent.

So, while you prepare for court by determining the expected direction of your testimony and carefully reviewing your client files, realize too that questions may arise that do not seem directly related to the client's treatment or your involvement with the client. In such situations, you must carefully decide whether you know the answer. Remember, witnesses can only testify about what they know.

Consider the following scenario. Let's suppose that, during treatment, Mr. Smith, a single father, reports that his drinking has been a problem for about 10 years. Among other things, he tells you that he is often hung over and that he often slips some whisky into his morning coffee while his 12-year-old son, Junior, is eating breakfast. Mr. Smith says his son is often with a babysitter while he is at a bar, and when he drinks at home, his son stays in his room. He also admits that he has missed a couple of Junior's school functions because he was drinking, which made his son angry. Mr. Smith says he feels bad about all of this and intends to make it up to Junior. Later, in court, you are asked about Mr. Smith.

Lawyer: *How has Mr. Smith's drinking problem interfered with his ability to be a good father to Junior?*

Witness: *I'm sorry. I can't answer that question. As Mr. Smith's addiction worker, I am not qualified to comment on his abilities as a father.*

The point is that you must consider the whole question and its implications, then decide whether you can answer it as asked. Mr. Smith provided plenty of information about his drinking and his son, but the question was about his "ability to be a good father." Carefully heed previous advice in the chapter about answering questions, and do not extrapolate pieces of information. For instance, the information in Mr. Smith's scenario speaks volumes about his alcohol problem, but really says nothing concrete about his ability to care for the child.

Another aspect of the special nature of testimony in family court involves the scope of the witness's testimony. As described elsewhere in this chapter, an ordinary witness is usually not permitted to testify as to opinions—such testimony is the province of the expert witness. However, addiction workers and other professionals may find that questions in family court often seem to fall in a grey area, eliciting testimony that falls somewhere between personal and expert knowledge. In this grey area, it is assumed that the witness has a certain amount of knowledge, based on overall experience and observations, as a result of employment in the profession. Questions and answers that call for this sort of opinion may need the assent of the court. Seeking that assent is often prompted by an objection from one lawyer to another lawyer's question, usually on the basis that it calls for an opinion or is not specific to the client.

If allowed, such questions are typically very general in nature and, unless the witness has a head full of statistics, result in an answer that is a sort of personal "semi-opinion" or conclusion. Examples of these types of questions are:

> *Based on your experience, is it common for a person's drinking problem to affect other family members?*

> *In the five years you have been employed as an addiction worker, what have you observed about . . .?*

Again, think before you answer, and try to avoid bias. No absolutes exist in the addiction field, so avoid the use of "never" or "always" in your answers. Start to answer with phrases like "It is my experience that . . ." or "I have observed that. . . ." Also, if need be, insert qualifiers such as "It is my experience that it is common for . . ., but that does not occur in every case."

Finally, a caution about "expert" status. It is typically reserved for people with significant experience, who have been advised prior to the case that they will testify as an expert. In such cases, the witness's status is established at the beginning of his or her testimony. However, a lawyer can also seek expert status for a witness, without prior warning, during the witness's testimony.

The testimony of addiction workers is often very important to judgments made in family court. Be prepared and take the responsibility seriously. Your expertise and confidence can help the court.

Conclusion

Although testifying in court will never be a delight, it need not be a dreaded, anxiety-filled experience. Understanding what is expected of you as a witness will make testifying less intimidating. Good preparation is even more important. While this may seem like a lot of work for a few minutes on the stand, the effort will be worthwhile. If you are prepared, you will feel more comfortable and be able to give your evidence in a relaxed, straightforward manner. This will enable you to make a better impression as a witness and to leave court feeling that you made a significant contribution to the administration of justice.

Resources

Publications

Brodsky, S.L. (2012). *Testifying in Court: Guidelines and Maxims for the Expert Witness* (2nd ed.). Washington, DC: American Psychological Association.

Vogl, R. & Bala, N. (2001). *Testifying on Behalf of Children: A Handbook for Canadian Professionals*. Toronto: Thompson Educational Publishing.

Internet

Children's Services Practice Notes: The Art of Testifying in Court
    www.practicenotes.org/vol12_no4/testifying.htm
Child Welfare Information Gateway: Testifying in Court
    www.childwelfare.gov/pubs/usermanuals/courts_92/courtsj.cfm

References

Ares v. Venner, 1970 SCR 608.

Canada Evidence Act, RSC 1985, c C-5.

Canadian Charter of Rights and Freedoms, s 2, Part I of the *Constitution Act, 1982*, being Schedule B to the *Canada Act 1982* (UK), 1982, c 11.

Evidence Act, RSO 1990, c E.23.

Sopinka, J., Lederman, S. & Bryant, A. (1999). *The Law of Evidence in Canada* (2nd ed.). Markham, ON: Butterworths.

Chapter 28

The Essential Ingredients for Clinical Supervision

Kirstin Bindseil, Marion Bogo and Jane Paterson

Juan just graduated from school and has successfully obtained his first job in the addiction field. He is happy with the job, but concerned about why, after he has been in the position for only two months, his work is being scrutinized by his supervisor, Janice. Although not all staff meet with their supervisor individually, Juan has already met with Janice five times. At their last meeting, she told him that she will observe videos of his group sessions starting next week and that he should be familiar with the consent procedure so the session can be taped for supervision. Juan is still not sure why he is going to supervision, and why he has to tape his sessions.

- What are some things Juan could say to get greater clarification about the role of supervision in his work?
- What could Janice do to provide greater clarification?

Henry is a new supervisor who has been asked to meet with Judy, an experienced addiction counsellor, after a client who was attending group therapy complained about her work. The client was upset that Judy had told Henry in an individual session that she did not see the benefit in Henry continuing group because he did not follow through with any group recommendations and she was "working harder than him" at his recovery. The client was offended by this comment and wonders if Judy is prejudiced against him for being a "crack addict."

When asked about the incident, Judy explains how frustrated she is with the client and is not surprised by the complaint. She reports that the client is always asking for letters of support and referrals to outside agencies and does not appear to be engaged in the work of the group. Furthermore, she is concerned that other clients are becoming overly invested in trying to help and support this client.

- What concerns might Henry have as a supervisor? What questions might Henry ask to further clarify the clinical situation?

- What concerns might Judy have as a supervisee? What might she contribute to the discussion to make the meeting useful to her?

Clinical supervision has come to play a key role in providing support, training and evaluation to both addiction counsellors and administrative staff in the addiction field. Although the research literature has not directly connected clinical supervision with client outcomes, clinicians anecdotally identify supervision as a key component to support their work with clients. Current research has focused on the impact of clinical supervision on staff burnout and emotional exhaustion. For example, in a study supported by the National Institute on Drug Abuse (Knudsen et al., 2008), administrators and staff from 262 treatment programs surveyed about the perceived impact of clinical supervision described supervision as strongly associated with health and well-being in the workplace: staff were less likely to want to leave their job and to feel emotionally exhausted. Furthermore, a positive supervision experience indirectly correlated with increased autonomy, procedural justice (staff have a voice in decision making) and distributive justice (fair distribution of job demands and rewards).

Project MERITS (Managing Effective Relationships in Treatment Services) surveyed 462 addiction counsellors in the United States about their perception of supervision (Eby et al., 2007). Counsellors who rated their clinical supervisor more favourably expressed greater job satisfaction, felt more committed to the organization and perceived more organizational support, and felt less overloaded and burned out in their roles. Despite the benefits of supervision, the supervisor and supervisee must work to address power differences; negotiate the dual role of supervisor being supporter and teacher on the one hand, and evaluator on the other; and be transparent and respectful.

This chapter outlines some key dimensions of clinical supervision, drawing on theoretical literature and emerging empirical findings in the field of addiction and concurrent disorders. While the literature on clinical supervision typically addresses supervisory functions, tasks and professional development (e.g., Bindseil et al., 2008; Powell & Brodsky, 2004), this chapter aims to help supervisees understand the key components of meaningful supervision and how to best benefit from the process. Although defined differently across professions, clinical supervision uniformly involves a senior staff member providing support, professional development and guidance to junior colleagues to ensure effective service to clients (Hall & Cox, 2009; Milne, 2007). Clinical supervision is referred to simply as *supervision* in this chapter.

The Organizational Context

An organization's commitment to the provision of clinical supervision is in essence a commitment to the organization's staff and clients. Clinicians need to receive formalized support for their clinical practice and can consult and receive guidance on their practice. Ideally through the supervision process, they will gain competencies and confidence and become better equipped to meet the needs of their clients; they will be able to identify areas for future development; and they will be guided on how to acquire the desired clinical skills. By providing good supervision, the organization indicates its commitment to the education and development of its staff. By committing to the advancement of clinicians' specialized current knowledge of best practices and clinical skills, an organization supports its goal of client-centred practice.

Supervision Models

Some supervision models are profession specific (see Jones, 2005, for nursing, and Bogo & McKnight, 2005, for social work); others are specific to client populations (see Pearlman & Saakvitne, 1997, for trauma-informed care); and still others are specific to a treatment (see Linehan, 1995, for dialectical behaviour therapy, and Martino et al., 2006, for motivational interviewing). This chapter describes the essential ingredients of supervision, which can be applied to various clinical settings in the addiction field. It also presents a general interprofessional approach to supervision, drawing from the literature and the authors' own supervision practice experience.

Common to the literature in nursing and social work is a three-factor model of supervision (Kadushin & Harkness, 2002; Proctor, 1986), which is experienced in the addiction field as comprehensive and easily adapted. The first factor is *administrative* or *normative* (managerial), and involves orienting clinicians, assigning cases and reviewing and evaluating work. The second factor is *educational* or *formative*, and includes developing and enhancing the clinician's practice capacity by teaching knowledge and skills, building on training and developing self-awareness. The third factor is *supportive* or *restorative*, and involves helping clinicians handle job-related stress by providing appropriate praise and encouragement, normalizing work-related reactions, affirming strengths, exploring personal triggers and sharing responsibility for difficult decisions.

Other supervision models discuss the importance of acknowledging developmental stages; for example, that a person new to the profession or even to the organization likely has greater need for support than a person with many years of experience. Supervisors can tailor their input to the features of the particular stage, and staff can gain support and training when needed and obtain greater autonomy as they progress through the developmental cycle.

Although several developmental models exist, that of Stoltenberg & McNeill (2010) is the model most often discussed in the substance use literature. It identifies three levels of development (see Table 29-1). The opportunity to match supervision to the level of development optimizes the work that is done in supervision.

TABLE 29-1

Developmental Approach to Clinical Supervision

STAGE OF DEVELOPMENT	CLINICIAN PRESENTS WITH	GOALS IN SUPERVISION	POSSIBLE STRATEGIES
Level 1	Taps into practice knowledge/skills Treatment may appear less focused and intentional Some skills used often, others under-used Treatment often driven by client crises	Help develop personal philosophies and approaches to counselling, integrating appropriate research and theory Reinforce areas of strength Highlight and support improvement in areas for development Help manage organization's expectations around workload	Observation Role play Case formulation Individual supervision
Level 2	Increased confusion and frustration Acknowledgment of gaps in learning Feelings of uncertainty with exposure to more challenges Greater challenges toward organizational practices	Help discover blind spots in practice Identify how current skills can be enhanced	Individual supervision with less frequency Case formulation Observation Group supervision

STAGE OF DEVELOPMENT	CLINICIAN PRESENTS WITH	GOALS IN SUPERVISION	POSSIBLE STRATEGIES
Level 3	Increased self-assurance and self-awareness in clinical work Skills adapted to better match client needs Greater comfort working within organizational context	Focus on issues before they become crises	Group supervision Consultation when needed Peer supervision

Adapted from Stoltenberg & McNeill (2010).

At the first level of development, clinicians may have gaps in knowledge or skills, so the treatment they provide may appear less focused and intentional, and more crisis-driven. Clinicians are not sure how to fit their skills to the range of client situations, and use some skills more and underuse others. Regular, frequent supervision sessions are recommended to help clinicians build their clinical knowledge, competence and professional style. Supervisors can provide performance feedback and engage supervisees in reflective discussion about the efficacy of what they have learned and how to develop personal philosophies of counselling. Observation, role plays and case formulations are key in this first phase of development. To be of greatest assistance, supervisors need to learn what the clinician is doing well in order to reinforce those strengths, while also providing guidance for further development. Supervision at this level also helps clinicians manage organizational expectations about workload.

Perhaps surprisingly, at the second level of development, the clinician may appear more confused and frustrated and less skilled and able in clinical work compared to a new supervisee. With more experience, the clinician may develop certain blind spots within clinical practice; the supervisor may need to challenge commonly held assumptions or ways of practising so the clinician can best serve the client population. This second phase may also be a time of uncertainty, as the clinician recognizes the complexities and common challenges of the work. The clinician focuses less on simple, prescribed responses and more on the client's narrative. He or she may challenge standard practice approaches, including issues regarding organizational systems. Supervision involves exploring alternative approaches through education. At this level, group supervision can be more effective, and individual sessions may be less important.

At the third level of development, clinicians are more self-assured and self-aware in their work. They are better able to fine-tune strategies to match client needs. There is a balanced approach to the work and a stronger ability to feel comfortable with limitations in the clinical and organizational contexts. By this time, clinicians are more aware of their subjective and emotional responses and are often able to ask for support before a crisis develops. Supervision continues to be part of the clinical realm and can be supplemented with peer consultation.

Importance of the Relationship between Supervisor and Supervisee

Consistent with the literature, our recent study of front-line addiction and mental health clinicians found that the quality of the relationship between supervisor and supervisee is paramount to the success of clinical practice (Bogo et al., 2011a). Supervisees want supportive, clinician-focused, content-oriented supervision offered by knowledgeable, skilled clinical experts. Regardless of the supervisor's profession, most important is the supervisor's expertise in treating the client population and his or her ability to help clinicians learn and achieve competence. In our study, some clinicians identified a tension between the supervisor's role in evaluating performance and the clinician's comfort in expressing a need for assistance with difficult client situations. This sentiment is reflected in the literature about the supervisor's dual role of evaluating and supporting staff. The reality in many mental health and addiction organizations is that the clinical supervisor has the authority to make administrative decisions, such as hiring or terminating staff, based on clinicians' performance (Powell & Brodsky, 2004; Roche et al., 2007). Effective supervisors balance the tensions inherent in the dual focus of their role.

Given this dual function, some clinicians may be reluctant to disclose aspects of their practice with which they need help. They may also question what is relevant to disclose and to what degree disclosure is important for their growth and development (Leszcz, 2011). In their book *What Therapists Don't Talk about and Why,* Pope and colleagues (2006) highlight 10 basic components for a successful supervision group:

1. Create an environment of safety and trust that encourages honesty, self-examination and risk taking.
2. Understand that this approach to learning requires self-direction.
3. Maintain readiness to disclose uncertain, uncomfortable and vulnerable thoughts and feelings, and to listen carefully to what others have to say.
4. Nurture respect for all participants.
5. Encourage active participation.
6. Acknowledge everyone's right to privacy.
7. Accept each person's disclosures as viable topics for discussion.
8. Maintain sensitive attention to the nuances of each participant's disclosures.
9. Communicate in a clear, honest manner.
10. Offer support for all participants as they engage in the process of learning and self-exploration.

It is important to establish clear expectations between supervisor and supervisee through contracting and re-contracting—a process that is useful for both parties. Contracting can be oral or written and can be requested by either person. The Center for Substance Abuse Treatment ([CSAT], 2009) has developed a clinical supervision protocol for addiction counsellors that outlines how contracts identify the purpose, goals, objectives and structure of supervision. Contracting can also clarify expectations of work in supervision (e.g., preparation of cases, frequency of observational work) and the evaluation process. It is important to clarify the process for non-compliance with expectations of conduct, clinical work or supervision. Through contracting, discussions occur about how to build trust and about related concerns around disclosures or risk taking. The following is an example of a contract that can be used in either individual or group supervision.

Clinical Supervision Contract

Date:_____

As clinician and clinical supervisor, we agree to:

- work together to facilitate in-depth reflection and enhanced expertise on issues affecting practice
- meet on average once per week as a group for one hour
- protect the time and space for clinical supervision by keeping to agreed appointments and time boundaries. Privacy will be respected and interruptions avoided
- provide a record for our employer, showing the times and the dates of the clinical supervision sessions
- work to the clinician's agenda within the framework and focus negotiated at the beginning of each session. However, the clinical supervisor reserves the right to highlight items apparently neglected or unnoticed by the clinician
- work respectfully, both of us being open to feedback about how we handle the clinical supervision sessions.

We both agree to challenge aspects of this agreement that may be in dispute.

As a clinician I agree to:

- prepare for the sessions, for example, by having an agenda or preparing notes, videos, observation opportunities, audiotapes
- take responsibility for making effective use of the time (including punctuality), the outcomes and any actions I may take as a result of clinical supervision
- be willing to learn, to develop my clinical skills and be open to receiving support and challenges.

As a clinical supervisor I agree to:

- keep all information you reveal in the clinical supervision sessions confidential, except for these exceptions:
  - you describe any unsafe, unethical or illegal practice that you are unwilling to go through the appropriate procedures to address
  - you repeatedly fail to attend sessions

- in the event of an exception arising, attempt to persuade and support you to deal appropriately with the issue directly yourself. If I remain concerned, I will reveal the information only after informing you that I am going to do so
- at all times work to protect your confidentiality
- not allow procedural issues of the work to monopolize the clinical supervision session
- offer you advice, support and supportive challenge to enable you to reflect in-depth on issues affecting your practice
- be committed to continually developing myself as a practising professional
- keep a record of our clinical supervision sessions
- ask for feedback for the purpose of evaluating the clinical supervision process
- use my own clinical supervision to support and develop my own abilities as a clinical supervisor and clinician, without breaking confidentiality.

Anything else?

Frequency of meetings: _____

Venue: _____

Duration of clinical supervision relationship: _____

Next review date: _____

Signed: _____ Signed: _____

(Clinician)   (Clinical supervisor)

Thank you for completing this questionnaire!

Source: Bolton Primary Care Trust. (2003). *Clinical Supervision (Professional Support) Policy & Guidance.* http://bolton.nhs.uk/ Library/policies/LDEV003.pdf. Adapted with permission.

Acknowledging power differences between supervisor and clinician is critical for the relationship. Even under ideal circumstances, with great trust and comfort, the fact that evaluation is an aspect of the supervisory role cannot be overlooked. Attending to power early and throughout supervision may help both supervisor and supervisee monitor the nature of their relationship and maintain sensitivity to this issue. Power exists on a continuum, and is influenced by factors such as the clinician's experience, knowledge and performance. For example, the power differential between supervisor and supervisee will likely be more pronounced with a newly graduated clinician who has little experience.

In other circumstances, the difference in power can be less pronounced, for example, when an Aboriginal clinician is working with an Aboriginal client and the supervisor does not belong to this population (Falender, 2010). In this case, the supervisee may have greater knowledge and cultural competence than the supervisor, and can therefore express a unique perspective and make suggestions with more power, tipping the balance in the opposite direction. Discussing these potential shifts in power enhances the supervisory relationship and deepens mutual respect.

Promote Culturally Informed Supervision

Cultural competence has emerged as a necessity in clinical practice. Although not all cities and towns across the country are seen as multicultural hubs, immigration patterns often shift the cultural landscape in unexpected ways. According to Statistics Canada's 2006 Census of Population, more than six million Canadians (about 20 per cent) were born outside the country (Statistics Canada, 2006). The Canadian Aboriginal population has also increased significantly: according to 2006 census data, the Aboriginal population increased by 45 per cent between 1996 and 2006 (Statistics Canada, 2006). These examples of changing population trends suggest that cultural differences between client, staff and supervisor will be more common. These differences can affect clinical practice positively or negatively, depending on whether differences are acknowledged and assessed.

Many organizations address client diversity through such strategies as increasing access to services, creating inclusivity and changing hiring practices. These strategies need to be backed up by similar processes at the front line. For example, clinicians' continuous reflection on their cultural competence is important for supervision (Srivastava, 2007). Developing clinical cultural competence is a process that evolves throughout one's career and involves learning how differences in self (clinician) and other (client) affect clinical outcomes. In relation to the self, supervision offers an opportunity to discuss the clinician's areas of privilege, which, if not addressed, can become a barrier to effective clinical care. Exploring our potential privilege based on age, gender, ability, income, education, sexual orientation, race and skin colour in relation to our clients can help to uncover potential "blind spots" in our understanding of the challenges our clients experience. For example, without understanding the financial impact of social assistance, we might erroneously assume that a client can afford to phone to make an appointment. Or without having lived in a part of the world where authorities are corrupt, we may not appreciate why a client would be mistrustful or worried about coming to a mainstream hospital or community centre for an appointment. These types of assumptions or misunderstandings create a divide between clinician and client, where empathy alone is not sufficient to promote a common understanding within the therapeutic relationships.

Furthermore, assessing the client's level of acculturation helps us to know what may or may not match with our own world view. The degree to which a client wishes to be connected to a cultural community is a rich area for discussion that can help clinicians determine how best to move toward effective change (Estrada et al., 2004).

Our natural tendency when working in difficult situations is to look for common ground, to find a place that is familiar in order to connect with the client and move forward together. However, it is also essential to discuss the differences between clinician and client in supervision in order to anticipate and understand tensions in the therapeutic relationship.

Promote Interprofessional Supervision

Interprofessional care and education are seen as important ways to manage resources and improve the quality of clinical care (Steinert, 2005). Interprofessional teamwork or collaborative practice values learning from different professional disciplines and applies to mutual learning among service providers (World Health Organization, 2010). Until about one decade ago, professional education took place in silos, so students did not fully learn about the roles and preparation of other mental health professionals or how to function effectively in interprofessional teams. Yet health care organizations expect practitioners from various disciplines to work together in teams. With minimal knowledge about team members' unique training, professional roles and capabilities, effective team functioning can be challenging.

Clinical supervision offered in a group format with professionals from various disciplines can serve as an important educational experience and opportunity to socialize. Supervisors can initiate discussions that address assumptions made about other disciplines and clarify expectations about members' ability to contribute to client care. Of extreme importance is helping team members communicate so that mistrust and power imbalances within the team can be examined openly (Orchard et al., 2005). While individual supervision sessions can also identify clinical concerns around team conflict or more effective collaboration, supervisors should bring such issues to the entire team and avoid discussions with individual members, which would undermine team cohesion.

Although not all addiction programs have staff from multiple disciplines on their teams, they can apply many principles of interprofessional care to help teams work together and to guide team supervision. In the addiction field, much debate has focused on differences between clinicians who are educated formally and those who have learned from personal recovery. (For a review of the literature, see Culbreth [2000].)

In our studies of interprofessional supervision at the Centre for Addiction and Mental Health, it was clear that staff work and live in their teams. Front-line clinicians spoke enthusiastically about the clinical assistance, professional and personal support and informal learning they gained from collaborative, cohesive, well-functioning teams (Bogo et al., 2011b). In interprofessional team supervision, learning from a range of disciplines occurred with the mutual respect of teammates.

Since well-functioning teams are important, it is useful to identify issues that can negatively affect team functioning and address them in group supervision sessions. Davoli (2004) poses the following questions for team members to consider when evaluating their individual performance and reflecting on the competencies of their team:

- Have you experienced communication problems with one or more members of the group?
- Have you taken action before consulting others just to get it done?
- Have you expected others to recognize the value of your contributions?
- Have you missed scheduled group or team meetings, even if it is for a good reason?

- Have you ever resented the limited co-operation or lack of productivity of some group members?

These questions offer an opportunity to reflect on current processes and assumptions about how team members relate to one another. Teams can then identify common areas of tension and agree to highlight areas that will enhance the team process. In group supervision, the ability to openly share the challenges and personal vulnerabilities of the work will be particularly difficult if members have not addressed how assumptions or misunderstanding others are affecting how the team functions.

When we first reviewed the clinical supervision literature and attended conferences, it immediately became apparent that different perceptions of supervision existed, based on histories and traditions in specific professions. For some, supervision was seen as a supportive process that took place almost weekly throughout one's career, while for others, supervision was part of a disciplinary action. These differences highlight the importance of discussing each profession's perspectives to arrive at a shared understanding of the current purpose of supervision, the value of each member's contribution and the expectations about sharing and jointly stepping back from the work to hear about and learn alternative viewpoints. The perspective from another discipline increases the chances of reflecting on our practice and improves our ability to expand our knowledge through the supervision process.

Observe and Be Observed

Supervision can be far more effective when the supervisor can actually observe our work and provide authentic, reality-based feedback. Yet a common reaction to being observed is to "run for the hills" or wish one could hide in an office and lock the door. For most, observation is very uncomfortable—at least in the beginning. We do not feel we can be our most relaxed self or provide the best care when we feel under the microscope. We fear being judged and showing vulnerability. We wonder whether the client will get the best care if we are nervous being observed. But clinicians who were observed as trainees may feel they learned a great deal from this observation and feedback. Observation provides an opportunity to improve clinical skills and increase confidence. Preparing for it can include expressing anxiety and concerns. Most supervisors will be able to normalize this feeling—and relate, since most have had their own experiences of being observed early in their careers.

Ideally, observation occurs regularly and is predictable. As with other aspects of the supervision relationship, it is important to feel that you are being observed for the purpose of facilitating your growth and development, not because of a complaint or concern. Observation should be consistent for all staff and not just a chosen few; however, staff new to the job may be observed more often than experienced clinicians. Clinicians have reported that both they and their clients feel more comfortable when the supervisor is in the room rather than when the interview is taped or observed behind a one-way mirror (Culbreth, 1999). Yet in children's mental health settings, observation by the team is a regular and accepted part of treatment services. Clinicians may request observation for an entire session or for more focused segments of their practice, for example, an assessment or education session.

Observing others is also useful for learning. Supervisees may wish to ask their supervisors whether they would be willing to be observed and participate in a post-session discussion where the supervisee could ask questions and provide feedback. Since our study found that clinicians wanted supervisors with clinical intervention knowledge and skill relevant to the setting (Bogo et al., 2011a), such observation opportunities are likely to facilitate learning.

Evaluate and Be Evaluated

The anxiety we experience in the observation process is clearly about having our work evaluated. Traditionally, evaluation of clinical work in the addiction field has been under-studied. The clinician was viewed as an expert—either a professional or person in recovery. Approaches to care focused on imparting our clinical wisdom to clients, who needed information, guidance and direction. However, with the emergence of collaborative and brief treatments, such as motivational interviewing (Miller & Rollnick, 2002) and narrative therapy (White, 2007; White & Epston, 1990), a shift has occurred toward the client and clinician co-constructing the therapeutic plan. As a result, clinicians are more active in obtaining ongoing feedback from clients about what is working and what could be changed, using standardized tools such as the Outcomes Rating Scale (Miller et al., 1997). From these clinical practices evolve other processes, in which clients are more likely to give feedback to clinicians and clinicians give feedback to supervisors. Clients also provide feedback to improve quality of care initiatives.

In the process of clinician evaluation by the supervisor, feedback is best received when it is continuous and regular. The supervisor can provide both formative and summative evaluations (CSAT, 2009). A formative evaluation involves ongoing feedback about a clinician's skill development and competencies, offered in regular supervision meetings and based on content that emerges from clinical observation. Summative evaluation is a more formal rating of overall job performance and fitness for the job. The summative review typically occurs in an annual performance review. Therefore, clinicians can expect to be provided with ongoing, frequent feedback about areas of strength and areas for further development. For the latter, supervisors should provide detailed, specific feedback to help the supervisee focus on enhancing particular skills needed to meet required competencies. Once we understand the landscape of our practice and how evaluation leads to focused supervision and clinical improvements, the clinician's confidence and efficacy increase.

Similar to observation, it is useful to have opportunities to evaluate the quality of supervision. As part of contracting with your supervisor, asking about what outcomes of supervision will be evaluated is another way to understand what you can expect to achieve in supervision. Although there does not seem to be a standard for when to evaluate supervision, requesting to evaluate often at first and more gradually over time allows for quick adjustments early in the process and ensures maximum benefit over time.

Student Field Instruction

The purpose of field instruction differs from staff supervision. Field instruction involves teaching students the generic knowledge and skill base of their profession as it is expressed in the specialized practice in addiction settings. The field instructor/staff member helps students to integrate the knowledge, values and skills they are learning in their academic program by discussing with them their practicum experience with clients. Since the practicum takes place in an organizational context, field instructors are accountable for the service students provide and must oversee or "supervise" students' work. The primary role, however, is that of educator; service is used in the context of teaching students. In contrast, the aim of staff supervision is to enhance client service through development and support of professional staff members' performance.

Many principles of supervision reviewed in this chapter are also important for field instruction, especially regarding the importance of the relationship, balancing autonomy and dependence with awareness of developmental stage, power dynamics and contracting, and culture and diversity; and being observed and observing others with opportunities to receive feedback and discuss interventions (Bogo, 2010). In their practicums, students apply what they have learned in academic courses to practice in the agency setting. Field instructors need to provide opportunities for reflective discussion, where observed practice can be linked to one or more conceptual frameworks. The knowledge base used in the setting may differ from that taught in the academic program. Students will need help examining practice through such a lens, as well as having opportunities to integrate concepts they are learning.

Revisiting the Case Studies

The case examples of Juan and Judy that began this chapter highlight how supervision is optimal if both supervisor and supervisee are engaged in the process.

> Juan is unclear about the purpose of observation and evaluation in his new job. For him, the first step in contracting is to clarify the expectations of supervision and address any concerns. Since Juan may identify with a Hispanic culture, there is an opportunity to explore any enhanced knowledge Juan might have, since many of the clients in the clinic where he works speak Spanish at home and English as their second language. In the absence of contracting expectations, Juan is likely to feel uneasy in the supervisory relationship.

Judy is a very experienced clinician. She reacted quickly to hearing about a client complaint, instead of considering how this feedback could help her reflect on her practice. Judy took a defensive stance, rather than being open to feedback. If this is a common reaction for her, she may need to develop new skills and be monitored through supervision and in her annual review. Since Judy is experienced, she can use her team to help explore this clinical challenge while still feeling supported. By affirming Judy's knowledge and experience, her supervisor, Henry, sets the stage for establishing a supportive supervisory relationship, where Judy can more openly examine and discuss potential gaps in knowledge or frustration she may have.

Conclusion

The educationally focused supervision experienced in student field instruction provides the foundation for ongoing growth and development of clinical skills and competencies. The essential ingredients of supervision discussed in this chapter are intended to extend clinicians' ability and confidence to provide high-quality clinical care, and to support clinicians so they may experience career growth and satisfaction.

Practice Tips

For supervisors:
- Take the time to clarify the organization's commitment to supervision.
- Establish a supervision contract with each supervisee.
- Discuss power and safety.
- Consider the level of development of each supervisee.
- Be open to being observed.
- Evaluate supervision regularly.

For supervisees:
- Discuss with your supervisor which type of supervision will be most effective.
- Be open to observation and evaluation.
- Recognize your role in contributing to the maintenance and development of healthy team dynamics.
- Identify your goals in terms of knowledge development, including ongoing cultural competence needs.

Resources

Publications

Bindseil, K., Bogo, M., Godden, T., Herie, M., Ingber, E., King, R. et al. (2008). *Clinical Supervision Handbook: A Guide for Clinical Supervisors for Addiction and Mental Health.* Toronto: Centre for Addiction and Mental Health.

Center for Substance Abuse Treatment. (2009). *Clinical Supervision and Professional Development of the Substance Abuse Counselor.* Treatment Improvement Protocol (TIP) series 52. Rockville, MD: Author. Retrieved from kap.samhsa.gov/products/manuals/tips/pdf/TIP52.pdf

Leszcz, M. (2011). Psychotherapy supervision and the development of the psychotherapist. In R. Klein, H. Bernard & V. Schermer (Eds.). *On Becoming a Psychotherapist: The Personal and Professional Journey* (pp. 114–143). Oxford, United Kingdom: Oxford University Press.

Internet

Australia's National Research Centre on Alcohol and Other Drugs Workforce Development
www.nceta.flinders.edu.au/projects/workforce_development/resources.html#A2

Ethnicity Online—Cultural Awareness in Health Care
www.ethnicityonline.net

University of Toronto Competency for Professional Practice Initiative
www.socialwork.utoronto.ca/research/initiatives/competency.htm

References

Bindseil, K., Bogo, M., Godden, T., Herie, M., Ingber, E., King, R. et al. (2008). *Clinical Supervision Handbook: A Guide for Clinical Supervisors for Addiction and Mental Health.* Toronto: Centre for Addiction and Mental Health.

Bogo, M. (2010). *Achieving Competence in Social Work through Field Education.* Toronto: University of Toronto Press.

Bogo, M. & McKnight, K. (2005). Clinical supervision in social work: A review of the research literature. *Clinical Supervisor, 24,* 49–67.

Bogo, M., Paterson, J., Tufford, L. & King, R. (2011a). Interprofessional clinical supervision in mental health and addiction: Toward identifying common elements. *Clinical Supervisor, 30,* 124–140.

Bogo, M., Paterson, J., Tufford, L. & King, R. (2011b). Supporting front-line practitioners' professional development and job satisfaction in mental health and addiction. *Journal of Interprofessional Care. 25,* 209–214.

Center for Substance Abuse Treatment (CSAT). (2009). *Clinical Supervision and Professional Development of the Substance Abuse Counselor.* Treatment Improvement Protocol (TIP) series 52. Rockville, MD: Substance Abuse and Mental Health Services Administration. Retrieved from kap.samhsa.gov/products/manuals/tips/pdf/TIP52.pdf

Culbreth, J.R. (1999). Clinical supervision of substance abuse counselors: Current and preferred practices, *Journal of Addictions & Offender Counseling, 20,* 15–25.

Culbreth, J.R. (2000). Substance abuse counselors with and without a personal history of chemical dependency: A review of the literature. *Alcoholism Treatment Quarterly, 18,* 67–82.

Davoli, G. (2004). Stacking the deck for success in interprofessional collaboration. *Health Promotion Practice, 5,* 266–270.

Eby, L.T., McCleese, C.S., Owen, C., Baranik, L. & Lance, C.E. (2007, October). *A process-oriented model of the relationship between clinical supervision, burnout, and turnover intentions among substance abuse counselors.* Poster session presented at the annual Addiction Health Services Research Conference, Athens, GA.

Estrada, D., Frame, M.W. & Williams, C.B. (2004). Cross-cultural supervision: Guiding the conversation toward race and ethnicity. *Journal of Multicultural Counseling and Development, 32,* 307–319.

Falender, C.A. (2010). Relationship and accountability: Tensions in feminist supervision. *Women & Therapy, 33,* 22–41.

Hall, T. & Cox, C. (2009). Clinical supervision: An appropriate term for physiotherapists? *Learning in Health and Social Care, 8,* 282–291.

Jones, J. (2005). Clinical supervision in nursing: What is it all about? *Clinical Supervisor, 24,* 149–162.

Kadushin, A. & Harkness, D. (2002). *Supervision in Social Work* (4th ed.). New York: Columbia University Press.

Knudsen, H.K., Ducharme, L.J. & Roman, P.M. (2008). Clinical supervision, emotional exhaustion, and turnover intention: A study of substance abuse treatment counselors in the Clinical Trials Network of the National Institute on Drug Abuse. *Journal of Substance Abuse Treatment, 35,* 387–395.

Leszcz, M. (2011). Psychotherapy supervision and the development of the psychotherapist. In R. Klein, H. Bernard & V. Schermer (Eds.), *On Becoming a Psychotherapist: The Personal and Professional Journey* (pp. 114–143). Oxford, United Kingdom: Oxford University Press.

Linehan, M.M. (1995). *Understanding Borderline Personality Disorder: The Dialectical Approach.* New York: Guilford Press.

Martino, S., Ball, S.A., Gallon, S.L., Hall, D., Garcia, M., Ceperich, S. et al. (2006). *Motivational Interviewing Assessment: Supervisory Tools for Enhancing Proficiency.* Salem, MA: National Institute on Drug Abuse.

Miller, S.D., Duncan, B.L. & Hubble, M.A. (1997). *Escape from Babel: Toward a Unifying Language for Psychotherapy Practice.* New York: Norton.

Miller, W.R. & Rollnick, S.P. (2002). *Motivational Interviewing: Preparing People for Change* (2nd ed.). New York: Guilford Press.

Milne, D. (2007). An empirical definition of clinical supervision. *British Journal of Clinical Psychology, 46,* 437–447.

Orchard, C.A.A., Curran, V. & Kabene, S. (2005). Creating a culture for interdisciplinary collaborative professional practice, *Medical Education Online, 10,* 1–13.

Pearlman L.A. & Saakvitne, K. (1997). *Trauma and the Therapist: Countertransference and Vicarious Traumatization in Psychotherapy with Incest Survivors.* New York: Norton.

Pope, K.S., Sonne, J.L. & Greene, B. (2006). *What Therapists Don't Talk about and Why: Understanding Taboos That Hurt Us and Our Clients.* Washington, DC: American Psychological Association.

Powell, D.J. & Brodsky, A. (2004). *Clinical Supervision in Alcohol and Drug Abuse Counseling: Principles, Models, Methods.* San Francisco: Jossey-Bass.

Proctor, B. (1986). Supervision: A co-operative exercise in accountability. In M. Marken & M. Payne (Eds.), *Enabling and Ensuring: Supervision in Practice* (pp. 21–34). Leicester, United Kingdom: National Youth Bureau and Council for Education and Training in Youth and Community Work.

Roche, A.M., Todd, C.L. & O'Connor, J. (2007). Clinical supervision in the alcohol and other drugs field: An imperative or an option? *Drug and Alcohol Review, 26,* 241–249.

Srivastava, R. (2007). *The Healthcare Professional's Guide to Clinical Cultural Competence.* Toronto: Mosby-Elsevier.

Statistics Canada. (2006). Aboriginal identity population, 2006 counts, percentage distribution, percentage change, 2006 counts for both sexes, for Canada, provinces and territories—20% sample data. Retrieved from www12.statcan.ca/census-recensement/2006/dp-pd/hlt/97-558/index.cfm?Lang=E

Steinert, Y. (2005). Learning together to teach together: Interprofessional education and faculty development. *Journal of Interprofessional Care, 19* (Suppl. 1), 60–75.

Stoltenberg, C.D. & McNeill, B.W. (2010). *IDM Supervision: An Integrative Developmental Model for Supervising Counselors and Therapists* (3rd ed.). New York: Routledge.

White, M. (2007). *Maps of Narrative Practice.* New York: Norton.

White, M. & Epston, D. (1990). *Narrative Means to Therapeutic Ends.* New York: Norton.

World Health Organization. (2010). *Framework for Action on Interprofessional Education and Collaborative Practice.* Geneva: Health Professionals Networks, Nursing and Midwifery.

Chapter 29

Care Pathways for Healing Journeys: Toward an Integrated System of Services and Supports

Rebecca Jesseman, David Brown and Wayne Skinner

Flora is an addiction worker in a specialized treatment setting. Most people she sees in assessment have severe substance use problems that qualify them for intensive treatment, including residential care. Many also have other health and social problems that are difficult to address through Flora's treatment service.

✦

Ali is a guidance counsellor in a high school. He sees most of the students who are having trouble meeting their academic requirements or adapting to the school's social environment. He is good at connecting with troubled teens, many of whom have substance use issues or spend too much time on gaming or other online activities that are distracting them from their studies.

✦

Ellen works as a probation officer. She has noticed that recidivism in the men and women she works with seems always to be related to substance use problems. But she doesn't know what she can do about it.

✦

Pierre works as a child protection intake worker at a child welfare agency. In at least half of the calls he investigates, one or both parents have substance use problems: this is always a key factor in deciding whether the children are safe from abuse or neglect.

✦

Ines is a nurse on a multi-service health team at a community health centre. When she follows up with clients who have experienced acute health events, such as heart attack, stroke or accidents, she has noticed that many have problems with tobacco, alcohol and prescription and illicit drug use. Their substance use appears to be not only a contributing factor in the health event that got them into care, but also a factor that interferes with rehabilitation and recovery.

The professionals introduced in these vignettes work across a range of sectors, and despite different job descriptions, each works with people experiencing challenges related to substance use. In some cases, substance use is the primary focus of their work. In others, it is part of the overall picture and may or may not be actively addressed. In each case, the ability to develop holistic, integrated programs of care is crucial to helping clients develop healthy behaviours. Unfortunately, problematic substance use and other addictive behaviours are features in the lives of many people who receive help in the health and social service systems. Other health and social problems have high rates of co-prevalence among clients whose substance use is affecting their functioning and health. Yet the systems in which these professionals work have historically done a poor job of identifying these other problems and of forging the collaborative connections needed to provide holistic care.

This chapter examines the clinical world at the systems level, shifting from a focus on particular practices to the broader contexts within which they take place. These contexts include the array of health and social services and supports that can be found in any community, region and province. They also include federal, provincial and territorial, regional and organizational policies, administration and practices that shape priorities and resource allocation. The chapter is a call to action for practitioners in the substance use field. Those on the inside are uniquely qualified to identify how the system is meeting clients' needs and where it is not. Everyone working in the system has a role to play in its development: this includes promoting or supporting collaboration, innovation, clinical research and evaluation.

As you read this chapter, consider the following questions in the course of your day-to-day clinical practice:

- What are my clients' needs and health goals? These might include:
  - particular specialized service needs
  - holistic needs that extend to other health and social sectors
  - continuity of care and system navigation
- How might these needs and goals change in different phases of my clients' healing journeys?
- How can I help my clients meet their needs when they require services and supports not provided by my agency?
- What new kinds of collaboration need to be forged with service and support providers to better meet the needs of clients? What current partnerships can we build on?
- What barriers prevent clients from experiencing real continuity of care across the multiple services and supports they may need to access? What strengths can we build on?
- How can we build on creative and innovative solutions to achieve broader system-level improvements?

Strengthening Local Care Pathways

Counsellors who work with people with substance use problems are seeing clients with increasingly complex problems and life circumstances. Many kinds of issues, and the interplay among them, are at the heart of each client's struggle. Together they make a daunting profile for any one practitioner—or any one kind of practitioner. Clients with complex problems will no doubt need help from a range of services and supports within the addiction treatment sector. They also will often need to access practitioners in primary medical care, mental health, housing and other sectors. Rather than offering therapeutic help to the client in an isolated way, counsellors need to help each client navigate between addiction treatment services and services the client may need before, during and after treatment.

Best practices literature points to the need for a continuum of services and supports connected through mechanisms such as co-location, case management, referrals and knowledge exchange. Clients benefit from effective care pathways between different kinds of services (e.g., withdrawal management, inpatient or outpatient treatment, supportive recovery, supportive housing). Certainly, examples of service collaborations and effective case management exist throughout Canada. Successful outcomes are enhanced and in part depend on clients' expectations of moving in a positive direction, rather than having to start over again and again—retelling their stories each time—as they continue to jump from one isolated service to another. However, as a whole, the "system" generally consists of independent and disconnected services and supports.

This kind of system fragmentation results in fragmentation at the client level. Clients pursue care journeys with the help of many kinds of services and supports, including family and community. People seeking services are whole persons who are hurting, and who are often dealing not only with complex problems, but also with their own failure to resolve them. The more fragmented the system is, the more clients are forced to break their own concerns into fragmented pieces.

Addiction has a huge impact on concerns addressed by other health and social sectors. The following impacts can't be ignored:

- Alcohol consumption is associated with liver disease, cancer and diabetes (Butt et al., 2011).
- Homeless youth and adults are more likely to use alcohol and other drugs in high-risk ways, and substance use is often a barrier to accessing stable housing (Patterson et al., 2007).
- A 2008 study of reported child abuse and neglect found that alcohol problems (21 per cent) and drug/solvent abuse (17 per cent) were among the most frequently noted concerns in substantiated maltreatment investigations (Public Health Agency of Canada, 2010).
- Stress, trauma and mental health are associated with substance use; among people seeking help for substance use problems, a considerable number—from up to 50 per cent (Canadian Centre on Substance Abuse, 2009) to up to 80 per cent (Rush et al., 2008)—also have mental health problems.

- Most provincially and federally incarcerated prisoners in Canada have histories of substance use. Problematic use is particularly high among Aboriginal men (Bouchard, 2004).
- Aboriginal people in Canada are more likely than the general population to experience challenges in the social determinants of health, many of which are predictive of substance use (Loppie Reading & Wien, 2009). These determinants, as well as cultural context (e.g., intergenerational trauma), should be considered in providing culturally appropriate services (Health Canada et al., 2011).

An Illustration: Common or Unusual?

Imagine a client with severe and complex substance use problems. Early on, you learn that he has been treated for an addiction. As you explore further, you find he also has been seen in psychiatric emergency departments for anxiety attacks, which have led to referrals for mental health counselling and prescriptions for anti-anxiety medication. You learn that the client has been involved with the criminal justice system, with charges for theft and public mischief leading to fines and probationary sentences. The client has lost his housing and is now living in a hostel. His last real job was more than one year ago. He has recently had physical health issues related to a persistent lung infection. He has been in and out of relationships, but is currently not involved with anyone. He reports being alienated from his family.

As a clinician, you may want more information about such a client, including more detail about his substance use (e.g., type of substances; last use; patterns of use—frequency, quantities; years of use; periods of abstinence or reduced use; age of first use; and what other addictive behaviours are creating risk or harm). Knowing these and other details, could you easily provide accessible, effective responses, or would you still feel overwhelmed, without the resources and the connections to offer someone with such diverse challenges the comprehensive care he or she needs? Would this kind of complexity be common or unusual in your work?

Given the prevalence of clients with complex issues, the helping system should have effective, routine ways of identifying complex problems and effective ways of addressing them. However, addiction providers are often trying to help people with complex problems who at the same time are trying to navigate complex systems.

One of the most crucial factors in determining what you can do and how you do it is the context within which you work. Where are you located in the array of health and social services that make up the "system" in your community?

A Tiered Model of Services and Supports

Over the past decade, national and international agencies have been exploring exactly what a comprehensive system of services and supports should look like—one that addresses the full spectrum of substance use problems through help from a broad spectrum of health and other services. The Mental Health Commission of Canada, following on *Out of the Shadows at Last*, a report of the Standing Senate Committee on Social Affairs, Science and Technology (2006), has highlighted how addiction and mental illness are intertwined. Around the same time, the National Treatment Strategy Working Group (2008), convened by the Canadian Centre on Substance Abuse (CCSA) and the Canadian Executive Council on Addiction, developed an approach to a model system that is being increasingly used to map current resources and to chart a course for system improvement. A key element of the emerging Canadian model is a strong consensus on the need to help people with substance use problems in ways that include, but that go beyond, the specialized addiction treatment system. The National Treatment Strategy Working Group (2008) report proposed a tiered model, identifying five sets of functions that all communities should have available to effectively respond to substance use.

A simple way of imagining the tiers is to think of the lower tiers (Tiers 1 and 2) as more community-based and broadly applicable, engaging the whole population, while the higher tiers are more specialized and able to provide more in-depth services and supports for the smaller set of people who have more severe and complex problems. Table 30-1 compares how different populations, functions and services might fall across the tiers. The tiers are intended to be groupings, not distinct or prescriptive categories. The idea is not to fit clients and services into tiers, but to look at the range of services available and the flow of clients through them. Many clients and services will have characteristics that can be located across more than one tier.

TABLE 30-1

Mapping Populations, Functions and Services across Tiers

TIER	POPULATION	FUNCTIONS	SERVICE EXAMPLES
1	Everyone	Prevention and health promotion	Community centre programming, information or awareness campaigns
2	Moderate risk	Early identification and intervention, referral, self-management	Screening and brief interventions by family physicians, peer support programs
3	Active risk, acute harm	Outreach, engagement, case management, risk/harm reduction	Assertive community outreach teams, needle exchange

TIER	POPULATION	FUNCTIONS	SERVICE EXAMPLES
4	High risk, chronic harm	Specialized, structured treatment	Assertive community outreach teams, pharmacotherapy, specialized outpatient or residential programs, outpatient withdrawal management
5	High risk, high severity, complex harm	Specialized, structured treatment for complex problems	Medical withdrawal management, concurrent disorders programs

Thinking visually, from the point of view of the system, the fifth tier is often presented at the top, and the first tier at the bottom. However, inverting that order illustrates that for the client, this progression represents a descent into the illness and disability that substance use can cause, especially at the severe end of the continuum.

Where would you locate your service, keeping in mind that one service can provide functions across many tiers? Can you identify services in your community that carry out functions that belong to each tier? How connected is your agency to services in other tiers? How does this make a difference for the clients with whom you work?

Most clients will need to access multiple services and supports as they work toward healing. Many of these services and supports will be part of local addiction treatment networks (e.g., withdrawal management, residential and other forms of treatment, supportive recovery), while others will be part of broader health and human services systems (e.g., primary medical care, mental health and housing services). Clients may have difficulty gaining access to or transitioning between any of these services. Some of these interrelated difficulties are outlined below.

Information: Clients often do not have the information they need about potential service providers, or they lack the personal means to readily get that information. This is compounded by the fact that providers themselves often do not have adequate information about what other providers are offering, or they lack access to a central clearinghouse that stores, updates and shares that information.

Referrals: Programs often get inappropriate referrals from other providers, which adds to delays in care, as well as frustrating clients and decreasing their motivation to get help. At the same time, providers who are frequently referral agents (e.g., withdrawal management centres and primary health services) often find that other treatment providers will not accept clients with more complex needs (e.g., people on methadone).

Access: Addiction treatment and support programs typically lack collaborative connections with mental health services. These collaborations would improve access through referrals between the two—ideally to access the concurrent care that the best practice literature suggests is needed to produce optimal outcomes (Health Canada, 2002). Instead of the services collaborating to meet the needs of the client, the client is often defined as ineligible by one or the other service, must prove that the other problem is in remission or is put on wait-lists.

Physical health issues such as chronic pain can also limit clients' successful recovery, but continuing medical care is often not easily available. The presence of other issues such as criminal justice involvement or unstable housing, which are common among people with addiction problems, further stigmatize the client and raise additional barriers to accessing needed resources.

Intake: Clients often experience the continuum of services and supports as a series of isolated programs, where each program requires that they start anew. This means that clients have to tell their story again and again, which can be demoralizing.

Housing: In some systems, clients may have to give up their stable housing to enter into a government-funded treatment program. Having to search for housing once residential phases are complete distracts clients from their care journeys. If they are unable to secure safe housing, they may return to situations that put them at increased risk for substance use problems.

Funding: Funding provisions (e.g., service restrictions) and guidelines may create technical barriers regarding eligibility, approval and access. These barriers may mean that when a client is ready for change a narrow window of opportunity is missed, making care pathways even more bumpy.

Communication: Even providers in the same geographic area often do not communicate about their respective services, potential partnerships or the specific clients they are working to help at the same time. Confidentiality, when introduced to explain why such disconnections are necessary, can be a red herring. There are ways to address privacy concerns without breaking confidentiality, for example, by introducing simple, standardized requests for consent during intake.

Oversimplification: Health funding authorities can have a simplistic understanding of programs, sometimes assuming that they can best manage the continuum of care as isolated providers rather than as an interactive team. For example, funding authorities may expect that all substance use treatment programs serve the same populations and in the same way. While this approach has some appeal at first glance, it can result in poorer care overall, as different populations have varying needs and levels of severity and complexity that require a range of care pathways.

Toward a Co-ordinated System

Policy-makers, planners, funders and the community itself often view the treatment system from a distance. But what does it look like to work within the system, working alongside clients who are struggling to deal with problems serious enough for them to seek professional help? This engaged view comes from being "within the system," being there because you want to help people affected by substance use and related problems to move toward change, recovery and healthier lives in supportive and caring communities.

For many workers and clients, there really doesn't seem to be a system. Specific services are available, both within the addiction field and across sectors, but these services don't seem to work together effectively, and they often don't respond in ways that are truly client centred.

This lack of co-ordination can be demoralizing. Workers are often good at making things happen because they are committed to helping their clients and because they have developed connections with other workers and services. However, most workers recognize that these connections should be part of a comprehensive, dependable system—not an informal network—in order to provide effective services able to respond to the needs of all clients.

The current trend toward substance use and mental health integration at the administrative level does not guarantee effective collaboration at the service delivery level (Rush & Nadeau, 2011). Integration, of course, does not call for substance services and supports to be taken over by mental health, medical practitioners or social service practitioners, although this is a real and valid concern within the substance use field. What integration *does* call for is the need for greater communication and collaboration between those working in the different sectors. Clearly, different practitioners will need to lead at different times in a client's healing journey, depending on their expertise and experience. In a co-ordinated, collaborative system, a range of practitioners would be engaged to some extent, for example, in working with a client whose complex problems include the challenges of diabetes, depression and substance use.

In a client-centred system, professionals in health, social service, housing and other areas contribute skills and expertise to form the overall continuum of services that will meet a person's needs. A key challenge in the field is developing mechanisms to recognize and promote collaboration rather than professional ownership of client care. The field has a unique opportunity to learn from the varied experiences of jurisdictions across Canada at different stages and using various models of integration between substance use, mental health and even primary care.

Elements of Integrated Care Pathways

Beyond personal and organizational commitment, the following examples illustrate how the substance use field can bring leadership to building integrated care pathways.

Central and Common Intake Processes

A referral system can be strengthened through a central (or common) intake process to allow for more co-operative service provision across sectors and less fragmented care journeys for clients. Family physicians, in particular, can benefit from having one access point in the system to initiate referrals for addiction or mental health services. Mechanisms for centralized intake can also help realize the principle that every door ought to be the right door for people seeking help with substance use and other health issues. Centralized intake can also reduce the likelihood of people being screened and assessed repeatedly. Clients should not have to tell their stories repeatedly before getting the help they seek.

Interdisciplinary Response Teams

People with more complex, severe substance-related problems often do not enter the continuum of care through routine appointments. Rather, their care journeys begin with crises that bring them into medical, mental health or policing acute response situations. Hospital emergency departments, for example, can be a revolving door for people with severe substance use problems. Such people often have many complex challenges, including lack of housing, mental illness and encounters with the justice system. They often also lack routine primary medical health care to address or prevent physical health conditions. Settings such as emergency departments, therefore, call for on-site collaborative interdisciplinary responses from different kinds of practitioners, including those who can initiate substance use screening, assessment and early treatment.

Shared Care Protocols

When a client seeks help from more than one kind of practitioner concurrently, uncertainties can arise as to how the providers should work together. On the one hand, when mental health or primary care practitioners are providing support to the client of a substance use treatment practitioner, concerns might emerge around protecting client confidentiality and choices. On the other hand, practitioners may find it challenging to keep one another informed about how their respective treatment processes are progressing with the same person, when it is important to do so. It is sometimes helpful to have a general shared care protocol established in advance to make the steps clearer when different kinds of practitioners find themselves working together with particular clients. These shared care protocols may need to be worked out at the organizational level between provider agencies, as well as at the clinical level for individual clients.

Planning Discussions

Whenever possible, we want to creatively address upstream challenges to have better downstream outcomes and positive client experiences. But prevention is difficult in systems that demand intense focus on a seemingly endless tide of challenging daily situations. The problem of planning for better systems is all the more daunting when we imagine trying to involve different sectors and different kinds of practitioners in the process. Nevertheless, getting planners and practitioners together from across the multi-sectoral continuum of care is likely essential for escaping fragmentation in how we respond to the needs of people in our communities. This requires a special form of leadership, one that bridges and connects with many sectors, needing addiction professionals from the ground up to become champions of collaboration and co-ordination. The more connections across sectors can be made, the better the outcome will be for the clients who receive addiction services, and who all too often have concurrent needs.

Knowledge Exchange

The purpose of knowledge exchange is to improve access to and use of relevant research, evidence and other information that can improve client care. One example of knowledge exchange is for different providers to simply come to a deeper understanding of how each works with people who have substance use problems. This understanding will help providers build complementarity and recognize common goals (thereby improving clients' care journeys and health outcomes) and overcome distractions caused by philosophical or other differences. At a more concrete level, different kinds of practitioners will often have insights and experience to share with one another about best practices; however, knowledge exchange will not happen unless practitioners are prepared to be engaged in the process and their organizations provide the necessary leadership and support.

Practice-Based Research

Front-line practitioners are well positioned to identify the kinds of information that will help others like themselves work more effectively with clients. Recent years have seen an increase in research in which practitioners themselves take on the role of research leads, sometimes in partnership with academic researchers. These practice-based inquiries often involve collaborations with clients, families and other stakeholders. A good example of this is the work of O'Grady and Skinner (2007, 2012) on partnering with families affected by addiction and co-occurring mental health problems. Since practice-based research takes place in actual service and support situations, it can provide important insights into real-world applicability, including barriers and opportunities for implementation.

Facilitating Access

Self-referral is a widely used means of accessing substance use treatment programs. However, even among self-referred clients, necessary access to information and the encouragement to follow through will often be provided by external sources of support. These sources can include other social service and health care providers, as well as families, friends and employers. Providers should ensure that the process of both formal and informal referral to treatment programs from outside providers is as effective as possible.

Similarly, substance use treatment providers may sometimes need to help clients link to these external service providers. While other kinds of providers offer services that focus on areas different from substance use, their contribution to the well-being of the same people may be critical. For example, clients with substance use problems often also face significant physical, mental and spiritual issues that go beyond the expertise of those who practise solely in the area of addictions. At the same time, substance use treatment providers are in a unique position to help educate other kinds of providers about the substance use-related issues clients may be experiencing.

Administrative and Policy Concerns

Structure

The current structure of services and supports for substance use in Canada is a result of forces at both political and professional levels. At the political level, responsibility for health and social service delivery rests with the province or territory. However, exceptions exist; for example, the federal government is responsible for providing services to people living in First Nations and Inuit communities, to people incarcerated in federal prisons and to those in the armed forces. Within provincial and territorial jurisdictions, health service delivery is usually further divested to the regional level, with anywhere from two (New Brunswick) to 18 (Quebec) administrative regions responsible for the planning and resourcing of local health care services. Most substance use services and supports are delivered within this publicly funded federal-provincial/territorial-regional structure.

Canada's diverse funding and planning structure is intended to provide greater local service integration, but it also presents a barrier to collaboration and consistency across jurisdictional boundaries. In recent years, increased attention has been paid to creating opportunities for collaboration across jurisdictions. At the national level this includes the Federal-Provincial-Territorial Liaison Committee on Problematic Substance Use, the Canadian Executive Council on Addictions and the National Framework for Action to Address the Harms Associated with Alcohol and Other Drugs and Substances in Canada. At the provincial level, this includes Ontario's Evidence Exchange Network and the B.C. Substance Use Network.

Private vs. Public

Privately funded services provide another option for accessing support for substance use problems in Canada. Like the publicly funded system, the services offered in the private sector vary considerably, creating both advantages and disadvantages for potential clients. Many private services follow a more traditional, abstinence-oriented model. Some provide truly innovative approaches, which may meet the needs of some clients, but which may not be supported by practice evidence. For people who can afford it, the private system can offer levels of privacy, personal attention and amenities that are not possible in the public system. But operating autonomously from the public system can also limit clients' access to other supports within the public service continuum, such as multi-sectoral, community-based and continuing care services. Because these private system services are not publicly accountable, less is known about their operations and outcomes. Increasing the dialogue between public and private systems is one way to increase awareness of the true range of choices available to clients.

Professional Recognition

The substance use field often faces considerable challenges advocating for resources and professional recognition. Substance use treatment is relatively young as a specialized health field. Professional and program-level standardization and accreditation are still in the developmental stage, and both vary greatly across Canada. Substance use also has a strong history of peer-led interventions not seen in most health fields, although they are growing in the mental health sector. Although a strong evidence base exists for the efficacy of certain treatment approaches, evaluation and data collection at the client, program and system levels have been inconsistent.

System Data

Good data are needed to promote evidence-based decisions at the political level (Pirie et al., 2013). Substance use has historically been a high-profile issue, associated with criminalization, media coverage, personal stigma and glamorization—from Al Capone, to the Temperance movement, to Mothers against Drunk Driving, to Lindsay Lohan. "Doing something about the scourge of addiction" is a popular political platform; however, it often focuses short-term resources on high-profile investments, such as tougher criminal sanctions, mandated treatment and residential beds, rather than on more strategic, evidence-based development with longer-term impacts.

When we think about services for substance use, we also tend to think about the specialized system—inpatient or intensive outpatient programs. However, only a small proportion of the population with substance use problems in fact requires this level of intervention. Better data about population needs, service use and service outcomes would support a system that is truly responsive to Canada's substance use profiles. Also important, however, is the recognition that working in non-specialized settings (whether, for example, community-based or multidisciplinary) often requires different but just as valuable skills and professionalism as working in more intensely specialized settings.

Factors Affecting Access

The fundamental purpose of the treatment system is to meet client needs. In order to do so, the system should be designed based on those needs—at both the population and individual levels.

Access and Availability

Only a minority of people who would benefit from substance use services and supports actually ever access them. Many barriers to service exist.

Geography

Canada's population is spread over a tremendous geographic area. Services are generally concentrated in urban centres, meaning that people living in rural or remote areas have access to limited options within their communities.

Physical accessibility

Clients may have difficulty accessing services that are not centrally located or easily accessible through public transport. Costs associated with transport, such as bus tickets or parking rates, can also be problematic for lower-income clients. High-intensity services targeting high-risk, high-need clients may also need to consider physical barriers to access, such as stairs and narrow doorways for clients whose concurrent health concerns limit mobility or require use of mobility aids.

Culture and language

Best practice tells us that services and supports need to be culturally informed to best meet client needs. Culturally informed services for Aboriginal people are available in some places in Canada, but are by no means broadly accessible due to distances, on- versus off-reserve jurisdictional boundaries and resources. As Canada's urban population becomes more ethnically diverse, services also face the challenge of responding to different linguistic and cultural needs. Improving accessibility and quality of service for people with limited English language skills extends beyond simple translation of materials to culturally appropriate outreach (e.g., materials that address cultural stigma around substance use, or health service access); service provider diversity; and culturally informed settings and practices (e.g., private waiting area, individual versus group treatment).

Gender and gender identity

Women are more likely than men to be primary care providers for children. Women who do not have access to child care, for social or financial reasons, may be unable to access services that do not incorporate or provide supervision for children. Ensuring that services are sensitive to gender and gender identity also goes beyond providing gender and lesbian, gay, transsexual and bisexual (LGTB)–specific programming. For example, women with substance use problems are more likely than men to have experienced trauma. Ensuring open space and open or unobstructed access to doors is a concrete way to make services more appropriate for clients with histories of trauma. Using LGTB-friendly symbols and messaging, as well as targeted services and staff training, can also contribute to a welcoming environment.

Stigma

Stigma and discrimination remain significant barriers for people accessing services. They also pose barriers at the system level. Medical professionals who are not familiar with or confident in substance use services and supports are unlikely to refer clients— either trying to address their clients' substance use themselves or simply ignoring it.

Addressing system barriers

System structure can play a key role in addressing barriers to service. Inter-jurisdictional agreements can help ensure that clients are able to access services as close to their communities as possible, even if that means within another province, territory or federal service envelope (e.g., National Native Alcohol and Drug Abuse Program [NNADAP]). Resources dedicated to knowledge exchange support the development and implementation of evidence-based services, including those that are culturally informed. Investments in standards for professional training and program accreditation can improve the level of service delivery and the perceived professionalism of the field.

Example 1: A community-based system

Healthy communities support and are supported by healthy families. Healthy families support and are supported by healthy individuals. Health promotion and illness prevention are therefore a primary concern at all three of these interconnected levels (community, family, individual). To the degree that we do not do a perfect job with prevention, the next best thing we can do at the system level involves early identification and intervention. Inevitably, there will be people who develop moderate to severe problems related to addictive behaviour who will need active treatment. These components are not enough. The evidence shows that better outcomes come not just from providing evidence-informed episodes of early intervention and active treatment, but also from providing continuing care. Think of these four components as elemental in structuring how to think about, design and deliver a feedback-driven system of care for people affected by addictions and related problems. In order to truly be responsive to diverse needs, add an effective understanding of the shaping role of culture, including the social determinants of health, at all levels. What begins to emerge is a system not just responsive to signs of illness, but proactive in building health and well-being at the individual, family and community levels, and driven by feedback to continuing quality improvement. Figure 29-1 illustrates our vision for such a system.

FIGURE 29-1: Care Pathways: A Community Systems Approach

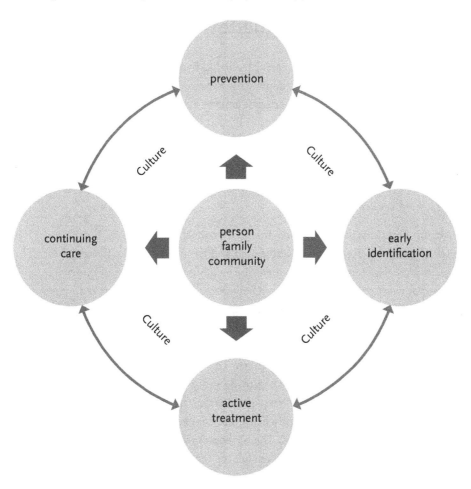

Example 2: Honouring Our Strengths framework

A promising development in conceptualizing care pathways and the ways they support healing journeys comes from the National Native Alcohol and Drug Abuse Program (NNADAP) renewal process championed by key partners across Canada. In addition to discussing tiers of service, the Honouring Our Strengths framework (Health Canada et al., 2011) also highlights interconnected elements that could be considered community capacities, starting with universal prevention and health promotion, supported by a set of functions related to early identification and intervention, not just for addictive behaviours, but also for the wide range of behavioural health issues. The "client" or the focus of concern in this model could be an individual, a family or the community itself. The elements model, and the NNADAP renewal as a whole, is intended to go beyond illness and disadvantage to focus on wellness and cultural rediscovery (See Chapter 24 on Aboriginal healing).

Revisiting the Case Vignettes

The vignettes that opened this chapter introduced five professionals who work in different settings, but who all deal with clients with substance use issues. Here we reintroduce each professional and provide scenarios of actions each could take to address the dilemmas he or she is facing at work.

> In her work at a specialized addiction treatment setting, Flora found that most people she was assessing had not only severe addiction problems, but also other health and social problems that are difficult to address at her treatment service.
>
> **Action:** Flora discusses with her team her concern that clients' health and social problems are not being addressed and the need to make things better for clients. The team uses the idea of a healing journey to map out better care pathways for complex clients. The journey includes an improved intake process, as well as a community-based, post-treatment care plan that will require more active communication with the agencies that refer clients to the program and the agencies the program refers out to, not just upon discharge, but also as treatment progresses. The team identifies and meets with the two community agencies that provide more than half of the program's referrals. The healing journey map provides a useful tool to demonstrate how collaboration will benefit their mutual clients, and both agencies sign formal partnership agreements. The agreements set aside time for weekly case planning discussions. If successful, the team hopes to adopt the model to work with other agencies to improve the family and social support services for program clients to increase retention and decrease relapse rates.

✦

As a high-school guidance counsellor, Ali notices that a high proportion of the troubled teens he sees have substance use issues, and a growing number are putting too much time into gaming or other online activities.

Action: Ali connects with an addiction service that focuses on youth prevention. He also arranges for an education session for teachers and guidance counsellors on gaming, and ways to identify risk and respond. Because of the parents' and community's growing interest in the topic, Ali then arranges, in partnership with the addiction agency, a series of evening information and education sessions on gaming, the Internet and risk factors for associated problems.

As a probation officer, Ellen has noticed that a lead cause of recidivism in the men and women she works with is their inability to avoid substance use.

Action: Ellen notices a workshop on relapse prevention for people with addictive behaviours. Her manager gives her the time to attend and covers the cost of registration. She learns that there are ways of identifying high-risk situations for people who are trying to stop substance use or other addictive behaviours, as well as ways of working with clients to reduce the risk of relapse. Ellen presents her findings to her team as a follow-up to the workshop. She is now piloting the tools she discovered, along with doing more routine screening of current and past addictive behaviour. She is also working with her manager to develop a protocol for all staff to identify risk and do relapse prevention work with clients.

In his work as a child protection intake worker in a child welfare agency, Pierre has noticed that in at least half of the calls he investigates, one and sometimes both parents have substance use problems.

Action: Pierre realizes that parents are often highly motivated to do what it takes to keep their families intact. He feels that if he had quick access to addiction assessment and counselling he could be more helpful to parents with addiction problems. Although there is a waiting list for the addiction assessment service, his manager and the manager for the addiction program have agreed to a pilot project offering immediate access to the service. They are tracking the impact so the results can be used to decide whether to continue or even extend this response. The agencies also agree to modify intake forms to obtain client consent to share information as a routine rather than exceptional practice for referrals. Pierre is also proposing that management recognize the use of the referral program in staff performance assessments as a way to promote its use.

✦

As a nurse in a community health centre, Ines notices that many of the people she follows up with after a heart attack, stroke, accident or other acute health problem have issues with substance use that are interfering with their rehabilitation and recovery.

Action: Ines feels that while she, and even more the doctor on the team, can flag concerns about substance use, their clinical times are so tightly scheduled they can't do more. Ines reaches out to one of the specialized substance use services in the area, and strikes an agreement to have one of its counsellors come into the centre on a weekly basis to provide brief interventions and referrals to clients with substance use concerns.

Conclusion

As these vignettes illustrate, practitioners can have a strong influence on the system in which they work. Innovation often results from front-line providers seeing a need and addressing it: this is simply part of providing client-centred care. Front-line providers know better than anyone the broad range of services needed to address the varying needs of clients they see every day. At a system level, we need to support these innovations and use them as building blocks to drive sustainable improvements in service. Practice-based research is already improving the connection between academia, policy and the needs of clients and practitioners. Increased engagement in system-level considerations can further this connection and accelerate movement toward a comprehensive, collaborative system of services and supports for substance use in Canada.

Practice Tips

Consider the following tips as you do the essential front-line work of finding, shaping and in some cases building the care pathways useful to people with addiction problems as they set out on their healing journeys.

- Identify the substance use issues that arise or are embedded in your work, whether you are in a health care, social service or education agency, in private practice or in a specialized substance use treatment setting. Consider how substance use issues have already affected your clients and the problems that have led these clients to you.
- Reflect on your personal scope of practice as a helping professional and the mandate of your work setting. Are they congruent? Why or why not?

- Understand the healing journeys of your clients. Where are the gaps, and what are their impacts?
- Identify the care pathways available to support people in their recovery goals, especially those with severe and complex problems.
- Locate the outreach and open access services and supports available for people who fail to respond successfully or who do not even become engaged in addiction treatment services.
- Look for opportunities to collaborate with other agencies that will help meet the complex needs of your clients.
- Work collaboratively with other service providers to build helping relationships based on client participation, engagement and commitment. The more complex the problems of your clients, the less you should be working alone, and the more you need to forge alliances that build the integrated care pathways that clients require.
- Never pass up an opportunity to build social support for your clients, including family involvement and support.
- Use your expert knowledge to advocate practical improvements that will benefit all clients. This could mean proposing innovative collaboration ideas to your colleagues and managers, championing pilot projects or leading and participating in clinical research and evaluation.

Resources

Publications

Mental Health Commission of Canada. (2009). *Toward Recovery and Well-Being: A Framework for a Mental Health Strategy for Canada*. Calgary, AB: Author. Retrieved from www.mentalhealthcommission.ca

Mikkonen, J. & Raphael, D. (2010). *Social Determinants of Health: The Canadian Facts*. Toronto: York University School of Health Policy and Management. Retrieved from www.thecanadianfacts.org

National Treatment Strategy Working Group. (2008). *A Systems Approach to Substance Use in Canada: Recommendations for a National Treatment Strategy*. Ottawa: Author. Retrieved from www.nts-snt.ca

Rush, B. (2010). Tiered frameworks for planning substance use service delivery systems: Origins and key principles. *Nordic Studies on Alcohol and Drugs, 27*, 617–636.

Internet

Canadian Centre on Substance Abuse
   www.ccsa.ca
Center for Substance Abuse Treatment—Treatment Improvement Protocol Series
   www.kap.samhsa.gov/products/manuals/tips/index.htm
Centre for Addiction and Mental Health Knowledge Exchange portal for professionals
   http://knowledgex.camh.net
Coalescing on Women and Substance Use
   www.coalescing-vc.org
Evidence Exchange Network
   www.eenet.ca
Implementation Science
   www.implementationscience.com

References

Bouchard, F. (2004). A health care needs assessment of federal inmates in Canada. *Canadian Journal of Public Health, 95* (Suppl. 1). Retrieved from http://journal.cpha.ca/index.php/cjph/article/view/1448/1637

Butt, P., Beirness, D., Gliksman, L., Paradis, C. & Stockwell, T. (2011). *Alcohol and Health in Canada: A Summary of Evidence and Guidelines for Low-Risk Drinking.* Ottawa: Canadian Centre on Substance Abuse. Retrieved from www.ccsa.ca

Canadian Centre on Substance Abuse (CCSA). (2009). *Competencies for Canada's Substance Abuse Workforce.* Retrieved from www.ccsa.ca/Eng/Priorities/Workforce/Competencies/Pages/default.aspx#resources

Health Canada. (2002). *Best Practices: Concurrent Mental Health and Substance Use Disorders.* Ottawa: Author. Retrieved from www.hc-sc.gc.ca

Health Canada, Assembly of First Nations & National Native Addictions Partnership Foundation. (2011). *Honouring Our Strengths: A Renewed Framework to Address Substance Use Issues among First Nations People in Canada.* Ottawa: Author. Retrieved from http://nnadaprenewal.ca/wp-content/uploads/2012/01/Honouring-Our-Strengths-2011_Eng1.pdf

Loppie Reading, C.L. & Wien, F. (2009). *Health Inequalities and Social Determinants of Aboriginal Peoples' Health.* Prince George, BC: National Collaborating Centre for Aboriginal Health. Retrieved from www.nccah-ccnsa.ca/docs/social%20determinates/nccah-loppie-wien_report.pdf

National Treatment Strategy Working Group. (2008). *A Systems Approach to Substance Use in Canada: Recommendations for a National Treatment Strategy.* Ottawa: Author. Retrieved from www.nts-snt.ca

O'Grady, C. & Skinner, W. (2007). *A Family Guide to Concurrent Disorders.* Toronto: Centre for Addiction and Mental Health.

O'Grady, C. & Skinner, W. (2012). Journey as destination: A recovery model for families affected by concurrent disorders. *Qualitative Health Research, 22,* 1047–1062.

Patterson, M., Somers, J., McIntosh, K., Shiell, A. & Frankish, C.J. (2007). *Housing and Support for Adults with Severe Addictions and/or Mental Illness in British Columbia.* Vancouver: Centre for Applied Research in Mental Health and Addictions. Retrieved from www.health.gov.bc.ca/library/publications/year/2007/Housing_Support_for_MHA_Adults.pdf

Pirie, T., Jesseman, R. & National Treatment Indicators Working Group. (2013). *National Treatment Indicators Report, 2010–11 Data.* Ottawa: Canadian Centre on Substance Abuse. Retrieved from www.ccsa.ca

Public Health Agency of Canada. (2010). *Canadian Incidence Study of Reported Child Abuse and Neglect, 2008: Major Findings.* Retrieved from www.phac-aspc.gc.ca/ncfv-cnivf/pdfs/nfnts-cis-2008-rprt-eng.pdf

Rush, B., Fogg, B., Nadeau, L. & Furlong, A. (2008). *On the Integration of Mental Health and Substance Use Services and Systems: Main Report.* Retrieved from www.ccsa.ca/ceca/pdf/Main-reportFINALa.pdf

Rush, B.R. & Nadeau, L. (2011). On the integration of mental health and substance use services and systems. In D.B. Cooper (Ed.), *Responding in Mental Health–Substance Use* (pp. 148–175). London, United Kingdom: Radcliffe Publishing.

Standing Senate Committee on Social Affairs, Science and Technology. (2006). *Out of the Shadows at Last: Transforming Mental Health, Mental Illness and Addiction Services in Canada.* Ottawa: Government of Canada. Retrieved from www.parl.gc.ca/Content/SEN/Committee/391/soci/rep/pdf/rep02may06part1-e.pdf

About the Editors

Marilyn Herie, PhD, RSW, is chair of community services at Centennial College in Toronto, and an assistant professor (status only) with the University of Toronto Factor-Inwentash Faculty of Social Work, where she has taught an online graduate course on addiction treatment for more than 10 years. Her past roles include director of the Collaborative Program in Addiction Studies at the University of Toronto, and director of a Faculty of Medicine–accredited interprofessional certificate program in tobacco dependence treatment and health behaviour change at the Centre for Addiction and Mental Health. She is a member of the International Motivational Interviewing Network of Trainers, and has published numerous books, chapters and journal articles on addiction, professional education and evidence-based practice, including the 2010 text *Substance Abuse in Canada*, with Oxford University Press. Marilyn's areas of interest and focus include e-learning and classroom teaching, curriculum and program development, motivational interviewing and health behaviour change, education research and evaluation, social media and interprofessional education.

W.J. Wayne Skinner, MSW, RSW, is head of the Problem Gambling Institute of Ontario at the Centre for Addiction and Mental Health (CAMH) in Toronto, as well as acting head of CAMH's Eating Disorders and Addiction Clinic and deputy clinical director of the Ambulatory Care and Structured Treatment Program. Between 1998 and 2005, he was clinical director of the Concurrent Disorders Program at CAMH. Wayne is involved in research about assessing and treating concurrent disorders, supporting families affected by addiction and mental health problems, and recovery processes based on mutual aid and peer support. He consults to and participates in policy initiatives related to addiction and mental health, including the National Treatment Strategy and the National Native Alcohol and Drug Abuse Program renewal. He is adjunct senior lecturer in the Factor-Inwentash Faculty of Social Work and an assistant professor in the Department of Psychiatry at the University of Toronto, and is a member of the Motivational Interviewing Network of Trainers. He edited *Treating Concurrent Disorders: A Guide for Counsellors* (CAMH, 2005) and is co-author of *A Family Guide to Concurrent Disorders* (CAMH, 2007) and *Substance Abuse in Canada* (Oxford University Press, 2010). Wayne is also associate editor (Canada) of the journal *Mental Health & Substance Use*.

About the Authors

Bruce Ballon, BSc, MD, ESP(C), FRPC, is director of education for SIM-one (Simulation Ontario Network of Excellence) and has helped develop mental health simulation capacity and programs at Mount Sinai Hospital and the Centre for Addiction and Mental Health (CAMH) in Toronto, as well as other organizations. He is an associate professor of psychiatry at the University of Toronto and an adjunct professor of health sciences at the University of Ontario Institute of Technology. He leads the Advanced Clinical and Educational Services for Problem Gambling, Gaming and Internet Use at CAMH. He has received many awards and grants for his work in medical simulation, addiction psychiatry, psychotherapy, education and the humanities, and for his writing.

Megan Barker, MA, has worked for the Centre for Addiction and Mental Health in Toronto since 2010 as the continuing medical education co-ordinator for the TEACH Project, a University of Toronto–accredited certificate program in smoking cessation counselling. In 2009 she graduated from the University of Guelph with an honours bachelor's degree in criminal justice and public policy, and women's studies. In 2010 she completed a master's degree in criminology and socio-legal studies at the University of Toronto. Megan has been a contributing author to peer-reviewed journal articles and book chapters focused on tobacco dependence treatment and knowledge translation in health care.

Jennifer Barr, BA, worked as a trainer, educator and community developer in the prevention and treatment of substance use and mental health problems with the Centre for Addiction and Mental Health (CAMH) in Toronto and its predecessor, the Addiction Research Foundation. She was the project leader of the CAMH Healthy Aging Project, which addressed mental health and addiction in older adults. Jennifer is now an independent consultant working with organizations in Ontario and across Canada in policy, research, training and program development. She is working on a master's degree in the School of Public Policy and Administration at Carleton University in Ottawa.

Kirstin Bindseil, MSW, RSW, is an advanced practice clinician at the Centre for Addiction and Mental Health in Toronto. She offers supervision, education and leadership to staff in the Addictions Program. Kirstin has worked as a clinical supervisor for nine years and has worked in mental health and addiction in both outpatient and inpatient services.

Marian Bogo, MSW, Adv. DipSW, is a professor, and former dean and field practicum co-ordinator at the Factor-Inwentash Faculty of Social Work at the University of Toronto. Her research focuses on social work field education and supervision, including the conceptualization and assessment of professional competence. She has published more than 100 journal articles and book chapters on field education and social work practice. Her most recent book is *Achieving Competence in Social Work through Field Education* (University of Toronto Press, 2010). She has lectured and consulted to schools of social work in Canada, the United States, Asia, Israel and the United Kingdom.

Nick Boyce, BSc, obtained his degree in psychology from Dalhousie University in Halifax, Nova Scotia. In 1999, he became a volunteer with the TRIP! Project, providing safer sex and safer drug use information and supplies in Toronto's rave and nightclub scenes. Subsequently, he was the gay men's harm reduction co-ordinator at the AIDS Committee of Toronto. Nick is provincial director of the Ontario HIV and Substance Use Training Program and has delivered training around HIV, hepatitis C, addiction, mental health and harm reduction. He was chair of the grant review panel for the City of Toronto's Drug Prevention Community Investment Program, and is currently vice-president of Addictions Ontario.

David Brown, PhD, has more than 20 years of experience in applied health research. He has expertise in organizational analysis, as well as in the use of multiple research methods, including community-based approaches. His background includes research director with the Addictions Foundation of Manitoba, scientist with the University of Wisconsin Faculty of Medicine and policy adviser with B.C. Mental Health and Addiction Services. David has worked extensively in the area of improving substance use screening and brief intervention practices in the context of primary health care settings.

Virginia Carver, PhD, has worked in the addiction field since the early 1970s. For most of that time she worked as a program consultant with the Addiction Research Foundation (now the Centre for Addiction and Mental Health) and Health Canada, and worked for a few years as a private contractor. She is now retired, but is still active as a volunteer. Her main areas of interest are substance use treatment and services for women and older adults.

Gloria Chaim, MSW, RSW, is deputy clinical director in the Child, Youth and Family Service at the Centre for Addiction and Mental Health in Toronto. She is an assistant professor in the Department of Psychiatry and an adjunct lecturer in the Factor-Inwentash Faculty of Social Work at the University of Toronto. Gloria's main interest is in developing service capacity for underserved populations, particularly women, children, youth and families where concurrent disorders are a concern. To foster opportunity for innovation, she has focused most recently has been on developing cross-sectoral networks and collaborations that provide a forum for knowledge exchange and joint service and research initiatives.

Robin Cuff, BComm, is manager of the Drug Treatment Court Program at the Centre for Addiction and Mental Health in Toronto. She has held various leadership positions in women's addiction treatment, withdrawal management, a young parents' resource centre, assessment and referral services and community capacity building. Robin has helped to develop provincial best practices for women's addiction treatment, as well as withdrawal management standards and guidelines for trauma-informed practices in substance use services. She obtained an honours bachelor of commerce (human resources) degree from Ryerson University. She is a faculty member with the Canadian branch of the William Glasser Institute.

Jim Cullen, PhD, RSW, is a social worker with a long history of working in mental health, health and addiction in clinical and leadership roles. He has worked primarily with vulnerable groups, such as the LGBTTIQ community, street-involved youth and First Nations in northern Ontario and British Columbia. Most recently Jim served as clinic head and manager of Rainbow Services at the Centre for Addiction and Mental Health in Toronto. He currently is a mental health consultant with the National Ballet School, and works in private practice, as well as providing training and consultation for organizations around the province. Jim holds an adjunct appointment at the University of Toronto.

John A. Cunningham, PhD, is the Canada Research Chair in Brief Interventions for Addictive Behaviours. In 1995, he received his doctorate in experimental psychology from the University of Toronto, where he is now a professor of psychology and public health sciences. He has spent his career at the Centre for Addiction and Mental Health, where his research is driven by the question, How do people change from addictive behaviours? To answer it, John has combined population research methods with clinical and other research traditions. His findings have been translated into brief interventions for problem drinkers and other drug users that can be applied in treatment or community settings.

Tony P. George, MD, FRCPC, is professor of psychiatry and co-director of the Division of Brain and Therapeutics in the Department of Psychiatry at the University of Toronto. He is medical director of the Complex Mental Illness Program and chief of the Schizophrenia Division at the Centre for Addiction and Mental Health. His research focuses on the neurobiology of tobacco and cannabis addiction in schizophrenia and other mental illness, and translation to addiction treatments in comorbid disorders. He is the author of more than 170 peer-reviewed research articles, reviews and book chapters, including the chapter on nicotine and tobacco in the 24th edition of *Goldman's Cecil Medicine* (Elsevier, 2011).

Tim Godden, BSc, MSW, RSW, is an advanced practice clinician at the Centre for Addiction and Mental Health (CAMH) in Toronto. He has worked in community mental health and addiction for 22 years. Since he joined CAMH's Addiction Program in 1999, Tim has worked in various roles, including as a therapist in the Youth, Brief Treatment and Concurrent Disorders services. He has provided supervision for several teams, including the Assessment, Aboriginal, Brief Treatment, Drug Treatment Court and Rainbow services. He has a strong interest in education and training in motivational interviewing, concurrent disorders and acquired brain injury.

Brian A. Grant, PhD, is director general of research for the Correctional Service Canada (CSC). The research branch conducts applied social science research in support of correctional operations and contributes to the safe reintegration of offenders into the community. He has worked as a researcher with CSC since 1992 and was the director of the Addictions Research Centre in Prince Edward Island before assuming his current position. He received his doctorate in social psychology in 1985 from Queen's University in Kingston, Ontario. He is an adjunct professor in psychology at Carleton University in Ottawa.

Sylvia Hagopian, BA, Dip. Creative Advertising, has managed the development and implementation of websites, psychoeducational resources and e-health solutions for more than a decade. Her portfolio includes interactive self-directed e-health tools, web communities of practice for professionals, diagnostic and treatment planning tools and mobile applications. She has also developed web and mobile versions of an addiction monitoring tool (MYGU: Monitor Your Gambling & Urges). She is the manager of communications and online services for the Problem Gambling Institute of Ontario at the Centre for Addiction and Mental Health in Toronto.

Susan Harrison, BA (Hon), BEd, MSW, RSW, has served as a child protection worker, family therapist, EAP consultant and trainer, project leader and senior manager. She has experience as an addiction counsellor, director of a women's addiction centre and social worker in two family health teams. She was the project leader for developing resources for women at the former Addiction Research Foundation and its successor, the Centre for Addiction and Mental Health, and for creating the conceptual framework for Ontario's Back on Track program for impaired drivers. Susan was co-editor of the first three editions of *Alcohol & Drug Problems*.

David C. Hodgins, PhD, is a professor of clinical psychology and head of the Department of Psychology at the University of Calgary in Alberta. He is a co-ordinator with the Alberta Gaming Research Institute. He received his BA (Hon) (1981) in psychology from Carleton University and his master's degree (1983) and doctorate (1987) in clinical psychology from Queen's University in Kingston, Ontario. He is registered as a clinical psychologist in Alberta. His research focuses on various aspects of addictive behaviours, including relapse and recovery from substance use problems and gambling disorders.

Keith Humphreys, PhD, is a professor of psychiatry and behavioral sciences at Stanford University in California and a senior research career scientist in the Veterans Health Administration. As a clinical and community psychologist by training, his research focuses on the prevention and treatment of addictive disorders, and on the extent to which medical research participants differ from people seen in everyday clinical practice. Since 2004, Keith has also volunteered as a consultant and teacher in the multinational humanitarian effort to rebuild the psychiatric care system of Iraq, for which he won the American Psychological Association's Award for Distinguished Contribution to the Public Interest.

Eva Ingber, MSW, RSW, has worked for more than 20 years in addiction and mental health. She was an advanced practice clinician at the Centre for Addiction and Mental Health in Toronto, where she provided training in concurrent disorders and motivational interviewing and managed a women's addiction program. She currently facilitates motivational interviewing training, provides clinical supervision and facilitates a group at an addiction agency for women who have family members with addiction or mental health issues. In private practice, Eva counsels people with addiction and mental health issues, as well as addressing relationship issues, self-care and behaviour change.

Rebecca Jesseman, MA, is a research and policy analyst with the Canadian Centre on Substance Abuse in Ottawa. Rebecca is the project lead for CCSA's Treatment Priority, and also works on issues that include criminal justice, legislative approaches to drug use, harm reduction and injection drug use. She has a master's degree in criminology from the University of Ottawa, where she also teaches as a sessional professor. Before joining CCSA in 2006, Rebecca worked for Public Safety Canada.

Meldon Kahan, MD CCFP, FRCPC, is an associate professor in the Department of Family Medicine at the University of Toronto, and medical director of the Substance Use Service at Women's College Hospital. Over the years, he has written a number of peer-reviewed articles, guidelines and educational publications on addiction-related topics. His main interests are primary care and addiction, methadone and buprenorphine treatment, and medical education in addiction.

John Kelly, PhD, is an associate professor in psychiatry at Harvard Medical School in Boston, founder and director of the Recovery Research Institute at the Massachusetts General Hospital (MGH), program director of the Addiction Recovery Management Service and associate director of the Center for Addiction Medicine at MGH. He is president elect of the American Psychological Association (APA) Society of Addiction Psychology. He has served as a consultant to U.S. federal agencies, non-federal institutions and foreign governments. His clinical and research work has focused on addiction treatment and the recovery process, including research on the effectiveness of mutual help groups as adjuncts to formal care.

Toula Kourgiantakis, MSW, RSW, RMFT, PhD candidate, is a couple and family therapist and social worker in the Problem Gambling Institute of Ontario at the Centre for Addiction and Mental Health in Toronto. She has worked with couples and families in many different settings for more than 20 years and is a clinical member of the American Association of Marriage and Family Therapy. Toula's doctoral research is examining the impact of problem gambling on families, as well as the role of the family in problem gambling treatment. Toula is a part-time faculty member at the School of Social Work at Ryerson University.

Dale Kuehl, MSW, RSW, is an advanced practice clinician in the Dual Diagnosis Service at the Centre for Addiction and Mental Health (CAMH) in Toronto, where he has worked since 2001. He is a sessional instructor at the School of Social Work programs at York and Ryerson University, and adjunct lecturer with the Factor-Inwentash Faculty of Social Work at the University of Toronto. He co-designed, developed and taught the first certificate program in harm reduction. He served on the board of directors for the Toronto Harm Reduction Task Force from 2004 to 2010 and has been on the John Howard Society of Toronto board since 2012.

Carolyn Lemsky, PhD, CPsych, ABPP-CN, is a board-certified neuropsychologist with 25 years of experience working in rehabilitation settings in the United States and Canada. For the past 15 years she has been clinical director at Community Head Injury Resource Services of Toronto—a Ministry of Health and Long-Term Care–funded agency designed to promote community reintegration of people with acquired brain injury. For the past eight years she has been director of the Substance Use and Brain Injury Bridging Project, a research and knowledge transfer initiative funded by the Ontario Neurotrauma Foundation.

Nina Littman-Sharp, MSW, RSW, is manager of the clinical program of the Problem Gambling Institute of Ontario at the Centre for Addiction and Mental Health in Toronto. She has worked in the problem gambling field since 1995. She has presented and written on various topics, including relapse prevention, family and couples work, gambling and attention-deficit/hyperactivity disorder, and gambling and fatigue. Nina is one of the authors of the Inventory of Gambling Situations, a relapse prevention instrument.

Tammy MacKenzie, MEd, has worked in the addiction field for 15 years in front-line and management roles. She is manager of the Concurrent Addiction Inpatient Treatment Service at the Centre for Addiction and Mental Health in Toronto. She has worked in women's treatment, child development, housing, harm reduction, assessment and community capacity development. Tammy has presented widely on fetal alcohol spectrum disorder, focusing on challenges and opportunities in treatment settings. She is co-author of a chapter about the unacknowledged grief of child apprehension in *Becoming Trauma Informed* (CAMH, 2012).

David C. Marsh, MD, CCSAM, ASAM, ISAM, joined the Northern Ontario School of Medicine as associate dean of community engagement in 2010. He was the physician leader for addiction medicine with Vancouver Coastal Health and Providence Health Care, and clinical associate professor in the School of Population and Public Health at the University of British Columbia. He held leadership roles at the Addiction Research Foundation and the Centre for Addiction and Mental Health in Toronto from 1996 until 2003. His research focuses on withdrawal management, methadone maintenance, heroin-assisted treatment and harm reduction interventions. In 2004, he received the Nyswander-Dole Award from the American Association for the Treatment of Opioid Dependence.

Gabor Maté, MD, is a physician and best-selling author whose books have been published in 20 languages internationally. His interests include child development, the mind-body unity in health and illness, and addiction treatment. He has worked in family practice, palliative care and addiction medicine. He regularly addresses professional and lay audiences throughout North America and has received various awards, including a Simon Fraser University Outstanding Alumnus Award and an honorary degree from the University of Northern British Columbia. His most recent book, *In the Realm of Hungry Ghosts: Close Encounters with Addiction*, won the Hubert Evans Prize for literary non-fiction.

Flora I. Matheson, PhD, BA, MA, is a sociologist who focuses on crime, deviance and socio-legal studies. She has extensive research experience with marginalized populations, specifically offenders and illicit drug users. She is a research scientist at the Centre for Research on Inner City Health at St. Michael's Hospital in Toronto, and an adjunct scientist in the Primary Care and Population Health and Mental Health and Addictions programs at the Institute for Clinical Evaluative Sciences. She is an assistant professor with the Dalla Lana School of Public Health at the University of Toronto and senior research associate with the Correctional Service of Canada.

Janet Mawhinney, MA, is manager for diversity and equity at the Centre for Addiction and Mental Health in Toronto. This role involves promoting the integration of equity and human rights into health service practices and systems. Her work includes human rights, employment equity, cultural competence, LGBTQ inclusion, harassment, bias in hiring, accessibility and health equity. Janet has developed and delivered various equity initiatives for front-line staff, management and board leadership in hospitals, universities, public health, community health centres and housing services. Her graduate work focused on equity pedagogies within organizational change strategies.

Peter Menzies, PhD, RSW, is a member of Sagamok Anishnawbek First Nation. He has spent 13 years at the Centre for Addiction and Mental Health (CAMH) in Toronto building culturally congruent mental health and addiction programs in partnership with Ontario's Aboriginal communities. He founded CAMH's Aboriginal Services program. Before joining CAMH, Peter held front-line and management positions at Native and mainstream agencies and worked with individuals and families in child welfare, family counselling, homelessness and income support programs. He won the Centre for Equity and Health in Society's Entrepreneurial Development and Integration of Services Award (2005) and the Kaiser Foundation's Excellence in Indigenous Programming Award (2011).

Andrea E. Moser, PhD, CPsych, is director of the Addictions Research Centre with the Correctional Service of Canada (CSC). She started her career with CSC in 1993 as a psychologist working with offenders with mental disorders at the Regional Treatment Centre in Ontario. She has been at CSC national headquarters since 1997 and has held various positions, including national manager of substance abuse programs, National Drug Strategy co-ordinator, national manager of violence prevention programs and national co-ordinator of institutional and community mental health initiatives. She has published articles and presented nationally and internationally on mental health, substance use treatment and correctional programming.

Caroline O'Grady, RN, MN, PhD, is an advanced practice nurse in the Ambulatory Care and Structured Treatments Program at the Centre for Addiction and Mental Health in Toronto, and an adjunct nursing professor at the University of Toronto. She is both principal and co-investigator on a number of research studies, including studies focusing on families and concurrent disorders, suicide prevention and women gamblers. Caroline is also a co-lead on the development of a new Registered Nurses' Association of Ontario best practice guideline, *Engaging Adults at Risk for Substance Use Disorders*.

Jane Paterson, MSW, RSW, is director of interprofessional practice at the Centre for Addiction and Mental Health in Toronto. Her clinical work focused on people with co-occurring substance use and mental health problems and on family treatment. In her current role, she has led practice change initiatives and established structures to support and mentor clinical staff. Her work involves clinical policy development and implementation, student education and training, and promoting optimal care and learning through interprofessional education and collaboration. She is cross-appointed to the Factor-Inwentash Faculty of Social Work at the University of Toronto and to Smith College School of Social Work in Northampton, Massachusetts.

Monique Peats, MTS-PC, OACCPP, MSW, RSW, is a psychotherapist, speaker and co-founder of the Life Recovery Program, an internationally awarded mental health and addiction online wellness program. Spanning more than 15 years, Monique's extensive career includes crisis and trauma intervention; family, couple and individual therapy in private practice; as well as work in hospital, church, university, corporate and agency settings. Her broad scope of experience and training enables her to provide an expansive range of expertise, perspective and skill from a holistic paradigm.

Cheryl Peever, BSc, MSW, received her degrees from the University of Toronto. She currently works at the Centre for Addiction and Mental Health in Toronto as manager of the Health, Safety and Wellness Program. In 2006, Cheryl received the Courage to Come Back Award after disclosing her past struggles with alcohol, cocaine addiction and depression. She speaks regularly in the media and to professional groups about the stigma surrounding mental health and addiction, particularly in the workplace.

Lisa Pont, BSW, MSW, received her degrees at Ryerson University and York University, respectively. In 2007 she joined the Problem Gambling Service at the Centre for Addiction and Mental Health (CAMH) in Toronto as the older adult specialist. Prior to that, she co-ordinated CAMH's telephone support line since its inception in 2003. Her experience in counselling, outreach, community work and training led to her position as a trainer and therapist with the Problem Gambling Project and Problem Gambling Service at CAMH. She is involved in training and counselling in the areas of gaming, gambling and Internet overuse.

Nancy Poole, MA, PhD candidate, works with the British Columbia Centre of Excellence for Women's Health on research and knowledge exchange related to girls' and women's health. She is a co-editor of two books published by the Centre for Addiction and Mental Health: *Highs & Lows: Canadian Perspectives on Women and Substance Use* (2007) and *Becoming Trauma Informed* (2012).

Anne Ptasznik, MSW, has worked in mental health and addiction for more than 20 years. She has worked with scientists and clinicians at the Centre for Addiction and Mental Health (CAMH) and other organizations to communicate health research and information to journalists and the public. She has written about mental health and addiction for *CrossCurrents: The Journal of Addiction and Mental Health*, *Reader's Digest* and other national publications. Her company, Creative Fusion, provides communications consulting, writing, media training and social media strategies for health care organizations. She co-organized the first Mental Health Camp in Toronto, which explored the use of social media in mental health.

Rachel A. Rabin, BSc, MSc, is a second-year PhD candidate at the Institute of Medical Science (IMS) at the University of Toronto. She is part of Dr. Tony George's Biobehavioural Addictions and Concurrent Disorders Research Laboratory, studying the effects of substance use on neurocognitive function in schizophrenia. She completed her bachelor's degree in psychology at McGill University in Montreal and earned her master's degree through IMS in 2011.

Paul Radkowski, MTS, is CEO and clinical director of the Life Recovery Program, and an internationally awarded psychotherapist and speaker. In addition to his extensive work in addiction, he has consulted with hospitals and other treatment agencies working with groups, families and individuals as a family and marriage therapist, crisis counsellor and trauma specialist. Paul is the recipient of the Outstanding Addictions Professional Award from the International Association of Addiction and Offender Counselors and the first recipient of the Ontario Association of Consultants, Counsellors, Psychometrists and Psychotherapists' Recognition Award for Outstanding Service and Contribution in the Field of Mental Health.

Peter Selby, MBBS, CCFP, FCFP, MHSc, DipABAM, is chief of the Addictions Program at the Centre for Addiction and Mental Health in Toronto. He is an associate professor in the Family and Community Medicine Department, the Psychiatry Department and the Dalla Lana School of Public Health at the University of Toronto. He created the TEACH project, a certificate program in smoking cessation counselling. He is a principal investigator with the Ontario Tobacco Research Unit, the STOP study and CAN-ADAPTT, a Canadian smoking cessation guideline development and dissemination project. He helped start the program for pregnant substance-using women at St. Joseph's Health Centre, and continues his clinical research with this population.

Joanne Shenfeld, MSW, RSW, is manager of outpatient and day treatment in the Youth Addiction and Concurrent Disorders Service at the Centre for Addiction and Mental Health in Toronto. She is an adjunct lecturer in the Factor-Inwentash Faculty of Social Work at the University of Toronto. She has extensive clinical experience in youth concurrent disorders, including individual, family and group work. Joanne was instrumental in developing CAMH's Family Addiction Service and day treatment services for youth, most recently focusing on a new day hospital program that combines intensive programming for inpatients and outpatients.

Linda Sibley, BA, CBS diploma, is executive director of Addiction Services of Thames Valley in London, Ontario, which specializes in screening, assessing and treating people with substance use and gambling problems and their families. She has more than 30 years of experience working in Ontario's addiction system and has provided workshops across Canada on a variety of topics. She has been a trainer for 20 years and is co-author of a clinical manual on standardized assessment for Ontario's addiction system.

Robert M. Solomon, LLB, LLM, is a professor in the Faculty of Law at the University of Western Ontario in London, and national director of legal policy for MADD Canada. He served on the board of directors of the Addiction Research Foundation (now part of the Centre for Addiction and Mental Health), and as a consultant to Health and Welfare Canada and other government departments. He has advised numerous addiction, health care and counselling agencies, and been retained by various law firms in this field. He is the author of *A Legal Guide for Social Workers* (Ontario Association of Social Workers, 2009).

Cate Sutherland, BA (Dist), MPA, is executive director of the Addictions Centre (Hastings/Prince Edward Counties) Inc., for which she has worked since 1978. She has worked extensively in the areas of mandatory clients, concurrent disorders and standardizing services. Cate is an alumnus of Queen's University in Kingston, Ontario, and has an undergraduate degree in psychology and a graduate degree in public administration.

Andrea Tsanos, MA, received her degree in psychology from McGill University in Montreal. She has worked at the Centre for Addiction and Mental Health (CAMH) in Toronto for 19 years, where she is an advanced practice clinician in the Addictions Program. Andrea has led concurrent disorders capacity-building initiatives, and has designed and delivered trainings for addiction and mental health professionals interested in developing their concurrent disorders clinical competency. Andrea's training efforts include facilitating face-to-face workshops and online courses. She has a long history of service delivery spanning concurrent disorders consultation and assessment, and individual and group therapy. She also provides individual and team-based clinical supervision.

Sydney J. Usprich is an emeritus professor in the Faculty of Law at the University of Western Ontario in London, where he taught criminal law and evidence since 1970. He was associate dean (academic) for the Faculty of Law between 1992 and 1995 and acting dean from 1995 to 1996. He received his law degree from the University of Toronto, followed by graduate work at Cambridge University as a Canada Council Fellow. He was director of the London Legal Clinic in London, Ontario, between 1982 and 1985. In addition to numerous articles on criminal law, he is co-author of *Evidence and Procedure in Canadian Labour Arbitration* (Carswell, 1991).

Lyn Watkin-Merek, RN, BScN, CPMHN, has worked at the Centre for Addiction and Mental Health (CAMH) in Toronto for more than 20 years, including as a staff nurse, discharge planner, assessment worker and therapist, and in program management. She was manager of the Structured Relapse Prevention Program, the Back on Track program for impaired drivers and the Youth Program. She is currently a unit manager in the Complex Mental Illness Program in CAMH's forensic division. Lyn co-authored the second edition of *Structured Relapse Prevention: An Outpatient Counselling Approach* (2006).

John R. Weekes, PhD, is a senior researcher with the Research Branch of the Correctional Service of Canada (CSC) in Ottawa and former acting director of CSC's Addictions Research Centre. He is an adjunct professor of forensic psychology and addictions at Carleton University. He has published extensively and has consulted widely on forensic addictions-related issues with correctional jurisdictions and agencies in Canada, as well as internationally, including the United Kingdom, the United States, Scandinavia and Ireland. His research interests include substance abuse assessment and treatment models, motivation for change, forensic psychology, clinical psychopathology, evidence-based treatment and treatment-outcome research.

Kathryn Weiser, MHSc, is a research analyst at the Problem Gambling Institute of Ontario at the Centre for Addiction and Mental Health (CAMH) in Toronto, where she brings a critical research lens to the development of education, prevention and policy resources. She provides evidence-based research to support her team's mandate in developing and implementing clinical training initiatives. She has held positions in research, policy and health promotion at CAMH, Toronto Public Health, the University Health Network and The Hospital for Sick Children. Kathryn has an honours BA in psychology from York University and a master's degree in health promotion from the University of Toronto.

Janis Wolfe, CPsych, is a psychologist in the Problem Gambling Treatment Service of the Problem Gambling Institute of Ontario at the Centre for Addiction and Mental Health in Toronto. She works with transitional-aged youth who have process addictions and/ or mental health concerns. She conducts psychoeducational assessments, and provides individual and group treatment for youth, as well as educational groups for parents of youth with process addictions. She has worked in this service since 2010.

Julie Yeterian, MA, PhD candidate, is a doctoral candidate in clinical psychology at Suffolk University and a clinical research co-ordinator at the Center for Addiction Medicine at Massachusetts General Hospital in Boston. Her research interests include exploring the role of religious and spiritual processes in recovery from drug and alcohol dependence. Julie has co-authored many articles and chapters on the role of mutual-help groups in supporting sustained recovery.

Rosanra Yoon, NP, MN, CPMHN(C), is an advanced practice nurse at the Addiction Medicine Service and Medical Withdrawal Service at the Centre for Addiction and Mental Health in Toronto. She provides interprofessional clinical supervision and support for clinicians in practice development and delivery of safe client care. Her background is in psychiatric mental health nursing and addictions nursing. She has worked with people who have concurrent disorders in various contexts, including inpatient acute care settings and intensive community case management and addiction medicine. She has a specific interest in concurrent disorders care delivery and the health needs of high-risk vulnerable populations.

Index

Note: f = figure, t = table

assessment and, 177, 282
benzodiazepines and, 148
brain injury and, 427, 437
cannabis and, 150
concurrent disorders and, 384, 385
definition of, 135
legal issues and, 690
methamphetamine and, 154
opioid addiction and, 69, 282
overdose and, 135
screening for, 168–169
solvents and, 152
Inuit people. *See* Aboriginal people
Inventory of Drug-Taking Situations (IDTS), 210,
215, 216–217f

J
Jaundice, 139

K
Ketamine, 156, 157, 553
Korsakoff's psychosis, 430

L
Learning disabilities, 431, 563t
Leeds Dependence Questionnaire (LDQ), 321
Legal issues
assessment and, 383, 676
confidentiality and disclosure of client information, 690–699, 710
consent, 678–684, 676–679
negligence, 684–690
treatment and, 676
Lesbians
AA and, 325, 327
aging and, 652
body image and, 651
care pathways and, 746
coming out for, 645–646, 647
concurrent disorders and, 375
crossdressers and, 662
diversity and health equity knowledge for, 49–50,
635–636
family issues and, 654
gender identity and, 643, 649, 746
HIV/AIDS and, 653–654
language and terminology for, 641, 662, 664,
666
marginalization of, 47–48
older adults and, 587
oppression of, 639–640, 650, 663
phobias and, 662, 664
relapse prevention and, 227
sexual orientation and, 643, 644f
sexuality and, 655
substance use and, 636–638, 649
trauma and, 403
women who have sex with women (WSW), 666
women-specific groups and, 537

LGBTTTIQ (lesbian, gay, bisexual, transgendered,
transsexual, two-spirit, intersex, queer) communities
519 Church Street Community Centre, Toronto, 652
anti-oppression framework, 639
biological sex and, 643f, 644f
biphobia, 639, 641, 650
body image in, 650–651, 661
clinicians and, 636, 641, 647–648, 649–650,
659–660, 661
coming out process in, 644–645, 646, 648, 661
confidentiality within, 653, 658
cultural competence in working with, 639
discrimination and, 649, 655, 661
diversity of, 641, 647, 656
DSM-5 terminology, 639
family and, 646, 654–655
Gay and Lesbian Medical Association (GLMA), 647
gender expression and, 643f, 644f
gender identity and, 642, 643f, 644f
gender privilege, 640, 648
genderism, 640
glossary of terms, 662–666
heterosexism, 640
heterosexual privilege, 640
HIV/AIDS and, 652–653, 661
homophobia, 639–641, 650
internalized oppression in, 649–650, 661
male-to-female (MtF), 638
men who have sex with men (MSM), 638, 644,
652, 653, 654
mental health problems in, 638–639
older adults in, 652
Pride celebrations, 657
racism and, 646
sensitivity to, 656–657
sexual orientation, 642–643f, 644f
sexuality in, 655–656
social activism and, 649
societal oppression of, 639, 661
specific services for, 657–658, 659–660
stigma and discrimination in, 639
substance use in, 636–637, 638, 644, 648, 649,
650, 654–655
terminology in, 641–642
transitioning in, 644–645, 649, 661
transphobia, 639–640, 641, 650
Librium. *See* chlordiazepoxide
Life Recovery Program (LRP), 349, 358–360
LifeRing, 41, 322, 324t, 334
Lorazepam (Ativan), 147
LRP. *See* Life Recovery Program
LSD, 154, 369, 553

M
MA. *See* Methadone Anonymous
Major depressive disorder, 338, 369–370, 371, 508,
526
Marijuana. *See* Cannabis